Cardiopulmonary Anatomy and Physiology for Respiratory Care Practitioners

Gregory P. Cottrell, BSc

Professor, Respiratory Therapy Program
School of Health Sciences
Health Technology Division
Fanshawe College
London, Ontario

F. A. DAVIS COMPANY • Philadelphia

F. A. Davis Company
1915 Arch Street
Philadelphia, PA 19103

Printed in the United States of America

Last digit indicates print number: 10 9 8 7 6 5 4 3 2 1

Publisher: Jean François Vilain
Senior Editor: Lynn Borders Caldwell
Developmental Editor: Christa Fratantoro
Designer: Bill Donnelly
Cover Designer: Louis J. Forgione

As new scientific information becomes available through basic and clinical research, recommended treatments and drug therapies undergo changes. The author(s) and publisher have done everything possible to make this book accurate, up to date, and in accord with accepted standards at the time of publication. The authors, editors, and publisher are not responsible for errors or omissions or for consequences from application of the book, and make no warranty, expressed or implied, in regard to the contents of the book. Any practice described in this book should be applied by the reader in accordance with professional standards of care used in regard to the unique circumstances that may apply in each situation. The reader is advised always to check product information (package inserts) for changes and new information regarding dose and contraindications before administering any drug. Caution is especially urged when using new or infrequently ordered drugs.

Library of Congress Cataloging-in-Publication Data

Cottrell, Gregory P.
    Cardiopulmonary anatomy and physiology for respiratory care practitioners / Gregory P. Cottrell.
        p. ; cm.
    Includes bibliographical references and index.
    ISBN 0-8036-0439-4
    1. Cardiopulmonary system—Physiology. 2. Cardiopulmonary system—Anatomy. 3. Respiratory therapists.
    [DNLM: 1. Respiratory Physiology. 2. Respiratory System—anatomy & histology. 3. Cardiovascular Physiology. 4. Cardiovascular System—anatomy & histology. WF 102 C851c2001] I. Title.
    QP121 C735 2001
    612.1—dc21   00-058982

Cover

The background, "The Lungs and Other Viscera" (c. 1508), is a pen and ink drawing by Leonardo da Vinci (1452–1519). The drawing is thought to be of pig lungs, a common subject for anatomical dissection through the ages. With the promise of animal heart-lung transplants used in humans, da Vinci's subject is particularly appropriate today. Computer-rendered illustrations and medical images of the thorax contrast with the 500-year-old drawing.

To Betty L. Sharick

Cardiopulmonary Anatomy and Physiology for Respiratory Care Practitioners is a specialty text that examines the structure and function of the cardiopulmonary system in depth. It is assumed that the reader has already studied introductory anatomy and physiology and is familiar with fundamental physiologic principles, such as homeostasis, as well as the general structure and function of body systems.

This book is designed to provide the reader with the solid physiologic fundamentals needed in subsequent clinical courses. The information in the book, while of an advanced nature, is still presented as preclinical information. In other words, information related to patient assessment, interpretation of clinical findings, and differential diagnosis is not given. Such information, although critical to the overall education of the respiratory care practitioner, is premature in a text designed to prepare students for their clinical experience.

The study of anatomy and physiology provides the theoretical underpinnings upon which many medical subjects are based. A solid understanding of these basic principles will make the study of clinical subjects and applied disciplines, such as pharmacology, pathophysiology, and pathology, more rewarding. The entire philosophy behind the text has been focused on this single goal.

Organization

The 24 chapters of the text are organized into three units that group chapters related to the same general topic in anatomy and physiology.

UNIT 1—THE RESPIRATORY SYSTEM

This extensive unit forms the backbone of the text by grouping 15 chapters that cover the anatomy and physiology of the entire age spectrum—from developmental aspects of the respiratory system to its inevitable decline with advancing years. Between these two extremes, the organization of conducting and respiratory zones of the lung is covered, as are the innervation and defense of the lung. An in-depth look at the structure of the thorax is presented as a prelude to the study of the statics of breathing, the dynamics of breathing, and pulmonary mechanics. A chapter providing a detailed study of the chemical and neural control of ventilation introduces newer concepts, such as central pattern generators and triphasic breathing. A chapter covering ventilation, perfusion, and metabolic function of the lung reminds the reader that the respiratory system is involved with several functions unrelated to gas exchange. A separate chapter covering ventilation-perfusion relationships is also presented in the unit.

UNIT 2—THE CARDIOVASCULAR SYSTEM

Because of the integral nature of the respiratory and cardiovascular systems, this unit of seven chapters is relatively detailed and is linked to the preceding unit. Following the same organization as that of the respiratory system unit, the cardiovascular unit begins with a chapter that discusses developmental aspects and ends with a chapter covering aging of the cardiovascular system. Chapters in this unit cover the gross anatomy of the heart, cardiac muscle and the cardiac conducting system, and the cardiac cycle and cardiac output. The unit also includes a chapter that introduces the basics of hemodynamic measurements and one that covers fundamentals related to flow, pressure, and resistance in blood vessels.

UNIT 3—THE URINARY SYSTEM AND ACID-BASE BALANCE

The final unit of the book consists of two chapters: one providing a review of renal structure and function, and the other covering the details of acid-base balance in the body.

APPENDICES

Information included in the appendices includes a list of symbols and abbreviations used in cardiopulmonary physiology and a table of body surface area data.

Pedagogical Aids

A variety of instructional aids of proven effectiveness are included in the text. These include chapter outlines, objectives, and summaries. Such aids help the reader locate information, associate related facts, and assess mastery of the material. To provide the reader with additional practice, an *electronic workbook on CD-ROM* contains review questions. Pedagogical aids are discussed in detail under the heading "To the Reader."

Readability

Cardiopulmonary Anatomy and Physiology for Respiratory Care Practitioners provides a highly organized, detailed description of the three body systems of most concern to respiratory care practitioners—respiratory, cardiovascular, and urinary systems. Consistent style, effective page layout design, and numerous tables and illustrations add to the enjoyment and readability of the book. Experts in cardiopulmonary anatomy and physiology extensively reviewed the original manuscript. The result is a concise and relevant text, focused on preclinical topics in the cardiopulmonary field.

Readability of the text is enhanced by the use of boldface type for key terms when they are first introduced and a phonetic pronunciation guide for new terms. Boxed information describing topics of historical, current, or future physiologic importance spark interest in the subject and add immensely to the readability of the text.

Supplementary Material for Instructors

On the CD-ROM in the back of this text, instructors will find both the students' electronic workbook and an *electronic Instructor's Guide*. This *Instructor's Guide* is designed to help the instructor in course design. Each chapter in the guide contains a Chapter

Synopsis, which provides a concise summary of textbook contents, and a section called Relationship to Other Chapters. The latter feature discusses how the chapter fits into the overall scheme of the book and helps link the chapter with those in related areas. This helps in course design, especially if the course length prevents a "cover-to-cover" approach. Suggestions concerning sections of text that can be minimized and those that are absolutely vital allow an instructor to custom-tailor the text material to individual course requirements.

Instructors who adopt *Cardiopulmonary Anatomy and Physiology for Respiratory Care Practitioners* will also receive a second CD-ROM that contains both a *computerized test bank* and *electronic art files*.

TO THE READER

Innovative learning aids have been incorporated into *Cardiopulmonary Anatomy and Physiology for Respiratory Care Practitioners*. These instructional aids are designed to reinforce the information and concepts presented in the book.

Chapters are grouped into three units. Each unit begins with a concise unit introduction that previews the general concepts to be introduced. The unit introduction briefly describes the common characteristics of the chapters that allow them to be grouped together as a unit. A chapter outline at the beginning of each chapter details major topics and subheadings to assist the reader in locating areas of interest. Chapter introductions provide a brief overview of chapter contents and relate the chapter to others in the unit.

The most important learning aid to the reader is the list of chapter objectives presented at the beginning of each chapter. These performance objectives detail the learning expectations of the chapter and are proven devices that promote mastery of the material. Performance objectives allow readers to assess their understanding of the information presented in the text. The reader is encouraged to study small segments of the text and then refer back to the appropriate chapter objectives to determine if the material has been understood. By using the chapter objectives as both study guide and feedback, the reader remains focused on a smaller amount of material before moving on to new topics.

Key terms unique to the topics introduced in the chapter are previewed at the beginning of each chapter and printed in bold type when they first appear in the text. Eponymous terms are those named after a person. Eponyms are usually nondescriptive and do not always indicate that the person whose name is used had anything to do with what was named. Nevertheless, eponyms are still in frequent use and have been included in the text, glossary, and index where appropriate. Eponyms commonly used clinically appear in parentheses, immediately following the current terms where they are used for the first time in a chapter [e.g. sternal angle (angle of Lewis) or glomerular capsule (Bowman's capsule)]. This dual nomenclature is presented to help the reader translate the clinical language often used in hospitals and on patients' charts.

Where applicable, a phonetic pronunciation guide is included with the list of key terms. Consult this list as often as necessary. If you cannot pronounce a word, you cannot remember it. The pronunciation guide uses the following format:

- The syllable that is most strongly accented is shown with a primary accent (′) symbol; syllables that are less strongly accented are shown with a secondary accent (″) symbol, as in physiology (fiz″ ē-ol′ ō-jē).
- Long vowels are indicated by a line (macron) over the letter and pronounced with the long sound, as in the following common words:

  ā   pain   (p ā n)
  ē   sleep   (s l ē p)
  ī   ripe   (r ī p)
  ō   sole   (s ō l)

- Short vowels are unmarked and are pronounced with a short sound, as in the following common words:

    | e | bed | (bed) |
    | i | lid | (lid) |
    | o | rot | (rot) |
    | u | tub | (tub) |

Extensive use of figures and tables helps reinforce important anatomical and physiologic concepts. Readers who are visual learners will appreciate this particular feature of the text. Some tables summarize text contents and are useful for quick reference. Others present additional information to enhance text material.

Most chapters include highlighted information in a boxed format. These perspectives, although not mandatory reading, provide interesting and enjoyable topics within the chapter narrative. Some topics are of historical interest, others relate text contents to clinical applications, while some offer a glimpse of future trends in physiology. These diversions provide insight into how anatomy and physiology affects our lives. A chapter summary at the end of each chapter succinctly reviews the major topics discussed in the chapter. Each chapter concludes with a bibliography. This collection of pertinent information serves as both a list of suggestions for additional reading and a reference for citations in the text narrative. The electronic workbook on CD-ROM provides you with review questions that reinforce the content of the chapters.

The appendices at the end of the book contain valuable reference information. Appendix A includes common abbreviations and symbols used in cardiopulmonary physiology. Appendix B presents the DuBois body surface area (BSA) chart used in many hemodynamic calculations. The index at the end of the book allows the reader to locate the page reference where specific terms, concepts, and mechanisms can be found. Use it often, especially when studying for exams. An extensive glossary at the end of the book provides a concise definition of the key terms introduced throughout the text.

Strive to be interactive with the text. Do not read the material passively. Go back and check off objectives as you achieve them. Study the figures and ask yourself what is being shown. Test yourself before moving on. Understand new terms and their pronunciation. Only by investing such time and effort can your study of cardiopulmonary anatomy and physiology reap the rewards you deserve.

ACKNOWLEDGMENTS

The editorial and production staffs at the F. A. Davis Company are gratefully acknowledged. My appreciation is especially extended to Christa Fratantoro and Marianne Fithian, Developmental Editors, who took on the myriad details and editorial tasks associated with this major work. Their guidance was welcomed and their patience was boundless. Lynn Borders Caldwell, Senior Editor, was not only enthusiastic and supportive when I first proposed the book, but was instrumental in overseeing the entire project. These editors were also responsible for recruiting an expert group of respiratory care reviewers and coordinating the efforts of those reviewers. Behind all of these editorial tasks at F. A. Davis the outstanding organizational efforts of Ona Kosmos, Editorial Assistant, are quietly carried out. As usual, her efforts are both recognized and appreciated. Organizational matters were also expertly handled by Elena Coler, who somehow kept track of the bewildering flow of manuscripts and illustrations during the final phase of this project. My thanks are extended to the Art Department at F. A. Davis, especially to Louis Forgione and Jack Brandt. Their efforts resulted in a graphical design and layout that adds immensely to the appearance, appeal, and readability of the book. I am also indebted to Rose Gabbay, Director of Production Services at UG/GGS Information Services. Her keen eye for detail helped eliminate errors and inconsistencies and add polish to the final product. I would like to thank Darlene Pedersen, who not only correlated much of the graphical material with the text, but was instrumental in securing permission to borrow excellent complementary artwork for the book from other sources. Those sources are gratefully acknowledged. Finally, I would like to thank Brian Howell, BSc, MRT(R), a valued colleague who provided invaluable technical guidance regarding the software I used for the computer-generated artwork.

REVIEWERS

An outstanding team of respiratory therapy educators was assembled to review the original manuscript for the book. Their critical comments and suggestions for improvement helped shape the final product. I am indebted to them for keeping the book focused and pointing out areas that could be clarified through rewriting. The entire manuscript was thoroughly reviewed for accuracy and respiratory relevance by:

Michael Wayne Cook, MA, RRT, Director
Associate Professor of Respiratory Care
Technologies Division
Mountain Empire Community College
Big Stone Gap, Virginia

Lawrence A. Dahl, EdD, RRT
Program Coordinator, Instructor
Department of Respiratory Therapy
Hawkeye Community College
Waterloo, Iowa

G. Woodard Gross, MA, RRT
Chair, Associate Professor
Department of Cardiopulmonary
  Sciences
School of Health Related Professions
University of Medicine and Dentistry
Blackwood, New Jersey

Donna M. Williams, RRT
Pulmonary Education Specialist
Children's Healthcare of Atlanta
Atlanta, Georgia

Portions of the original proposal and manuscript were reviewed by:

James Joseph Bierl, MS, RRT
Associate Professor
Department of Respiratory Care
Erie Community College
Buffalo, New York

Lisa Ramfjord Elstun, BS, RRT
Education Management and Accreditation
  Consulting
Dallas, Texas

Patricia G. Hyland, BS, RRT
Program Director
Department of Respiratory Care
Hudson Valley Community College
Troy, New York

Beverly L. Tabor, BHS, RRT
Program Chair
Department of Respiratory Care
Florida Community College at
  Jacksonville
Jacksonville, Florida

CONTENTS

UNIT ONE • The Respiratory System 1

UNIT TWO • The Cardiovascular System 235

UNIT THREE • THE URINARY SYSTEM AND ACID-BASE BALANCE 321

COLOR PLATES

COLOR PLATES

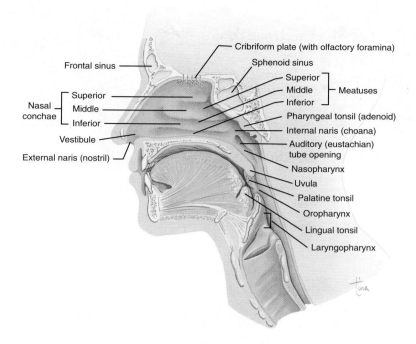

COLOR PLATE 1. Upper respiratory tract (midsagittal view). Nasal septum has been removed to show detail of the right lateral wall of the nasal cavity. (Adapted from Scanlon VC and Sanders T: Essentials of Anatomy and Physiology, ed. 3. FA Davis, Philadelphia, 1999, p 327, with permission.)

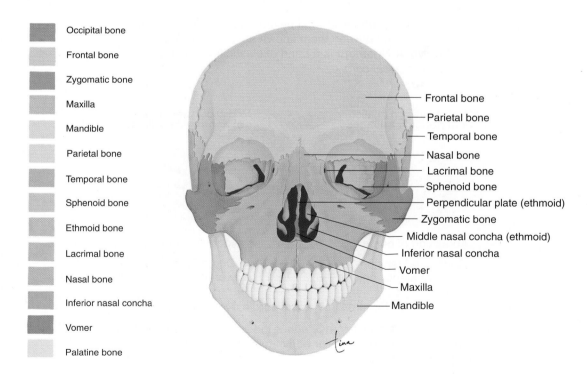

COLOR PLATE 2. Skull (anterior view). (Adapted from Scanlon VC and Sanders T: Essentials of Anatomy and Physiology, ed. 3. FA Davis, Philadelphia, 1999, p 107, with permission.)

COLOR PLATES

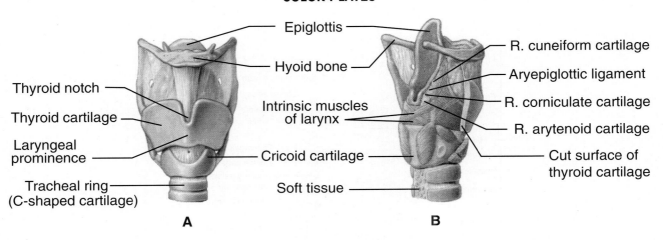

Epiglottis

Hyoid bone

Thyroid notch

Thyroid cartilage

Laryngeal prominence

Tracheal ring (C-shaped cartilage)

Intrinsic muscles of larynx

Cricoid cartilage

Soft tissue

R. cuneiform cartilage

Aryepiglottic ligament

R. corniculate cartilage

R. arytenoid cartilage

Cut surface of thyroid cartilage

A

B

COLOR PLATE 3. Larynx. (A) Anterior view; (B) posterolateral view.

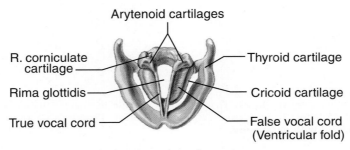

Arytenoid cartilages

R. corniculate cartilage

Rima glottidis

True vocal cord

Thyroid cartilage

Cricoid cartilage

False vocal cord (Ventricular fold)

A. Laryngeal cartilages

Note: The **glottis** is formed by the *true vocal cords* plus the opening between them known as the *rima glottidis*. The **vocal ligament** is a band of elastic tissue lying within the *true vocal cord*.

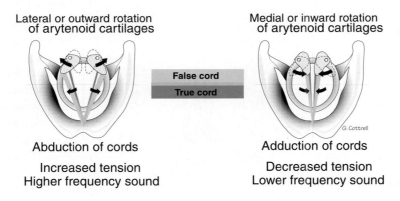

Lateral or outward rotation of arytenoid cartilages

Medial or inward rotation of arytenoid cartilages

False cord

True cord

Abduction of cords

Increased tension
Higher frequency sound

Adduction of cords

Decreased tension
Lower frequency sound

B. Schematic of vocal cord movement

Note that the false vocal cord is *above* the true vocal cord and that both pairs of cords have similar bony attachments on the thyroid and arytenoid cartilages.

COLOR PLATE 4. Vocal apparatus of the larynx (superior view). (A) Laryngeal cartilages; (B) schematic of vocal cord movement.

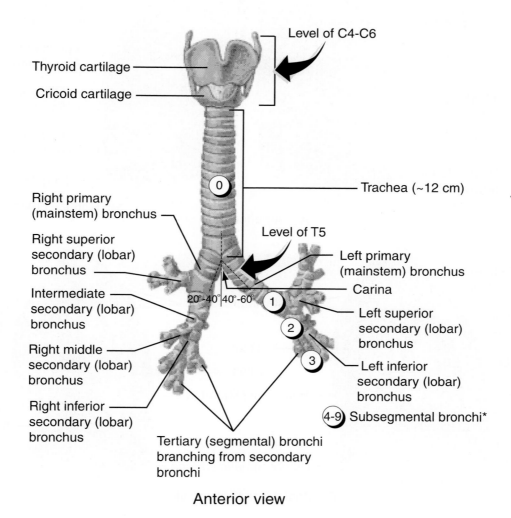

Level of C4-C6

Thyroid cartilage

Cricoid cartilage

Trachea (~12 cm)

Right primary
(mainstem) bronchus

Level of T5

Right superior
secondary (lobar)
bronchus

Left primary
(mainstem) bronchus

Carina

Intermediate
secondary (lobar)
bronchus

20°-40°|40°-60°

Left superior
secondary (lobar)
bronchus

Right middle
secondary (lobar)
bronchus

Left inferior
secondary (lobar)
bronchus

Right inferior
secondary (lobar)
bronchus

Subsegmental bronchi*

Tertiary (segmental) bronchi
branching from secondary
bronchi

Anterior view

COLOR PLATE 5. Cartilaginous airways and the tracheobronchial tree. Subsegmental bronchi are small-diameter (1-mm) cartilaginous airways that continue as distal branches of the segmental bronchi. Airway generations are designated by a numbered circle. Note the vertical orientation of the two mainstem bronchi at the bifurcation of the trachea.

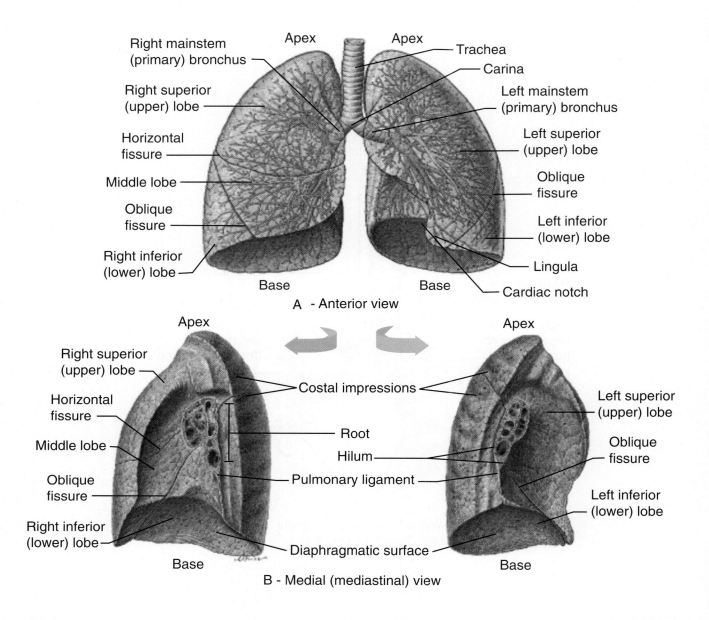

Right mainstem (primary) bronchus
Right superior (upper) lobe
Horizontal fissure
Middle lobe
Oblique fissure
Right inferior (lower) lobe
Apex
Base
Trachea
Carina
Left mainstem (primary) bronchus
Left superior (upper) lobe
Oblique fissure
Left inferior (lower) lobe
Lingula
Cardiac notch
Apex
Base

A - Anterior view

Right superior (upper) lobe
Horizontal fissure
Middle lobe
Oblique fissure
Right inferior (lower) lobe
Apex
Base
Costal impressions
Root
Hilum
Pulmonary ligament
Diaphragmatic surface
Apex
Base
Left superior (upper) lobe
Oblique fissure
Left inferior (lower) lobe

B - Medial (mediastinal) view

Note: Due to the diagonal orientation of the **oblique fissures**, the **inferior lobes** of the lung are much larger than they appear when viewed from the front (see Fig. 2-11).

COLOR PLATE 6. Lung surface features.

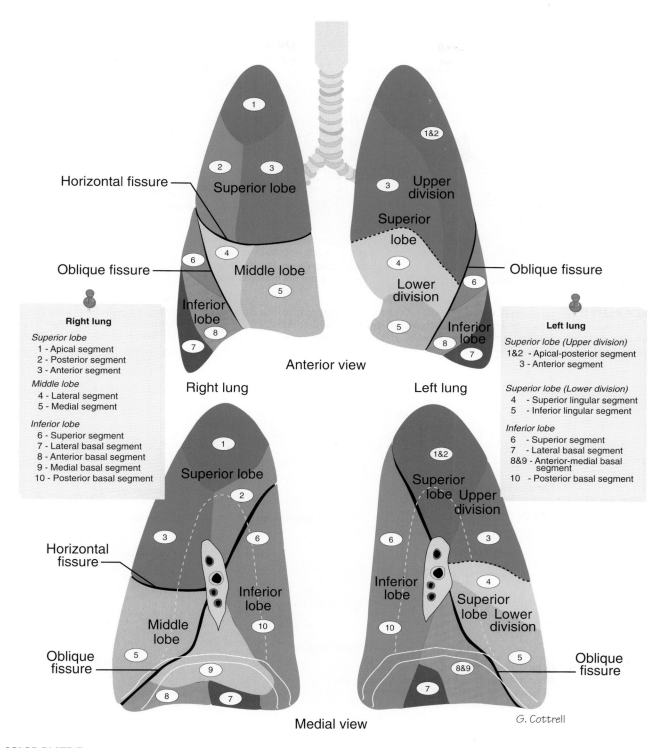

Horizontal fissure

Oblique fissure

Right lung

Superior lobe
 1 - Apical segment
 2 - Posterior segment
 3 - Anterior segment

Middle lobe
 4 - Lateral segment
 5 - Medial segment

Inferior lobe
 6 - Superior segment
 7 - Lateral basal segment
 8 - Anterior basal segment
 9 - Medial basal segment
 10 - Posterior basal segment

Superior lobe

Middle lobe

Inferior lobe

Anterior view

Right lung

Left lung

Upper division

Superior lobe

Lower division

Inferior lobe

Oblique fissure

Left lung

Superior lobe (Upper division)
 1&2 - Apical-posterior segment
 3 - Anterior segment

Superior lobe (Lower division)
 4 - Superior lingular segment
 5 - Inferior lingular segment

Inferior lobe
 6 - Superior segment
 7 - Lateral basal segment
 8&9 - Anterior-medial basal segment
 10 - Posterior basal segment

Horizontal fissure

Superior lobe

Middle lobe

Inferior lobe

Oblique fissure

Superior lobe Upper division

Inferior lobe

Superior lobe Lower division

Oblique fissure

Medial view

G. Cottrell

COLOR PLATE 7. Bronchopulmonary segments. Bronchopulmonary segments are supplied by tertiary (segmental) bronchi. Note that there are 10 segments in the right lung and 8 in the left. Most sources agree that this is due to the fusing of lung segments: the *apical-posterior segment* and the *anterior-medial basal segment.*

COLOR PLATES

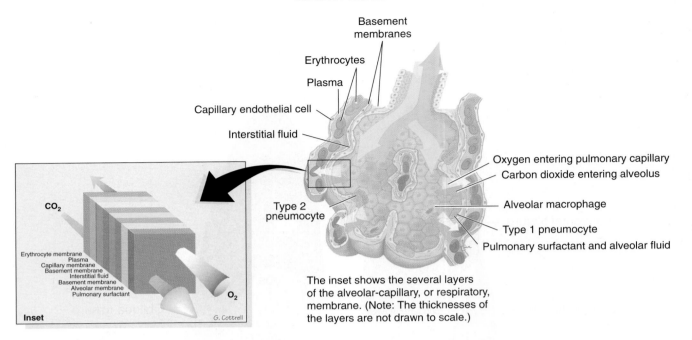

The inset shows the several layers of the alveolar-capillary, or respiratory, membrane. (Note: The thicknesses of the layers are not drawn to scale.)

COLOR PLATE 8. Alveolar-capillary membrane. At the site of external respiration, simple squamous epithelium provides the smallest possible separation between the airstream and the bloodstream. The alveolar membrane consists of a single type 1 pneumocyte; the capillary membrane consists of a single endothelial cell. (Adapted from Scanlon VC and Sanders T: Essentials of Anatomy and Physiology, ed. 3. FA Davis, Philadelphia, 1999, p 332, with permission.)

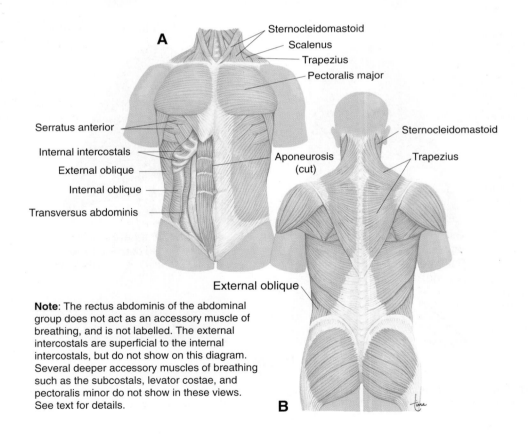

Note: The rectus abdominis of the abdominal group does not act as an accessory muscle of breathing, and is not labelled. The external intercostals are superficial to the internal intercostals, but do not show on this diagram. Several deeper accessory muscles of breathing such as the subcostals, levator costae, and pectoralis minor do not show in these views. See text for details.

COLOR PLATE 9. Accessory muscles of breathing. (A) Anterior view; (B) superior view. (Adapted from Scanlon VC and Sanders T: Essentials of Anatomy and Physiology, ed. 3. FA Davis, Philadelphia, 1999, p 145, with permission.)

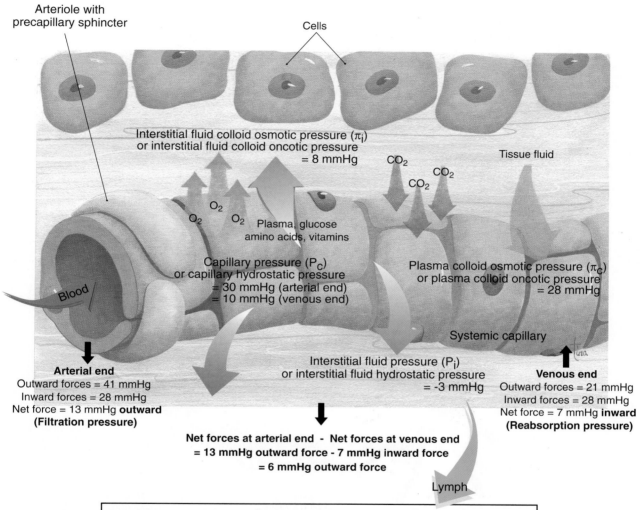

Arteriole with precapillary sphincter

Cells

Interstitial fluid colloid osmotic pressure (π_i) or interstitial fluid colloid oncotic pressure = 8 mmHg

CO_2
CO_2
CO_2

Tissue fluid

O_2
O_2
O_2

Plasma, glucose amino acids, vitamins

Capillary pressure (P_C) or capillary hydrostatic pressure = 30 mmHg (arterial end) = 10 mmHg (venous end)

Plasma colloid osmotic pressure (π_C) or plasma colloid oncotic pressure = 28 mmHg

Blood

Systemic capillary

Arterial end
Outward forces = 41 mmHg
Inward forces = 28 mmHg
Net force = 13 mmHg **outward**
(Filtration pressure)

Interstitial fluid pressure (P_i) or interstitial fluid hydrostatic pressure = -3 mmHg

Venous end
Outward forces = 21 mmHg
Inward forces = 28 mmHg
Net force = 7 mmHg **inward**
(Reabsorption pressure)

Net forces at arterial end - Net forces at venous end
= 13 mmHg outward force - 7 mmHg inward force
= 6 mmHg outward force

Lymph

Note: Because of the "pumping" action of the pulmonary lymphatics, a slight negative pressure is generated in the tissue spaces of loose connective tissue. The interstitial fluid hydrostatic pressure is typically around -3 mmHg, thus causing fluid to "flow" in the tissue spaces from the arterial end to the venous end of the blood capillaries, and be scavenged by the lymph capillaries.

COLOR PLATE 10. Starling forces acting at the capillary wall. Arrows depict the direction of movement of fluid between the vascular and tissue fluid compartments. (Adapted from Scanlon VC and Sanders T: Essentials of Anatomy and Physiology, ed. 3. FA Davis, Philadelphia, 1999, p 279, with permission.)

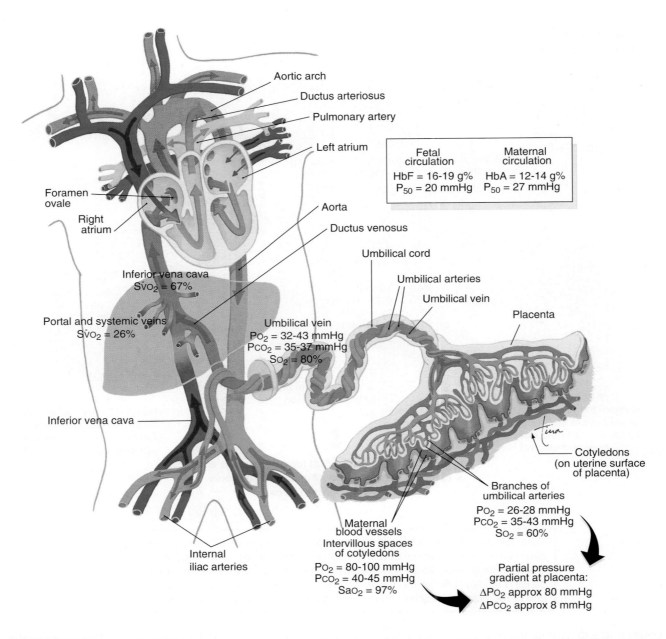

COLOR PLATE 11. Fetal circulation. (Adapted from Scanlon VC and Sanders T: Essentials of Anatomy and Physiology, ed. 3. FA Davis, Philadelphia, 1999, p 290, with permission.)

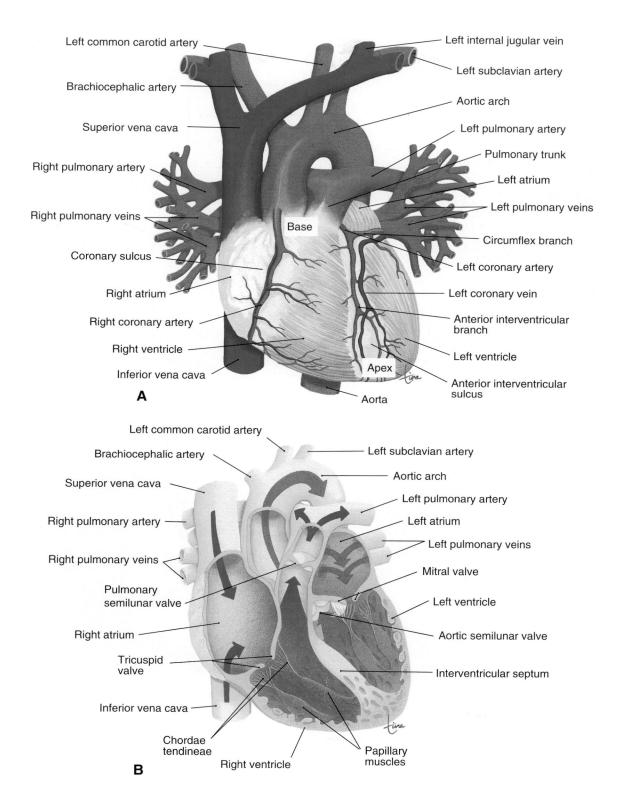

COLOR PLATE 12. Cardiac structures. (A) Surface features of the heart (anterior view). (B) Internal features of the heart (coronal view). (Adapted from Scanlon VC and Sanders T: Essentials of Anatomy and Physiology, ed. 3. FA Davis, Philadelphia, 1999, p 260, with permission.)

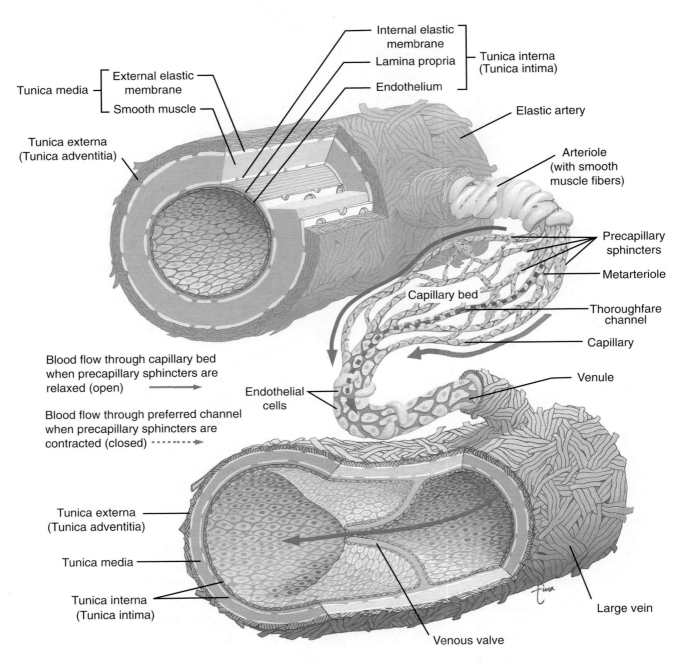

COLOR PLATE 13. Blood vessel structure. (Adapted from Scanlon VC and Sanders T: Essentials of Anatomy and Physiology, ed. 3. FA Davis, Philadelphia, 1999, p 277, with permission.)

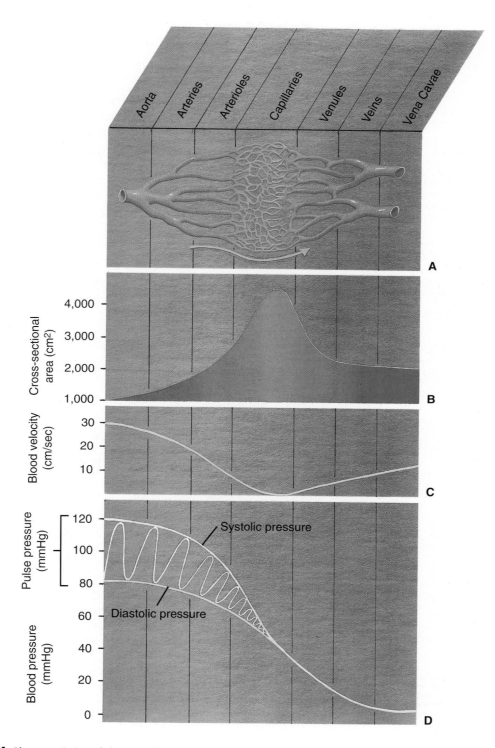

COLOR PLATE 14. Characteristics of the vascular system. (A) Schematic of the branching vessels. (B) Cross-sectional area. (C) Blood velocity. (D) Systemic blood pressure changes. (Adapted from Scanlon VC and Sanders T: Essentials of Anatomy and Physiology, ed. 3. FA Davis, Philadelphia, 1999, p 291, with permission.)

COLOR PLATES

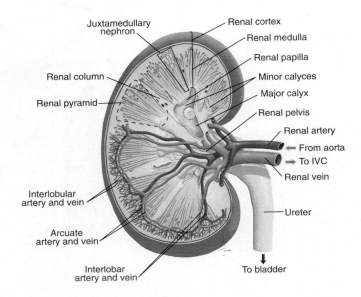

COLOR PLATE 15. Structural features of the kidney. (Adapted from Scanlon VC and Sanders T: Essentials of Anatomy and Physiology, ed. 3. FA Davis, Philadelphia, 1999, p 405, with permission.)

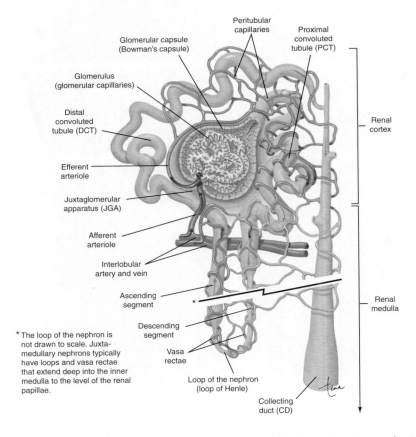

*The loop of the nephron is not drawn to scale. Juxtamedullary nephrons typically have loops and vasa rectae that extend deep into the inner medulla to the level of the renal papillae.

COLOR PLATE 16. Nephron. Juxtamedullary nephron with its associated blood vessels. Arrows depict the direction of flow of blood and of glomerular filtrate. (Adapted from Scanlon VC and Sanders T: Essentials of Anatomy and Physiology, ed. 3. FA Davis, Philadelphia, 1999, p 406, with permission.)

The Respiratory System

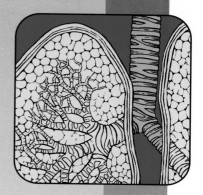

The following unit covers the structure, function, and the entire age spectrum of the respiratory system—from its embryonic beginnings to its inevitable decline. In this unit we examine the astounding transition of the embryonic lung from its dependent existence in a fluid environment to its independent, air-filled state. The unit provides a review of the gross and microscopic anatomy of the respiratory system and associated thoracic structures and muscles, and explores the physiologic mechanisms of ventilatory control, external and internal respiration, gas transport, and lung defense. The unit concludes with a brief discussion of the effects of aging on the structure and function of the respiratory system.

CHAPTER 1

Development of the Respiratory System

chapter objectives

After studying this chapter the reader should be able to:

☐ Explain the functional role of vascularized, wet epithelial linings in respiration.

☐ Summarize the embryologic events that characterize the following periods in the development of the primitive respiratory tube:
   Glandular period, canalicular period, alveolar period.

☐ Summarize the embryologic events that characterize the development of the following structures as they relate to the respiratory system:
   Ventral body cavity, diaphragm, pleural cavity, mediastinum, alveolar-capillary membrane, type II pneumocytes, pulmonary surfactant.

☐ Define the following terms:
   Compliance, elastic forces.

☐ Discuss the structure and function of the connective tissue fibers of the lung and explain how they contribute to instability of the infant lung.

☐ Define the following terms:
   Surface tension, distending (collapse) pressure.

☐ State the LaPlace equation and explain how surface tension and the radius of a sphere affect the pressure of the sphere.

☐ Describe how surface tension contributes to instability of the infant lung.

☐ Explain the concept of interdependence of alveoli and describe how the phenomenon helps stabilize the lung.

☐ State the source of pulmonary surfactant.

☐ Explain how pulmonary surfactant contributes to lung stability of the infant by describing its mechanism of action on liquid films.

☐ Describe the effect of pulmonary surfactant on alveolar radius, surface tension, and inspiratory pressures by summarizing the sequence of events involved in an infant's first breath.

☐ Explain how the ratio of lecithin to sphingomyelin (L/S) is used to assess fetal lung maturity.

☐ Describe the postnatal changes that occur in alveoli.

☐ Correlate the first breath with postnatal circulatory adjustments.

key terms

alveolar-capillary membrane	lobar buds
alveolar period; terminal sac period	lung bud
bronchial buds (brong' ke-al)	mediastinum (mē"dē-as-tī' num)
canalicular period (kan" a-lik' ū -lar)	pleurae (ploo' rī)
coelom (sē' lom)	parietal pleura
extraembryonic coelom	visceral pleura
intraembryonic coelom	pleural canals
pleuroperitoneal coelom	pleural cavity
compliance	pleuropericardial folds
diaphragm	pleuroperitoneal folds
elastic forces	primitive respiratory tube
embryology	pulmonary surfactant; surfactant
glandular period	surface tension (ST)
interdependence of alveoli	trachea (trā' kē-a)
laryngotracheal tube (la-ring" gō-trā' kē-al)	transverse septum
larynx (lar' inks)	

A few weeks after conception one of the most dramatic transformations in the development of body systems is initiated. The amazing process begins with an inconspicuous tubular structure that is slowly converted over a period of 9 months into a mature respiratory system capable of exchanging atmospheric gases with the circulatory system, thus sustaining a newborn infant. The respiratory system is unique among body systems in that it undergoes continuous development throughout the gestation period but remains *nonfunctional* right up to the time a newborn takes his or her first breath. In that brief instant, the respiratory system must become fully functional and assume its life-supporting role in gaseous exchange. The importance of the transition cannot be overemphasized—survival depends upon it. The embryonic development of all other body systems will have been in vain if the structural and functional development of the respiratory system is unable to support the transition from a fluid to an air environment—from dependent intrauterine life to an independent extrauterine existence.

The Human Respiratory System

A MIRROR OF VERTEBRATE DEVELOPMENT

Stages in development of the human respiratory system introduce the reader to the entire range of development of respiratory structures in vertebrates. For example, some stages resemble the simple respiratory structures of amphibians; hence, an early stage in the development of human lungs is referred to as the "amphibian stage." With increasing structural complexity, the developing human lung passes through a "reptilian stage" of development. This is not to say that our complex respiratory system, when completed, has traces or evidence of fish, amphibian, reptilian, or avian respiratory structures, merely that certain stages in the embryologic development of mammalian lungs closely resemble the final form of the respiratory system of lower animals. In spite of amazing variety in the gross anatomic features of vertebrate respiratory structures, the microscopic structures that make external respiration possible are strikingly similar. Namely, all vertebrates, whether they breathe with gills or with lungs, depend on *wet epithelial linings* that are *highly vascularized* to provide an effective surface area and interface for gaseous exchange between the external environment and the bloodstream.

EMBRYOLOGY: THE ELUSIVE "BIG PICTURE"

One of the difficulties in the field of **embryology**—the study of the origin and development of an individual—is that many events are occurring simultaneously and in rapid fashion. At this point we encounter our first challenge in understanding the overall process. The individual mechanisms occur in an orderly and sequential fashion, but because multiple processes are occurring at the same time, the overall scheme of embryologic development resembles a virtual explosion of activity on several fronts—a form of "controlled chaos"—as select groups of cells in different parts of the developing body migrate to different regions, or differentiate and organize into sheets of tissues that may fold inward or bulge outward to form entirely new structures. The result is a dynamic, constantly changing form. For example, at the time when the future lungs are differentiating and expanding as small buds from a simple hollow tubular structure, the developing tube itself is pushing into a future body cavity that has not yet completely formed. The pleural membranes also must invade the developing cavity but must do so in advance of the incoming lung structures to both line the cavity and cover the primitive lung. In addition, complex partitioning is required to separate the thoracic cavity from the abdominopelvic cavity and to further subdivide the thoracic cavity into separate compartments for each lung and for the heart. Meanwhile, precursors of thoracic cage structures such as undifferentiated bone and primitive muscle fibers continue their development as they push into the region. All of these morphologic and functional changes contribute to the development of the respiratory system.

Herein lies the challenge: the reader needs a *global view* of the complex developmental events that are under way in the embryo even though the individual events are presented in the text in a *sequential* manner. It should be pointed out that a sequential description of these events, as previewed in the chapter outline, is an oversimplification. Keep in mind the multifaceted nature of embryonic development as you read the following chronologic and sequential description of the transformation of the human respiratory system. To further appreciate the structural and functional complexity of the interrelated events, remember that we are discussing introductory embryologic concepts re-

lated to a *single* body system and that simultaneous development is also occurring in the cardiovascular, neuroendocrine, urinary, digestive, musculoskeletal, and reproductive systems, and that the development of all of these systems is well under way a mere 8 weeks after conception.

The reader wishing to learn more about developmental anatomy is encouraged to consult the embryology sources cited at the end of the chapter. For our purposes, the overview presented in this chapter, plus an appreciation of the simultaneous and complex events that accompany development of the respiratory system, will suffice.

Embryologic Development of the Primitive Respiratory Tube

Development of the respiratory system from a **primitive respiratory tube** is divided into several periods concerned first with development of the various classes of airways comprising the *conducting zone,* followed by a *transitional stage,* and concluding with development of the gas-exchange structures of the *respiratory zone.* Table 1–1 is a time line of significant events occurring in the development of the primitive respiratory tube.

NOTE: Different reference sources often describe the following developmental periods in slightly different ways.

GLANDULAR (PSEUDOGLANDULAR) PERIOD

During the developmental period known as the **glandular period,** the primitive respiratory tube differentiates and successively branches into the tracheobronchial tree. This development of the conducting zone of the respiratory system continues from fertilization to approximately 16 weeks gestation and results in the production of approximately the first 17 to 20 orders of branches. Recall from general anatomy of the respiratory system that each time a respiratory tube branches, a new *order,* or *generation,* of airway is produced. For example, the bifurcation, or branching of the trachea, represents the first order of branches.

During the first one-third of the glandular period, from fertilization to approximately 5 weeks gestation, the first two orders of branches arise, resulting in the formation of the trachea, as well as primitive mainstem and lobar bronchi. This initial period is referred to as the "embryonic period" (Des Jardins, 1998). The period begins with the development of the **laryngotra-**

TABLE 1-1	**Time Line of Development of the Primitive Respiratory Tube**
Glandular Period General comments	Fertilization to approximately 16 weeks Differentiation and branching of tracheobronchial tree into approximately the first 17–20 orders of branches
Embryonic Period (fertilization to 5 weeks)	Laryngotracheal tube develops from primitive pharynx Cranial part of tube becomes larynx Caudal part of tube becomes trachea Primitive lung bud developes from distal end of tracheal tube 4 weeks: right and left bronchial (primary) buds develop from long bud ("amphibian stage")
Pseudoglandular Period (5–16 weeks)	5 weeks: lobar (secondary) buds develop from bronchial buds 7 weeks: segmental (tertiary) branches develop from lobar buds Subsegmental branches develop from segmental branches Connective tissue and blood vessel ingrowth into the developing terminal air sacs ("reptilian stage") 10 weeks: goblet cells develop 12–26 weeks: tracheobronchial glands develop 12–13 weeks: ciliated epithelium develops 14 weeks: mucus production begins
Canalicular period General comments	17–24 weeks Transitional period between development of distal parts of the conducting zone and development of the proximal parts of the respiratory zone Continued development of terminal bronchioles as well as initial development of respiratory bronchioles
Alveolar period *(terminal sac period)* General comments	24 weeks to birth (approximately 38–41 weeks) Final development of functional units of the lung Total number of alveoli continues to increase until approximately 8 years (i.e., alveolar period extends *postnatally*) Primitive respiratory bronchioles (from canalicular period) continue to develop 34 weeks: respiratory units (acini) composed of alveolar ducts, alveolar sacs, and alveoli develop from respiratory bronchioles Type I alveolar cells (type I pneumocytes) develop as squamous epithelial cells at the future alveolar-capillary membrane Type II alveolar cells (type II pneumocytes) become increasingly active in surfactant production during late stages of alveolar period leading up to birth

Note: All time periods given above are approximate.

cheal tube located on the floor of the primitive pharynx (Fig. 1–1). The cranial portion of the tube grows to become the **larynx** and the caudal portion develops into the **trachea.** Further development of the caudal end of the tubelike structure is evident as a single conspicuous outpouching that becomes the **lung bud** (see Fig. 1–1). Around 28 days gestation, **right** and **left bronchial buds** branch from the embryonic lung bud (see Fig. 1–1). These bronchial buds are the precursors of the right and left primary, or mainstem, bronchi. The final orientation and shape of these structures are discussed in the next chapter, but even at this early developmental stage 1 month after conception, the morphologic differences between the right and left primary bronchi are apparent. The development of the paired bronchial buds represents the so-called amphibian stage

of lung development because of its resemblance to the simple lung structure of amphibians—a structure that consists essentially of two air sacs, each with a single large lumen.

Approximately 1 week after the bronchial buds develop from the primitive lung bud, two **lobar buds** develop from each bronchial bud (see Fig. 1–1). These small outpouchings develop secondary branches that will connect to the future lobes of the lung—a superior, middle, and inferior lobe on the right and a superior and inferior lobe on the left.

The embryonic phase of the glandular period ends around 5 weeks after conception but blends seamlessly into the final phase of the glandular period. This final phase covers the gestation period from 5 weeks to approximately 16 weeks and is referred to as the

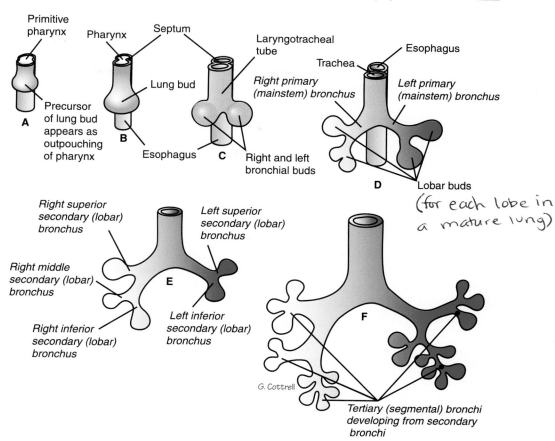

FIGURE 1–1. Primitive lung bud, bronchial buds, and lobar buds (anterior view). (Structures are not drawn to scale. Buds shown are the precursors of the bronchial branches *labeled in italics.*)

"pseudoglandular period" by Des Jardins (1998). As the lobar buds continue to develop, tertiary branches appear at around 7 weeks gestation (see Fig. 1–1). These branches (*segmental bronchi*) will supply the bronchopulmonary segments of the lung: 10 in the right lung and 8 in the left lung (see Fig. 2–11). Additional branching results in development of *subsegmental bronchi* that continue to proliferate throughout the balance of the glandular period. The developing segments become isolated by connective tissue into separate, distinguishable units, each with accompanying pulmonary blood vessels. This phase of the glandular period is referred to as the "reptilian stage" of development because of its resemblance to the final form of the reptilian respiratory system, a system of branching tubes that end in terminal sacs similar to primitive alveoli (Netter, 1979).

The development of future secretory and clearance structures such as *tracheobronchial glands* and ciliated airways is a hallmark of the glandular period. (The structure and function of these components are discussed in later chapters.) *Goblet cells* begin to appear in the trachea and expanding orders of bronchi at approximately the 10th week of gestation, and *bronchial mucous glands* develop a short time later at around 12 weeks gestation, and begin producing mucus by 14 weeks. Bronchial glands continue to form until 25 or 26 weeks gestation. Ciliated epithelium is found in the lining of the mainstem bronchi at approximately 12 weeks and in the lining of the segmental bronchi around 13 weeks gestation.

CANALICULAR (TRANSITIONAL) PERIOD

The **canalicular period** is a *transitional* period in fetal lung development that covers the gestation period from 17 to approximately 24 weeks. This period includes changes characteristic of the final stages of conducting zone development as well as the initial stages of respiratory zone development. The period is marked by continued division of the *terminal bronchioles* of the conducting zone and the first appearance of primitive *respiratory bronchioles* of the respiratory zone (see Table 1–1).

ALVEOLAR (TERMINAL SAC) PERIOD

The final period in the development of the tracheobronchial tree structures is the **alveolar period,** also known as the terminal sac period. This period is concerned with the final structural development of the respiratory zone, which began during the latter portion of the preceding canalicular period. In terms of fetal development of the respiratory system, the alveolar period of development extends from 24 weeks to birth, with birth occurring between 38 and 41 weeks in a normal gestation period (see Table 1–1). However, since the total number of alveoli are not formed by the time of birth, and continue to be formed for several more years, the alveolar period can be viewed as an extended period of development reaching from the late fetal period until approximately the eighth year of life. The postnatal development of alveoli is briefly discussed at the end of this chapter. Primitive respiratory bronchioles that first made their appearance in the canalicular period each divide into three to six *alveolar ducts,* which, in turn, end in a terminal *alveolar sac* that possesses separate *alveoli.* By 34 weeks, this entire *respiratory unit* becomes well defined. The respiratory unit is also known as the *acinus,* a collective term used to describe a single respiratory bronchiole with all of its distal branches—alveolar ducts, alveolar sacs, and alveoli.

The cellular architecture of the respiratory zone continues to be refined throughout the alveolar period. *Type I alveolar cells,* also known as *type I pneumocytes,* become well defined as squamous epithelial cells at the future *alveolar-capillary membrane.* Such flattened cells, although they are outnumbered by the secretory cells of the alveoli, comprise 25 times the surface area compared to that of the secretory cells and are, therefore, well suited to their role in gas exchange at the future air-blood interface (Taylor et al, 1989). Secretory cells called *type II alveolar cells,* or *type II pneumocytes,* are much larger and more numerous than the type I pneumocytes making up the developing alveolar walls.

These secretory cells become increasingly active throughout the latter stage of respiratory tube development and are responsible for the production of *pulmonary surfactant,* a complex chemical substance necessary for infant survival. The critical role of pulmonary surfactant is explored at the end of this chapter.

Embryologic Development of Other Respiratory System Structures

VENTRAL BODY CAVITY

An undifferentiated embryonic body cavity is known as a **coelom.** The **extraembryonic coelom** is associated with the amnion and yolk sac, whereas the **intraembryonic coelom** develops into the future body cavities of the embryo. Human embryos have two parallel intraembryonic coelomic cavities that run the length of the embryo (Fig. 1–2). The pericardial, pleural, and peritoneal cavities develop as subdivisions of these intraembryonic cavities. At approximately week two, the paired intraembryonic cavities in the vicinity of the developing heart fuse into a single pericardial cavity that will ultimately enclose the heart (see Fig. 1–2). While the pericardial cavity is forming, it is still in communication with the paired intraembryonic coeloms extending into the future abdominopelvic region.

Although the scale and the relative locations of the infantile structures differ from those of the adult, the reader is urged to develop a mental image of these

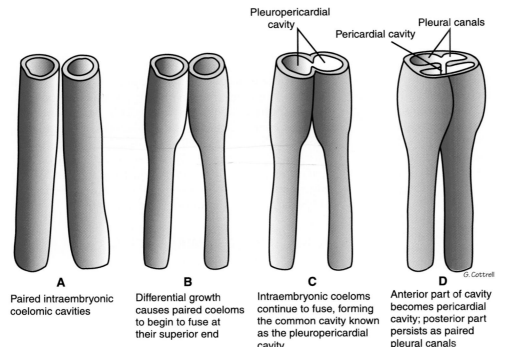

Pleuropericardial cavity

Pericardial cavity

Pleural canals

G. Cottrell

A
Paired intraembryonic coelomic cavities

B
Differential growth causes paired coeloms to begin to fuse at their superior end

C
Intraembryonic coeloms continue to fuse, forming the common cavity known as the pleuropericardial cavity

D
Anterior part of cavity becomes pericardial cavity; posterior part persists as paired pleural canals

FIGURE 1–2. Schematic—fusion and partitioning of intraembryonic coeloms (anterior view).

events as they unfold. For example, picture the various spatial relationships of the structures at this point in time: The relatively large, developing heart is positioned anteriorly and is being enclosed within the protective pericardial cavity, a cavity that still opens to the abdominal cavity. Furthermore, the relatively small, primitive lungs have not completely pushed into the future thoracic space, nor are they yet partitioned from the heart or from each other at this early stage. In simplest terms, what is required at this point in development is a sequence of partitioning, or "wall-building," that will divide the cavity, separating it from top to bottom and from right to left—a transverse as well as a sagittal partition. The transverse partition will develop from several folds to become the future diaphragm separating the thoracic and abdominopelvic cavities; the sagittal partition will develop from a series of folds that will ultimately separate the right and left lung as well as isolate the heart in the midline of the body.

Partitioning of the developing pericardial coelom from the two primitive intraembryonic coeloms occurs with the growth of a horizontally directed **transverse septum** (Fig. 1–3). The direction of growth of the transverse septum occurs posteriorly toward the dorsal body wall of the embryo, but the septum does not reach the dorsal wall. Instead, communication between the pericardial coelom and the paired primitive coeloms is maintained for a while longer as paired **pleural canals** (see Fig. 1–3). The primitive lung buds discussed earlier with the development of the respiratory tube will grow into these pleural canals.

The common cavity consisting of the pericardial coelom and the paired pleural canals is divided by the growth of the **pleuropericardial folds** (Fig. 1–4). These vertically oriented folds of tissue project as ridges from the lateral sidewalls of the body. As the right and left pleuropericardial folds grow medially into the cavity they bulge into the pleural canals and finally fuse along the midline. This partition in the frontal plane completely separates the pericardial cavity from the pleural canals at a level superior to the developing diaphragm. At this point the pleural canals are still in communication with the peritoneal cavity. The resulting common cavity is known as the **pleuroperitoneal coelom** (see Fig. 1–4).

The partitioning process continues with the development of a transverse structure that will separate the thorax from the peritoneal cavity. Ultimately the lungs will be isolated in the thoracic cavity by the diaphragm, a muscular partition created through the continued growth of the transverse septum and two horizontally-oriented **pleuroperitoneal folds** (Fig. 1–5). The pleuroperitoneal folds are internal ridges of the dorsolateral body wall that grow anteriorly and medially to fuse with the advancing transverse septum. As the three contributing structures of the diaphragm grow toward each other, they effectively "surround," or encase, structures already located in the midline of the cavity. These structures include the aorta, esophagus, inferior vena cava, thoracic duct, and nerves (see Fig. 1–5). At this point in time, the two embryonic pleural cavities superior to the diaphragm have been walled off from the peritoneal cavity below. Eventually, muscle and nerve fibers migrate into the newly formed diaphragm to make it functional, thus transforming a simple partition into the dome-shaped muscular floor of the thoracic cavity.

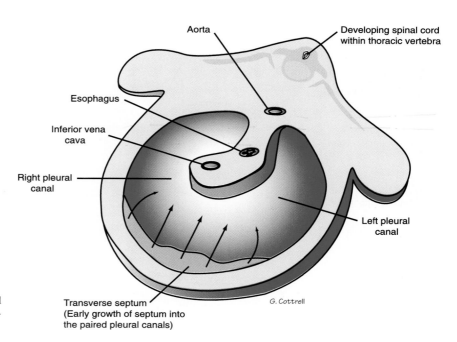

FIGURE 1–3. Transverse septum and pleural canals (transverse section at the level of the developing diaphragm).

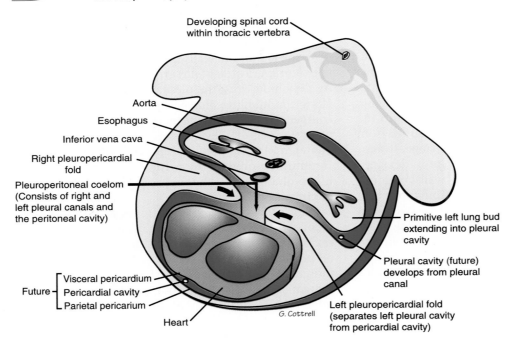

Developing spinal cord within thoracic vertebra

Aorta

Esophagus

Inferior vena cava

Right pleuropericardial fold

Pleuroperitoneal coelom (Consists of right and left pleural canals and the peritoneal cavity)

Future —[Visceral pericardium / Pericardial cavity / Parietal pericarium

Heart

Primitive left lung bud extending into pleural cavity

Pleural cavity (future) develops from pleural canal

Left pleuropericardial fold (separates left pleural cavity from pericardial cavity)

G. Cottrell

FIGURE 1–4. Pleuropericardial folds (transverse section at a level superior to the developing diaphragm).

DIAPHRAGM

Following fusion of the transverse septum with the right and left pleuroperitoneal folds, the middle portion of the **diaphragm** develops a tough, membranous structure called the *central tendon* (Fig. 1–6). Structures such as the aorta, inferior vena cava, thoracic duct, and esophagus pass through the central tendon, along with smaller blood vessels and nerves. The periphery of the circular diaphragm is transformed into a strong sheet of muscle by the migration of striated muscle fibers (see Fig. 1–5). In addition, branches of the third, fourth, and fifth cervical spinal nerves, precursors of the phrenic nerve, innervate the newly arrived muscle fibers to provide the sole motor control for diaphragmatic movement. Simple contractions in the form of hiccup-like actions begin soon after and serve to prepare the respiratory muscle for an extrauterine existence. Upon contraction, the radially oriented muscle fibers of the diaphragm apply tension to the dome-shaped central tendon and cause it to flatten, thus increasing the length of the thorax and pro-

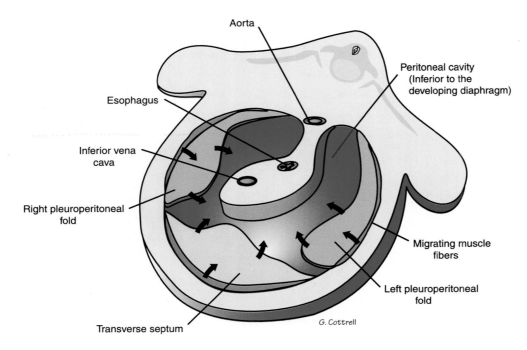

Aorta

Esophagus

Inferior vena cava

Right pleuroperitoneal fold

Transverse septum

Peritoneal cavity (Inferior to the developing diaphragm)

Migrating muscle fibers

Left pleuroperitoneal fold

G. Cottrell

FIGURE 1–5. Pleuroperitoneal folds (transverse section at the level of the developing diaphragm).

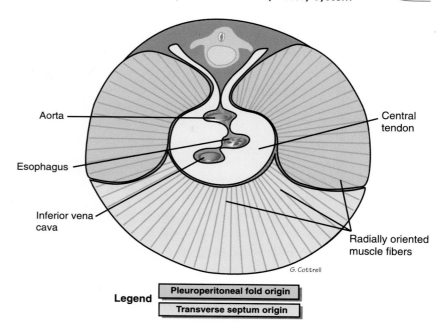

Aorta

Esophagus

Inferior vena cava

Central tendon

Radially oriented muscle fibers

G. Cottrell

FIGURE 1–6. Schematic—components for the diaphragm (superior view).

Legend

| Pleuroperitoneal fold origin |
| Transverse septum origin |

ducing a negative intrapleural pressure. Diaphragmatic movements, as well as volume and pressure changes in the thorax and lung, are examined in Chapter 7. Differential growth in the thoracic cage structures result in an apparent "migration" of the diaphragm caudally so that its inferior attachments ultimately are found at approximately the level of the first lumbar vertebra. The phrenic nerves lengthen to accommodate this "new" location of the diaphragm.

PLEURAL CAVITY AND MEDIASTINUM

The pace of development and growth in the respiratory and cardiovascular systems is uneven, thus affecting not only overall size, but relative positions of the organs. For example, at 6 to 7 weeks gestation, the anteriorly situated heart dwarfs the relatively small and primitive lungs (Fig. 1–7). By 8 weeks, however, the situation has changed considerably. For instance, the membrane-lined, paired pleural canals, which are the precursors of the **pleural cavities,** have grown to nearly surround the heart and are now located more anteriorly (see Fig. 1–7). This development of the pleural canals is slightly in advance of the lungs that will grow into the newly created spaces on either side of the heart. The other consequence of early development of the pleural canals is that they effectively isolate other developing thoracic structures such as the heart, great vessels, and esophagus in a midline septum called the **mediastinum** that extends from the vertebral column ventrally to the sternum (see Fig. 1–7). The right pleural cavity, even at this early stage of respiratory system development, is larger than the left. The size difference is related to the shift of the heart from the midline to the left side of the thorax, with the

heart ultimately occupying the cardiac notch of the left lung.

As the lungs migrate into the pleural spaces, they push into the thin tissue lining the cavity and become covered by the membrane, just as one's fist is tightly covered by clinging plastic film when the fist is pushed into a sheet of thin plastic wrap. The layer of material that contacts and adheres to the lung surface is known as the **visceral pleura;** the membranous layer that remains as the lining of the wall of the developing pleural cavity is called the **parietal pleura.** The visceral pleura reflects off the lung's surface at the root of the lung and continues as the parietal pleura (see Fig. 1–7). These two layers are separated by a fluid-filled potential space known as the pleural cavity, or pleural space. The role of the pleural space and pleural fluid in the mechanics of breathing is examined further in Chapter 7.

ALVEOLAR-CAPILLARY MEMBRANE

The **alveolar-capillary membrane** is composed of a type I pneumocyte and a capillary endothelial cell plus their respective basement membranes. The extremely thin membrane is the interface between the airstream and the bloodstream and thus serves as the site of gas exchange between the external environment and the blood. Overall, the function of the alveolar-capillary system is to expose the blood to an optimal external surface area for the effective exchange of gas. In general, the alveolar-capillary system consists of an extensively vascularized, wet epithelial lining common to all animals, terrestrial as well as aquatic species. The structure and function of the individual components of the respiratory membrane are examined in Chapters 11 and 12, but at this stage it will suffice to point out that

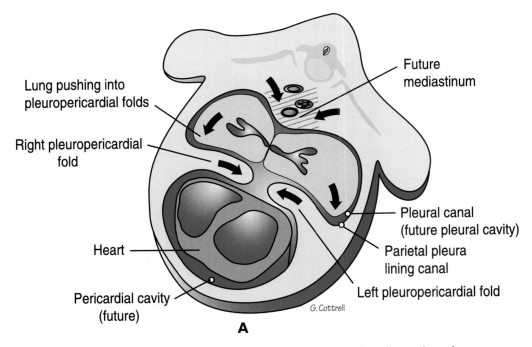

Lung pushing into pleuropericardial folds

Right pleuropericardial fold

Heart

Pericardial cavity (future)

Future mediastinum

Pleural canal (future pleural cavity)

Parietal pleura lining canal

Left pleuropericardial fold

G. Cottrell

A

Early stage – Lungs expand into the pleural canals, distorting the pleuropericardial folds. *Mediastinum* begins development as a bulge in the dorsal body wall (shown as the cross hatched area).

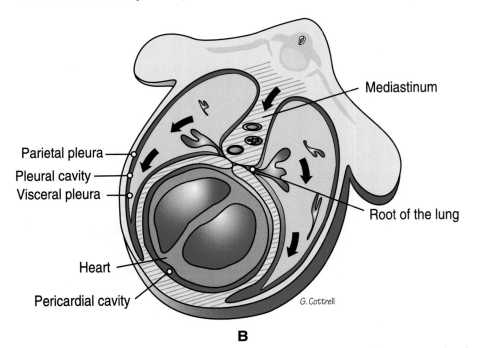

Parietal pleura

Pleural cavity

Visceral pleura

Heart

Pericardial cavity

Mediastinum

Root of the lung

G. Cottrell

B

Late stage – *Parietal pleura* lining the pleural canals adheres to the lung surfaces as they expand into the future pleural cavities. The covering of the lungs becomes the *visceral pleura*. The *mediastinum* develops as a semirigid partition between the lungs extending from the vertebra to the sternum, and encasing the esophagus, great vessels, and heart.

FIGURE 1–7. Pleural cavities and mediastinum (transverse section).

embryonic development of this gas exchange system results in the formation of approximately 24 million primitive alveoli by the time of birth (Netter, 1979). At birth these primitive alveoli, produced during the alveolar period of respiratory tube development, are present as inconspicuous bulges of the walls of terminal sacs and respiratory bronchioles; but they become more defined and conspicuous immediately following birth. Their thickness at birth is approximately 0.4 μm (1 μm = 1 micrometer = 1×10^{-6} m), which is within the range of adult values (0.1 μm to 2.5 μm). The thickness is acceptable for supporting functional gas exchange. Furthermore these primitive alveoli are capable of supporting respiration because sufficient pulmonary surfactant is present to stabilize the alveoli and prevent atelectasis, or collapse, of the lung (Netter, 1979).

TYPE II PNEUMOCYTES AND PULMONARY SURFACTANT

At approximately the 23rd week of gestation lamellar inclusion bodies become well defined in the type II pneumocytes of the lining of the terminal sacs. Lamellar inclusion bodies in type II pneumocytes are the precursors of pulmonary surfactant, a secretory substance critical in the stability of alveoli. The appearance of this morphologic change is of vital importance because it heralds the start of surfactant production. Pulmonary surfactant is a lipoprotein rich in phospholipids. Surfactant functions to reduce the surface tension present in the fluid layer lining primitive alveoli. Surface tension is discussed in detail in the following section. By reducing the surface tension of the monomolecular layer at the interface between air and the alveolar lining fluid, pulmonary surfactant helps stablize alveoli and thereby act as an antiatelectasis factor to prevent collapse of alveoli at the end of expiration. It should be noted, however, that even though surfactant may be detected in the lungs as early as 23 weeks, the lungs are unable to retain air and tend to collapse completely before 28 to 32 weeks (Netter, 1979). Surfactant has a half-life of 14 to 24 hours; therefore it must be produced throughout our lives in order to maintain the low surface tension necessary to keep the alveoli inflated. The importance of its life-supporting role in the immediate postnatal period cannot be overemphasized.

Pulmonary surfactant is produced in increasing quantity toward the end of a full-term pregnancy; therefore, older fetuses have a better chance of survival when spontaneous ventilation and respiration must occur. Failure of the type II pneumocytes to produce sufficient quantities of pulmonary surfactant prior to birth is associated with infant respiratory distress syndrome (IRDS), also known as surfactant deficiency disease (SDD). In this pulmonary condition, large numbers of alveoli collapse due to the high surface tension of the fluid lining the alveoli, leaving too few to support neonatal respiration. Immature lungs are very unstable for this reason. Postmortem changes in the lining of the alveoli cause the production of a glassy, proteinaceous, membranelike deposit containing large numbers of epithelial cells shed from the walls of the alveoli. Hence IRDS is also referred to as hyaline membrane disease (HMD) (Greek *hyalos,* glass). The survival of many premature infants has been greatly enhanced through the use of exogenous pulmonary surfactant administered shortly after birth. Surfactant derived from calf lung and from synthetic sources has proven effective in the management of these high-risk infants (Box 1–1).

Table 1–2 shows a time line of significant events occurring in the development of respiratory system structures.

The First Breath—Changes from Intrauterine to Extrauterine Life

As previously noted, the respiratory system is the only organ system that remains completely nonfunctional right up until the moment of birth. At that instant, the morphologic and functional development of the preceding 9 months immediately come into play to allow the newborn to breathe spontaneously and thus complete the transformation from a liquid to a gaseous environment. The normal infant will exert an incredible physical effort to inflate the lungs for the first time, a feat that will not be matched again with subsequent breaths. Why is this initial inspiratory effort so demanding and what factors in the infant lung make such an extraordinary feat possible?

INSTABILITY OF THE LUNG

Concepts such as lung compliance and lung elasticity are related to the forces operating in the newborn lung and need to be briefly introduced at this point. The details of the concepts, however, is examined with the topic of pulmonary ventilation of the adult lung (see Chap. 9). We will see that different types of lung compliance can be measured, but for our present purposes, **compliance** can be defined as the degree to which the lungs expand for each unit increase in the transpulmonary pressure. Transpulmonary pressure is the difference between the alveolar pressure and the pleural pressure, or the difference between the pressure in the alveoli and the pressure at the outer surface of the lung. The transpulmonary pressure can be thought of as the *recoil pressure* of the lungs, or the tendency of the

P E R S P E C T I V E S

BOX 1-1

Extending Infant Survivability

Observations made of the nature of edematous foam issuing from the lungs of animals experimentally exposed to noxious gases helped lead the way to the eventual discovery of pulmonary surfactant, the remarkable surface active agent produced by the lung. West (1998) notes that researchers working with the animals "noticed that the tiny air bubbles of the foam were extremely stable." Since it was known that the collapse tendency of small spheres is normally quite high, it was obvious that these small air bubbles of "tracheal froth" derived from the animals' lungs were being affected by some condition or factor that substantially lowered the surface tension of the fluid in the bubbles.

Naturally produced pulmonary surfactant consists of several phospholipids, proteins, and ions. *Surfactant apoproteins* and *calcium ions* (Ca^{2+}) function to facilitate the spread of phospholipids across the surface of the fluid lining of the alveoli. The most important phospholipid synthesized by the type II alveolar epithelial cells of the lung is colfosceril palmitate, which is also known as *1,2-dipalmitoylphosphatidylcholine* (DPPC). This substance disrupts the strong intermolecular binding forces present in the surface molecules of the fluid lining the alveoli, thus reducing the surface tension of the film and decreasing the work of breathing. Surfactant deficiency is most often associated with premature infants and with infants born to mothers with diabetes. Without sufficient surfactant production, newborns quickly fatigue and are at considerable risk for developing widespread atelectasis and pulmonary edema. Severe respiratory distress may develop a few hours to several days after birth (Guyton and Hall, 1996). Without supportive measures, infants in respiratory distress generally die of suffocation as more and more regions of the lungs progressively collapse.

Exogenous surfactant, or pulmonary surfactant derived from an external source, is available as a replacement surface active agent for prophylactic use in babies who are at risk for developing infant respiratory distress syndrome (IRDS), and for the rescue treatment of newborns who have developed IRDS. Exogenous surfactant is available as a synthetic drug and as a drug derived from an animal source. The synthetic version, known as Exosurf Neonatal, is composed of *colfosceril palmitate, cetyl alcohol,* and *tyloxapol.* Cetyl alcohol and tyloxapol serve as spreading agents for the distribution of DPPC, the surface active agent. Beractant (Survanta) is a modified DPPC extract derived from bovine lungs, rather than from a synthetic source. Exogenous surfactant is instilled directly into the infant's trachea where it disperses rapidly onto the airway surfaces. Both Exosurf and Survanta typically cause an immediate decrease in alveolar surface tension to result in improved lung compliance and oxygenation. These life-saving drugs have played a pivotal role in extending the survivability of some infants. The drugs are indicated in the prophylactic treatment of premature infants of very low birth weight (1250 to 1350 g) who are at risk for developing IRDS (Liechty et al, 1991; Long et al, 1992) and in the prophylactic treatment of larger babies who have evidence of lung immaturity (Long et al, 1991). Exogenous surfactants have also proven invaluable in the rescue treatment of infants who have developed IRDS.

- Cottrell GP and Surkin HB: Pharmacology for Respiratory Care Practitioners. FA Davis, Philadelphia, 1995.
- Guyton AC and Hall JE: Textbook of Medical Physiology, ed 9. WB Saunders, Philadelphia, 1996.
- Liechty EA et al: Reduction of neonatal mortality after multiple doses of bovine surfactant in low birth weight neonates with respiratory distress syndrome. Pediatrics 88:19–28, 1991.
- Long J: Surfactant replacement therapy. In Aloan CA and Hill TV: Respiratory Care of the Newborn and Child. JB Lippincott, Philadelphia, 1997.
- Long W et al: Retrospective search for bleeding diathesis among premature newborn infants with pulmonary hemmorhage after synthetic surfactant treatment. The American Exosurf Neonatal Study Group I, and the Canadian Exosurf Neonatal Study Group. J Pediatr 120:S45-S48, 1992.
- Long W et al: A controlled trial of synthetic surfactant in infants weighing 1250 g or more with respiratory distress syndrome. The American Exosurf Neonatal Study Group I, and the Canadian Exosurf Neonatal Study Group. N Engl J Med 325:1696–1703, 1991.
- West JB: Respiratory Physiology: The Essentials, ed 6. Williams & Wilkins, Baltimore, 1998.

TABLE 1–2	Time Line of Development of Various Respiratory System Structures
Birth to 2 weeks	*Glandular period* begins (*embryonic period*)
	Intraembryonic coeloms develop
3 weeks	Development of diaphragm begins
3–4 weeks	Laryngotracheal groove (precursor of laryngotracheal tube) appears
4 weeks	Primitive right and left nasal cavities develop
	Pharynx develops
	Phrenic nerves develop
5 weeks	*Pseudoglandular period* begins
	Pulmonary artery and vein develop
6 weeks	Larynx continues to develop
7 weeks	Oropharynx develops
	Tracheal cartilages begin to develop
	Bronchial smooth muscle develops
8 weeks	Vocal cords appear
9 weeks	Bronchial arteries develop
10 weeks	Mucous glands, goblet cells, and cilia begin to develop
	Cartilaginous rings of trachea continue to develop
11 weeks	Pulmonary lymphatic tissue develops
16–17 weeks	*Canalicular period* begins
24 weeks	*Alveolar (terminal sac) period* begins
26–28 weeks	Alveolar-capillary surface area and surfactant production is sufficient to support extrauterine life
36 weeks	Mature alveoli present

Note: All time period given above are approximate.
Source: Modified from Tomashefski and Richmond (1988).

lungs to collapse at each point of expansion (Guyton and Hall, 1996). Lung compliance, then, is a measure of *distensibility* of the lungs. Lungs with high compliance are those that expand easily with each incremental rise in pressure, whereas stiff lungs that inflate with difficulty are said to lack compliance. **Elastic forces** determine the recoil pressure of the lung, thereby affecting lung compliance. Lungs that lack compliance and exhibit high collapse tendencies due to unusually strong elastic forces are inherently unstable. The compliance of the lung is attributed to two separate factors: (1) *elastic forces of the lung connective tissue,* and (2) *elastic forces caused by the surface tension of the fluid lining the alveoli.* These factors affect both neonatal and adult lungs but are especially important in the newborn struggling with the critical first few breaths.

CONNECTIVE TISSUE

Collagen and elastin fibers surround blood vessels and bronchi and are found throughout the interstitium of the lung. These structural proteins are interwoven among the lung parenchyma, or functional units, and serve as a fibrous meshwork to support the gas-exchange elements. When the lungs are deflated, the collagen and elastin fibers are in a partially contracted state, but when the lungs are inflated, the fibers are stretched and straightened. West (1998) suggests that the geometric arrangement of structural fibers in the lung resembles a nylon stocking, noting that such material is very distensible because of its knitted makeup, even though the individual nylon fibers are difficult to stretch. This analogy is especially appropriate because it helps the reader visualize the lung's ability to both expand and return to its resting volume. Tissue elastic forces are generated when the lung is expanded, thus increasing the recoil pressure and the collapse tendency of the air-filled lung. This structural feature of connective tissue contributes to lung instability. Guyton and Hall (1996) states that such forces account for only about one-third of the total elasticity of the lung. The balance of lung elasticity is produced through the effect of surface tension.

SURFACE TENSION

An important factor contributing to the instability of the lung is the effect of surface tension of the fluid lining the alveoli and small air passages. *Atelectasis* refers to the collapse of alveoli, either in a localized area of the lung, an individual lobe, or an entire lung. What is surface tension and how does it increase lung elasticity and recoil pressure to bring about atelectasis?

Surface tension (ST) is the force (expressed in dynes) acting across 1 cm of the surface of a liquid. It is responsible for holding the liquid surface intact at a liquid-gas interface. By acting parallel to the surface of a fluid, this contractile force decreases the area of the interface. ST is caused by the cohesion that binds similar molecules together at the surface of a fluid and pulls the molecules toward the interior. It is generated by powerful intermolecular forces that produce the membranelike properties seen at the surface of water. Such a monomolecular film is strong enough to support a flat razor blade carefully floated on its side in a dish of water or an insect on the surface of a pond. ST also holds raindrops together and is responsible for the characteristic shape of a soap bubble. In this commonplace structure, the thin layer of soap molecules assumes a spherical shape, the most efficient shape for equally distributing the forces acting at the film interface (Fig. 1–8). The pressure required to keep the bubble open is called the *distending pressure*, and the relationship between the distending pressure and the surface tension of the sphere when there are two liquid-gas interfaces present is given by the *LaPlace equation:*

$$\text{Pressure} = \frac{4 \times \text{surface tension}}{\text{radius}}$$

However, when one liquid-gas interface is present, as in a fluid-lined alveolus (or a bubble blown underwater from a tube), a factor of two is used in the LaPlace equation; therefore:

$$\text{Pressure} = \frac{2 \times \text{surface tension}}{\text{radius}}$$

From the LaPlace equation two characteristics of alveolar structure are evident:

- The distending pressure required to maintain the patency of a sphere is directly proportional to the surface tension of the film.
- The distending pressure is inversely proportional to the radius of the sphere.

In actual fact, alveoli are not true spherical structures, but as an approximation, the relationship between pressure and radius is valid. For instance, at a constant surface tension the distending pressure of an alveolus with a radius of 50 μm is double that of an alveolus with a radius of 100 μm. Thus as the radius of an alveolus decreases, the distending pressure required to hold the alveolus open increases. Since the pressure needed to expand a sphere is exactly balanced by the pressure required to deflate a sphere, the distending pressure may also be referred to as the *collapse pressure* of a sphere. The radius of the alveoli in many premature infants may be as little as one-quarter of the radius of normal alveoli. Therefore, the collapse pressures in such small-radius alveoli are extremely high, further contributing to the instability of the immature

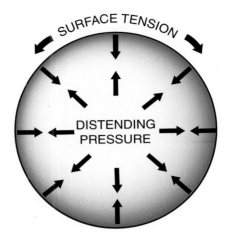

The relationship between the distending pressure and the surface tension required to keep the sphere inflated is given by the law of LaPlace:

$$\text{Pressure} = \frac{2 \times \text{surface tension}}{\text{radius}} \quad \text{or} \quad P = \frac{2\,ST}{r}$$

where　r = radius of the sphere when there is one
liquid-gas interface (e.g., fluid-lined alveolus)

FIGURE 1–8. Forces at the surface of a sphere.

lung. To illustrate this point consider the branched airway model shown in Figure 1–9. Two spherical "alveoli" are connected to a Y-shaped length of tubing. Limb A of the tube ends at a sphere inflated to produce a radius of 1 cm; limb B is connected to an inflated sphere of 2 cm. When the clamps are opened on both limbs of the branched tube, gas immediately flows from the smaller sphere to the larger sphere, inflating the larger sphere further. This simple procedure clearly shows that the collapse pressure in the smaller sphere is higher than that in the larger sphere. Because alveoli are found in several sizes in the lung, and because they have extensive interconnections, the tendency for smaller-radius alveoli to overinflate adjacent larger-radius alveoli contributes to the inherent instability of the lung. However, as we will see, both the infant and the adult lung have structural features that counter this tendency.

STABILITY OF THE LUNG

The stability of alveoli, and thus the stability of the lung, is maintained by factors that minimize the destabilizing factors discussed above. The elastic forces generated by the collagen and elastin meshwork when it is distended and the powerful elastic forces produced by surface tension effects in the fluid lining the alveoli are countered by the actual structural arrangement of adjacent alveoli and by the action of a potent surface-active agent within the alveoli. These factors—one mechanical, the other biochemical—are examined in the following section.

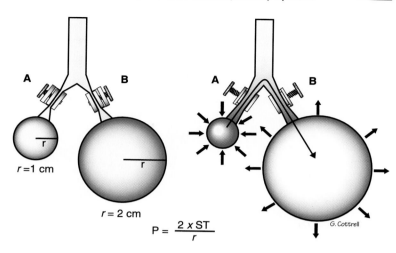

$$P = \frac{2 \times ST}{r}$$

The *distending pressure* of a sphere is also known as the *collapse pressure*. A smaller sphere has a higher collapse pressure than a larger sphere, as shown by the LaPlace relationship (P = 2 x ST / r). Therefore, a small sphere connected to a larger sphere will inflate the larger sphere.

FIGURE 1–9. Branched airway model showing different collapse pressures.

INTERDEPENDENCE OF ALVEOLI

With the exception of those alveoli at the surface of the lung, immediately adjacent to the visceral pleura, all alveoli in the lung are totally surrounded by other alveoli (West, 1998). In fact, many alveolar structural arrangements involve shared septa so that the alveoli support each other (Fig. 1–10). The woven arrangement of elastin and collagen interstitial fibers discussed previously penetrates from the lung surface and forms fibrous septa around the individual functional units of the lungs. These 50,000 functional units each consist of one or a few alveolar ducts and associated alveoli; therefore, the presence of fibrous elements provides additional mechanical links that support, or "splint," the various alveoli, alveolar ducts, and other air spaces to maintain patency (Guyton and Hall, 1996). Because of these structural features, individual alveoli in the lung are not totally independent. Such a communal arrangement results in a complex system of mutually supported and interconnected alveoli. In this arrangement called **interdependence of alveoli,** any tendency of an alveolus or a group of alveoli to change volume relative to that of the other units in the structure is automatically opposed. Consider the following example: If a small-radius alveolus (having a high collapse pressure) begins to deflate, thus inflating an adjacent larger-radius alveolus to which it is connected, the alveolar collapse is immediately minimized. This stabilizing effect occurs because of the interdependence of alveoli. As the larger alveolus distends, its mechanical interconnections with surrounding alveolar units exert a powerful expanding force on the collapsing alveolus to limit the amount of deflation (see Fig. 1–10).

A system of interconnected structural units in the lung parenchyma counters the tendency of alveoli to collapse, thus opposing regional atelectasis and contributing to lung stability. In summary, the interdependence of alveoli opposes nonuniform changes in lung volume (Taylor et al, 1989).

PULMONARY SURFACTANT

Composition

Pulmonary surfactant is a complex chemical formed from precursors released from the microvilli of type II pneumocytes. Alveolar transformations change the precursor molecules into the active substance which forms a thin monomolecular layer on the luminal surface of the fluid lining the alveoli (Fig. 1–11). Surfactant is a *surface active agent* that spreads over the surface of a fluid and effectively lowers the ST of the fluid. Recall that surface tension produces substantial elastic forces in the lung and contributes to lung instability. Pulmonary surfactant plays a prominent role in the reduction of those forces and, therefore, contributes to alveolar stability.

Surfactant is a complex fluid composed of several phospholipids, proteins, and ions. The proteins and ions in the surfactant complex do not lower surface tension themselves but are essential because they act as "spreading agents" to promote the rapid distribution of surface-active phospholipids over the surface of alveolar lining fluid. The most important phospholipid in surfactant is *1,2-dipalmitoylphosphatidylcholine,* or *DPPC.* This phospholipid is synthesized in the lung from fatty acids and, as mentioned previously, the synthesis is carried out on a continuous basis because of a relatively short half-life (14–24 h).

The molecules of DPPC align themselves systematically on the surface of the alveolar lining fluid because

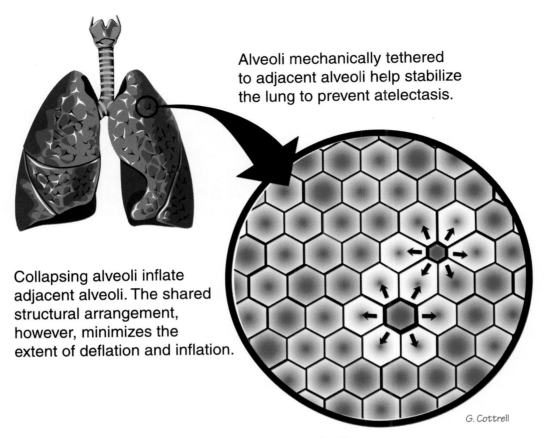

Alveoli mechanically tethered to adjacent alveoli help stabilize the lung to prevent atelectasis.

Collapsing alveoli inflate adjacent alveoli. The shared structural arrangement, however, minimizes the extent of deflation and inflation.

G. Cottrell

FIGURE 1–10. Interdependence of alveoli.

they are composed of a hydrophilic and a hydrophobic end (see Fig. 1–11). With the hydophilic head of the molecule oriented with the fluid layer on the alveolar surface, the hydrophobic tail of the phospholipid molecule is directed toward the interior of the alveolus. Thus a lipid hydrophobic surface is exposed to the air in the alveolus. At the hydrophilic head end of the DPPC molecules, intermolecular repulsive forces of the DPPC molecules disrupt the attractive forces of the surface molecules responsible for generating the surface tension of the liquid film (West, 1998). As a result of this action the surface tension of the alveolar lining fluid ranges from one-twelfth to one-half the surface tension of pure water (Guyton and Hall, 1996). Does surfactant work equally well in small- and large-radius alveoli to promote their stability?

Function

Pulmonary surfactant lowers surface tension in alveoli of differing radii, and does so with the same effectiveness. However, surfactant exhibits varying degrees of activity, depending on the size of the alveolus. Compare this unique action with the activity of artificial surface active agents such as detergents. When a drop of liquid detergent is placed on the surface of a liquid such as water or

saline, the surface tension of the fluid is reduced irrespective of the area of its surface. In other words, a measurement of surface tension will be the same no matter what the surface area. By contrast, when surfactant is added to a small surface, there is a large reduction in surface tension, but when surfactant is added to a larger surface, the reduction in surface tension is not as great. How does surfactant exhibit this dual-mode action?

In a small alveolus, the liquid film lining the sphere is greatly compressed; therefore, the DPPC molecules aligned on its surface are more closely crowded together, thus increasing their concentration and causing more repulsive forces to be directed at the surface molecules of the film (Fig. 1–12A). The result of the DPPC molecules being squeezed together is that the surface tension in the small sphere is reduced further. This effect offsets the greater collapse tendency of a smaller sphere and promotes alveolar stability. As alveoli enlarge, the DPPC layer covering their fluid lining becomes somewhat "stretched" with the individual molecules moving further apart (Fig. 1–12B). This separation reduces the concentration of phospholipid molecules and decreases their ability to lower surface tension. As a result, the surface tension increases, which limits further expansion of large alveoli. Through this dual action on surface tension, surfactant helps prevent atelectasis of

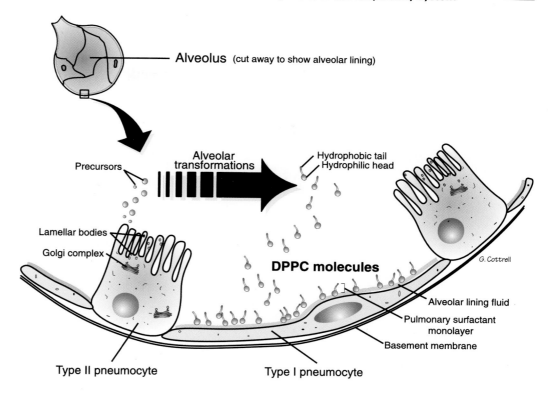

Although other substances are found in pulmonary surfactant, 1, 2-dipalmitoyl phosphatidylcholine (DPPC) molecules make up most of the phospholipid content of the layer.

FIGURE 1–11. Surfactant layer on alveolar fluid within alveolus.

small alveoli and overdistension of large alveoli to result in further stabilization of the lung.

Surfactant and the First Breath

Recall that surfactant has the ability to increase its activity as its surface area is reduced. The result of this action is that at end-expiration, when alveoli are at their smallest, surfactant lowers the surface tension so that air can be retained in the alveoli. Without adequate surfactant, small-radius alveoli are especially prone to collapse. Figure 1–13 compares what can occur in a newborn when pulmonary surfactant is absent and present. In both cases intense inspiratory effort is required to initiate the first breath when the airways are fluid filled. Typically, a collapsed alveolus of 25 μm radius will require a negative pressure of 40 to 100 cm H_2O in order to be inflated to a radius of 100 μm. In the infant with normal type II pneumocyte development and normal surfactant production, the inflation of the alveolus stimulates the release of additional surfactant, which forms an air-surfactant interface that has several times less surface tension than an air-water interface. Consequently, the alveoli (which are now air filled, rather than fluid filled) deflate to a radius of approximately 50 μm after the end of the first breath, and exhibit a surface tension of 5 dynes/cm or less. A negative inspira-

tory pressure of only 2 cm H_2O is required to reinflate these alveoli during subsequent breaths. By contrast, the surfactant-deficient alveolus will collapse back to its preinspiratory radius of 25 μm after the end of the first breath because it is subjected to an extremely high surface tension of 50 dynes/cm. Reinflation of this collapsed air-filled alveolus requires the infant to generate a negative inspiratory pressure as high as 20 cm H_2O (Netter, 1979). Such ventilatory effort cannot be maintained by a newborn. Without mechanical ventilation, pharmacologic intervention using exogenous surfactant, or a combination of both measures, exhaustion of the infant will occur.

Surfactant and Lung Maturity

Because of the critical role played by pulmonary surfactant in infant survival, the embryologic development of type II alveolar epithelial cells and their ability to synthesize the surface active agent provides a valuable biologic marker to assess fetal lung maturity. In the prenatal procedure known as *amniocentesis* a needle is inserted transabdominally with ultrasound guidance into the amniotic cavity within the uterus and a small quantity of amniotic fluid is withdrawn for chemical and cytologic analysis. This diagnostic procedure carries with it some degree of risk: it is not performed earlier

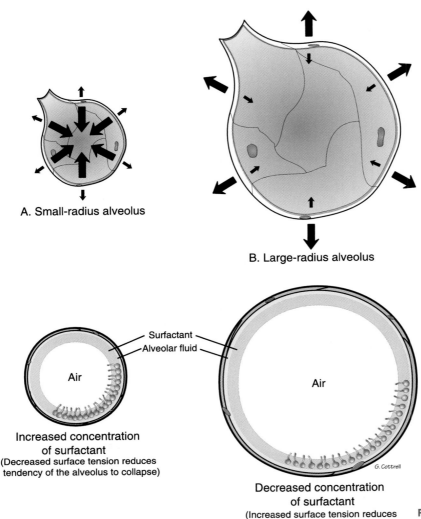

A. Small-radius alveolus

B. Large-radius alveolus

Surfactant
Alveolar fluid

Air

Air

Increased concentration
of surfactant
(Decreased surface tension reduces
tendency of the alveolus to collapse)

Decreased concentration
of surfactant
(Increased surface tension reduces
tendency of the alveolus to distend)

G. Cottrell

FIGURE 1–12. Surfactant concentration in alveoli.
(A) Small-radius alveolus. (B) Large-radius alveolus.

than 14 weeks gestation, nor is it routinely carried out with all pregnancies. The fluid sample is studied to detect genetic and biochemical disorders, maternal-fetal blood incompatibilities, and fetal maturity.

Amniotic fluid is produced by the fetal kidneys and by the amniotic membranes. The volume of amniotic fluid produced by the fetus is normally between 500 mL and 1 liter, but wide variation exists (Guyton and Hall, 1996). Absorption is via amniotic membranes as well as the gastrointestinal tract and lungs of the fetus. Once the fluid reaches the fetal bloodstream it is sent to the placenta where it enters maternal circulation to be eliminated by the mother's kidneys. A small number of fetal cells is continually shed from the skin, gastrointestinal tract, and lungs and normally suspended in the amniotic fluid. In the amniocentesis procedure these cells are separated from the fluid and cultured for several weeks in the laboratory in order to obtain enough cells on which to perform genetic tests that include assessment of chromosome morphology and number.

Amniotic fluid also contains chemicals that give an indication of fetal lung maturity. Some of the fluid in the fetal respiratory system is brought in by the "practice" respiratory movements of the diaphragm, but up to 120 mL per hour near term is produced by the glands lining of the fetal respiratory tract (Netter, 1979). The continual replenishment of pulmonary fluid serves to isolate and protect the delicate lining of the respiratory tract from substances that may be present in the amniotic fluid, including meconium derived from the fetal intestines. Fetal pulmonary fluid contains key phospholipids. This fluid passes out of the oral and nasal cavities of the fetus and mixes with amniotic fluid. When amniocentesis is performed before the 35th week, analysis of the fluid reveals a ratio of *lecithin* to *sphingomyelin* (L/S) that is less than or equal to one, indicating that the fetus is immature in relation to pulmonary surfactant production and respiratory distress is likely (Aloan and Hill, 1997). However, as the pregnancy proceeds, the type II pneumocytes in-

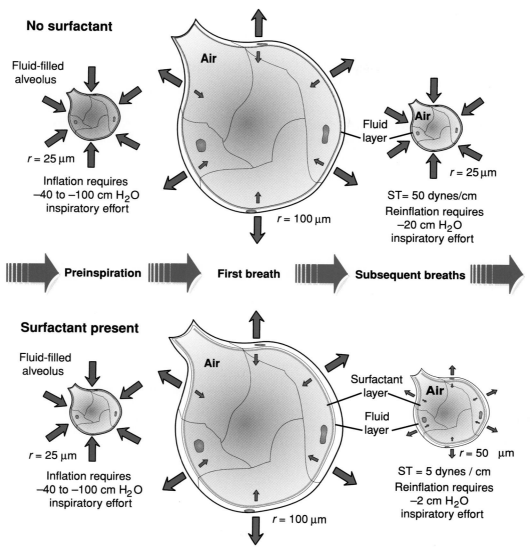

FIGURE 1–13. Schematic—infant's first breath (normal surfactant versus deficient surfactant).

crease their production of surfactant, thus increasing the amount of lecithin released into the pulmonary fluid. Sphingomyelin production is constant throughout the gestation; therefore, an L/S ratio of more than 2:1 indicates that the fetal lungs are mature in relation to surfactant production and the risk for development of respiratory distress in the infant is minimal. If the L/S ratio is between 1.0 and 2.0, respiratory distress may or may not develop (Aloan and Hill, 1997).

POSTNATAL CHANGES IN ALVEOLI

The entire lung does not inflate as soon as spontaneous respiration begins in a newborn. Instead, the alveoli within the lungs gradually inflate over the first week to 10 days after birth (Netter, 1979). From birth to around 3 years of age the increase in the size of the lung is due to multiplication of alveoli rather than to an increase in the size of alveoli, but from age 3 to 8 alveoli increase in both size and number, finally totaling approximately 300 million and providing an extensive surface area of 70 to 80 m². After the eighth year alveoli become larger after the chest wall stops growing, ultimately reaching a mature diameter of 100 to 300 μm (Netter, 1979).

SPONTANEOUS BREATHING AND POSTNATAL CIRCULATORY ADJUSTMENTS

The pivotal event at birth is the inflation of the lungs with the infant's first breath. Prior to birth the collapsed, fluid-filled lung causes widespread compression of pulmonary blood vessels. As a result of this condition in the pulmonary microcirculation, relatively little blood leaves the fetal heart to enter the high-resistance vascular beds in the lung. Sudden expansion of the lungs, however, induces vasodilation and relieves much of the vascular resistance in the pulmonary circuit. This in turn allows more blood to enter the lung from the right ventricle and helps establish the normal postnatal circulatory pattern. Chapter 16 examines the development of the cardiovascular system and further explores the correlation between respiratory and cardiovascular events occurring in the perinatal period.

Summary

This chapter has traced the development of the respiratory system from its embryologic beginnings as an undifferentiated series of primitive branching tubes to its critical role in supporting gas exchange in an air-breathing infant. We have examined the transformation of both the conducting zone and the respiratory zone of the lung and briefly discussed the development of associated structures such as body cavities, the diaphragm, pleural membranes, and the mediastinum. The chapter also presented an overview of the elastic forces that contribute to the instability of the lung and discussed the mechanical and biochemical features that help stabilize the lung. Finally, the chapter examined the changes that accompany an infant's first breath—the final transformation from an intrauterine to an extrauterine existence.

BIBLIOGRAPHY

Aloan CA and Hill TV: Respiratory Care of the Newborn and Child, ed 2. JB Lippincott, Philadelphia, 1997.

Cottrell GP and Surkin HB: Pharmacology for Respiratory Care Practitioners. FA Davis, Philadelphia, 1995.

Des Jardins T: Cardiopulmonary Anatomy and Physiology: Essentials for Respiratory Care, ed 3. Delmar Publishers, Albany, NY, 1998.

Guyton AC and Hall JE: Textbook of Medical Physiology, ed 9. WB Saunders, Philadelphia, 1996.

Koff PB: Development of the cardiopulmonary system. In Koff PB, Eitzman D, and Neu J (eds): Neonatal and Pediatric Respiratory Care, ed 2. Mosby-Year Book, St. Louis, 1993.

Matsumura G and England MA: Embryology Colouring Book. Wolfe Publishing (Mosby-Year Book Europe), Barcelona, 1992.

Netter FH: Respiratory System, Vol 7. In Divertie, MB (ed): The CIBA Collection of Medical Illustrations. CIBA Pharmaceutical Co, Division of CIBA-GEIGY Corp, Summit, NJ, 1979.

Schnapf B and Kirley S: Fetal lung development. In Barnhart SL and Czervinske MP (eds): Perinatal and Pediatric Respiratory Care. WB Saunders, Philadelphia, 1995.

Taylor AE et al: Clinical Respiratory Physiology. WB Saunders, Philadelphia, 1989.

Tomashefski JF and Richmond B: Development of the respiratory system. In Carlo WA and Chatburn RL (eds): Neonatal Respiratory Care. Year Book Medical Publishers, Chicago, 1988.

West JB: Respiratory Physiology: The Essentials, ed 6. Williams & Wilkins, Baltimore, 1998.

CHAPTER 2

Conducting Zone and Gross Anatomy of the Lung

chapter objectives

After studying this chapter the reader should be able to:

☐ Differentiate between the conducting zone and the respiratory zone of the respiratory system.

☐ Define the following terms:
   External respiration, internal respiration, ventilation.

☐ Explain the relationship between surface area and volume of an object and relate this to cellular metabolism.

☐ Describe the organization of the conducting zone into an upper and lower respiratory tract, identifying the borders of each division.

☐ Describe the structure and function of the following nasal cavity structures:
   Paranasal ducts, nasolacrimal ducts, auditory (eustachian) tubes.

☐ Name the bony and cartilaginous elements of the nose and nasal cavity, explaining how they contribute to the structure of the:
   Bridge of the nose, roof of the nasal cavity, lateral walls of the nasal cavity, floor of the nasal cavity, nasal septum, external nose.

☐ Describe how the turbinates contribute to filtration of inspired air.

☐ Identify the histologic types of epithelium present in the nasal cavity.

☐ Describe how the lining of the nasal cavity is suited to its functions.

☐ Explain how the following functions of the nasal cavity are accomplished:
   Conditioning of incoming air, olfaction, phonation.

☐ Describe the role of the oral cavity in relation to the respiratory system.

☐ Identify the three regions of the pharynx and describe the function of each.

☐ Differentiate between cartilaginous and noncartilaginous airways.

☐ Describe the structure and function of laryngeal cartilages.

☐ Describe the structure and function of the vocal apparatus.

- ☐ Briefly discuss sound production in the larynx.
- ☐ Explain how extrinsic laryngeal muscles protect the airway from aspiration.
- ☐ Compare and contrast the function of suprahyoid and infrahyoid muscle groups.
- ☐ Identify the following regarding the tracheobronchial tree:
    Number of generations of airway, airway diameter, organization of smooth muscle and cartilage components, epithelial lining.
- ☐ Describe the structure and function of the following tracheobronchial tree elements:
    Trachea, primary (mainstem) bronchi, secondary (lobar) bronchi, tertiary (segmental) bronchi, subsegmental bronchi, bronchioles, terminal bronchioles.
- ☐ Discuss how bronchioles and terminal bronchioles are supported to maintain airway patency.
- ☐ Define the following terms:
    Peribronchial connective tissue sheath, parenchyma, Clara cells, canals of Lambert, interbronchial connections, collateral ventilation.
- ☐ Identify the compartments of the thorax.
- ☐ Describe the structure and function of the pleural membranes and pleural space.
- ☐ Define the following terms:
    Pulmonary ligament, root, hilum, interlobar fissures, lobes, cardiac notch, lingua, costal impressions.
- ☐ Describe the following surface features of the lung:
    Apex, base (diaphragmatic surface), mediastinal surface, costal surface.
- ☐ Identify the bronchopulmonary segments of each lung.

key terms

adenoid (ad′ e-noyd)
alar cartilages (â′ lar) **(greater and lesser alar cartilages)**
apex
arytenoid cartilages (ar″ i-tē′ noyd)
auditory tube; eustachian tube (ū-stā′-shen)
base (diaphragmatic surface)
bronchiole (brong″ kē-ol)
bronchopulmonary segments
canals of Lambert
cardiac notch
carina (ka-rī′ na)
cartilaginous airways
choana (kō′ a-na)
Clara cells
conducting zone
corniculate cartilages (kōr-nik′ ū-lāt)
costal impressions
costal (lateral) surface
cribriform plate (krib′ ri-form); **horizontal plate**
cricoid cartilages (krī′ koyd)
cuneiform cartilages (kū-nē′ i-form)
epiglottis cartilage (ep″ i-glot′ is)
ethmoid bone (eth′ moyd)
extrinsic laryngeal muscles
  infrahyoid group
  suprahyoid group

frontal bone
glottis (glot′ is)
hard palate
hilum (hī′ lum)
inferior nasal conchae (kong′ kē)
interbronchial connections
interlobar fissures (horizontal, oblique)
intrinsic laryngeal muscles
lacrimal bones
laryngopharynx (lar-in″ gō-far′ inks)
larynx (lar′ inks)
lateral cartilages
lingua
lingual tonsils (ling′ gwal)
lobar bronchi; secondary bronchi (superior, intermediate, middle, inferior)
lobes (inferior, middle, superior)
lower respiratory tract
mainstem bronchi; primary bronchi
maxilla
meatus
mediastinal (medial) surface
mediastinum
nasal bones
nasal cavity
nasal fossae
nasolacrimal duct

nasopharynx (nā″ zō-far′-inks)
noncartilaginous airways
nostril; external nares
oral cavity
oropharynx (ōr″ ō-far′-inks)
palate
palatine bones
palatine tonsils
paranasal ducts
paranasal sinuses (frontal, maxillary, sphenoidal, ethmoidal)
perpendicular plate (of ethmoid bone)
pharyngeal tonsils (far-in′ jē-al)
pharynx (far′ inks)
pleura
   parietal pleura
   visceral pleura
pleural cavity; pleural space; intrapleural space
pleural fluid
pulmonary ligament
respiratory zone

rima glottidis (rī′ ma glot′ id-is)
root
segmental bronchi; tertiary bronchi
septal cartilage
soft palate
subsegmental bronchi
terminal bronchiole
thyroid cartilage
thyroid notch
trachea
tracheobronchial tree; respiratory tree
turbinates
upper respiratory tract
uvula (ū′ vū-la)
vestibule
vibrissae (vī-bris′ ē)
vocal cords
   false vocal cords; ventricular folds
   true vocal cords
vocal ligament
vomer

In this chapter we discuss how a complex structure such as the human body is able to meet the considerable gaseous requirements needed for metabolism, in spite of having a limited surface area for gas exchange. We will also review the general structure and function of the conducting passages found in the respiratory system. The embryologic development of these structures was examined in the previous chapter, but here we discuss in more depth the gross anatomy of the various classes of airway that convey gas to and from the lung. We also examine the gross anatomy of the lung itself.

General Structural Plan

CONDUCTING ZONE AND RESPIRATORY ZONE

The respiratory tract can be viewed as an organ system composed of an elaborate arrangement of branching tubes that comprise the *conducting zone,* and an enormous interconnected complex of microscopic saclike structures called alveoli making up the *respiratory zone.*

The **conducting zone** consists of air passages of varying diameter and number whose function is to convey air between the external environment and the gas-exchange units of the lungs. Large structures such as the nasal cavity as well as tubular passages such as the trachea are part of the conducting zone. The various passageways described subsequently are lined with different types of epithelial cells that provide filtration, secretion, protection, and clearance functions. Patency is maintained in most of the conducting passages by muscle, bone, or cartilaginous tissue associated with the wall of the structures.

The exchange of gas between the air and the circulatory system is called *external respiration,* and this action is in contradistinction to *ventilation,* which refers to the rhythmic movement of the chest and the mechanics of breathing. External respiration takes place in the **respiratory zone** of the lung, a highly perfused region exposed to the air delivered through the passages of the conducting zone. (*Internal respiration* refers to gas exchange between the bloodstream and cells of the body other than those involved in external respiration.) The structures of the respiratory zone are examined in Chapter 3, and the mechanisms of gas exchange in the respiratory zone are covered in Chapter 12. How does the general structural plan of the human respiratory system accommodate the exchange of substantial volumes of oxygen and carbon dioxide with the external environment when the surface area of the body is relatively small?

OPTIMIZATION OF SURFACE AREA

Metabolism is the sum total of all of the biochemical reactions occurring in the body at any given time. Many of them involve the utilization of oxygen or the production of carbon dioxide. Large amounts of oxygen are consumed and large amounts of carbon dioxide are produced during normal metabolism in a complex organism. How are these gases exchanged between the air and the blood when the metabolic needs and volume of the organism are large but its external surface area is small?

The transfer of substances through cell membranes to support cellular metabolism is accomplished by a variety of transport mechanisms such as diffusion, osmosis, filtration, endocytosis, and exocytosis, with each cell employing some combination of processes to get the job done. Since the same processes must be repeated *by each cell* to move certain substances through membranes, why aren't tissues simply composed of fewer but larger cells, thus eliminating wasteful duplication of function? Stated another way, *Why are cells so microscopic?* The answer to this question is found in a very basic relationship concerning the surface area of an object and its volume. This biologic principle is involved in the development of an optimal size for cells, the efficiency of heating and cooling responses, gas exchange in the lung and tissues, and is a factor in the determination of overall body size.

As an object increases in size, its volume changes at a faster rate than its area, as shown by the simple formulas:

$$\text{Area} = \text{length} \times \text{width}$$

$$\text{Volume} = \text{length} \times \text{width} \times \text{height}$$

The proportion of surface area to volume is smaller with a large object compared to a small object. Put another way, a small object has an ideal, or optimal, ratio of surface area to volume for the exchange of gases, nutrients, and wastes. The small volume of the cell and the metabolic activity carried out within it are effectively matched by the cell's surface area. Figure 2–1, however, shows what happens to this surface area-volume ratio when an object doubles in size. For simplicity's sake, imagine a perfect cube-shaped cell that is one centimeter (1 cm) on each side. The surface area of such a cell would be 1 cm² (1 cm × 1 cm = 1 cm²) per side, for a total surface area of 6 cm² (6 × 1 cm² = 6 cm²). The volume of such a cell is 1 cm³ (1 cm × 1 cm × 1 cm = 1 cm³).

Now consider the cell that is twice as large (see Fig. 2–1). Its surface area per side has quadrupled to 4 cm² (2 cm × 2 cm = 4 cm²), and its total surface area is now 24 cm² (6 × 4 cm² = 24 cm²). The volume, however, has increased dramatically and is now *eight times* as large, soaring from 1 cm³ to 8 cm³ (2 cm × 2 cm × 2 cm = 8 cm³). Comparing the two cells shows that when a cell doubles in size, its surface area increases by a factor of 4, but its volume increases by a factor of 8. The ratio of surface area to volume, therefore, decreases drastically as an object increases in size. At some critical point, the surface area of our fictitious cell will not be optimally matched to its volume. In other words, the surface area of the cell membrane will not be large enough to meet the gaseous, nutrient, and waste exchange requirements of the large cytoplasmic volume of the cell. By remaining small a cell maintains an ideal ratio of surface area to volume. Another reason cells are small is that the cell nucleus has a limited amount of genetic material with which to control cellular activities such as protein synthesis. The nucleus in a fictitious large cell would not be able to influence cellular activities to any great extent if the volume of the cytoplasm was large. The nucleus would simply be too far removed from the metabolic machinery of the cell.

If constructing a complex organism from tissues composed of just a few large cells does not work, as we have seen, how *do* large organisms consisting of billions of cells cope with the limits imposed by area-volume relationships?

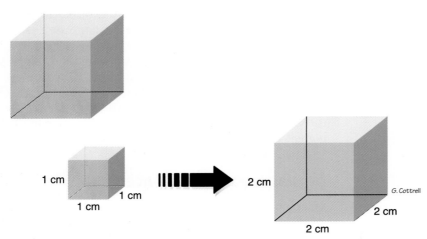

Area per side = 1 cm x 1 cm = 1 cm²
Total surface area = 6 x 1 cm² = 6 cm²
Volume = 1 cm x 1 cm x 1 cm = 1 cm³
Ratio of surface area to volume = **6:1**

Area per side = 2 cm x 2 cm = 4 cm²
Total surface area = 6 x 4 cm² = 24 cm²
Volume = 2 cm x 2 cm x 2 cm = 8 cm³
Ratio of surface area to volume = **3:1**

FIGURE 2–1. Surface area to volume relationships.

Complex multicellular organisms solve the problem of scale in similar ways. Since the volume of such organisms is relatively fixed, the only way to maintain an acceptable ratio between area and volume in a large organism is to increase the surface area of the organism, either by extending its exterior or "hollowing out" its interior. Trees have extensive *external* branching that increases the surface area of their leaf canopy. This in turn promotes increased photosynthesis to support the metabolic needs of their large volume. The tree's extended exterior provides an improved surface area for gas exchange and nutrient production. Large animals have developed a similar system to increase the surface area exposed to the external environment. The branching, of course, is carried out *internally* by an extensive respiratory tree that ends with millions of fluid-lined functional units that interface with a vast network of blood vessels. Recall from the discussion of embryologic development that highly vascularized wet epithelial linings are common in the respiratory systems of complex animals. Because the airways of our respiratory system communicate directly with the external environment, the internal branching arrangement of the tracheobronchial tree increases the body's actual 1.7 m^2–1.8 m^2 surface area to an apparent "external" surface area of approximately 70 m^2–80 m^2, an area about half the size of a tennis court. This increased surface area dramatically improves the area-volume relationship that is so crucial in the metabolism of larger organisms (Box 2–1). By exposing the bloodstream to a larger area of the external environment, more efficient exchange of oxygen and carbon dioxide occurs and higher levels of metabolism can be supported.

Upper Respiratory Tract

NASAL CAVITY

The **upper respiratory tract** consists of the *nasal cavity, oral cavity,* and *pharynx.* These structures are part of the conducting zone of the respiratory system. Because of the functional importance of the nasal cavity in the conditioning of incoming air, and the clinical importance of the nasal cavity in certain respiratory care procedures such as the use of nasal cannulae for the delivery of therapeutic oxygen, we will begin our study of the respiratory system at the point where outside air normally enters the body and begins its journey to the lungs. The **nasal cavity** is a space in the midline of the skull directly above the oral cavity. The anterior portion of the cavity functions solely as a respiratory system structure, whereas the posterior portion has subdivisions that serve both respiratory and digestive system functions. The nasal cavity communicates anteriorly with the external environment through the pliable cartilaginous portion of the nose that projects distally from the face. Posteriorly, the communication is with the pharynx. Several internal openings are located in the nasal cavity and pharynx (Box 2–2):

- **Paranasal ducts** connect the nasal cavity with mucous membrane-lined air spaces in the skull called **paranasal sinuses.** Ciliated epithelium that is continuous with the mucosa of the nasal cavity functions to transport mucus produced by the glands of the paranasal sinuses into the nasal cavity. Upper respiratory infections (URIs), sinusitis, and allergic responses may cause excess production of fluid by the paranasal sinuses, often with retention of secretions. Paranasal sinuses are named according to the skull bone in which they are located (e.g., frontal, maxillary, sphenoid, ethmoid) and function to warm and humidify incoming air, add a resonance quality to the voice, and reduce the overall mass of the skull (Fig. 2–2; see also Color Plate 1).
- The **nasolacrimal ducts** are small-diameter tubes that pass through the lacrimal canals of the lacrimal bones. These canals lead from the medial margin of the orbit to the lateral walls of the nasal cavity. Tear production from the lacrimal glands passes into the nasolacrimal ducts and is directed into the nasal cavity through these small passageways.
- **Auditory (eustachian) tubes** extend medially from the middle ear and communicate with the lateral walls of the posterior pharynx. These tubes function to equalize air pressure in the middle ear with that of the external environment (see Fig. 2–2).

Bone and Cartilage Framework of the Nose and Nasal Cavity

The structure of the nasal cavity and nose consists of a combination of cartilaginous and bony support elements that form the bridge of the nose, the lateral walls, roof, floor, and nasal septum of the nasal cavity, and the framework of the external nose.

Paired **nasal bones** and the unpaired **maxilla** are classified as facial bones. The frontal processes of the maxilla on either side of the nasal bones, plus a small portion of the **frontal bone** (a cranial bone), form the bony *bridge* of the nose (Fig. 2–3; see also Color Plate 2).

The *lateral walls* of the nasal cavity are formed by the maxilla, the paired **lacrimal bones,** and the paired **inferior nasal conchae** of the face, plus the superior and middle nasal conchae attached to the unpaired **ethmoid bone** of the cranium (see Fig. 2–3). The nasal conchae are composed of very thin, delicate bones that form convoluted passageways that cause incoming air to swirl around as it passes through the nasal cavity. This turbulent air flow causes heavier particulate matter such as inhaled dusts to settle before

PERSPECTIVES

BOX 2-1

Why Brobdingnagians Were Short (of Breath)

In 1735 an imaginative book relating fantastic stories of adventures in faraway and strange lands was written by Jonathan Swift. The book was a thinly veiled political satire titled *Gulliver's Travels (Travels into Several Remote Nations of the World, In Four Parts)*. Gulliver is probably best known for his encounter with the Lilliputians, a race of diminutive people, but he also visited a race of giant people in "Part II—A Voyage to Brobdingnag." The Brobdingnagians had humanlike proportions but "appeared as Tall as an ordinary Spire-steeple; and took about ten Yards at every Stride." When the hapless Gulliver was picked up by one of the giants, he was "held in the Air above sixty Foot from the Ground." A 9-year-old girl was described as being "very good natured, and not above forty Foot high, being little for her Age." Could normally proportioned, 60-foot tall beings have walked about in Brobdingnag? More important, would they have been able to breathe?

As the volume of a body increases, so does its mass. The cross-section of a bone determines, in part, its weight-bearing capabilities. Therefore, to support the bulk of a Brobdingnagian, femurs would have to be as big as tree trunks. Clearly, humanlike proportions for a Brobdingnagian would not be possible from a *bioengineering* standpoint. From a *physiologic* standpoint, Gulliver's voyage to Brobdingnag is even more fantastic. As the volume of a body increases, its external surface area does not keep pace. Animals cope with this volume-area mismatch by developing a greatly expanded internal surface area for gas exchange. If the surface area of the Brobdingnagian lung expanded to match the massive volume of the body, the giant could not have had a thoracic cavity proportioned like that of a human. Since Jonathan Swift described the residents of Brobdingnag as having normal proportions, we have to conclude that their lungs could not have had sufficient surface area to support the metabolism required by their great bulk. Brobdingnagians, therefore, probably suffered shortness of breath as well as multiple compression fractures of weight-bearing bones. Unfortunately, Jonathan Swift didn't confirm these minor details in his intriguing account of Captain Lemuel Gulliver's voyages.

• Greenberg RA and Piper WB (eds): The Writings of Jonathan Swift. WW Norton & Co, New York, 1973.
• Swift J: Gulliver's Travels, edited by Davis H. Basil Blackwell and Mott, Ltd, Oxford, 1959. (Originally published as Volume III of the Author's Works containing *Travels into Several Remote Nations of the World, In Four Parts*, printed by and for George Faulkner, Dublin, 1735.)

they enter deeper parts of the respiratory tract. In this way the **turbinates,** as these bony structures are collectively called, function as a crude filtration system. The openings between conchae are called **meatuses** (see Fig. 2–2).

The *roof* of the nasal cavity is formed anteriorly by the bridge structures described earlier and superiorly by the frontal bone and the horizontally oriented **cribriform plate** of the ethmoid bone (Fig. 2–4). This thumbnail-sized thin plate of bone is perforated by olfactory foramina that give it a sievelike appearance that resembles the top of a salt shaker (Greek *ethmos*, sieve, +*eidos*, form, shape; Latin *cribrum*, a sieve, +*forma*, form). The foramina allow branches of the olfactory nerve to leave the nasal cavity, enter the olfac-

tory bulb, and carry electrical impulses directly to the brain via the olfactory tract. These impulses are concerned with the sense of smell.

The *floor* of the nasal cavity is formed anteriorly by the palatine process of the maxilla and posteriorly by the paired **palatine bones** (see Fig. 2–4). These horizontally directed bony structures form the **hard palate.** The **soft palate,** composed of flexible connective tissue, lies directly behind the palatine bones of the hard palate and also contributes to the floor of the nasal cavity (see Fig. 2–4).

When studying skull anatomy, the reader should note that many structures serve a dual purpose because of their close proximity to each other, thereby contributing to shared structures such as partitions. For

P E R S P E C T I V E S

BOX 2–2   **Unwanted Communication**

Although various tubular structures (e.g., nasolacrimal ducts, paranasal ducts, and auditory tubes) are essential to allow communication between compartments in the skull, these passageways also permit upper respiratory infections (URIs) to spread easily from one area to another. Among the more serious complications of this intercavity communication is the potential for the development of purulent otitis media infections following a URI. Inflammatory conditions of the middle ear often accompany infections and may recur in young children because of a child's increased susceptibility to infection and because of anatomic characteristics of the immature skull. The auditory (eustachian) tube is generally short and oriented more or less horizontally as it passes from the middle ear to the nasopharynx. As a child matures, however, the proportions of the skull change, primarily due to differential growth in the maxilla. As the typical "rounded" appearance of a child's skull takes on a more vertically oriented shape, the angle and length of the auditory tube changes. This change in the auditory tube reduces the chance of infectious material from the nasal cavity entering the middle ear cavity as a result of a forceful sneeze or cough. If middle ear infections progress to an inflammatory stage, the auditory tube closes and drainage is impaired. This, in turn, causes intense earache as a result of the increase in pressure. In severe cases the pressure from inflammation may cause rupture of the tympanic membrane (eardrum).

A very serious complication of middle ear infections is mastoiditis, an inflammation of the air spaces within the mastoid process of the temporal bone. Mastoidal air cells do not drain into the nasal cavity as do the paranasal sinuses. Therefore, if infectious material enters the mastoid air cells from the inner ear, it may accumulate and destroy the thin bony partition separating the mastoid air cells from the cranial cavity, resulting in potentially serious complications such as inflammation of the coverings of the brain (meningitis) or of the brain itself (encephalitis).

Occasionally URIs can "seed" lower respiratory infections (LRIs) to result in inflammatory conditions in organs that are far removed from the original location. For example, recurrent bronchitis in some patients may be traced to chronic sinusitis conditions. Material from the paranasal sinuses enters the nasal cavity and from here, may reach the bronchi, especially in patients with compromised cough or mucociliary transport mechanisms. These clearance mechanisms normally function to remove material from the airways.

- Thibodeau GA and Patton KT: Anatomy and Physiology, ed 3. Mosby–Year Book, St Louis, 1996.
- Van De Graaff KM: Human Anatomy, ed 3. Wm C Brown, Dubuque, IA, 1992.

example, consider the structures we have already discussed in association with the nasal cavity: (1) the lateral walls of the nasal cavity are also the medial walls of the orbits, (2) the roof of the nasal cavity serves as a small area of the cranial floor, and (3) the floor of the nasal cavity is also the bony partition that forms the roof of the mouth. Strive to produce mental images of these three-dimensional structural relationships, rather than simply trying to memorize the names and locations of the bones and their topographic features.

The *nasal septum* subdivides the nasal cavity into two air channels called the **nasal fossae.** Each nasal fossa opens anteriorly into an expanded portion called the

vestibule, which in turn, opens anteriorly through the **external naris (nostril)** (see Figs. 2–2 and 2–4). Posteriorly, each nasal fossa communicates with the nasopharynx through the **choana,** also known as the **internal naris** (see Figs. 2–2 and 2–4). The nasal septum is formed by a combination of bony and cartilaginous structures. The superior portion of the septum is formed by the **perpendicular plate** of the ethmoid bone; the inferior part of the septum is formed by an unpaired facial bone called the **vomer.** The vomer articulates with the hard palate formed by the maxilla and the palatine bones. The anterior portion of the nasal septum is composed of the **septal cartilage,** a vertical plate of carti-

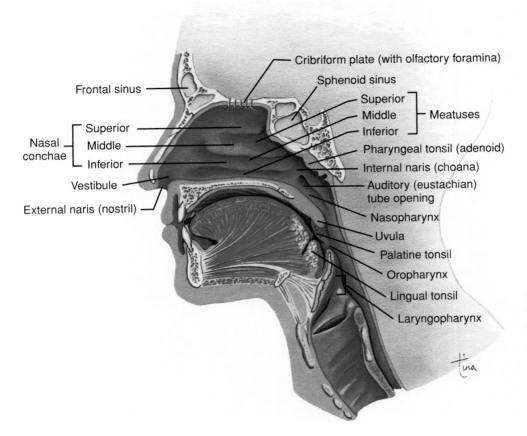

FIGURE 2–2. Upper respiratory tract (midsagittal view). Nasal septum has been removed to show detail of the right lateral wall of the nasal cavity. (Adapted from Scanlon VC and Sanders T: Essentials of Anatomy and Physiology, ed. 3. FA Davis, Philadelphia, 1999, p 327, with permission.) (See also Color Plate 1.)

lage that articulates with the bony septum (see Fig. 2–4). Cartilaginous and bony structures in the nasal cavity are covered by a mucosal epithelial lining that is highly vascularized. The nature of this lining contributes to the warming and humidification functions of the nasal cavity (discussed subsequently).

Finally, *supporting cartilages* contribute to the distinctive shape of the external nose (see Fig. 2–4). These flexible cartilages include paired **lateral cartilages** that articulate with the nasal bones and extend distally to articulate with several **alar cartilages** that form the framework around the nostrils (greater and lesser alar cartilages).

Epithelial Lining

The epithelial lining of the nasal cavity is well suited to the functions carried out by the cavity. Recall from basic histologic studies in anatomy that epithelium is one of the four basic types of tissues found in the body and that it is found lining hollow structures or covering surfaces of organs or the body itself. In regions exposed to the external environment (such as the organs of the respiratory system), noxious materials and environmental conditions cause rapid destruction of cell lay-

ers. Epithelial tissue is an ideal building material in such locations because it characteristically exhibits a rapid rate of cell replacement. This high cell turnover rate minimizes the "wear-and-tear" conditions that are typical in tubular structures of the respiratory, digestive, and genitourinary systems exposed to the outside. The anterior portion of the nasal cavity is lined with *stratified squamous epithelium,* an arrangement of flattened cells that are stacked, or layered, on top of one another. The posterior portion of the nasal cavity is lined with *pseudostratified ciliated columnar epithelium,* the type of lining described earlier in conjunction with the lining of the paranasal sinuses. In this distinctive arrangement, tall rectangular cells, sometimes with a tapering shape, extend from a basement membrane to the luminal surface. The nonuniform arrangement of nuclei in the cells gives them the appearance of being arranged in layers, or strata, but no actual layering is evident on closer inspection. Mucus-producing cells are squeezed between the columnar epithelial cells. The free border of the columnar epithelial cells is equipped with numerous cilia that beat rhythmically to propel mucus posteriorly toward the nasopharynx. The mucus is produced by the glands of both the nasal cavity and the paranasal sinuses.

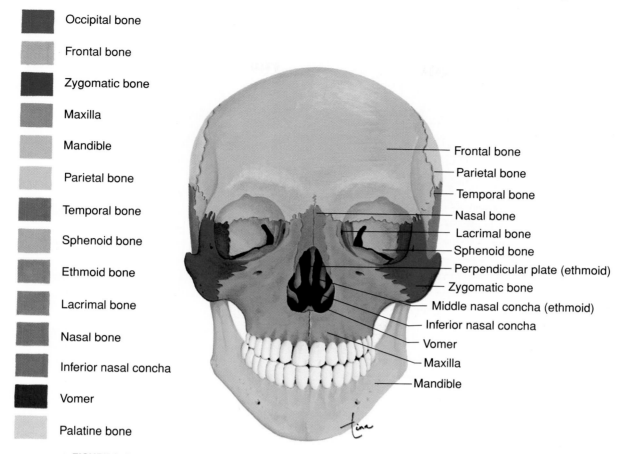

Occipital bone

Frontal bone

Zygomatic bone

Maxilla

Mandible

Parietal bone

Temporal bone

Sphenoid bone

Ethmoid bone

Lacrimal bone

Nasal bone

Inferior nasal concha

Vomer

Palatine bone

Frontal bone
Parietal bone
Temporal bone
Nasal bone
Lacrimal bone
Sphenoid bone
Perpendicular plate (ethmoid)
Zygomatic bone
Middle nasal concha (ethmoid)
Inferior nasal concha
Vomer
Maxilla
Mandible

FIGURE 2–3. Skull (anterior view). In this view showing the anterior structures of the nasal cavity, the superior nasal conchae of the ethmoid bone are not visible because they are located in the upper part of the nasal cavity. The superior and middle nasal conchae of the ethmoid, along with the paired facial bones known as the inferior nasal conchae, form the *turbinates,* an integral part of the nasal cavity walls. These structures disrupt the incoming air stream, changing it to a turbulent type of flow pattern. (Adapted from Scanlon VC and Sanders T: Essentials of Anatomy and Physiology, ed. 3. FA Davis, Philadelphia, 1999, p 107, with permission.) (See also Color Plate 2.)

Functions of the Nasal Cavity

Conditioning of Inspired Air

The epithelial lining described previously is ideally suited to the functions carried out by the nasal cavity. For example, the nasal epithelium that covers the conchae on the side walls of the nasal cavity and lines the paranasal sinuses is highly vascularized and aids in the *warming* of incoming air. The mucus added to the surface of the epithelial lining by the glands of the nasal cavity and the paranasal sinuses serves to *humidify* this air, while the combined action of the turbinates and **vibrissae,** or nasal hairs, functions to *filter* inhaled dusts, smoke, and pollen from the inspired air and cause these particles to be trapped in the moist mucous lining of the cavity. As inspired gas passes over the surfaces of the turbinates, the turbulent air flow produced causes noxious gases such as sulfur dioxide (SO_2) to deposit and dissolve in nasal cavity mucus (Taylor et al, 1989). In-

spired gas must be warmed to 37°C and fully saturated with water vapor before it is presented to the alveoli. Warming to approximately 33°C occurs by the time gas reaches the posterior pharynx, and it is further warmed to 37°C by the time it reaches the distal airways. Approximately 120 mL of water per day is added to inspired dry gas in order to sufficiently humidify it and prevent damage to the fragile alveoli (Taylor et al, 1989). These functions—warming, humidification, and filtration—help prepare, or condition, incoming air before it reaches the more delicate and vulnerable portions of the respiratory system. Gases that are warm and moist exchange more effectively than those that are cold and dry, therefore, conditioning of air in the nasal cavity improves the efficiency of gas exchange in the lung.

Olfaction

The olfactory sense, or the sense of smell, is an example of a nonrespiratory function of the nasal cavity. The

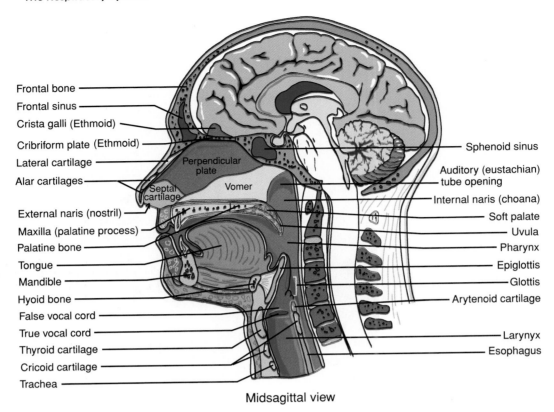

Frontal bone
Frontal sinus
Crista galli (Ethmoid)
Cribriform plate (Ethmoid)
Lateral cartilage
Alar cartilages
Perpendicular plate
Septal cartilage
Vomer
External naris (nostril)
Maxilla (palatine process)
Palatine bone
Tongue
Mandible
Hyoid bone
False vocal cord
True vocal cord
Thyroid cartilage
Cricoid cartilage
Trachea

Sphenoid sinus
Auditory (eustachian) tube opening
Internal naris (choana)
Soft palate
Uvula
Pharynx
Epiglottis
Glottis
Arytenoid cartilage
Larynyx
Esophagus

Midsagittal view

FIGURE 2–4. Head and neck. The nasal septum is formed by the *perpendicular plate* of the ethmoid bone, the *vomer,* and the *septal cartilage.* The pharynx is subdivided into three areas: (1) the *nasopharynx* extends from the choana to the soft palate; (2) The *oropharynx* extends from the soft palate to the hyoid bone; and (3) the *laryngopharynx* extends from the hyoid bone to the larynx.

sense is dependent on the action of olfactory receptor cells found in the upper medial portion of the roof of the nasal cavity on either side of the nasal septum. These sensory cells are continually moistened by mucus and supported by adjacent glandular and columnar epithelial cells. Axons from the cells form the branches of the olfactory nerve (cranial nerve I). These branches pass through the olfactory foramina of the cribriform plate of the ethmoid bone to enter the brain.

Phonation

The production and modification of sounds is another nonrespiratory function of the nasal cavity and paranasal sinuses. A quality of richness or resonance is added to the voice as exhaled air passes through these hollow chambers.

ORAL CAVITY

The **oral cavity** is normally studied with the digestive system because of the mechanical function of chewing and the enzymatic action of saliva released into the cavity, but it is also considered a *secondary* or *accessory respiratory passage.* Because of the clinical importance of certain oral cavity structures in respiratory care proce-

dures such as endotracheal intubation, we will briefly examine the major landmarks and functions of the oral cavity.

The tongue is a prominent structure occupying most of the floor of the oral cavity. It is composed of muscle and is attached posteriorly to the *hyoid bone* (see Figs. 2–2 and 2–4). Embryologically, the anterior part of the hard palate is formed by the fusion of right and left maxillary bones to form the palatine process of the maxilla. The resulting horizontal plate articulates with horizontal structures of the paired palatine bones to form the roof of the mouth (see Fig. 2–2). Failure of the right and left maxillary bones to join together results in a structural defect known as a *cleft palate,* a communication between the nasal and oral cavities. The posterior part of the roof of the oral cavity is formed by the soft palate, a flexible mass of collagen and adipose connective tissue. The lining of the oral cavity consists of *stratified squamous epithelium,* which is the same as that of the anterior part of the nasal cavity.

PHARYNX

The **pharynx,** commonly called the throat, is a funnel-shaped structure that carries out both respiratory and digestive functions. It is subdivided into three regions on the basis of location and function (see Fig. 2–2):

Nasopharynx

The **nasopharynx** is the superior region of the pharynx. It performs a respiratory role and is located posterior to the nasal cavity and immediately above the soft palate. The nasopharynx is lined with *pseudostratified ciliated columnar epithelium* that is continuous with the lining of the posterior portion of the nasal cavity. This mucous membrane helps entrap particulate matter so that the ciliated border can transport the mucus to the back of the throat where it is swallowed or expelled. The lateral walls of the nasopharynx contain the openings of the auditory tubes leading medially from the middle ear cavities. The **pharyngeal tonsils,** also known as **adenoids,** are located on the posterior wall of the nasopharynx (see Fig. 2–2). A small pendulous mass of soft tissue called the **uvula** (Latin *uvula*, small grape) hangs downward from the posterior margin of the soft palate (see Fig. 2–4). During swallowing, the soft palate and uvula are raised to block the posterior entrance to the nasal cavity. In this way, food and liquids are normally prevented from passing through the choanae (internal nares) into the nasal cavity (see Fig. 2–4).

Oropharynx

The middle region of the pharynx is known as the **oropharynx** and is located between the soft palate and the hyoid bone. This region plays both a digestive and respiratory system function. Paired masses of lymphoid tissue called **lingual tonsils** are found at the base of the tongue, which forms the anterior wall of the oropharynx. At the posterior lateral margins of the oropharynx are found the paired **palatine tonsils** which, like other tonsils, are masses of lymphoid tissues that function in protection (see Fig. 2–2). The lining of the oropharynx is continuous with that of the oral cavity and is composed of *stratified squamous epithelium.*

Laryngopharynx

The most inferior of the pharyngeal regions, and the distal structure of the upper respiratory tract, is the **laryngopharynx.** This subdivision continues from the level of the hyoid bone to the entrance into the proximal end of the *larynx.* The upper end of the laryngopharynx functions as a common respiratory and digestive system passageway, but at its lower end, air is diverted anteriorly into the trachea and food posteriorly into the esophagus. We now examine how the larynx separates inspired air from swallowed food and liquids.

Lower Respiratory Tract

The **lower respiratory tract** begins with the larynx and continues as multiple generations of different-sized airways. These structures, like those of the upper respiratory tract, are part of the conducting zone of the respiratory system. The proximal structures of the lower respiratory tract are supported by external cartilages that provide rigidity, patency, and flexibility. Flexibility is required because many of the airways are contained *within* the lung and are, therefore, subjected to expansion and stretching as the lung changes shape during ventilatory movements. These proximal elements of the lower respiratory tract comprise the **cartilaginous airways** of the conducting zone and include the larynx and most classes of airway. The most distal structures of the conducting zone lack cartilage in their walls and are known as **noncartilaginous airways.**

LARYNX

The **larynx** ("voicebox") is a triangular-shaped structure located on the anterior midline of the neck between the fourth and sixth cervical vertebrae (C4-C6). The framework of the larynx is composed of a series of flexible cartilages connected by ligaments and membranes that give it a semirigid structure (Fig. 2–5; see also Color Plate 3). This cartilaginous arrangement keeps the larynx patent but still allows the neck to be flexed, extended, and rotated. Three large unpaired cartilages plus three pairs of smaller cartilages are found in the larynx. Collectively they allow the larynx to (1) conduct air to and from the lungs, (2) prevent the aspiration of liquids and solids during swallowing, and (3) generate sounds.

Laryngeal Cartilages and Vocal Cords

The largest of the nine laryngeal cartilages is the shield-shaped **thyroid cartilage** located anteriorly and forming the apex of the triangular larynx (see Fig. 2–5A). The thyroid cartilage is easily palpated on the midline of the neck, especially the **thyroid notch** on the superior border and the vertical ridge on the anterior surface that is known as the *laryngeal prominence* ("Adam's apple"). This surface landmark is most noticeable in mature males.

The **cricoid cartilage** is another of the unpaired cartilages of the larynx (see Fig. 2–5A and B). Unlike the thyroid cartilage, the cricoid cartilage forms a complete circular structure when viewed from above (Fig. 2–6A and B; see also Color Plate 4). This ring-shaped cartilage connects the thyroid cartilage with the trachea.

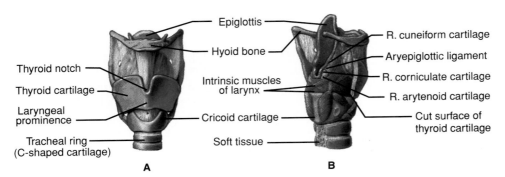

Epiglottis

Hyoid bone

Thyroid notch

Thyroid cartilage

Laryngeal prominence

Intrinsic muscles of larynx

Tracheal ring (C-shaped cartilage)

Cricoid cartilage

Soft tissue

R. cuneiform cartilage

Aryepiglottic ligament

R. corniculate cartilage

R. arytenoid cartilage

Cut surface of thyroid cartilage

A   B

FIGURE 2–5. Larynx. (A) Anterior view; (B) posterolateral view. (See also Color Plate 3.)

The **epiglottis cartilage** is a large, unpaired spoon-shaped cartilage of the larynx (see Figs. 2–2, 2–4, and 2–5). It is anchored just behind the root of the tongue and aids in closing the glottis during the action of swallowing to prevent the aspiration of foreign materials. The term **glottis** refers to the true vocal cords plus the **rima glottidis,** the slitlike space between the true vocal cords that opens into the upper end of the larynx (see Fig. 2–6A). The rima glottidis is the narrowest part of the adult larynx (Thibodeau and Patton, 1996). Foreign objects obstructing the airway or edema of the laryngeal mucosa covering the vocal cords or laryngeal walls can rapidly become a life-threatening emergency because of the narrowness of this passageway. During swallowing a reflex is evoked that causes the extrinsic muscles of the larynx to contract and rapidly elevate the larynx so that the glottal opening is pressed tightly against the lower surface of the epiglottis cartilage. In this way, solids or liquids being swallowed are directed posteriorly into the esophagus, instead of anteriorly into the open larynx and trachea.

The paired **arytenoid cartilages** are pyramidal shaped cartilages that are moveable and articulate with the cricoid cartilage posteriorly (see Fig. 2–5B). The arytenoids are located behind the thyroid and superior to the cricoid cartilage. As can be seen in Figure 2–6B, the arytenoids articulate with the cricoid, but rotate medially and laterally in an asymmetrical manner, much like a cam being rotated back and forth.

The arytenoid cartilages serve as the posterior attachment for two pairs of connective tissue bands called the **true vocal cords** and the **false vocal cords,** or **ventricular folds** (see Fig. 2–6). The ventricular folds are located directly above the true vocal cords. They strengthen the true vocal cords but do not contribute to sound production. Both sets of cords are anchored anteriorly to the inner (luminal) surface of the thyroid cartilage, therefore, any movement of the arytenoids will change the length and tension of the cords, thus changing their frequency when expired air passes over and vibrates them. Inward (medial) rotation of the arytenoid cartilages adducts the vocal cords, reduces their tension, and causes a lower frequency

sound to be produced. Lateral (outward) rotation of the arytenoids abducts the vocal cords, increases their tension, and raises the frequency and pitch of the sound produced (see Fig. 2–6B). The actual intensity of the sound generated by the vibratory action of the vocal cords as expired air passes over the **vocal ligament** on their medial margins is not very great. This feeble sound is amplified and modified by other structures such as the lips, tongue, teeth, and nasal cavity. Because of the vibrating action, vocal cord structures are covered with nonciliated lining of the *stratified squamous epithelium* type, whereas other laryngeal structures are covered with *pseudostratified ciliated columnar epithelium* forming the mucous membrane lining of the larynx. This lining continues downward into the trachea and the first few orders of branches of bronchi.

Two pairs of small accessory cartilages are found closely associated with the arytenoid cartilages. The **corniculate cartilages** are very small, triangular shaped cartilages that are attached to the upper surface of the arytenoid cartilages (see Figs. 2–5B and 2–6A). The corniculate and **cuneiform cartilages** stabilize and strengthen the lateral folds of tissue that connect the arytenoid cartilages to the epiglottis (see Fig. 2–5B).

Laryngeal Muscles

Two groups of laryngeal muscles are associated with the larynx: (1) the **intrinsic laryngeal muscles** responsible for rotating the arytenoid cartilages and thus changing the tension on the vocal cords, and (2) the **extrinsic laryngeal muscles** responsible for elevating and depressing the larynx during swallowing and for assisting the opening of the mandible.

The extrinsic group of laryngeal muscles consists of the **suprahyoid group** of muscles, some of which act to pull the hyoid bone upwards. Other muscles in this group cause retraction (movement posteriorly) or protraction (movement anteriorly) of the hyoid bone. The larynx, through its attachments to the hyoid bone, is also moved by the actions of the suprahyoid group of muscles. In addition, when the larynx and hyoid bone are stabilized by contraction of the infrahyoid group of

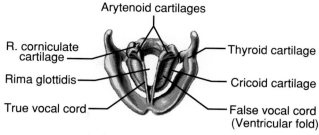

R. corniculate cartilage

Rima glottidis

True vocal cord

Arytenoid cartilages

Thyroid cartilage

Cricoid cartilage

False vocal cord (Ventricular fold)

A. Laryngeal cartilages

Note: The **glottis** is formed by the *true vocal cords* plus the opening between them known as the *rima glottidis.* The **vocal ligament** is a band of elastic tissue lying within the *true vocal cord.*

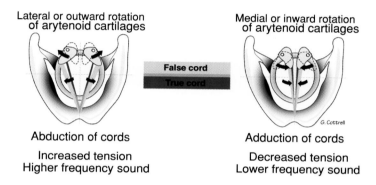

Lateral or outward rotation of arytenoid cartilages

Medial or inward rotation of arytenoid cartilages

False cord

True cord

Abduction of cords

Increased tension
Higher frequency sound

Adduction of cords

Decreased tension
Lower frequency sound

G. Cottrell

B. Schematic of vocal cord movement

FIGURE 2–6. Vocal apparatus of the larynx (superior view). (A) Laryngeal cartilages; (B) schematic of vocal cord movement. (See also Color Plate 4.)

Note that the false vocal cord is *above* the true vocal cord and that both pairs of cords have similar bony attachments on the thyroid and arytenoid cartilages.

muscles, contraction of the suprahyoid group is directed to the mandible to assist in opening the jaw.

The **infrahyoid group** of muscles typically have attachments on thoracic cage structures such as the sternum; therefore, contraction of these muscles results in the hyoid bone and larynx being lowered. When the suprahyoid group stabilizes the hyoid bone and larynx, contraction of the infrahyoid group causes a slight elevation of the sternum. The action, however, is not very powerful because of the small size of the muscles of infrahyoid group.

TRACHEOBRONCHIAL TREE

The lower respiratory tract distal to the larynx consists of passageways that are clearly *tubular* structures. Each leads into successively more and smaller-diameter air passages that collectively make up the extensively branched **tracheobronchial tree,** or **respiratory tree.** Several general trends regarding airway numbers, diameters, and other structural features are evident in the tracheobronchial tree going from proximal to distal regions. These features are summarized in Table 2–1.

Trachea

The **trachea** ("windpipe") is composed of 16 to 20 C-shaped cartilages. These hyaline cartilages are incomplete on their posterior side, but the space is filled in by connective tissue and smooth muscle (see Fig. 2–5B). The cartilaginous nature of the trachea provides both flexibility and patency. The trachea is approximately 2.5 cm in diameter and extends roughly 12 cm distally into the thoracic cage from the cricoid cartilage of the larynx (see Fig. 2–5A). At the level of the sternal notch, at approximately the fifth thoracic vertebra, the trachea divides into a *right* and *left primary bronchus.* The tracheal bifurcation (branching) into the bronchi is reinforced by a keel-like cartilage called the **carina** (Fig. 2–7; see also Color Plate 5). The trachea is lined with *pseudostratified ciliated columnar epithelium* containing numerous *submucosal glands* and mucus-secreting *goblet cells.* These secretory cells and tissues, and the clear-

TABLE 2-1	**Structural Features of the Tracheobronchial Tree**				
	Generation Number	**Diameter**	**Supporting Elements**	**Epithelial Lining**	**Secretory Tissue**
Cartilaginous Airways					
Trachea	0	2.5 cm	C-shaped cartilages	Pseudostratified ciliated columnar	Submocosal glands Goblet cells
Mainstem bronchi	1	—	C-shaped cartilages	Pseudostratified ciliated columnar	Submocosal glands Goblet cells
Lobar bronchi	2	—	Cartilaginous plates	Pseudostratified ciliated columnar	Submucosal glands Goblet cells
Segmental bronchi	3	—	Small cartilaginous plates	Ciliated columnar (height of cells decreases)	Submucosal glands Goblet cells decrease in number
Subsegmental bronchi	4–9	1 mm	Very small fragments of cartilage Peribronchial connective tissue sheaths	Ciliated columnar (height of cells decreases through generations 4–9)	Submucosal glands Goblet cells decrease in number
Noncartilaginous Airways					
Bronchioles	10–15	<1 mm	No cartilage Mechanical tethering to parenchyma ("radial traction") Peribronchial connective tissue sheaths	Ciliated columnar (height of cells decreases through generations 10–15)	Secretory tissue gradually decreases through generations 10–15
Terminal bronchioles	16–19	0.5 mm (avg.)	No Cartilage Mechanical tethering to parenchyma ("radial traction") Peribronchial connective tissue sheaths	Transition from ciliated columnar to nonciliated cuboidal through generations 16–19	Goblet cells gradually disappear Clara cells scattered throughout epithelium

There are several general trends to note in the various passageways of the tracheobronchial tree, going from the proximal to the distal airways: (1) an increase in the number of branches of airways; (2) a decrease in the diameter of individual airways; (3) an increase in the *total* cross-sectional area of the air passages; (4) a decrease in the percentage composition of supporting cartilage in the walls of the airways; (5) an increase in the percentage composition of smooth muscle in the walls of airways; (6) a decrease in the thickness of epithelial cell layering arrangements and in the thickness of the epithelial cells themselves (e.g., columnar to cuboidal); and (7) a decrease in the amount of secretory tissue present in the airway.

ance mechanisms for defense of the lung, are examined in Chapter 5.

Primary Bronchi

Each branch of the tracheobronchial tree is considered a new *generation,* or *class,* of airway (see Table 2–1). The trachea is designated as the "zero" generation of airways; therefore, the bifurcation producing the right and left **primary bronchi** represents the first generation of airway in the respiratory tree. Primary bronchi are also known as **mainstem bronchi** (see Fig. 2–7). The mainstem bronchi are relatively large diameter cartilaginous airways, complete with C-shaped hyaline cartilages to maintain airway patency. As discussed in the developmental anatomy chapter, the orientation of the two mainstem bronchi is slightly different. The right mainstem bronchus splits from the trachea and is directed more vertically, has a slightly larger diameter, and is somewhat shorter than the left mainstem bronchus (see Fig. 1–1). Figure 2–7 shows the approximate angles the two bronchi make with the trachea— the right mainstem bronchus is oriented approximately 20 to 40 degrees from the vertical, and the left mainstem bronchus splits from the trachea at an angle of approximately 40 to 60 degrees from the vertical. As a result of this structural difference, foreign objects that are aspirated tend to lodge more commonly in the right primary bronchus (Taylor et al, 1989; Van De Graaff, 1992).

Secondary Bronchi

Each mainstem bronchus divides into **secondary bronchi,** also known as **lobar bronchi** (see Fig. 2–7). The lobar bronchi represent the second generation of

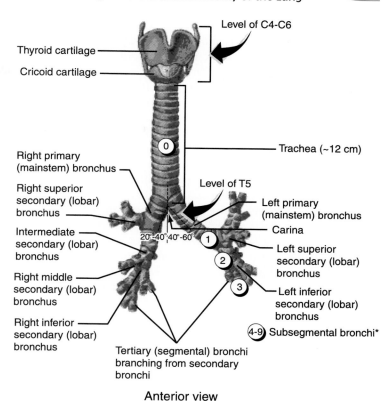

FIGURE 2–7. Cartilaginous airways and the tracheo-bronchial tree. Subsegmental bronchi are small-diameter (1-mm) cartilaginous airways that continue as distal branches of the segmental bronchi. Airway generations are designated by a numbered circle. Note the vertical orientation of the two mainstem bronchi at the bifurcation of the trachea. (See also Color Plate 5.)

airway and function to connect the primary bronchi with the *lobes* of the lungs. The right lung has three lobes that are supplied by the right mainstem bronchus. This bronchus initially divides into the *superior lobar bronchus* and the *intermediate lobar bronchus;* however, the intermediate lobar bronchus extends but a short distance into the lung and then immediately divides again into the *middle lobar bronchus* and the *inferior lobar bronchus* to serve lung lobes of the same name. The left lung has two lobes and is supplied by a *superior lobar bronchus* and an *inferior lobar bronchus.* Smaller plates of hyaline cartilage, rather than more complete C-shaped cartilages, provide the external support for the secondary bronchi.

Tertiary Bronchi

After a lobar bronchus enters a lobe of the lung, it gives off branches classified as third-generation airways. These are the **tertiary bronchi** that supply individual **bronchopulmonary segments,** which are subdivisions within each lobe of the lung. Because of the association of these airways with the lung's bronchopulmonary *segments,* they are also known as **segmental bronchi.** The right lung has a total of 10 segmental bronchi supplying its bronchopulmonary segments; the left lung has 8 segmental bronchi corresponding to its 8 bronchopulmonary segments (see Fig. 2–11).

It should be noted that there is lack of agreement on

the way in which names should be applied to bronchopulmonary segments in the left lung. A few reference sources recognize *10* segments. The majority of sources, however, identify only eight segments in the left lung, using combination names such as *apical-posterior segment* and *anterior-medial basal segment* (see Fig. 2–11).

Subsegmental Bronchi

Distal branches of the segmental bronchi comprise the fourth through ninth generation of airway and are referred to as **subsegmental bronchi** (see Table 2–1). The walls of these small diameter (1 mm) airways contain small fragments of cartilage and are, therefore, still considered cartilaginous airways of the conducting zone. Much of the structural support for the subsegmental bronchi is provided by external cuffs of tissue called *peribronchial connective tissue sheaths.*

Bronchioles

The noncartilaginous airways of the conducting zone begin with the **bronchioles** and form approximately the 10th through the 15th generation of airways (see Table 2–1). These very-small-diameter (less than 1 mm) airways lack both cartilage and peribronchial connective tissue sheaths for support. External support to maintain patency of the noncartilaginous airways is provided mainly by the connection of such airways to the surrounding parenchyma of the lung (Fig. 2–8). (*Parenchyma* refers to the functional units of an organ rather than to its supporting elements.) We will examine the functional units of the lung in the next chapter. Briefly, lung parenchyma consists of tens of thousands of closely packed thin-walled gas exchange units attached to each other, as well as to an elaborate meshwork of elastic connective tissue (see Fig. 1–10). These interwoven elastic fibers exert *radial traction* on the gas exchange units and help keep them open.

Understanding this concept can be challenging. To aid in the process, first review the concept of *interdependence of alveoli* discussed in the previous chapter and try to visualize a delivery system of *collapsible* tubes that is embedded in the organ being served. Since these airways become an integral part of the organ itself, owing to the interconnections described above, any change in pressure or volume of the organ will have an immediate effect on the diameter of thin-walled conducting tubes that lack intrinsic supporting structures such as cartilage. Essentially, the lung functions as an air pump with the delivery tubes contained within the pump itself and subject to the pressures generated by the pump. We examine this phenomenon further in subsequent chapters where we discuss changes in the lung parenchyma and the effect that these changes have on airway patency.

Bronchioles have a high percentage composition of smooth muscle in their walls, which makes their diameters very sensitive to the amount of tension developed by the airway muscle. Bronchiolar smooth muscle is present in a unique double spiral arrangement of fibers wound around the outside of the tube (see Fig. 3–2). The absence of cartilaginous support renders these small airways susceptible to changes in the lung parenchyma and changes in *bronchomotor tone* developed by the smooth muscle fibers. The lining of the bronchioles is composed of *ciliated columnar epithelium*, but the height of the columnar cells and the number of glandular cells steadily decreases through the several generations of bronchioles.

Terminal Bronchioles

The distal branches of bronchioles subdivide further to give rise to the **terminal bronchioles.** Terminal bronchioles form the 16th to 19th generation of airways of the tracheobronchial tree and represent the final elements of the conducting zone of the respiratory system (see Table 2–1). The respiratory zone and gas exchange begins beyond this point. Terminal bronchioles, like the bronchioles that supply them, are supported by external interconnections to the lung parenchyma. Typical diameters of terminal bronchioles are approximately 0.5 mm; therefore, this class of airway is exquisitely sensitive to changes in bronchomotor tone as well as to changes in lung size and pressure.

To appreciate just how small these air passages are, consider the writing point of most technical pens or mechanical pencils. The replacement lead used in a typical mechanical pencil is usually 0.3, 0.5, or 0.7 mm in diameter. Take a look at the opening in the tip of one of these mechanical pencils and you are looking at a diameter that is close to that found in most of the terminal bronchioles of the lung. It is truly amazing that such a small-diameter, collapsible passageway can be kept open within an organ that is constantly changing its size, shape, and pressure 8 to 10 times each minute.

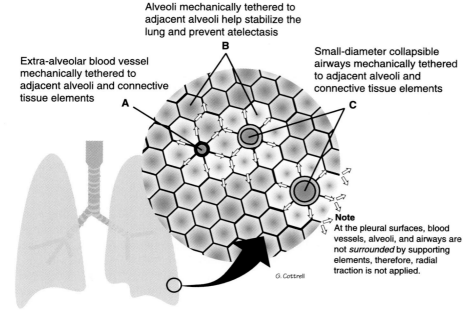

Alveoli mechanically tethered to adjacent alveoli help stabilize the lung and prevent atelectasis

B

Small-diameter collapsible airways mechanically tethered to adjacent alveoli and connective tissue elements

Extra-alveolar blood vessel mechanically tethered to adjacent alveoli and connective tissue elements

A

C

Note
At the pleural surfaces, blood vessels, alveoli, and airways are not *surrounded* by supporting elements, therefore, radial traction is not applied.

G. Cottrell

FIGURE 2–8. Patency. (A) Extra-alveolar blood vessel; (B) alveoli; (C) noncartilaginous airways. Radial traction exerted on the walls of the blood vessels, alveoli, and collapsible airways helps maintain patency of the structures and is most noticeable at higher lung volumes.

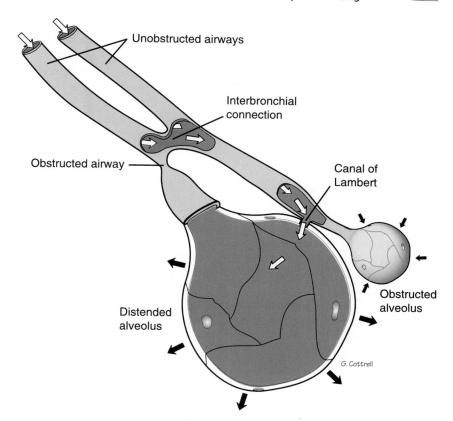

FIGURE 2–9. Schematic—collateral ventilation. Interbronchial connections provide collateral ventilation in the conducting zone; canals of Lambert allow collateral ventilation to occur between the conducting and respiratory zones of the lung. Interalveolar structures called pores of Kohn provide collateral ventilation within the respiratory zone (see Fig. 3–1).

The lining of the various orders of terminal bronchioles gradually changes from *ciliated columnar epithelium* to *nonciliated cuboidal epithelium.* Mucus-producing goblet cells also gradually disappear in the distal branches. **Clara cells** are found in the surface epithelium of the terminal bronchioles where they synthesize a protein that coats and protects the lining. Bronchioalveolar communication is provided by **canals of Lambert** (Fig. 2–9). These small passages (30-μm diameter) connect terminal bronchioles with adjacent alveoli, thereby providing collateral ventilation that helps prevent atelectasis of the lung. Similarly, **interbronchial connections** are large passages (80- to 150-μm diameter) that link adjacent bronchi (see Fig. 2–9). *Collateral ventilation* refers to a system of alternate pathways that permits air to get into and out of a particular part of the lung. Such a system provides communication between ventilated and occluded regions of the lung (Taylor et al, 1989).

Structural features of the tracheobronchial tree are summarized in Table 2–1.

Lung

COMPARTMENTS OF THE THORAX

The thoracic cavity is subdivided into four separate *compartments* that serve to isolate and protect the various thoracic organs from the effects of trauma or infectious disease. Each lung is contained in its own *pleural cavity,* and the heart is housed in a separate *pericardial cavity* within the *mediastinum.* The **mediastinum** is a semirigid compartment located between the two lungs, extending from the thoracic vertebrae to the sternum (see Fig. 1–7). The compartment contains organs situated in the midline of the chest, such as the trachea, the heart and its great vessels (aorta and vena cavae), esophagus, thoracic duct, lymphatics, and nerves. In young children the thymus gland is also found within the mediastinum.

PLEURAL MEMBRANES

The pleural membrane that adheres to and becomes an integral part of the lung's surface is called the **visceral pleura.** The membrane that originally lined the primitive pleural canal in the embryo is called the **parietal pleura** (see Fig. 1–7). This membrane forms the outer layer of the **pleural cavity,** a cavity also known as the **pleural space** or **intrapleural space.** The actual size of the space is quite small. In fact, it is usually referred to as a *potential space,* implying that only under extraordinary circumstances is an actual gap found between the visceral and parietal pleurae. Such a gap may accompany a *pneumothorax,* a condition caused by a penetrating chest wound that allows air to enter the intrapleural space. Nevertheless, a very small amount of

pleural fluid is present in the pleural cavity and serves to moisten the adjacent surfaces of the two membranes. This serous (watery) fluid is produced by the cells that line the cavity. Cohesion effectively binds the two pleural membranes together by nature of powerful intermolecular attractive forces. Through such a "fluid coupling," movement of the chest wall lined by parietal pleura is transmitted to the viscera pleura to cause movement of the lung. The natural tendency of the lung is to recoil, or collapse, whereas the tendency of the thoracic cage is to expand. The dynamic balance maintained between these two static forces is the subject of Chapter 7 (see Fig. 7–2).

The parietal pleurae cover not only the lateral (costal) surface of the thoracic cavity but also the concave upper surface of the diaphragm and the medial (mediastinal) surface of the thoracic cavity. At the *root* of the lung, which is the collective term for the structures such as bronchi and blood vessels that enter and exit the lung, each parietal pleura *reflects* back upon itself as the visceral pleura. The reflection (folding) of the pleural membranes upon themselves forms a

strengthened region around the root called the **pulmonary ligament** (Fig. 2–10B; see also Color Plate 6). This structure aids in support of the lung. The visceral pleurae cover all surfaces of the lung and also extend into the *interlobar fissures* (discussed below).

SURFACE FEATURES OF THE LUNG

Several topographic features are evident on an anterior view of the lung (see Fig. 2–10A). The right lung is larger than the left and both are divided by **interlobar fissures** into distinct lobes, or subdivisions. The *horizontal fissure* of the right lung separates the **superior lobe** and the **middle lobe.** The middle lobe is separated from the **inferior lobe** by the *oblique fissure* that starts on the anterior surface and spirals around the lung at an angle. The left lung possesses a **superior lobe** separated from an **inferior lobe** by a single *oblique fissure.* Viewed from the front the inferior lobe of each lung appears as a small triangular structure. However, the apparent size and shape is misleading because the oblique fissure slices diagonally across the

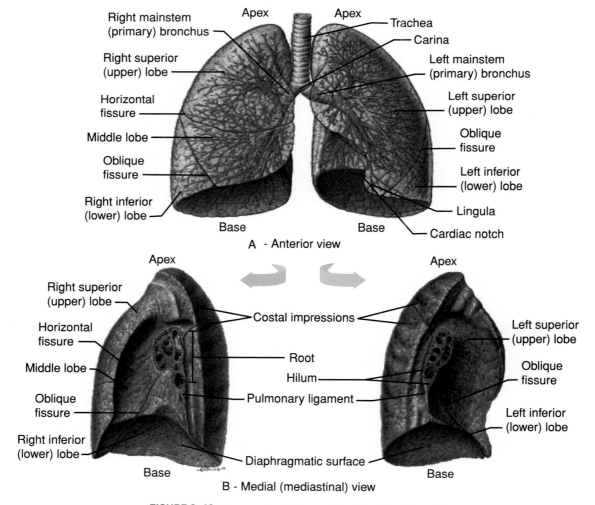

FIGURE 2–10. Lung surface features. (See also Color Plate 6.)

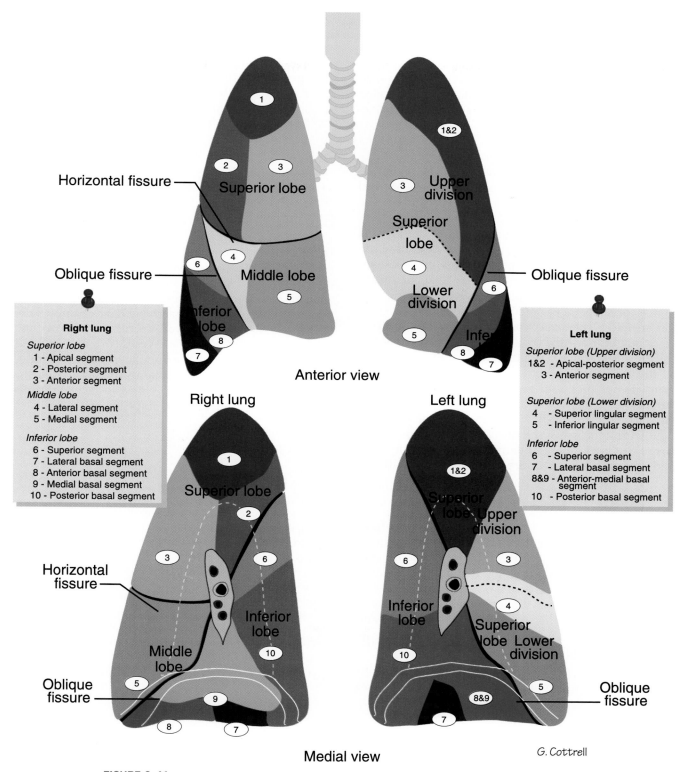

Anterior view

Right lung

Horizontal fissure

Oblique fissure

Superior lobe

Middle lobe

Inferior lobe

Right lung

Superior lobe
1 - Apical segment
2 - Posterior segment
3 - Anterior segment

Middle lobe
4 - Lateral segment
5 - Medial segment

Inferior lobe
6 - Superior segment
7 - Lateral basal segment
8 - Anterior basal segment
9 - Medial basal segment
10 - Posterior basal segment

Left lung

Upper division

Superior lobe

Lower division

Inferior lobe

Oblique fissure

Left lung

Superior lobe (Upper division)
1&2 - Apical-posterior segment
3 - Anterior segment

Superior lobe (Lower division)
4 - Superior lingular segment
5 - Inferior lingular segment

Inferior lobe
6 - Superior segment
7 - Lateral basal segment
8&9 - Anterior-medial basal segment
10 - Posterior basal segment

Right lung

Superior lobe

Horizontal fissure

Middle lobe

Inferior lobe

Oblique fissure

Left lung

Superior lobe Upper division

Inferior lobe

Superior lobe Lower division

Oblique fissure

Medial view

G. Cottrell

FIGURE 2–11. Bronchopulmonary segments. Bronchopulmonary segments are supplied by tertiary (segmental) bronchi. Note that there are 10 segments in the right lung and 8 in the left. Most sources agree that this is due to the fusing of left lung segments: the *apical-posterior segment* and the *anterior-medial basal segment*. (See also Color Plate 7.)

surface to separate the inferior lobe from the rest of the lung (see Fig. 2–10B). The left lung is distinguished on its anterior side by the **cardiac notch,** an indentation on the medial margin of the lung that accommodates the location of the heart to the left of the midline. The lowermost strip of tissue of the cardiac notch is called the **lingua** because it resembles a tongue (see Fig. 2–10A).

Additional surface features include the **apex,** a pointed superior part that projects to approximately the level of the clavicle, and the **base,** the diaphragmatic surface of the lung that conforms to the domed contour of the diaphragm (see Figs. 2–10A and B). The anterior margin of the base of the lung is found at approximately the sixth rib, at the level of the xiphoid process of the sternum, but posteriorly, the lung extends downward so that its posterior margin lies at approximately the eleventh rib. The medial, or **mediastinal surface** of the lungs is slightly concave to match the shape of the mediastinum (see Fig. 2–10B). The surface is characterized by a vertical slit-like structure called the **hilum** that accommodates the **root** of the lung. The root of the lung includes structures such as the mainstem bronchus, pulmonary arteries and veins, lymphatics, and nerves. The lateral, or **costal surface** of the lung is slightly convex to fit the concave curvature on the inside of the rib cage. The lungs are tightly pressed against the ribs, and distinct **costal impressions** are visible as indentations on both the costal and posterior surfaces of the lung (see Fig. 2–10B).

BRONCHOPULMONARY SEGMENTS

Segmental bronchi supply the 10 **bronchopulmonary segments** of the right lung and the 8 bronchopulmonary segments of the left lung. Bronchopulmonary segments are subdivisions within the lobes of the lungs and, as can be seen in Figure 2–11 (see also Color Plate 7), there are structural similarities and differences in the organization of the segments within the right and left lung. Two features should be noted when comparing the bronchopulmonary segments of the lungs:

- The left lung does not have a true middle lobe. Instead, it is organized as a superior lobe having two divisions: an *upper division* and a *lower* or *lingular division.* (The lingular division is so named because of its proximity to the lingua of the lung.)
- The left lung has fewer bronchopulmonary segments than the right (8 segments in the left lung compared with 10 segments in the right). The difference is a result of the presence of *fused* segments in the left lung (e.g., the upper division of the superior lobe has a combined *apical-posterior segment* and the inferior lobe has a combined *anterior-medial basal segment*).

Summary

In this chapter we explored the problem of scale and the optimization of surface area encountered in large, complex organisms. We have seen how the conducting zone of the respiratory system is organized into the upper and lower respiratory tracts and have examined the structure and function of various components making up the conducting zone. We have also briefly examined how the distal parts of the conducting zone are integrated into the respiratory zone of the lung. This discussion, and an in-depth look at the gas-exchange units of the lung, continues in the next chapter.

BIBLIOGRAPHY

Cottrell GP and Surkin HB: Pharmacology for Respiratory Care Practitioners. FA Davis, Philadelphia, 1995.

Des Jardins T: Cardiopulmonary Anatomy and Physiology: Essentials for Respiratory Care, ed 3. Delmar Publishers, Albany, NY, 1998.

Saladin KS: Anatomy and Physiology: The Unity of Form and Function. WCB/McGraw-Hill, Boston, 1998.

Shier D, Butler J, and Lewis R: Hole's Human Anatomy and Physiology, ed 7. Wm C Brown, Dubuque, IA, 1996.

Taylor AE et al: Clinical Respiratory Physiology. WB Saunders, Philadelphia, 1989.

Thibodeau GA and Patton KT: Anatomy and Physiology, ed 3. Mosby-Year Book, St Louis, 1996.

Van De Graaff KM: Human Anatomy, ed 3. Wm C Brown, Dubuque, IA, 1992.

West JB: Respiratory Physiology: The Essentials, ed 6. Williams & Wilkins, Baltimore, 1998.

CHAPTER 3

Respiratory Zone and Microscopic Anatomy of the Lung

chapter objectives

After studying this chapter the reader should be able to:

☐ Differentiate between lung parenchyma and lung interstitium.

☐ Describe the organization of a primary lobule of the lung.

☐ Explain the organization of alveoli by describing the structure of respiratory bronchioles, alveolar ducts, and alveolar sacs.

☐ Discuss how alveoli are stabilized through interdependence.

☐ State Poiseuille's law and describe the relationship between airway resistance and radius.

☐ Explain the changes in cross-sectional area observed in the respiratory system going from the conducting zone to the respiratory zone.

☐ Discuss the concept of collateral ventilation by describing the structure and function of interbronchial connections, canals of Lambert, and pores of Kohn.

☐ Describe how pores of Kohn are formed in interalveolar septa.

☐ Describe the structural organization of the alveolar-capillary system.

☐ Compare and contrast type 1 pneumocytes and type 2 pneumocytes on the basis of morphology, function, location, and number.

☐ Describe the role of alveolar macrophages.

☐ Explain how the interstitium of the lung is organized to support the parenchyma.

key terms

acinus; acini (as' i-nus; as' i-nī)
alveolar-capillary membrane; respiratory
    membrane

alveolar duct
alveolar macrophage
alveolar sac

alveolus; alveoli (al-vē′ ō-lus; al-vē′ ō-lī)
canals of Lambert
Hagen-Poiseuille Law; Poiseuille's law
interstitium (in″ ter-stish′ ē-um)
parenchyma (par-en′ ki-ma)
pores of Kohn (kōn)

primary lobule; terminal respiratory
   unit
respiratory bronchiole
respiratory zone
type 1 pneumocyte; type 1 alveolar cell
type 2 pneumocyte; type 2 alveolar cell

The microscopic organization of the lung is the subject of this chapter. In it we review how the respiratory zone communicates with the conducting zone and examine how various structural configurations of alveoli are arranged to form the functional portion, or parenchyma, of the lung. We also examine how the interstitium of the lung supports the functional elements embedded within it and how the entire structure remains patent during both inspiration and expiration. This chapter also introduces the microscopic structures that comprise the interface between the air stream and bloodstream—the site of gas exchange between the body and the external environment. The functional significance of this alveolar-capillary system is studied in subsequent chapters.

Lung Parenchyma

RELATIONSHIP BETWEEN CONDUCTING AND RESPIRATORY ZONES

Recall that the conducting zone of the respiratory system is composed of a series of branched passageways that end with the distal terminal bronchioles at approximately the 19th generation of airways (see Table 2–1). At this level the airway diameters have decreased to approximately 0.5 mm or less, supporting cartilage is largely absent but bronchiolar smooth muscle is conspicuous in the walls of the airways, and the lining of the passageways is composed of simple low cuboidal epithelial cells with relatively few mucus-secreting cells. Patency in these small-caliber airways is maintained by a combination of bronchomotor tone and by attachments of the airways to the surrounding lung *parenchyma*.

Parenchyma refers to the functional part of an organ, rather than to its structural, or supporting, elements. Lung parenchyma is composed of all the sac-like structures, or *alveoli*, found distal to the terminal bronchioles. Collectively these units have a volume of about 3000 mL and make up the **respiratory zone** of the lung, the site of external respiration. These parenchymal structures are referred to variously as **acini, terminal respiratory units,** or **primary lobules.** Acini have extensive interconnections with each other, with adjacent

conducting zone structures, and with the surrounding interstitial structures of the lung that support them. The resulting interdependence formed by these connections helps maintain patency of the alveoli.

ALVEOLAR ORGANIZATION

The overall design of the respiratory system provides an optimal surface area for exchange of gases between the bloodstream and the external environment. Efficiency is achieved by an arrangement of millions of thin-walled gas exchange units called **alveoli** that expose the air to a highly perfused vascular bed. Alveoli are polyhedral in shape like the units of a honeycomb and are approximately 0.25 mm to 0.50 mm in diameter (Van De Graaff, 1992). They comprise the lung parenchyma and are arranged in several different configurations as shown in Figure 3–1. Each terminal bronchiole of the conducting zone branches into approximately three generations of **respiratory bronchioles,** each of which has several alveolar buds arranged as outpouchings from the wall of the respiratory bronchiole. Respiratory bronchioles, in turn, branch into approximately three generations of **alveolar ducts,** consisting of alveoli connected in a linear fashion to each other to form a short passageway. Finally, the alveolar ducts terminate in clusters of 15 to 20 **alveolar sacs.** Note that alveolar sacs share a common wall, whereas alveoli are separate budlike structures (see Fig. 3–1).

These different morphologic arrangements of alveoli have the same function—to bring the air and blood as close as possible to each other. The various alveolar structures that branch from a terminal bronchiole comprise a single acinus of the lung. The distance from a terminal bronchiole to the most distal alveoli in the acinus is only a few millimeters, but because of the extensive branching of alveolar structures, the respiratory zone contributes to most of the substance of the lung. Approximately 130,000 primary lobules containing a total of 300 million alveoli make up the lung parenchyma.

The interconnections of adjacent alveoli impart stability to the lung to counteract the recoil pressure generated by the static elastic forces of the lung connective tissue. Shared alveolar septa, plus the interconnections provided by elastin and collagen fibers

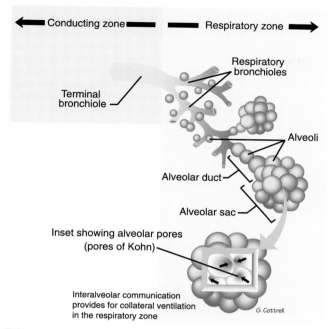

FIGURE 3–1. Primary lobule. The primary lobules (also known as the acini or respiratory units) make up the *parenchyma,* or functional area of the lung. Several alveolar configurations are found in the lobule: (1) alveolar buds attached to the respiratory bronchiole, (2) alveoli lined up end to end to form the alveolar duct, and (3) clusters of 15–20 alveoli, which share septal walls to form the alveolar sac (see inset). Several generations of respiratory bronchioles branch from each terminal bronchiole.

that penetrate from the lung surface to the septa, function to support the alveoli and keep them open. Because of the resulting interdependence, if a single alveolus begins to deflate as a result of a high collapse pressure, it fills adjacent alveoli which, in turn, exert a strong expanding force on the deflating alveolus to counteract the collapse and maintain patency (see Figs. 1–9 and 1–10). Through this mutual support arrangement, all of the alveoli within a primary lobule resist nonuniform changes in lung volume to maintain lung stability.

CROSS-SECTIONAL AREA

Because of the relationships between laminar flow, length and radius of a tube, and the viscosity of a gas, the resistance to flow of a gas in a *single* airway increases dramatically with decreasing radius of the tube. The concept that links these variables is known as the **Hagen-Poiseuille law,** named after Heinrich Gotthilf Hagen, a German civil engineer, and Jean Marie Poiseuille, a French physiologist. Their findings concerning the laminar flow behavior of fluids in pipes were documented between 1839 and 1841 (Dupuis, 1992). The relationship is usually referred to simply as *Poiseuille's law,* and can be shown by the following equation:

$$\dot{V} = \frac{\pi \, \Delta P \, r^4}{8\eta l}$$

where:

$\dot{V}$ = flowrate of the gas
π = mathematical constant (*pi*)
ΔP = pressure gradient (driving pressure)
r = radius of the tube
η = viscosity (*eta*) of the gas
l = length of the tube

Conductance (C) refers to the ability of a substance to pass through a tube, and in the above equation, conductance can be expressed as:

$$C = \frac{\pi r^4}{8\eta l}$$

Furthermore, conductance is the reciprocal of *resistance* (R), therefore:

$$R = \frac{8\eta l}{\pi r^4}$$

From the above relationship it is clear that resistance to laminar flow is directly proportional to the viscosity of a gas and the length of a tube, but it is inversely proportional to the *fourth power of the radius* of a tube. If the viscosity of a gas and the length of an airway is assumed to be constant, it follows that small changes in airway radius will result in sizable changes in airway resistance. For example, in an airway with one-half the radius of another, the airflow resistance in the smaller airway will be sixteen times as great (Fig. 3–2). These statements based on Poiseuille's law refer to laminar flow in a single airway, but it must be remembered that the *total number* of small-diameter structures distal to the terminal bronchioles is very large; therefore, the total cross-sectional area of the respiratory zone is enormous compared with that of the conducting zone (Fig. 3–3). As a result, very little resistance to flow is encountered by air traveling in the most distal parts of the respiratory system. In fact, the forward velocity of the air mass in the respiratory zone is essentially reduced to zero. Diffusion of gas within the acini, therefore, becomes the primary mechanism for ventilation in the respiratory zone distal to the terminal bronchioles (West, 1998).

COLLATERAL VENTILATION IN THE RESPIRATORY ZONE

A number of microscopic structures exist to permit air to move from occluded to ventilated regions of the lung. These alternative air passageways are called collateral air channels and include the *interbronchial connections* (80 to 150 µm) in the terminal airways; the **canals of Lambert** (30 µm) that connect terminal bronchioles with alveoli (see Fig. 2–9); and the **pores**

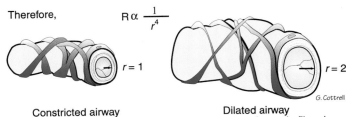

Resistance to laminar flow in a single airway

$$R = \frac{8\,l}{\eta r^4}$$

Where R = resistance

η = viscosity (eta) of the gas

l = length of the airway

π = mathematical constant (pi)

r = radius of the airway

If the viscosity of the gas and the length of the airway are held constant, resistance to flow is inversely proportional to the fourth power of the tube radius,

Therefore, $R \propto \dfrac{1}{r^4}$

$r = 1$

$r = 2$

G. Cottrell

Constricted airway
(due to contracted muscle fibers)

$R \propto \dfrac{1}{1^4}$

$R \propto \dfrac{1}{1}$ Resistance 1

Dilated airway
(due to relaxed muscle fibers)

$R \propto \dfrac{1}{2^4}$

$R \propto \dfrac{1}{16}$ Resistance 1/16

FIGURE 3–2. Airway resistance. Notice the spirally arranged smooth muscle fibers and lack of cartilage support elements in these collapsible airways. The resistance equation (above) is derived from the Hagen-Poiseuille law, which describes the relationship between flow and pressure in a tube with fixed dimensions, under conditions of laminar flow. See text for full explanation.

of Kohn (3 to 13 μm) that connect adjacent alveoli (see Fig. 3–1). Pores of Kohn are formed in the interalveolar septa through several mechanisms:

1. The "shedding" of alveolar epithelial cells, a process called *desquamation*
2. The *degeneration* of cells
3. The *movement* of alveolar macrophages
4. A *combination* of these events, all of which leave an opening in the alveolar wall (Des Jardins, 1998)

The number of pores increases with age and with pathophysiologic states such as chronic obstructive pulmonary disease (COPD). Collateral ventilation is especially important in providing alternate air passageways in the lungs of patients with COPDs such as emphysema. The interbronchial connections provide collateral ventilation within the conducting zone, the canals of Lambert allow for collateral air movement between the conducting and respiratory zones of the lung, and the pores of Kohn perform as collateral air channels within the respiratory zone. In this way, air can be shunted around obstructions in the conducting zone, the respiratory zone, or both, to reach alveoli of the lung that are perfused with blood.

Alveolar-Capillary System

Individual alveoli are extensively covered by pulmonary capillaries, creating the equivalent of a thin "film" of blood in continual contact with the air contained in the alveoli. This air is being constantly exchanged with the external environment; therefore, the continuously replenished "film" of blood forms an effective air-blood interface that is part of the **alveolar-capillary membrane** or **respiratory membrane** (Fig. 3–4; see also Color Plate 8). An artificial device such as a membrane oxygenator is designed in a similar fashion to bring the bloodstream as close as possible to a gas source over the largest possible surface area (Box 3–1).

Of course, in such gas-blood exchange devices, whether natural or artificial, there is no actual physical contact between the air and blood. In the lung, the airstream and bloodstream are separated by a very narrow distance of approximately 0.35 μm. Taylor et al (1989) describe this thickness as about 1/50 that of thin airmail stationery. The thinner the membrane for gas exchange, the more efficient the diffusion of gas (see Chap. 12). Fick's law of diffusion relates the diffusion of gas, membrane thickness, and the surface area of membranes. Simply stated, the volume of gas that diffuses across a sheet of tissue is directly proportional to the surface area of the sheet but inversely proportional to its thickness (West, 1998). Clearly, an alveolar-capillary membrane with a thickness much less than that of tissue paper and a huge surface area about half the size of an average bungalow (approximately 750 ft² or 80 m²) will be conducive to efficient gas diffusion, allowing gaseous equilibrium in the blood and air to be reached very quickly.

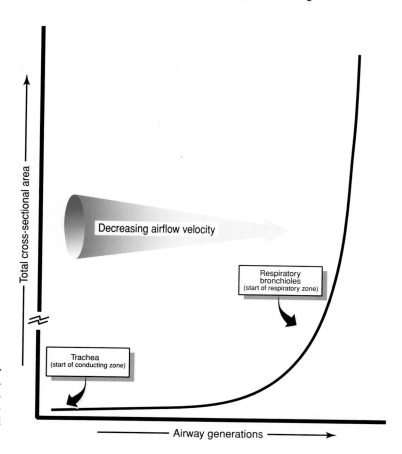

FIGURE 3–3. Total cross-sectional area of the respiratory system. The total cross-sectional area of the respiratory system increases dramatically in the distal parts of the lung because of the large numbers of small-diameter airways. Average airflow velocity decreases as the total cross-sectional area of the respiratory system increases.

The structures of the alveolar-capillary system include the squamous epithelial cell of the alveolar wall, two basement membranes separated by a narrow interstitial space, and the squamous endothelial cell of the pulmonary capillary (see Fig. 3–4). In terms of functional tissue barriers, the cytoplasmic membrane of the erythrocyte represents an additional layer through which gases must diffuse. The average diameter of a mature erythrocyte is about 7 μm, which is slightly *less than* that of most pulmonary capillaries. Consequently, erythrocytes must fold or bend slightly and must line up in single file to be pushed through the narrow vessels of the pulmonary circuit. As described in Chapter 12, this action slows the transit of erythrocytes past the alveolus, further improving the efficiency of gas exchange.

Cells of the Respiratory Zone

The general trend that has been discussed in relation to the epithelial lining of the respiratory tract is a gradual reduction in the thickness of the lining, both in layering arrangements and in cell morphology. The transition includes changes from stratified (multiple layers) to simple (single layer) organization, and from columnar to cuboidal to squamous morphological types of cells (see Table 2–1). In the alveoli of the respiratory zone, two types of epithelial cells are arranged in a single layer comprising the wall structure: the flattened *type 1 pneumocytes* and the cube-shaped *type 2 pneumocytes*.

The number of **type 1 pneumocytes,** also known as **type 1 alveolar cells,** present in the alveolar walls is only about one-half that of the type 2 pneumocytes. The surface area of the alveolus, however, is comprised mainly (95%) of type 1 cells that provide the thin alveolar barrier needed for effective gas exchange. The squamous morphology and slight bulge where the nucleus is located gives the cells a "fried egg" appearance (West, 1998) (see Fig. 1–11). In spite of the relatively few numbers of type 1 cells, their luminal surface is approximately 25 times that of the type 2 pneumocytes. The drawback to such a thin shape for cells is one of fragility. Type 1 pneumocytes are virtually incapable of supporting themselves. Further, they are prone to collapse as a result of powerful surface tension forces produced by the alveolar fluid that lines them and by pressure and volume changes generated in the lung during ventilation. Type 1 pneumocytes do not replicate themselves but are replaced by type 2 pneumocytes that have divided and differentiated into type 1 cells.

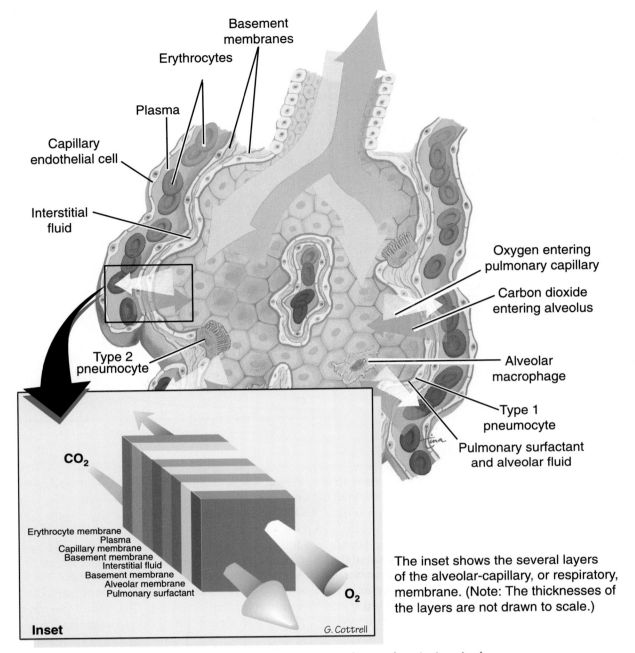

FIGURE 3–4. Alveolar-capillary membrane. At the site of external respiration, simple squamous epithelium provides the smallest possible separation between the airstream and the bloodstream. The alveolar membrane consists of a single type 1 pneumocyte; the capillary membrane consists of a single endothelial cell. (Adapted from Scanlon VC and Sanders T: Essentials of Anatomy and Physiology, ed. 3. FA Davis, Philadelphia, 1999, p 332, with permission.) (See also Color Plate 8.)

Type 2 pneumocytes are also known as **type 2 alveolar cells.** These cube-shaped cells play a crucial role in lung maturity because of their production of pulmonary surfactant. This complex phospholipid is secreted onto the alveolar surface where it reduces alveolar surface tension and thereby contributes to lung stability (see Fig. 1–11). The secretory nature of type 2 cells is characterized by the presence of (1) conspicuous microvilli on the free border for the release of secretory product; (2) numerous mitochondria and Golgi complexes to support high metabolic activity associated with synthesis and packaging of product; and (3) the presence in the cytoplasm of conspicuous lamellar bodies, which are the storage form of the precursors of pulmonary surfactant. As pointed out previously, type 2 pneumocytes are numerous in the walls of alveoli but do not contribute significantly to the alveolar surface area because of their compact, cuboidal shape.

P E R S P E C T I V E S

BOX 3–1

ECMO and Artificial Alveolar-capillary Membranes

In patients unable to properly oxygenate the blood, a biomedical device called an oxygenator is sometimes indicated. Various oxygenator designs exist that employ tubes, plates, or membranes to provide a large surface area for gas exchange between the bloodstream and a gas source. Membrane oxygenators are among the most efficient devices and are used in a procedure known as extracorporeal membrane oxygenation, or ECMO. In this process, the membrane oxygenator simulates the role of the alveolar-capillary system in external respiration by providing the interface for gas exchange. ECMO procedures are sometimes used to reduce pulmonary vascular resistance (PVR) in an infant. *Extracorporeal* refers to a location "outside the body" and is used to describe that portion of the bloodstream that is pumped externally to devices such as heart-lung machines, hemodialysis machines, or oxygenators.

Although other treatment modalities such as high-frequency ventilation, surfactant replacement, liquid ventilation, and nitric oxide therapy have a present or future role in treating neonatal and pediatric respiratory failure, ECMO remains an effective therapy responsible for increasing infant survival rates (Arensman et al, 1996).

- Arensman RM et al: Modern treatment modalities for neonatal and pediatric respiratory failure. Am J Surg. 172(1):41–47, 1996.
- Cottrell GP and Surkin HB: Pharmacology for Respiratory Care Practitioners. FA Davis, Philadelphia, 1995.
- O'Rourke PP: ECMO: Where have we been? Where are we going? Respiratory Care. 36:683–692, 1991.

Type 1 and type 2 pneumocytes are the *fixed* cells of the alveoli; in other words, their numbers may vary somewhat but their locations are stable. In contrast to this stationary structural arrangement is the *mobile* cell population of the alveoli—the **alveolar macrophages.** These large, motile phagocytic cells are free to slowly move via amoeboid movement to ingest bacteria, cellular debris, and particulate matter that enters the alveoli. Alveolar macrophages are part of the body's nonspecific defense mechanism. Alveolar macrophages are derived from stem cells in bone marrow that initially give rise to monocytes in the bloodstream. Monocytes, which are a type of leukocyte, then undergo specialization, migrating to the lung to take up residence in the alveoli as alveolar macrophages.

Lung Interstitium

The **interstitium** of the lung is the network of supporting structures that maintains the integrity of the functional elements. Recall that the maintenance of a thin alveolar membrane and a large total alveolar surface area is crucial in gas exchange, but that such a structural arrangement is inherently fragile and unstable as a result of the high collapse tendency of small spheres and the elastic recoil of lung structures. Strong collagen and elastin connective tissue fibers weave around the pulmonary capillaries to provide support. These fibers are attached on one end to the connective tissue fibers that penetrate into the lung parenchyma from the pleura. The other end of the fibers that support the alveolar septa is attached to fibers associated with the pulmonary artery and bronchi. Through this interwoven support arrangement the interdependent alveolar walls are maintained under tension during inspiration, thus causing them to stretch out and produce a large surface area ideal for gas exchange.

Lung interstitium also supports and contains lymphatics and nerve branches. The loosely arranged collagen fibers of the interstitium serve to limit alveolar distention during inspiration. Inflation beyond the limits imposed by these interstitial fibers can cause occlusion of pulmonary capillaries, damage to alveolar walls, or both. In subsequent chapters we discuss the effect that pathologic changes in the lung interstitium have on gas exchange and on ventilation.

Summary

In this chapter we have examined the microscopic anatomy of the respiratory zone of the lung by discussing the organization of both the parenchyma and the interstitium. Collateral air channels and interconnecting support fibers were presented as structures that connect the conducting and respiratory zones. Different morphologic arrangements of alveoli comprising the lung parenchyma were introduced, and the concept of interdependence of alveoli was reviewed through a discussion of the support role of the lung interstitium. In addition, the cells of the respiratory zone were discussed as well as the microscopic structure of the alveolar-capillary system as a prelude to an examination of its functional role in gas exchange in subsequent chapters.

BIBLIOGRAPHY

Des Jardins T: Cardiopulmonary Anatomy and Physiology: Essentials for Respiratory Care, ed 3. Delmar Publishers, Albany, NY, 1998.

Dupuis YG: Ventilators: Theory and Clinical Application, ed 2. Mosby–Year Book, St. Louis, 1992.

Taylor AE et al: Clinical Respiratory Physiology. WB Saunders, Philadelphia, 1989.

Thibodeau GA and Patton KT: Anatomy and Physiology, ed 3. Mosby–Year Book, St Louis, 1996.

Van De Graaff KM: Human Anatomy, ed 3. Wm C Brown, Dubuque, IA, 1992.

West JB: Respiratory Physiology: The Essentials, ed 6. Williams & Wilkins, Baltimore, 1998.

CHAPTER 4

Innervation of the Tracheobronchial Tree and Lung

chapter objectives

After studying this chapter the reader should be able to:

☐ Describe the organization of the nervous system into central (CNS) and peripheral (PNS) divisions.

☐ Review neurochemical transmission by defining the following terms:
Afferent, efferent, neurotransmitter, receptor, adrenergic, norepinephrine, cholinergic, acetylcholine, secondary messenger.

☐ Explain the function of the following receptors in the airways and lungs:
α_1-adrenergic, β_1-adrenergic, β_2-adrenergic, M_3-muscarinic, N_1-nicotinic, nitric oxide (NO), vasoactive intestinal peptide (VIP).

☐ Summarize how the smooth muscle, glands, and blood vessels of the tracheobronchial tree and lung are controlled through the adrenergic, cholinergic, and inhibitory nonadrenergic noncholinergic (i-NANC) systems.

key terms

adrenergic receptors (ad-ren-er' jik); adrenoceptors
α_1-adrenergic receptors; α_1-adrenoceptors
β_1-adrenergic receptors; β_1-adrenoceptors
β_2-adrenergic receptors; β_2-adrenoceptors
autonomic nervous system (ANS)
parasympathetic division
sympathetic division

cholinergic receptors (kō″ lin-er' jik); cholinoceptors
M_3-muscarinic cholinergic receptor
N_1-nicotinic cholinergic receptor
N_2-nicotinic cholinergic receptor
nonadrenergic noncholinergic (NANC) neurotransmission

The neural control of the tracheobronchial tree and lung is the topic of this chapter. The material is designed to provide review and reinforcement of basic principles of autonomic control introduced in general anatomy and physiology courses. The focus of the chapter is on the neurotransmitters and receptors involved in adrenergic control, cholinergic control, and inhibitory nonadreneric noncholinergic (i-NANC) control of airway smooth muscle and glands.

Control of the Tracheobronchial Tree and Lung

BACKGROUND INFORMATION

Various structures such as bronchiolar smooth muscle, submucosal airway glands, and vascular smooth muscle found in the tracheobronchial tree and lung, as well as functions such as the production of histamine and other autacoids, are controlled either directly or indirectly by neural impulses. (*Autacoids,* or allergic mediators, are covered with defense of the lung in Chapter 5.) The nervous control of respiratory system structure and function occurs below the level of consciousness and is mediated by elements of the *peripheral nervous system* (PNS). The peripheral nervous system is made up of components that are not part of the brain or spinal cord, the two organs that comprise the *central nervous system* (CNS) (Fig. 4–1). The reader is encouraged to review appropriate sections of the peripheral nervous system that were introduced in general anatomy and physiology courses. However, it can be stated briefly that the PNS is made up of an *afferent system* composed of the various receptors of the body and the sensory pathways that connect such receptors to the CNS, and an *efferent system* that handles the motor outflow from the CNS to the muscles and glands of the body (Fig. 4–2).

The efferent system is divided into the *somatic nervous system,* which carries motor impulses to the skeletal muscles, and the **autonomic nervous system (ANS),** which controls the smooth muscle, cardiac muscle, and glandular tissue of the body. The ANS is further divided into the **sympathetic division** and the **parasympathetic division**. Nerve fibers from one or both of these two ANS divisions innervate not only the tracheobronchial tree and lung structures listed previously but also other organs such as the heart, blood vessels, and gastrointestinal tract (Table 4–1). In addition, some of these structures are controlled by the *nonadrenergic noncholinergic* (NANC) nervous system. We now review the organization and distribution of sympathetic, parasympathetic, and NANC nervous system components as they relate to the neurotransmitters released, receptors involved, and the mechanisms of action responsible for producing changes in the tracheobronchial tree and lung. For additional details of the structural, functional, and neurochemical features of the sympathetic and parasympathetic divisions of the ANS, and an overview of the NANC system, see Cottrell and Surkin (1995).

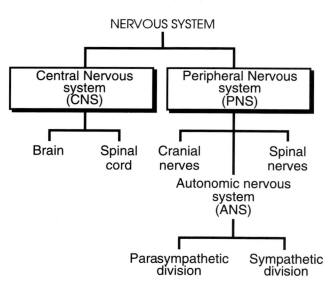

FIGURE 4–1. Conceptual divisions of the nervous system. (From Cottrell GP and Surkin HB: Pharmacology for Respiratory Care Practitioners. FA Davis, Philadelphia, 1995, p 74, with permission.)

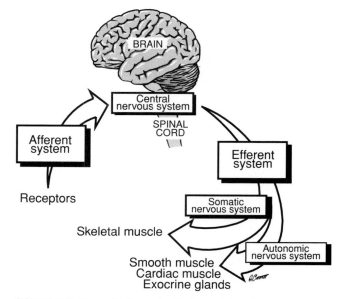

FIGURE 4–2. Flow of information in the peripheral nervous system. (From Cottrell GP and Surkin HB: Pharmacology for Respiratory Care Practitioners. FA Davis, Philadelphia, 1995, p 75, with permission.)

TABLE 4–1	Autonomic Stimulation of Organs	
Organ	**Sympathetic**	**Parasympathetic**
Eye	Dilation	Constriction
Iris	Decrease	Decreased
Intraocular pressure	—	Increased
Tear gland secretion		
Glands		
Salivary	Viscous secretion	Watery secretion
Sweat	Secretion, palms	Generalized secretion*
Piloerectors	Contraction	—
Bronchioles		
Secretions	Mixed response	Increased
Smooth muscle	Relaxation†	Contraction
Heart		
Rate	Acceleration	Deceleration
Force	Increased	Decreased
Gastrointestinal tract		
Muscle wall (motility)	Relaxation	Contraction
Sphincters	Contraction	Relaxation
Secretion	—	Increased
Spleen	Contraction	—
Urinary bladder		
Fundus	Relaxation	Contraction
Trigone and sphincter	Contraction	Relaxation
Blood vessels (arterioles)		
Skeletal muscle	Dilation	Dilation‡
Coronary	Dilation (β_2)	Dilation
Skin, viscera	Constriction	—

*Many sweat glands have receptors that are stimulated by acetylcholine-like drugs and blocked by atropine-like drugs. The anatomic origin of these nerves is sympathetic; therefore, they are called *cholinergic sympathetic*.

†Sympathetic neurons do not innervate smooth muscle found in bronchioles. However, β_2-adrenoceptors are located on airway smooth muscle. When such receptors are stimulated, bronchodilation results.

‡Parasympathetic neurons do not innervate vascular beds found in skeletal muscle, but muscarinic receptors are located on the vascular smooth muscle membranes. When such receptors are stimulated, vasodilation results.

Source: Adapted from Long (1989).

Adrenergic Control

To discuss the role of the sympathetic division of the nervous system in the control of the tracheobronchial tree and lung, a few basic terms need to be reviewed. The term *adrenergic* is used in association with *norepinephrine (noradrenalin)*, a naturally produced substance that functions as a chemical messenger in both the nervous system and the endocrine system. Nerve fibers that release norepinephrine (NE) are classified as *adrenergic* fibers. Membrane receptors that interact with nor-

epinephrine, or substances that closely resemble it, are known as *adrenergic* receptors. Finally, drugs that structurally resemble norepinephrine are classified as *adrenergic* drugs. Most, but not all, sympathetic fibers release NE and are classified as adrenergic fibers. A few sympathetic fibers, such as those innervating the adrenal medulla and autonomic ganglia, release *acetylcholine* (ACh) and are referred to as *cholinergic* fibers.

If we confine our review of the autonomic nervous system to postjunctional receptors, that is, to the membrane receptors found on the postsynaptic side of a synapse, two functional classifications of adrenergic receptors are recognized:

- Alpha$_1$-adrenergic receptors (α_1-adrenoceptors)— When norepinephrine from an adrenergic nerve fiber interacts with α_1-adrenergic receptors, it produces excitatory or stimulatory changes such as contraction of vascular smooth muscle.
- Beta-adrenergic receptors (β-adrenoceptors)— Norepinephrine released from adrenergic nerve fibers interacts with β-adrenergic receptors to cause characteristic changes at different locations. Norepinephrine complexes with β_2-adrenergic receptors to cause inhibitory or depressive changes in the effector cell, such as relaxation of bronchiolar smooth muscle or relaxation of vascular smooth muscle. By contrast, norepinephrine causes stimulation of β_1-adrenergic receptors, such as those found on cardiac muscle, resulting in excitatory changes such as an increase in heart rate and force. Note that it is the receptor *response*, not the chemical messenger, that determines whether a neurotransmitter is considered "excitatory" or "inhibitory."

How is the sympathetic division of the ANS involved in the nervous control of the tracheobronchial tree and lung? Pulmonary vasculature is under direct sympathetic control with most of the pulmonary blood vessels controlled by α_1-adrenergic receptors. The degree of α_1-adrenergic stimulation of pulmonary blood vessels, therefore, determines the degree of contraction of vascular smooth muscle, thereby helping regulate vascular tone and pulmonary perfusion. Bronchiolar smooth muscle, by contrast, is *not* under direct sympathetic control. There are no sympathetic nerve fibers innervating airway smooth muscle in the human respiratory system. Adrenergic receptors, however, exist in several locations in the tracheobronchial tree and lung and are affected both by endogenous catecholamines such as circulating norepinephrine or *epinephrine (adrenalin)* secreted by the adrenal medulla, and by exogenous catecholamines such as adrenergic drugs used to control bronchial asthma symptoms. (*Catecholamines* are chemical entities that possess a unique six-carbon-ring structure that has a characteristic hydrocarbon side chain.

Most of the catecholamines and catecholamine derivatives exhibit similar biochemical and clinical properties because of their close resemblance to native catecholamines such as norepinephrine and epinephrine.)

β_2-Adrenergic receptors are found on bronchiolar smooth muscle throughout the respiratory tree, but are most numerous in the smaller-diameter peripheral airways. Airway epithelium and some vascular smooth muscle in the lung is equipped with β_2-adrenergic receptors. Stimulation of such receptors relaxes vascular smooth muscle, thereby reducing vasomotor tone and blood pressure. Bronchial submucosal glands and alveolar walls possess both β_1- and β_2-adrenergic receptors, but the β_2 subtype outnumbers the β_1-adrenergic receptors by a ratio of approximately 3:1 (Howder, 1993). The complete role of β_1-adrenergic receptors in the lung is not fully understood. Bronchiolar smooth muscle in the smaller airways has a number of α_1-adrenergic receptors, but the dominant type of adrenergic receptor in the airways is the β_2-adrenoceptor. Because α_1-adrenergic receptors are located on airway smooth muscle, vascular smooth muscle, and submucosal glands, selective stimulation of α_1-adrenergic receptors causes bronchoconstriction, vasoconstriction, and glandular secretion.

The mechanism of action of catecholamines such as norepinephrine at β_2-adrenoceptors in the lung depends on the activation of an intracellular enzyme controlling the production of an intracellular messenger. This *secondary messenger,* in turn, relaxes bronchiolar smooth muscle, reduces glandular secretion, and inhibits histamine release from target cells such as sensitized mast cells. Catecholamine or catecholamine derivatives such as albuterol (salbutamol) and salmeterol are commonly employed as therapeutic β_2-adrenoceptor bronchodilators in the treatment of acute bronchospasm. The widespread use and effectiveness of such bronchodilators is due in part to their ability to promote the rapid production of secondary messengers in effectors such as bronchiolar smooth muscle cells.

The effects of adrenergic stimulation of the tracheobronchial tree and lung are summarized in Table 4–2.

Cholinergic Control

Following the same format used previously to review the sympathetic division in relation to adrenergic activity, we briefly turn our attention to the parasympathetic division of the autonomic nervous system to understand how this ANS division affects the tracheobronchial tree and lung. The term *cholinergic* is derived from ACh, a neurotransmitter operating in several locations in the nervous system, including the ANS, somatic nervous system, and CNS (Fig. 4–3). *Cholinergic* fibers are those that release acetylcholine. Most parasympathetic fibers are classified as cholinergic fibers but, as we have already seen, some sympathetic fibers are also classified as cholinergic nerve fibers. Receptors that complex with acetylcholine or with substances that resemble acetylcholine are classified as **cholinergic receptors** or **cholinoceptors.** Similarly, *cholinergic* drugs are those having a molecular structure that resembles that of acetylcholine and thus are able to interact at cholinergic receptors. Postjunctional cholinergic receptors can be categorized on the basis of their location in the body, as follows:

- **M_3-muscarinic cholinergic receptors**—These postsynaptic cholinergic receptors get their unusual name because they are stimulated by *muscarine,* a poisonous alkaloid substance used experimentally. The designation "M_3" indicates that these muscarinic receptors are at the terminal synapse of parasympathetic pathways. In other words, they are located on the postjunctional side of cholinergic synapses at the connection between parasympathetic postganglionic fibers and neuroeffector organs (see Fig. 4–3). Other muscarinic receptor locations exist at prejunctional sites (M_2) and at autonomic ganglia (M_1), but do not concern us in this discussion.

- **Nicotinic cholinergic receptors**—Nicotinic receptors are stimulated by *nicotine,* the poisonous alkaloid found in tobacco. A convenient way of remembering the distribution of the *postjunctional* cholinergic receptors in the PNS is to remember that the terminal synapse in parasympathetic pathways is mediated by M_3-muscarinic receptors, and that all other postjunctional cholinergic receptors are designated as nicotinic receptors. Within the nicotinic receptor category, two subtypes of postjunctional receptor exist: **N_1-nicotinic receptors** located at autonomic ganglia (sympathetic *and* parasympathetic) and **N_2-nicotinic receptors** found at neuromuscular junctions (NMJs) for the control of skeletal muscle (see Fig. 4–3).

The parasympathetic division contributes to the direct control of the tracheobronchial tree and lung by (1) regulating the degree of bronchomotor tone that develops in airway smooth muscle, (2) determining the amount and nature of the secretions produced by the respiratory tract, and (3) by controlling the production and release of allergic mediators such as histamine. Therefore, an increase in the amount of cholinergic activity has a profound effect on airway caliber, glandular activity, and inflammatory responses in the respiratory system.

Vagal efferent nerves release ACh when they are stimulated. Acetylcholine, in turn, complexes with M_3-muscarinic receptors and initiates a chain of events within the effector cell that result in the characteristic responses listed previously. The large-diameter central

| TABLE 4–2 | Control of the Tracheobronchial Tree and Lung |

Organ	Adrenergic Receptors (NE)			Cholinergic Receptors (ACh)[1]		i-NANC Receptors (NO)
	α_1- Adrenergic	β_1- Adrenergic	β_2- Adrenergic	M_3- Muscarinic	N_2- Nicotinic	NO
Bronchiolar Smooth Muscle	Contraction and increased bronchomotor tone (slight)[2]	?[3]	Relaxation and decreased bronchomotor tone (e.g., small-diameter peripheral bronchioles)[4]	Contraction and increased bronchomotor tone (e.g., large-diameter central bronchioles)	—	Relaxation and decreased bronchomotor tone
Pulmonary Blood Vessels	Contraction and increased vasomotor tone	?	Relaxation and decreased vasomotor tone	Contraction and increased vasomotor tone[5]	—	Relaxation and decreased vasomotor tone
Submucosal Glands	Increased secretion	?	Decreased secretion	Increased volume and viscosity of secretions; increased release of inflammatory mediators (e.g., histamine)	—	?
Respiratory Muscles	—	—	Slight stimulation (as a result of the small number of β_2 receptors present)	—	Contraction of skeletal muscle	—

? = Unknown effect

[1]N_1-Nicotinic receptors are found at autonomic ganglia of *both* ANS divisions; therefore, it is difficult to predict the effects produced in the tracheobronchial tree and lung. Such ganglionic effects have been omitted from the table. In most instances, adrenergic effects predominate at effectors such as vascular smooth muscle (sympathetic dominance).

[2]Very few α_1-adrenergic receptors are present in the airways.

[3]Relatively few β_1-adrenergic receptors are present in the airways (e.g., β_2 receptors outnumber β_1 receptors 3:1).

[4]β_2-Adrenergic receptors respond to circulating native catecholamines (e.g., adrenaline) and to exogenous catecholamines (e.g., inhaled β_2-agonist drugs); bronchiolar smooth muscle is not controlled by adrenergic nerve fibers.

[5]Most blood vessels are controlled through the adrenergic system; relatively few vascular beds in the body receive cholinergic nerve fibers.

bronchioles have a high density of M_3-muscarinic receptors, whereas the smaller-diameter peripheral airways have relatively few M_3-muscarinic receptors. (Recall that the arrangement of β_2-adrenergic receptors is essentially the reverse of this situation.) Because of the location of these muscarinic receptors, the excitatory reaction elicited by ACh results in bronchial smooth muscle contraction, an increase in bronchial gland secretion, and an increase in the viscosity of the bronchial mucus produced. In addition, ACh triggers the release of inflammatory mediators such as histamine and chemotactic factors from target cells and initiates the production of arachidonic acid metabolites. These mediators bring about the inflammatory response in the lung and are examined in Chapter 5. Clearly, inhibition of vagal activity in the lung is potentially beneficial in the control of certain kinds of bronchospasm.

The mechanism of action of acetylcholine at M_3-muscarinic receptors involves the activation of an intracellular enzyme that controls the production of a secondary messenger different from the one activated by adrenergic stimulation. This messenger produces antagonistic actions such as bronchospasm, hypersecretion, and mucosal edema—cardinal signs of the inflammatory response in the lung.

Table 4–2 summarizes the effects of cholinergic stimulation of the tracheobronchial tree and lung.

Nonadrenergic Noncholinergic (NANC) Control

If airway smooth muscle is devoid of sympathetic innervation as we have seen, and parasympathetic effects produce a baseline amount of bronchomotor tone, what mechanism functions to modify the bron-

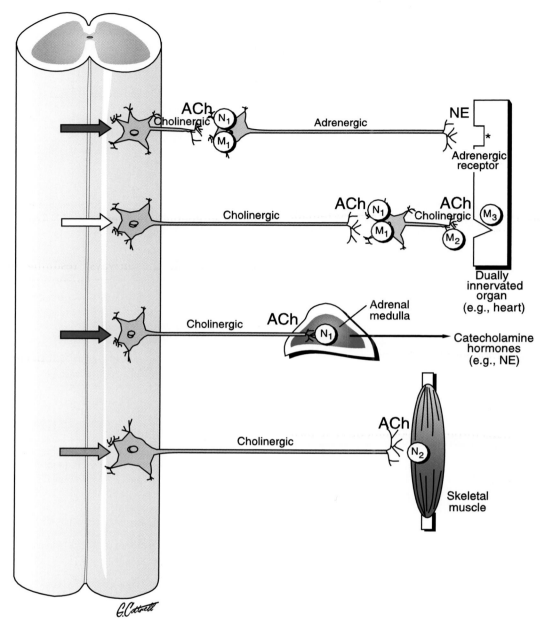

FIGURE 4–3. Neurotransmitters and receptors of the peripheral nervous system. Large blue arrow = sympathetic division, autonomic nervous system; large white arrow = parasympathetic division, autonomic nervous system; large gray arrow = somatic nervous system; ACh = acetylcholine; NE = norepinephrine. Receptors: N_1 = N_1-nicotinic; N_2 = N_2-nicotinic; M_1 = M_1-muscarinic; M_2 = M_2-muscarinic; M_3 = M_3-muscarinic. (From Cottrell GP and Surkin HB: Pharmacology for Respiratory Care Practitioners. FA Davis, Philadelphia, 1995, p 81, with permission.)

*Adrenergic receptors are classified functionally into alpha (α) and beta (β) subtypes on the basis of their response to norepinephrine.

choconstriction brought about by M_3-muscarinic stimulation? As pointed out previously, airway smooth muscle possesses β_2-adrenergic receptors even though it lacks sympathetic nerves. Furthermore, circulating catecholamines such as neurotransmitters, hormones, or drugs stimulate such receptors to cause relaxation of bronchiolar smooth muscle. But what of *neural control*

to reverse bronchoconstriction? Researchers point to a third controlling system of airway diameter called **nonadrenergic noncholinergic (NANC) neurotransmission.** More precisely, we are interested in a system that functionally opposes the parasympathetic (vagal) effects in the tracheobronchial tree and lung—an *inhibitory* NANC mechanism, or *i-NANC system.*

Several regulatory substances including *vasoactive intestinal peptide* (VIP), *nitric oxide* (NO), and *adenosine triphosphate* (ATP) are being investigated as i-NANC neurotransmitters in the relaxation response of smooth muscle in the airways and gastrointestinal tract. When known mechanisms of airway function—such as stimulation of β_2-adrenergic receptors (bronchodilation) or stimulation of M_3-muscarinic receptors (bronchoconstriction)—are selectively blocked, and when known mediators of airway function such as prostaglandins are inhibited, chemical or electrical stimulation of the airways continues to cause bronchodilation through the i-NANC mechanism (Barnes, 1992; Barnes, 1993; Belvisi et al, 1992). Furthermore, when systematic blockade of suspected i-NANC mediators such as VIP and ATP is carried out, the bronchodilator response persists.

These findings point to NO as the mediator responsible for the inhibitory effect on bronchiolar smooth muscle contraction. What happens if NO is not available at bronchiolar smooth muscle? Inhibition of NO causes the i-NANC bronchodilator response to disappear and allows unopposed cholinergic effects to increase bronchomotor tone. Additionally, the administration of a precursor needed in the synthesis of NO results in restoration of inhibitory NANC-mediated bronchodilation. Finally, NO is rapidly removed in physiologic solutions through a spontaneous chemical breakdown. These findings—*specificity, reversibility,* and *rapidity*—are key features of neurotransmitters and are exhibited by nitric oxide in the i-NANC control of airway function. In addition, NO appears to play an important role in regulation of blood vessel diameter.

Nitric oxide was originally known as endothelium-derived relaxing factor (EDRF), so named because it is released from the lining of blood vessels, where it promotes relaxation of vascular smooth muscle. For this reason inhaled NO is being used as a *selective* vasodilator to treat pulmonary hypertension. As a vasodilator, NO activates a secondary messenger, which decreases free calcium ions (Ca^{2+}) in smooth muscle cells. Because Ca^{2+} is required to initiate muscle contraction, a decrease in the concentration of Ca^{2+} promotes relaxation of vascular smooth muscle to bring about selective vasodilation of pulmonary blood vessels.

Other substances such as VIP and ATP may play a neuromodulator, or modifying, role in the control of airway caliber. For example, functional VIP receptors have been found on airway smooth muscle, epithelial cells, and submucosal glands. Stimulation of such receptors by VIP initiates an enzyme sequence to result in relaxation of bronchiolar smooth muscle (Howder, 1992).

The effects of inhibitory nonadrenergic noncholinergic control of the tracheobronchial tree and lung are summarized in Table 4–2.

Summary

We have seen that neural control of the tracheobronchial tree and lung is the result of a delicate balance among adrenergic, cholinergic, and NANC components. A defect or disturbance in the inhibitory NANC system (i-NANC) allows vagally mediated cholinergic effects to predominate in the airways, resulting in bronchoconstriction. Conversely, introduction of β_2-adrenergic drugs activates specific β-adrenergic receptors to promote bronchodilation and prevent histamine release. Cholinergic stimulation via the vagal nerves, or pharmacologic stimulation by means of cholinergic drugs, results in increased glandular secretion, elevated bronchomotor tone, and histamine release.

BIBLIOGRAPHY

Barnes PJ: Autonomic pharmacology of the airways. In Chung KF and Barnes PJ (eds): Pharmacology of the Respiratory Tract: Experimental and Clinical Research. Marcel Dekker, New York, 1993.

Barnes PJ: Neural mechanisms in asthma. Br Med Bull. 48: 149–168, 1992.

Belvisi MG et al: Inhibitory NANC nerves in human tracheal smooth muscle: A quest for the neurotransmitter. J Appl Physiol. 73: 2502–2510, 1992.

Cottrell GP and Surkin HB: Pharmacology for Respiratory Care Practitioners. FA Davis, Philadelphia, 1995.

Howder CL: Antimuscarinic and β_2-adrenoceptor bronchodilators in obstructive airways disease. Respiratory Care 38:1364–1388, 1993.

Lammers JW, Barnes PJ, and Chung KF: Nonadrenergic, noncholinergic airway inhibitory nerves. Eur Respir J. 5:239–246, 1992.

Long JP: Drugs acting on the peripheral nervous system. In Conn PM and Gebhart GF (eds): Essentials of Pharmacology. FA Davis, Philadelphia, 1989.

Sanders KM and Ward SM: Nitric oxide as a mediator of nonadrenergic noncholinergic neurotransmission. Am J Physiol. 262: G379–392, 1992.

Shier D, Butler J, and Lewis R: Hole's Human Anatomy and Physiology, ed 7. Wm C Brown, Dubuque, IA, 1996.

Thibodeau GA and Patton KT: Anatomy and Physiology, ed 3. Mosby–Year Book, St Louis, 1996.

CHAPTER 5

Defense of the Lung

chapter objectives

After studying this chapter the reader should be able to:

☐ Differentiate between natural resistance factors and acquired resistance factors.

☐ Define the first, second, and third lines of defense.

☐ Discuss the protection of the respiratory system by describing the structure and function of the epithelial cells lining the airways.

☐ Describe how the fluid lining of the airway is produced and list the functions of the fluid layer.

☐ Discuss the functions of bronchial mucus.

☐ Name the sources of mucous secretions in the respiratory system and describe how these secretions can be stimulated and inhibited by various conditions and drugs.

☐ Explain how the macromolecular structure of mucus results in it exhibiting properties of both solids and liquids.

☐ Define the following terms:
Dipeptide links, disulfide links, hydrogen bonds, gel phase, sol phase.

☐ Define rheology and explain the concepts of elasticity and viscosity as they apply to solids and liquids.

☐ Apply the concepts of viscoelasticity to explain how the gel phase of bronchial mucus is affected by the beating action of respiratory tract cilia.

☐ Explain what occurs to mucous transport when the viscosity of mucus is increased and what occurs when it is decreased.

☐ Describe the operation of the bronchoconstriction reflex, the mucociliary transport mechanism, the sneeze reflex, and the cough reflex by describing the stimuli involved, the sensory and motor pathways that are operative, and the response that is evoked.

☐ Explain how the phagocyte defenses of the respiratory system function to provide protection.

☐ Define the following terms:
Antigen, antibody, immunoglobulin.

☐ Explain the role of mast cells, leukocytes (basophils, eosinophils, neutrophils), and thrombocytes in the inflammatory response of tissues.

☐ Define the term autacoid and describe the action of the following allergic mediators:

Histamine, chemoattractants (neutrophil chemotactic factor of anaphylaxis, eosinophil chemotactic factor of anaphylaxis, platelet activation factor), eicosanoids (prostanoids, leukotrienes), kinins.

key terms

acquired resistance
antibody
antigen; allergen
autacoid
   eicosanoids (ī kō'-sa noyd) (prostanoids, leukotrienes)
   eosinophil chemotactic factor of anaphylaxis (ECF-A)
   histamine
   kinins
   neutrophil chemotactic factor of anaphylaxis (NCF-A)
   platelet activation factor (PAF)
bronchoconstriction reflex; irritant reflex
elasticity
immunoglobulin; gamma globulin (γ-globulin)
lines of defense
   first line of defense

second line of defense
third line of defense
mucociliary escalator; ciliary transport mechanism
mucus
   gel phase
   sol phase
natural resistance
rheology (rē-ol' ô-jē)
subepithelial irritant receptors; rapidly adapting receptors (RAR)
target cells
   basophils
   eosinophils
   mast cells; tissue basophils
   neutrophils
   platelets; thrombocytes
viscosity

The defense of the lung presents a special challenge. The respiratory system, because it is designed to expose a very large surface area to the external environment, puts the entire body at risk because the external environment is not always benign. In addition to natural challenges such as the inspiration of air that is dusty, dry, hot, or cold, the environment is becoming increasingly hostile due to the presence of atmospheric pollutants. To put this challenge in perspective, consider that the surface area of the lungs is about 50 times greater than that of the skin and easily represents the greatest exposure to the external environment of any organ in the body. The resulting risk is formidable. The structures and mechanisms outlined in this chapter represent the lung defenses that help minimize this risk.

Defense Against a Hostile Environment

The body has several lines of defense to protect against the entry of noxious substances such as irritating chemicals, dusts, allergens, and microorganisms. Two broad categories of defense exist: *natural resistance* factors made up of structures and mechanisms that are present at birth, and *acquired resistance* factors that are developed postnatally. **Natural resistance** factors are *nonspecific* mechanisms that include the **first line of defense,** a mechanical barrier imposed collectively by the intact skin, epithelial and mucous membranes, and chemical environments such as tears and gastric juice; and the **second line of defense,** a cellular defense that includes the phagocytic cells of the body that ingest cellular debris and microorganisms. **Acquired resistance** is a *specific* mechanism provided by the **third line of defense,** the body's immune mechanism of antibody production activated by antigenic stimuli from the external environment. We now examine each of these defenses as they apply to protection of the respiratory system.

Mechanical and Chemical Defenses

EPITHELIAL AND FLUID BARRIERS

Epithelial Lining of the Airways

Epithelial tissue is found as coverings and linings and is a major component of the body's first line of defense.

Epithelium covers the body as a protective layer of skin and also provides a covering for many internal organs. Epithelial barriers are also found lining hollow structures such as body cavities and the tubular organs of the digestive, urinary, reproductive, and respiratory systems that communicate with the external environment. In general, epithelium is made up of densely packed cells that resist the entry of noxious substance such as microorganisms. In addition, some epithelium such as that of the nasal cavity is layered to produce multiple strata of protective cells. Epithelium has a high rate of cell turnover, or mitotic activity. Therefore, when epithelial cells are damaged or worn out, they can be replaced at a relatively rapid rate to maintain the protective nature of the barrier. Some epithelial cells such as type 2 pneumocytes are modified for a secretory function with extensive microvilli on their surface; others such as the ciliated columnar epithelial cells of the upper respiratory tract are modified for the transport of **mucus** past the cells' surface.

Many of the general features of epithelium are evident in the morphologic changes seen in the transition from large-diameter to small-diameter airways (see Table 2–1). The lining of larger airways is characterized by ciliated columnar epithelium, goblet cells, a basement membrane, small submucosal glands, and large interstitial spaces with smooth muscle and supporting cartilage. Terminal bronchioles possess smaller, cuboidal epithelial cells, Clara cells, goblet cells, a basement membrane, and a relatively large amount of smooth muscle with supporting cartilage largely absent. Finally, alveoli are composed of epithelial cells, designated as type 1 pneumocytes, forming the squamous cell lining, with type 2 pneumocytes serving a secretory role in the production and release of pulmonary surfactant (see Fig. 3–4).

Fluid Lining of the Airways

The epithelial cells of the airways are covered by a thin layer of fluid that removes inhaled noxious particles and gases such as sulfur dioxide (SO_2) and serves as an impervious layer to combat desiccation (drying) of the airway membranes. The fluid is produced by a cotransport, or symporter, mechanism whereby an active chloride ion (Cl^-) secretory process moves Cl^- extracellularly from the epithelial cells. Sodium ions (Na^+) passively follow. As these ions accumulate in the extracellular fluid immediately adjacent to the airway epithelial cells, they create an osmotic pressure that draws water across the cell membranes, producing an isotonic fluid layer on the luminal surface of the epithelial cells (Taylor et al, 1989). Serous secretions from submucosal glands also add to this fluid layer, known as the **sol phase** of bronchial mucus (Fig. 5–1). The isotonic fluid layer provides water for humidifica-

tion of inspired gas and also provides a low-viscosity medium in which the cilia of airway cells beat. Goblet cells and mucous cells within submucosal glands secrete a mucous layer, which floats on top of the watery sol layer. The mucous layer becomes the viscous **gel phase** of bronchial mucus (see Fig. 5–1).

The epithelial membrane of alveoli is relatively impermeable to the entry of small molecules as a result of tightly packed type 1 epithelial cells and the presence of a fluid lining. Water tends to enter the alveolar space because of surface tension effects, but alveolar epithelial cells actively transport Na^+ and Cl^- out of alveoli into the interstitium to balance this tendency and prevent accumulation of water in the alveoli. The net result is the maintenance of a very thin layer of fluid lining the alveoli.

BRONCHIAL MUCUS

Functions

Mucus lining the respiratory tract is produced by glands found in the paranasal sinuses, nasal cavity, trachea, and bronchi. In the tracheobronchial tree, as well as in locations in the upper respiratory tract, the primary function of mucus is to entrap inhaled particulate matter to prevent it from reaching deeper, and more vulnerable, levels of the respiratory system. Once material is embedded in the surface layer of mucus, the layer is propelled superiorly toward the oropharynx by the rhythmic action of ciliated epithelial cells. Bronchial mucus, like the fluid lining of the airways, provides a relatively impervious layer at the epithelial cells. Mucus also contains antioxidants to reduce oxidant-induced lung injury caused by inhaled noxious substances (Taylor et al, 1989).

Source of Mucus Secretions

Respiratory tract secretions are produced from two groups of cells that include mucus-secreting *goblet cells* lining the airways and secretory cells found within *submucosal glands*. Cup-shaped goblet cells are found scattered among pseudostratified columnar epithelial cells lining the airways from the nasal cavity to the terminal bronchioles (see Fig. 5–1). Goblet cells are stimulated by inhaled irritants such as smoke, dust, and chemicals.

Tracheal glands and bronchial glands are subtypes of submucosal glands. As indicated by the name, these glands are located below the mucous lining of the conducting passageways. Submucosal glands contain secretory cells known as mucous cells and serous cells (see Fig. 5–1). The mucous cells produce a thick secretion, whereas the serous cells release a thin, watery secretion. The secretions are carried to the luminal surface

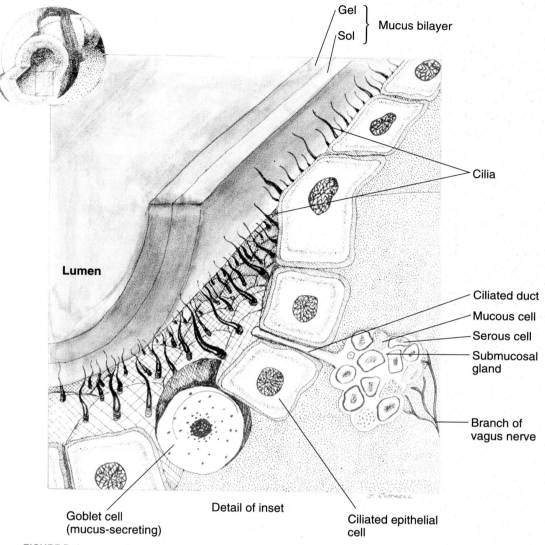

Gel ⎫
Sol ⎬ Mucus bilayer

Cilia

Lumen

Ciliated duct

Mucous cell

Serous cell

Submucosal gland

Branch of vagus nerve

Goblet cell (mucus-secreting)

Detail of inset

Ciliated epithelial cell

FIGURE 5–1. Cells producing tracheobronchial secretions. Note that the cilia project onto the sol layer of mucus. Rhythmic ciliary action propels the "cylinder" of protective mucus toward the oral cavity. (From Cottrell GP and Surkin HB: Pharmacology for Respiratory Care Practitioners. FA Davis, Philadelphia, 1995, p 203, with permission.)

of the airways by small-diameter ciliated ducts. The secretory output from the submucosal glands greatly exceeds the mucus output from the combined goblet cell population. Profuse secretions from the submucosal glands result when the glands are stimulated by parasympathetic nerve impulses (vagus nerve) or by cholinergic drugs that mimic such stimulation.

Characteristics of Mucus

Mucus is a complex fluid created by the combined action of the goblet cells and tracheobronchial secretory cells. It is composed of about 95% water, with the balance of 5% made up of glycoproteins, carbohydrates, lipids, DNA, and cellular debris. Glycoproteins are

macromolecules consisting of long chains of amino acids with shorter attached side chains of carbohydrates (Fig. 5–2). The long mucus strands are stabilized by a variety of chemical bonds, including intramolecular bonds that form the molecular backbone of the protein strands, and intermolecular bonds that cross-link adjacent macromolecules to provide an interconnected latticework (see Fig. 5–2).

The appearance of a glycoprotein molecule is similar to that of a narrow test tube brush, with the protein as the central twisted wire of the brush and the attached carbohydrate molecules represented by the side bristles of the brush. The macromolecular structure of bronchial mucus is represented in such a model by an interwoven arrangement of these bottle brushes, each

Two Interconnected Glycoprotein Strands

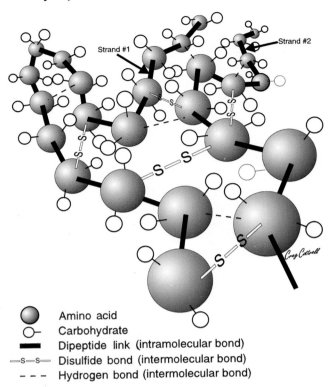

Strand #1

Strand #2

- ⬤ Amino acid
- ◯— Carbohydrate
- ▬ Dipeptide link (intramolecular bond)
- —s═s— Disulfide bond (intermolecular bond)
- - - - Hydrogen bond (intermolecular bond)

FIGURE 5–2. Glycoprotein macromolecule of mucus. (From Cottrell GP and Surkin HB: Pharmacology for Respiratory Care Practitioners. FA Davis, Philadelphia, 1995, p 204, with permission.)

connected through adjacent bonds and forming a tapestry of complex molecules. Mucus is present as a two-phase blanket of material resting on the ciliated epithelial lining of the airways (see Fig. 5–1). This mucous blanket is part of the *mucociliary escalator* and is composed of two distinct layers. The mucoid gel phase is relatively viscous and elastic and is present at the luminal surface of the passageway to entrap inhaled particulate matter. This is the layer produced by the combined secretory output of goblet cells and mucous glands. The less viscous sol phase contacts the beating cilia of the surface epithelial cells and is produced as an isotonic fluid layer by the Cl^- and Na^+ transport mechanism and by serous secretions from submucosal glands.

Rheologic Properties of Mucus

The study of the deformation and flow of matter when forces are applied and removed is called **rheology.** The interconnected chemical bonds of mucus give it the rheologic properties of both a solid and a liquid, physiochemical characteristics crucial to its movement.

Elasticity is a property of *solids* and is a measurement of the ability of a solid to deform, or change

shape, when a force is applied. In an "ideal elastic solid" the energy of deformation is temporarily stored, and the solid returns to its original shape when the force is removed, much as a spring recoils after being stretched (Fig. 5–3A). This rheologic character of elasticity is evident in mucus gel when it is stretched. Mucus has a tendency to deform and flow, and then return to its original shape once a force is removed. The propulsive force causing the deformation of mucus gel is provided by the rhythmic action of cilia, an action critical in the clearance of respiratory tract secretions.

Viscosity is a property of *liquids* and is a measurement of the resistance of a fluid to flow when a force is applied. A shock absorber is a good mechanical model of a viscous system that resists movement (Fig. 5–3B). The more viscous the fluid, the greater its resistance to flow. A greater force must be applied to move a liquid with high viscosity, much as a greater force must be applied to move a large shock absorber compared to a smaller shock absorber.

The flow characteristics of the gel phase of bronchial mucus can be shown by a mechanical model made up of a coil spring representing elasticity and *connected in series* to a shock absorber representing viscosity (Fig. 5–4). Movement in the spring affects the piston of the shock absorber because one end of the spring is fas-

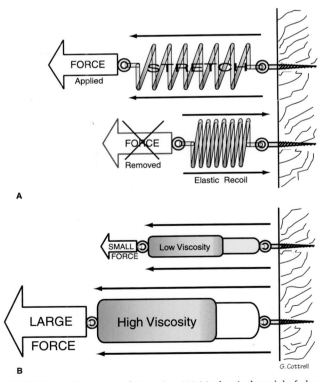

FIGURE 5–3. Elasticity and viscosity. (A) Mechanical model of elasticity (coil spring); (B) mechanical model of viscosity (shock absorber). (From Cottrell GP and Surkin HB: Pharmacology for Respiratory Care Practitioners. FA Davis, Philadelphia, 1995, p 205, with permission.)

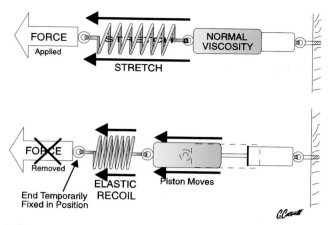

FIGURE 5–4. Normal viscoelasticity of mucus (mechanical model). (From Cottrell GP and Surkin HB: Pharmacology for Respiratory Care Practitioners. FA Davis, Philadelphia, 1995, p 205, with permission.)

tened to the movable piston of the shock absorber, and the other end of the shock absorber is anchored in place. As a constant force is applied to the free end of the coil spring, the spring elongates proportionally, storing the energy of the deformation. If the force is removed when the spring is fully extended, and the end of the spring is temporarily fixed in place, the piston is pulled toward the spring by the recoil action of the spring. The stored energy of the spring overcomes the resistance of the shock absorber and continues to move the piston until the spring reaches its original unextended length and is totally relaxed (see Fig. 5–4).

When mucus is deformed, a similar sequence of events is set in motion. The beating cilia at the gel surface provide the constant force that causes the chemical bonds of mucus to be stretched. The stretching action of the bonds temporarily stores energy, as in the stretching of the mechanical spring. As a cilium finishes its power stroke, the force is briefly removed, thus allowing the elastic recoil of the mucus strands to overcome the viscosity inherent in the mucus gel, just as the viscosity of the shock absorber is overcome by the elastic recoil of the mechanical spring. As a result of its intrinsic viscoelastic properties, the gel phase of the mucus blanket is propelled superiorly toward the oral cavity by the combined action of millions of cilia. The degree of stretch of the mucus strands and the duration of the applied force is determined by the power stroke of the cilia as they contact the bottom of the gel layer. Beating cilia exert a ratchetlike action on the gel layer that continually propels the mucus blanket upwards.

REFLEXES AND CLEARANCE MECHANISMS

Restricting Entry

In addition to filtration of incoming air within the nasal cavity, and the presence of epithelial cells, airway fluid,

and mucous linings that restrict the entry of noxious substances into the respiratory system, certain reflexes perform restrictive functions that contribute to overall defense of the lung. The protective **bronchoconstriction reflex,** or **irritant reflex,** results in rapid bronchospasm of small airways to prevent the inhalation of potentially damaging substances into the deeper parts of the respiratory system. The inhalation of cold air, atmospheric pollutants, irritating chemical vapors, allergic substances (allergens), or pathogenic microorganisms (pathogens) serves as a stimulus that activates **subepithelial irritant receptors** located beneath epithelial cells of the airways. The resulting sensory impulse is transmitted by an afferent branch of the vagus nerve into the central nervous system. The motor impulse of the reflex loop is carried by an efferent branch of the vagus nerve that distributes parasympathetic fibers to bronchiolar smooth muscle, mucous glands, and target cells containing stored **histamine** (Fig. 5–5). Motor activity arriving through these pathways causes rapid bronchoconstriction, glandular secretion, and possible release of histamine from storage sites.

Although mild bronchospasm clearly serves a protective role in lung defense, the usefulness of increased glandular secretion and histamine release is less clear. For example, stimuli such as allergens and pathogens

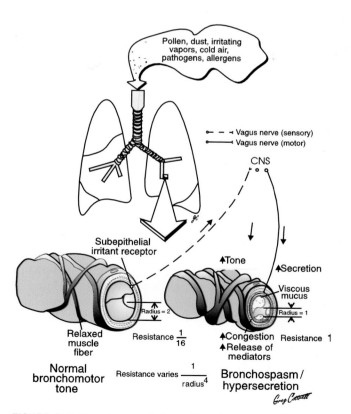

FIGURE 5–5. Bronchoconstriction reflex. (From Cottrell GP and Surkin HB: Pharmacology for Respiratory Care Practitioners. FA Davis, Philadelphia, 1995, p 151, with permission.)

may cause the release of allergic mediators, especially in individuals with a prior history of allergic reactions. Histamine is a powerful bronchoconstrictor that also stimulates increased submucosal gland activity. These responses of bronchospasm and hypersecretion decrease airway diameter further and may result in the clinical symptoms of wheezing, coughing, and dyspnea. West (1998) points out that stimulation of irritant receptors and the histamine-releasing mechanism may play a role in bronchoconstriction associated with asthma attacks. Subepithelial irritant receptors are referred to as **rapidly adapting receptors** by some physiologists because the receptors exhibit a characteristically rapid adaptation to stimuli and seem to be involved in mechanoreceptor functions in addition to their role in the airway response to inhaled irritant stimuli (West, 1998).

Promoting Removal

Mucociliary Transport

The removal of noxious substances such as smoke and dust particles from the airways is achieved through the combined action of filtration in the nasal cavity, phagocytosis in the alveoli, and the operation of the cough reflex and the **mucociliary escalator** or **ciliary transport system.** When stretched, the unique physiochemical properties of mucus gel enable it to flow upward toward the oropharynx, carrying embedded particulate matter that is subsequently swallowed or expectorated. The propulsive force to move the blanket of mucus is provided by rhythmic ciliary action of the epithelial cells found from the nasal cavity down to the terminal bronchioles. Propulsion of physiologically normal mucus occurs as small clawlike structures on the distal ends of a cilium contact the gel layer on their forward power stroke and cause the gel layer to deform. This action allows elastic recoil of the protein strands to pull the blanket along, thus overcoming the resistance to flow inherent in the viscosity of the mucus gel. Normal mucus has a relatively low viscosity but a sufficiently high elasticity to flow in response to the forward propulsion provided by the beating cilia.

Cilia contact the bottom surface of the mucus gel and move very rapidly at a rate of approximately 1000 to 1500 times per minute in the low-viscosity, sol layer of mucus (see Fig. 5–1). Mucus is moved out of the airways by this action at a velocity of about 10 to 15 mm/min (Taylor et al, 1989). The ciliary beat frequency and the rheologic properties of mucus determine the transport rate and, therefore, the rate of mucociliary clearance. The ciliary beat frequency, however, can be decreased by factors such as the administration of antimuscarinic and general anesthetic drugs, advancing age, cigarette smoking, and atmospheric pollutants such as SO_2 and ozone (Pedersen, 1990).

Rheologic properties of mucus are not static, but are changed by temporary conditions such as dehydration that increase the viscosity of bronchial mucus, or by mucus-regulating drugs that decrease the viscosity (Box 5–1). Respiratory cilia, therefore, are normally exposed to a wide range of viscous loadings. Surprisingly, they exhibit very little change in beat frequency or amplitude in response to changes in viscosity of bronchial mucus. Instead, they auto-regulate their activity by increasing the force generated during their power stroke. As a result of this activity, cilia are able to maintain normal mucus transport rates in spite of different viscous loadings (Johnson et al, 1991).

Cough Reflex

The mucociliary escalator is very effective in clearing material from the airways. As a result, coughing does not occur very frequently under normal physiologic conditions. Occasionally, however, the production of respiratory tract secretions may surpass the ability of the ciliary transport system to clear the secretions. Such a situation may occur in cases of severe bronchitis. In other instances, the mucociliary transport system itself is damaged, as occurs in the airways of cigarette smokers. In these examples coughing becomes more frequent and, therefore, serves an important defense role in the removal of irritant substances.

The cough reflex consists of a reflex loop made up of sensory cells, a sensory nervous pathway, a central processing center, a motor nervous pathway, and effector cells. The sensory cells are subepithelial irritant receptors located in the larynx, trachea, and bronchi (see Fig. 5–5). Such receptors respond to chemical and mechanical stimuli such as inhaled smoke or noxious chemicals and relay sensory impulses into an afferent pathway in the vagus, glossopharyngeal, or trigeminal nerve. Functional groupings of neurons in the medulla and pons of the hindbrain act as a cough control center that transmits motor impulses through the vagus nerve to the muscles of ventilation.

Three distinct phases of the cough are recognized: First, with the arrival of the motor impulse from the central nervous system, ventilatory muscles are stimulated to contract rapidly, causing an abrupt *inspiratory phase*. This is immediately followed by a *compression phase* as intra-alveolar pressures rise dramatically. Finally, an explosive *expiratory phase* occurs, which generates the velocity required to clear material from the airways. An ineffective cough may result from muscles that are weakened by drugs or disease, as occurs with neuromuscular blockers, bronchial asthma, chronic obstructive pulmonary disease, spinal cord trauma, surgical pain, or neuromuscular disease such as myasthenia gravis.

P E R S P E C T I V E S

BOX 5-1 When Is Mucolysis Not Mucokinesis?

Mobilization, or movement, of airway secretions is termed *mucokinesis* and is affected by a variety of conditions that alter the viscoelasticity of mucus. These conditions include cholinergic nerve impulses and cholinergic drugs that stimulate submucosal glands, and antimuscarinic drugs such as atropine that reduce secretory activity by blocking the vagal impulses going to the glands. In addition, pathophysiologic conditions such as chronic bronchitis, bronchial asthma, or respiratory tract infections may dramatically increase the viscosity of secretions.

To maintain mucokinesis under these conditions, specific drugs called *mucokinetic agents* are employed. The pharmacologic action of most mucokinetic drugs modifies the structure of bronchial mucus. This alteration, in turn, changes the physical characteristics of mucus to enhance its clearance by the mucociliary transport system. Several different pharmacologic mechanisms of action are capable of altering the viscoelasticity of mucus—most involve changes in the chemical bonds found in mucus. For example, *N*-acetylcysteine (Mucomyst), a common mucokinetic agent, weakens the intermolecular forces binding adjacent glycoprotein chains together by splitting disulfide (–S–S–) bonds and replacing them with sulfhydryl (-SH) groups (see Fig. 5–2). Other mechanisms of action include the rupture of hydrogen bonds to weaken the intermolecular binding of adjacent macromolecules (e.g., *propylene glycol*); alteration of pH to weaken the saccharide side chains of glycoproteins (e.g., *sodium bicarbonate*); and destruction of protein contained in the glycoprotein core of macromolecules through the action of proteolytic enzymes (e.g., *seaprose*).

Most of these mechanisms reduce the viscosity of the gel phase of mucus by splitting, or lysing, the secretions in some way (mucolysis). However, mucokinetic drugs of the future may exhibit mechanisms of action other than that of mucolysis. Therefore, descriptive terms such as "mucoregulatory," "mucoactive," or "mucus-controlling" are preferable to *mucolytic* when describing drugs used to mobilize secretions.

- Braga PC et al: In vitro rheological assessment of mucolytic activity induced by seaprose. Pharmacol Res. 22:611–617, Sep–Oct 1990.
- Braga PC et al: Rheological profile of nesosteine: A new mucoactive agent. Int J Clin Pharmacol Res. 9:77–83, 1989.
- Cottrell GP and Surkin HB: Pharmacology for Respiratory Care Practitioners. FA Davis, Philadelphia, 1995.
- Majima Y et al: Effects of orally administered drugs on dynamic viscoelasticity of human nasal mucus. Am Rev Respir Dis. 141:79–83, 1990.
- Marchioni CF et al: Effects of erdosteine on sputum biochemical and rheologic properties: Pharmacokinetics in chronic obstructive lung disease. Lung. 168:285–293, 1990.

Cellular Defenses

PHAGOCYTIC CELLS OF THE RESPIRATORY SYSTEM

Although the epithelial cells, mucous lining, and cilia of the airways prevent the entry into the lungs of many potentially damaging agents, the macrophage defenses of the distal airways and alveoli provide the main protection in these regions against noxious agents, microorganisms, and foreign particles. *Alveolar macrophages* within the alveoli ingest noxious substances and pro-vide an invaluable second line of defense in the lung (see Fig. 3–4). These phagocytic cells possess numerous lysosomes to break down ingested material. Pulmonary lymphatics remove particulate matter directly and in the form of alveolar macrophages contained in lymph. Substances that cross the epithelial barrier of the airways are attacked by *tissue macrophages* as well as by blood *polymorphonuclear leukocytes* that have migrated to the vicinity of the lungs (Taylor et al, 1989). (Polymorphonuclear cells are so named because of the varied shape of their nuclei, a distinctive morphologic arrangement of two or more interconnected lobes.)

This type of granulocytic white blood cell includes neutrophils, basophils, and eosinophils (Table 5–1). Collectively the phagocytic cells of the respiratory system play a crucial role in maintaining the normally sterile condition of the lung in spite of exposure of its large surface area to an unsterile and hostile environment.

Humoral Defenses

ANTIGENS AND ANTIBODIES

Antigens, or **allergens,** are foreign materials that have the capability to stimulate the body's immune system. Most antigens are high-molecular-weight proteins and include many common substances with which we come into contact daily. These include substances encountered in the diet as well as antigenic substances of plant, animal, or microbial origin. Many of these etiologic (causative) factors are capable of triggering an allergic response in the respiratory system of susceptible individuals (Table 5–2). In addition, some drugs introduced into the body combine with plasma proteins and gain antigenic capabilities, a mechanism that may be responsible for some drug allergies.

Following an antigenic challenge the immune system responds to the presence of very small quantities of antigen by producing very specific proteins called **antibodies,** which are released from cells of lymphoid tissue. Two distinctive features of the immune response, therefore, are the *high sensitivity* and the *high specificity* of the reaction. Plasma proteins are converted into antibodies by immune system cells. The proteins serving as "raw materials" are called **gamma globulins (γ-globulins)** or **immunoglobulins.** The specific immunoglobulin serving as an antibody in allergic reactions is called immunoglobulin E (IgE). The spatial configuration of an IgE antibody is such that it precisely matches that of a specific antigen. When such a close three-dimensional match exists, host antibodies are able to bridge, or connect with, a foreign antigen (Fig. 5–6). The resulting antigen-antibody complex serves to neutralize the antigen, thus providing the humoral antibody response that serves as the body's third line of defense. The lung is especially well endowed with cells called mast cells that serve as target sites for antigen-antibody reactions.

Typically there is a latent interval, or lag period, ranging from a few days to several months between the *primary exposure,* or *sensitizing dose,* and the appearance of host antibodies. Sensitization can occur as a result of an initial exposure to a particular antigen, or as a result of repeated exposure to the same antigen. Figure 5–7 shows the long lag period and relatively few antibodies produced following initial exposure to a specific antigen. The immune system is equipped with special memory cells called B lymphocytes that retain a genetic record of the spatial configuration of the specific antibody produced following the initial exposure. These remarkable cells direct the rapid synthesis of antibodies following subsequent exposure to the same antigen. This *secondary exposure* to an identical antigen is called the *shocking dose,* or *challenge reaction.* Such exposure results in a rapid and dramatic rise in the plasma level of antibodies because the immune system already has the necessary genetic blueprint with which to synthesize large numbers of specific antibodies (see Fig. 5–7).

TARGET CELLS

Neutralization reactions between antigens and antibodies take place at the surface of **target cells,** which also function in the synthesis and storage of allergic mediators. When an antigen is bound by two IgE antibodies, as occurs in allergic reactions, calcium (Ca^{2+}) channels in the cell membrane of target cells open and extracellular calcium ions flow into the cell (see Fig. 5–6). Calcium ion influx causes the target cell to degranulate, releasing its stored allergic mediators. A variety of target cells and allergic mediators exist in the body and are summarized in Table 5–1.

The most common target cell is the **mast cell,** or **tissue basophil.** These cells are derived from the basophils of the bloodstream, which form a small population of target cells. Mast cells are commonly found next to small blood vessels and scattered in loose connective tissue. They are also found in the mucosal linings of small caliber airways and are common in the interstitium of the lung, where they are exposed to antigens present in the bloodstream as well as in the conducting passageways (see Fig. 5–6). Mast cells contain histamine, *chemoattractants* that cause other target cells to migrate to the site of an allergic reaction, and histaminelike mediators that are activated following an antigen-antibody reaction.

White blood cells, or leukocytes, such as **basophils, eosinophils,** and **neutrophils** also function as target cells and contain small quantities of histamine. **Platelets (thrombocytes)** produce a mediator known as thromboxane and also serve as targets of antigen-antibody reactions (see Table 5–1). Leukocytes and thrombocytes migrate to areas of tissue inflammation as a result of the action of chemoattractants released from mast cells.

AUTACOIDS

Allergic mediators are chemicals either released or produced as a result of an antigen-antibody reaction at a target cell. Such a chemical is classified as a tissue hormone, or **autacoid** (Gr. *self-remedy* or *self-medicinal*).

TABLE 5-1	Target Cells and Allergic Mediators

Mast Cells

Mediators	Actions	Comments
Histamine	Capillary leakage	Mast cells are largest storage pool of histamine
	Vasodilation	Mast cells (tissue basophils) are derived from circulating basophils
	Bronchoconstriction	
	Glandular secretion	Lung is well endowed with mast cells
ECF-A	Accumulation of eosinophils	Amplification effect
		Eosinophilia in airway exudate indicates allergic response
NCF-A	Accumulation of neutrophils	Amplification effect
PAF	Accumulation of thrombocytes (platelets)	Amplification effect
Arachidonic acid metabolites	Conversion to eicosanoids (histaminelike mediators)	Eicosanoids yield prostanoids through cyclooxygenase - metabolism and leukotrienes through lipoxygenase metabolism

Basophils

Mediators	Actions	Comments
Histamine	Same as for mast cells	These granulocytes ("base-loving" cells) are stained by a basic, or alkaline, differential stain
		Make up a small fraction of total number of granulocytes
		Converted to tissue basophils (mast cells)
		Largest non–mast cell source of histamine

Eosinophils

Mediators	Actions	Comments
Histamine	Same as for mast cells	Eosinophils are attracted by ECF-A
		These granulocytes ("eosin-loving" cells) are stained by eosin, an acidic differential stain
		Contain small amounts of histamine
		Make up small fraction of total number of granulocytes
LTB_4	Accumulation of additional eosinophils	Amplification effect
	Accumulation of additional neutrophils	Amplification effect
		LTB_4 produced through lipoxygenase pathway

Neutrophils

Mediators	Actions	Comments
Histamine	Same as for mast cells	Neutrophils are attracted by NCF-A
		These granulocytes ("neutral-loving" cells) have a neutral staining reaction
		Contain small amounts of histamine but form the largest fraction of granulocytes in the blood
PAF	Same as for mast cells	Amplification effect

Thrombocytes (Platelets)

Mediators	Actions	Comments
Histamine	Same as for mast cells	Attracted by PAF
		Contain small amounts of histamine
TXA_2	Histamine-like actions	TXA_2 produced through the cyclooxygenase pathway
	Accumulation of additional platelets	Amplification effect

ECF-A = eosinophil chemotactic factor of anaphylaxis; LTB_4 = leukotriene B_4; NCF-A = neutrophil chemotactic factor of anaphylaxis; PAF = platelet activation factor; TXA_2 = thromboxane A_2.

Source: From Cottrell GP and Surkin HB: Pharmacology for Respiratory Care Practitioners. FA Davis, Philadelphia, 1995, p 130, with permission.

TABLE 5–2	Allergic Reactions of the Respiratory System	
Reaction	**Causative Factors**	**Remarks**
Hay fever (allergic or seasonal rhinitis)	Plant pollens Molds	Seasonal
Bronchial asthma (reactive airways disease)	(See subtypes below.)	Acute or chronic Reversible
Extrinsic asthma (allergic or atopic asthma)	IgE-associated (dusts, plant pollens, foods, or drugs)	Most common in children and adolescents
Intrinsic asthma (idiopathic, infective, or nonatropic asthma)	Non–IgE-associated (respiratory tract infections, exercise)	Most common in middle-aged adults
Status asthmaticus	Any of the above	Intense symptoms unrelieved by maximal doses of drugs
Anaphylaxis (anaphylactic shock)	Large amount of antigen (insect or snake venom, blood type mismatch, drug injection in a previously sensitized person)	True anaphylaxis is uncommon (compared with hay fever or bronchial asthma)

IgE = immunoglubulin E.
Source: Modified from Cottrell GP and Surkin HB: Pharmacology for Respiratory Care Practitioners. FA Davis, Philadelphia, 1995, p 128, with permission.

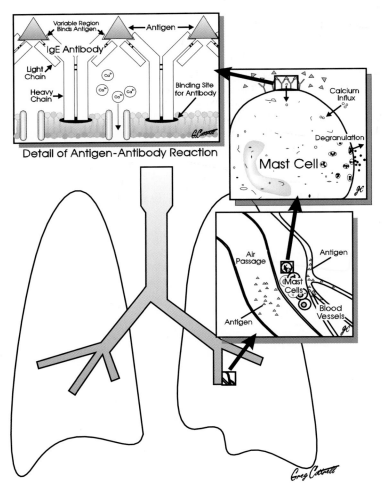

FIGURE 5–6. Antigen-antibody reaction at target cell. (From Cottrell GP and Surkin HB: Pharmacology for Respiratory Care Practitioners. FA Davis, Philadelphia, 1995, p 126, with permission.)

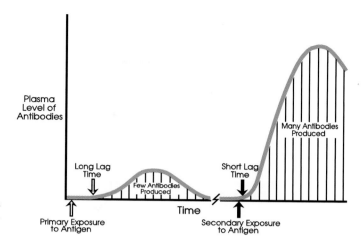

Plasma Level of Antibodies

Long Lag Time

Few Antibodies Produced

Short Lag Time

Many Antibodies Produced

Time

Primary Exposure to Antigen

Secondary Exposure to Antigen

FIGURE 5–7. Antibody response. (From Cottrell GP and Surkin HB: Pharmacology for Respiratory Care Practitioners. FA Davis, Philadelphia, 1995, p 127, with permission.)

Unlike conventional hormones produced by the endocrine glands, autacoids produce their effects close to the point where they are synthesized.

The protective role of histamine in the defense of the body is seen when it is released in small quantities following an antigenic stimulus. In small amounts it prevents the systemic spread of material such as microorganisms by promoting edema formation in tissue. Histamine increases capillary permeability and causes fluid to be transferred into interstitial spaces. The resulting swelling slows the dissemination of potentially damaging material into the rest of the body. Histamine also causes vasodilation of arterioles to result in the delivery of more blood to affected tissue, along with additional leukocytes and nutrients. Unfortunately, amplification effects with allergic mediators, as well as a predisposition to allergy seen in some individuals, lead to an exaggeration of histamine's effects. These effects can include the contraction of nonvascular smooth muscle such as bronchiolar smooth muscle. Table 5–3

summarizes the effect of the release of a small quantity and a large quantity of histamine on various tissues.

Chemoattractants are autacoids that do not exhibit any bronchospastic activity on their own but, instead, promote the migration (*chemotaxis*) of target cells to sensitized tissue, thus expanding the overall pool of histamine-containing cells. This amplification effect is an example of a positive feedback mechanism and is promoted by autacoids such as **neutrophil chemotactic factor of anaphylaxis (NCF-A), eosinophil chemotactic factor of anaphylaxis (ECF-A),** and **platelet activation factor (PAF).**

Histamine and *kinins* cause cell membrane phospholipids in target cells to release *arachidonic acid* (see Fig. 5–8). This substance is an inactive precursor of a group of 20-carbon autacoids known as the **eicosanoids** (Gr. *eicosa,* meaning 20). Arachidonic acid is converted by the enzyme cyclooxygenase into intermediates that become the **prostanoids.** This group of compounds includes the *prostaglandins* and *thromboxane.* Some of the prostaglandins, such as $PGF_{2\alpha}$ and PGD_2, cause vaso-

TABLE 5–3	Histamine Effects	
Tissue Effect	**Outcome of a Small Release of Histamine**	**Outcome of a Large Release of Histamine**
Increased capillary permeability	Localized edema to limit systemic spread of noxious substances	Widespread and severe tissue edema Migration of leukocytes into tissues
Vasodilation	Local increase in blood flow to deliver nutrients and leukocytes to the area	Hyperemia Peripheral vasodilation Systemic hypotension Accumulation of large numbers of leukocytes in inflammatory exudate leading to amplification effect
Bronchoconstriction	Increased bronchomotor tone	Intense bronchospasm Wheeze, dyspnea
Glandular secretion	Increase in glandular activity	Hypersecretion of tracheobronchial glands; cough Hypersecretion of gastric acid

Source: From Cottrell GP and Surkin HB: Pharmacology for Respiratory Care Practitioners. FA Davis, Philadelphia, 1995, p 131, with permission.

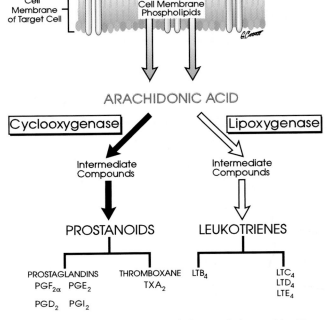

FIGURE 5–8. Arachidonic acid metabolism and eicosanoids. (From Cottrell GP and Surkin HB: Pharmacology for Respiratory Care Practitioners. FA Davis, Philadelphia, 1995, p 131, with permission.)

constriction and bronchoconstriction, whereas other members of the prostaglandin series such as PGE_2 and PGI_2 promote vasodilation and bronchodilation. Thromboxane (TXA_2) causes vasoconstriction, bronchoconstriction, and platelet aggregation. Arachidonic acid can be converted into different intermediate compounds by the enzyme action of lipoxygenase. These intermediates are further converted into mediators known as the **leukotrienes (LTs).** Leukotriene B_4 (LTB_4) functions as a leukocyte chemoattractant, whereas other leukotrienes such as LTC_4, LTD_4, and LTE_4 exhibit histaminelike actions.

Kinins such as *bradykinin* exhibit potent histamine-like effects in the tissues following tissue trauma. The kinins are not found in a preformed state in target cells, but are produced in traumatized tissues following cell injury.

NOTE: Glucocorticoid drugs exert some of their powerful anti-inflammatory actions by inhibiting the cyclooxygenase and lipoxygenase pathway of arachidonic acid metabolism, and by blocking the production of bradykinin.

In general, the presence of autacoids, *in small amounts,* serves to localize offending substances through the

promotion of mild tissue edema, thus providing a defensive role. It should be noted, however, that the reaction to allergic mediators in some individuals can result in pathophysiologic responses such as a fall in blood pressure as a result of widespread vasodilation, bronchoconstriction caused by contraction of airway smooth muscle, hypersecretion as a result of excessive glandular secretion, or a combination of these unwanted complications.

Summary

In this chapter we examined the various natural and acquired resistance factors that protect the lung. In view of the considerable surface area of the lung exposed to a hostile environment, the effectiveness of the defense mechanisms is truly remarkable. The role of physical and chemical barriers, reflexes and clearance mechanisms, and cellular and antibody defenses was discussed in relation to protection of the respiratory system. In addition, the function of target cells and allergic mediators was briefly outlined in an overview of the humoral antibody response.

BIBLIOGRAPHY

Burkhalter A, Julius D, and Frick OL: Histamine, serotonin, and the ergot alkaloids: In Katzung BD (ed): Basic and Clinical Pharmacology, ed 6. Appleton & Lange, Norwalk, CT, 1995.

Clark WG, Brater DC, and Johnson AR: Goth's Medical Pharmacology, ed 13. Mosby–Year Book, St. Louis, 1992.

Clarke SW: Rationale of airway clearance. Eur Respir J (Suppl) 7:599s–603s, 1989.

Cottrell GP and Surkin HB: Pharmacology for Respiratory Care Practitioners. FA Davis, Philadelphia, 1995.

Hecker M, Foegh ML, and Ramwell PW: The eicosanoids: Prostaglandins, thromboxane, leukotrienes, and related compounds. In Katzung BD (ed): Basic and Clinical Pharmacology, ed 6. Appleton & Lange, Norwalk, CT, 1995.

Holgate ST and Kay AB: Mast cells, mediators and asthma. Clinical Allergy. 15:221–234, 1985.

Johnson NT et al: Autoregulation of beat frequency in respiratory ciliated cells: Demonstration by viscous loading. Am Rev Respir Dis. 144:1091–1094, 1991.

Pedersen M: Ciliary activity and pollution. Lung. 168 (Suppl): 368–376, 1990.

Shires TK: Anti-Inflammatory Drugs: In Conn PM and Gebhart GF (eds): Essentials of Pharmacology. FA Davis, Philadelphia, 1989.

Taylor AE et al: Clinical Respiratory Physiology. WB Saunders, Philadelphia, 1989.

West JB: Respiratory Physiology: The Essentials, ed 6. Williams & Wilkins, Baltimore, 1998.

CHAPTER 6

The Thorax

chapter objectives

After studying this chapter the reader should be able to:

☐ Name the basic parts of a generalized vertebra.

☐ Describe the development and orientation of the vertebral column curves.

☐ Describe the basic parts of a thoracic vertebra.

☐ List the boundaries of the thoracic inlet and the thoracic outlet.

☐ Identify the following parts of a typical rib:
    Head, neck, tubercle, angle, body, costal groove, costal cartilage.

☐ Differentiate between true ribs and false ribs and describe the attachments of floating ribs.

☐ Name the thorax topographical features used to locate the following structures:
    Apex of lung, carina of trachea, base of the lung.

☐ Identify the following structures and parts of the sternum and briefly describe their function:
    Manubrium, jugular notch, clavicular notches, costal notches, sternal angle, body, xiphoid, infrasternal angle.

☐ Describe the structure and function of the following joints of the thorax:
    Intervertebral, costovertebral, costochondral, interchondral, sternochondral, sternal.

☐ Describe the biomechanics of the thorax by explaining the axis of rotation of the ribs responsible for pump-handle movement of the sternum and bucket-handle movement of the ribs.

☐ Explain why expiration is passive during normal, quiet breathing.

☐ Describe the structure and function of the following diaphragmatic structures:
    Central tendon, hemidiaphragms, crura.

☐ Describe the innervation of the diaphragm, its range of movement, and the pressure changes generated in the thorax by diaphragmatic movements.

☐ Explain in general terms how the accessory inspiratory group of muscles assists the diaphragm.

☐ Describe the origin, insertion, and action of the following accessory muscles of inspiration:

External intercostals, internal intercostals—interchondral parts, subcostals, levator costae, sternocleidomastoids, scalenus, serratus anterior, pectoralis major, pectoralis minor, trapezius.

☐ Describe the origin, insertion, and action of the following accessory muscles of expiration:

Internal intercostals, external obliques, internal obliques, transversus abdominis.

key terms

accessory expiratory group
  abdominals (external obliques, internal obliques, transversus abdominis)
  internal intercostals
accessory inspiratory group
  external intercostals
  internal intercostals—interchondral parts
  levator costae (lē-vā′ tor kos′ tē)
  pectoralis major (pek″ tō-rā′ lis)
  pectoralis minor
  scalenus (skā-lē′ nus)
  serratus anterior (ser-ā′-tus)
  sternocleidomastoids
    (ster″ nō-klī″ dō-mas′ toyd)
  subcostals
  trapezius (tra-pē′ zē-us)
bucket-handle movement
costal cartilage
costal margin
costochondral junction; costochondral joint
diaphragm
  central tendon
  costal part
  crura (kroo′ ra)
  hemidiaphragm
  lumbar part; vertebral part
  sternal part
pump-handle movement
ribs (false ribs, floating ribs, true ribs)

  angle
  body; shaft
  costal groove
  head
  neck
  tubercle
sternum
  body
  clavicular notches
  costal notches
  infrasternal angle
  jugular notch; suprasternal notch
  manubrium (ma-nū′ brē-um)
  sternal angle; angle of Lewis
  xiphoid (zif′ oyd)
thoracic inlet; superior thoracic aperture
thoracic joints
  costochondral joints
  costovertebral joints
  costotransverse joints
  interchondral joints
  intervertebral joints
  manubriosternal joint
  sternochondral joints; sternocostal joints
  xiphisternal joint
thoracic outlet; inferior thoracic aperture
thoracic vertebrae
thorax

S triated muscle is not found in the lungs; therefore, the organs are incapable of active, spontaneous movement. Instead, they must be made to move to transport air into and out of the alveoli to support gas exchange. This chapter examines the musculoskeletal structures and movements of the thorax that passively move the lung to make alveolar ventilation possible.

Function of the Thorax

The **thorax** (Gr., *chest*) is defined by *Taber's Cyclopedic Medical Dictionary* as "That part of the body between the base of the neck superiorly and the diaphragm inferiorly." This definition includes not only the traditional skeletal structures—the thoracic vertebrae, ribs, and sternum—but also associated soft tissues such as costal cartilages, muscles, mediastinal structures, the heart enclosed in the pericardium, and the lungs covered by pleura. Such a sweeping definition is very close to the original definition of the thorax developed by Galen, the famous Greek physician:

> . . . all that cavity bounded by the ribs on both sides, extending to the sternum and the diaphragm in front and curving down to the spine in the rear is customarily called the Thorax by the physician.
> Galen–*On the Usefulness of Parts,* Book VI, 300
> (Roussos, 1995). As quoted by Roussos C: Prologue:
> The Thorax through History into Medicine.
> In Roussos C (ed): The Thorax—Part A: Physiology, ed 2.
> Marcel Dekker, New York, 1995.

The cagelike structure of the thorax provides the paradoxic functions of *protection* and *flexibility.* Protection is essential because of the vital functions performed by the heart and lungs sheltered within the cage. Flexibility is made possible by the natural elasticity and articulations of the thoracic cage. Muscle contractions and flexibility of the thoracic structures allow the chest to assume different shapes and volumes which, in turn, permit different pressures to be produced. Different pressures are essential to move the lungs passively within the thorax. We now examine the bones, joints, and muscles responsible for movement of the thorax.

Bones of the Thorax

VERTEBRAL COLUMN

Recall from general anatomy that the vertebral column consists of 26 irregularly shaped *vertebrae* that (1) pro-

vide attachments for the shoulder and pelvic girdles, (2) permit an upright stance for bipedal movement, and (3) form a bony channel called the *spinal (vertebral) canal* for protection of the spinal cord. The vertebral column consists of a series of alternating curves that provide stability to help maintain the upright posture, counter the tendency of the abdominal organs to pull the vertebral column anteriorly, and provide shock absorption to help cushion the spinal cord housed within the spinal canal (Fig. 6–1). In the fetal and neonatal spine, the vertebral column curves of the four basic regions—cervical, thoracic, lumbar, and sacral—are all oriented as anterior concave curves, and are designated *primary curves.* Around age 3 months, the cervical curve changes into an anterior convex curve that allows the infant's head to be raised. Such an anterior convex curve is called a *secondary curve.* When a child is approximately 1 year old, the lumbar curve is also converted into a secondary curve, tilting the pelvic structures posteriorly and increasing the volume of the pelvic cavity. This biomechanical change also positions the center of gravity of the body directly beneath the head and allows the pelvic limbs to provide locomotion for the child. The alternating arrangement of vertebral column curves is retained in the adult. Figure 6–1 shows the primary (anterior concave) curvature of the thoracic region and the resulting depth, or anteroposterior (A-P) diameter, of the thorax that results from this orientation of thoracic vertebrae.

THORACIC VERTEBRAE

A typical vertebra possesses a weight-bearing *body,* a prominent *dorsal spine* (*spinous process*) projecting pos-

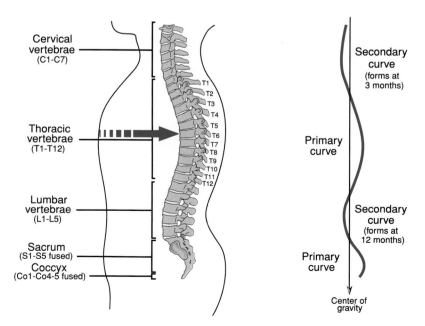

FIGURE 6–1. Vertebral column curves (lateral view of left side). The large arrow shows the increased anteroposterior dimension of the thorax that results from the orientation of the primary curvature of the thoracic vertebrae (T1-T12).

teriorly, a *vertebral foramen* encasing the spinal cord, a pair of *transverse processes,* a pair of *superior articular processes,* and a pair of *inferior articular processes* (Fig. 6–2). Most of the deviation from this general morphologic plan is seen in the unique vertebrae of the neck region. The **thoracic vertebrae** closely follow this generalized description but are further modified to carry out the specific functions of the thoracic region, such as providing the posterior pivoting attachment for the ribs.

The twelve thoracic vertebrae possess relatively small bodies that show a slight increase in size going from T1 to T12. They are, however, considerably larger than those of the cervical region. The delicate dorsal spines of typical thoracic vertebrae are relatively long and slender and are oriented inferiorly (see Fig. 6–1). The vertebral foramina show a slight decrease in diameter from T1 through T12, reflecting the reduced diameter of the spinal cord that results as pairs of spinal nerves exit through *intervertebral foramina* formed by notchlike structures on the lateral sides of adjacent vertebrae (see Fig. 6–2). Superior and inferior articular processes are typical and form the joints between adjacent vertebrae in the column. The unique structural feature of thoracic vertebrae is the presence of *articular facets* that allow the 12 pairs of ribs to join the vertebrae. All thoracic vertebrae (T1 to T12) have a *superior costal facet* and an *inferior costal facet* located on the lateral side of the body, at the junction with an adjacent vertebra (see

Fig. 6–2). These facets, when in contact with the intervertebral disc, accommodate the head of the rib and permit a small range of motion. In addition to these articular facets, the uppermost nine thoracic vertebrae (T1 to T9) possess an *articular facet* on the lateral side of the right and left transverse process (see Fig. 6–2). These facets articulate with the tubercle of the rib, a small knoblike process found just distal to the head of the rib. The function of these rib structures in the movement of the thoracic cage is outlined in the next section.

RIBS AND COSTAL CARTILAGES

Much of the overall shape of the thorax is determined by the shape and orientation of the **ribs.** In the adult the thorax is elliptical, or "flattened," in horizontal section, with its transverse diameter greater than its anteroposterior diameter (Fig. 6–3). The **thoracic inlet,** or **superior thoracic aperture,** is the narrowed superior opening into the thorax (Fig. 6–4). It is bounded by the upper margin of the sternum ventrally, the paired first ribs laterally, and the first thoracic vertebra dorsally. The downward slope of the clavicles and first pair of ribs allows the *apex* of the lung to protrude superiorly into the thoracic inlet. Clinically, this orientation has important consequences because penetrating injuries at the base of the neck, above the clavicle, may puncture the pleura or the lung itself and admit air into

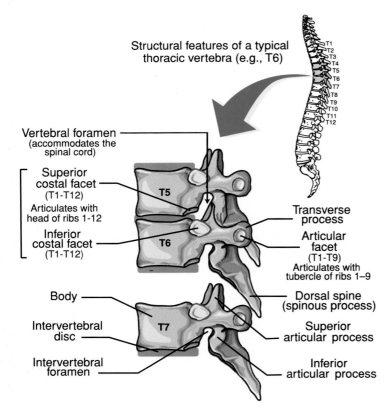

Structural features of a typical thoracic vertebra (e.g., T6)

Vertebral foramen (accommodates the spinal cord)

Superior costal facet (T1-T12) Articulates with head of ribs 1-12

Inferior costal facet (T1-T12)

Body

Intervertebral disc

Intervertebral foramen

Transverse process

Articular facet (T1-T9) Articulates with tubercle of ribs 1–9

Dorsal spine (spinous process)

Superior articular process

Inferior articular process

FIGURE 6–2. Thoracic vertebrae (lateral view of left side showing major surface features).

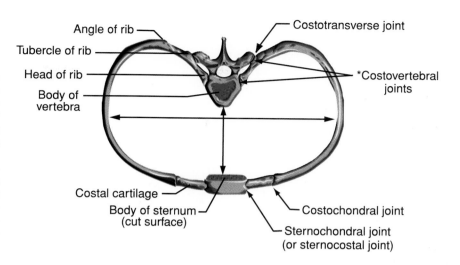

Angle of rib — Tubercle of rib — Head of rib — Body of vertebra — Costotransverse joint — *Costovertebral joints — Costal cartilage — Body of sternum (cut surface) — Costochondral joint — Sternochondral joint (or sternocostal joint)

FIGURE 6–3. Elliptical shape of the thorax (superior view). Notice that the transverse dimension of the thorax is greater than the anteroposterior (AP) dimension, producing a "flattened" appearance of the thorax when viewed from above. Several thoracic joints are visible in this view.

*Costovertebral joints include the joint between the head of the rib and the costal facets of the bodies of thoracic vertebrae, as well as the joint between the tubercle of the rib and the articular facet of the transverse process of the corresponding vertebra, forming the costotransverse joint (see Fig. 6–2).

the pleural space to cause a *pneumothorax*. The inferior opening of the thorax is called the **thoracic outlet,** or the **inferior thoracic aperture** (see Fig. 6–4). This large-diameter opening is limited by the costal cartilages, the anterolateral abdominal wall, and the lower thoracic vertebrae. The 12 pairs of ribs have a graceful, curved shape and increase in length from the first rib to approximately the seventh rib, and then become progressively shorter to the twelfth rib (see Fig. 6–4).

As shown in Figure 6–4, the ribs have a unique orientation. Instead of forming the circular shape of the thorax by connecting a thoracic vertebra with the sternum *in the horizontal plane,* like hoops on a barrel, each rib is "slung" in a downward position from its corresponding vertebra. The superior seven pairs of ribs curve dorsally a very short distance from the thoracic vertebrae (T1 to T7), and then curve downward and laterally before curving abruptly upward and medially to connect with the sternum (see Figs. 6–3 and 6–4). The result of this orientation is that the thoracic articulation of a rib is superior to its sternal articulation. More importantly, the angle of the rib points downward and is *below* the two pivot points that allow its movement. The angle is the point where the shaft of the rib abruptly curves forward and laterally (see Fig. 6–3). Elevating the curved rib will produce a wider lateral diameter of the thorax—the so-called **bucket-handle movement** explained in the section on movements of the thorax. Elevation of the ribs from their downward-slung position, therefore, is an effective way to increase the overall volume of the thorax. This change has an important bearing on the pressures produced within the cavity and are discussed in a later section.

The third through the ninth rib have basic characteristics in common and are often referred to as *typical ribs.* The proximal end of a typical rib possesses a rounded **head** that articulates with the shallow depression formed by the superior and inferior costal articular facet found on the bodies of adjacent thoracic vertebrae (Fig. 6–5). The lower part of the head of the rib articulates with the superior costal facet of the thoracic vertebra corresponding to the number of the rib; the upper part of the head of the rib articulates with the inferior costal facet of the thoracic vertebra located immediately above (the superjacent vertebra). The **neck** of the rib is a narrowed region that separates the head from a knoblike protrusion called the **tubercle.** The *articular surface* of the tubercle joins the articular facet found on the transverse process of a thoracic vertebra (see Figs. 6–3 and 6–5).

The joints formed by the attachment of the head and the tubercle of the rib with the bodies and transverse processes of thoracic vertebrae are classified functionally as slightly movable, or *amphiarthrotic joints.* The articulation of the ribs allows an eccentric movement that results in the rib cage's assuming a wider dimension when the ribs are elevated by muscles of inspiration. The curved portion of the rib is the **body,** or **shaft,** of the bone. The point where the shaft turns abruptly forward, just distal to the tubercle, is called the **angle** of the rib (see Fig. 6–3). The lower margin of the shaft is marked by the shallow **costal groove** that contains and protects the intercostal neurovascular bundle, a collective term for the intercostal nerve, artery, and vein (NAV). The ribs are classified morphologically as *flat bones,* a designation based on the profile of their cross-section (see Fig. 6–5). In adults the flat bones of the thorax, including the ribs, serve as the primary sites of hemopoiesis, or blood cell production.

The uppermost 10 pairs of ribs each possess a **costal cartilage** that articulates with a cup-shaped depression on the anterior end of the shaft of the rib at the **costochondral junction (costochondral joint)** (see Fig. 6–5). The cartilages also articulate with each other anteriorly. These hyaline cartilages provide for flexible,

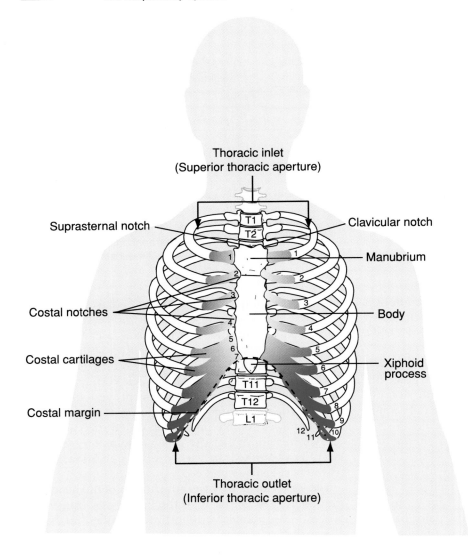

Thoracic inlet
(Superior thoracic aperture)

Suprasternal notch

Clavicular notch

Manubrium

Costal notches

Body

Costal cartilages

Xiphoid
process

Costal margin

Thoracic outlet
(Inferior thoracic aperture)

FIGURE 6–4. Bony thorax (anterior view). Costal cartilages and ribs are numbered at their medial ends. The costal margin is shown as a dotted line. The apex of the lung projects superiorly above the clavicles and rib 1. Note that the downward slope of the ribs from the thoracic vertebrae to the sternum is greater for ribs in the middle and lower parts of the thorax (e.g., rib 6), but that the ribs in the upper part of the thorax are directed in a more horizontal plane (e.g., rib 1). The orientation of these planes affects the biomechanics of the thorax during ventilation of the chest.

resilient attachments at the sternum to allow the ribs to be raised and lowered. The inferior margin of the fused costal cartilages is called the **costal margin** (see Fig. 6–4).

All the ribs of the bony thorax have posterior thoracic vertebrae (T1 to T12) attachments but can be classified on the basis of their anterior attachments. The superior seven pairs of ribs possess a direct sternal attachment through individual and separate costal cartilages and are called **true ribs.** Ribs 8 through 12 are designated **false ribs** because they lack a *direct* sternal attachment. Within this group, ribs 8 through 10 attach *indirectly* to the sternum through the costal cartilage of the seventh rib. Ribs 11 and 12, the **floating ribs,** do not attach to the sternum at all (Table 6–1). The name of these ribs is a misnomer of sorts because the distal ends of the "floating ribs" are stabilized between muscles of the abdominal wall and, therefore, do not actually "float." These free, or floating, ribs provide protection posteriorly and laterally for the

inferior lobes of the lungs and for organs such as the kidneys.

Figure 6–6 shows the general structural features of the thorax, as well as several important topographical (surface) landmarks related to the respiratory system. For example, the medial end of the clavicle and the sternoclavicular joint can be easily palpated at the superior end of the sternum. The first rib lies immediately below the clavicle and marks the approximate location of the *apex* of the lung. The second costal cartilage lies at about the level of the *carina* of the trachea. Deep palpation at the inferior end of the sternum reveals the seventh rib. Immediately above this rib is the sixth rib at approximately the level of the *base* of the lung, as viewed from the front. On the posterior chest, an important topographical feature is the apex, or inferior angle, of the scapula. With the arms in anatomic position, the apex is at the level of the dorsal spine of the seventh thoracic vertebra. With the spine of C7 identified, the vertebrae can be counted by palpating their

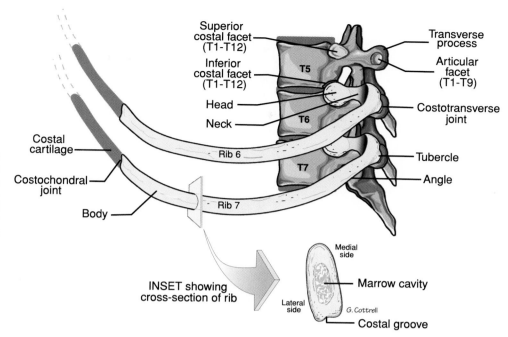

FIGURE 6–5. Structural features of a typical rib (lateral view of left side showing costovertebral joints). Ribs 3–9 have very similar structural features and are called *typical ribs*. Heads articulate with superior and inferior costal facets of adjacent vertebrae; tubercles articulate with the articular facet of the transverse process of the vertebra. (Ribs 1–2 and 10–12 do not have tubercles.) The number of the rib is the same as that of the thoracic vertebra forming the costotransverse joint.

respective spines, and the corresponding ribs can be identified. For example, the 11th rib (four ribs below the apex of the scapula) lies at approximately the level of the base of the lung, viewed from behind.

STERNUM

The "dagger-shaped" **sternum** is classified morphologically as a flat bone. Through the right and left *sternoclavicular joints,* it articulates with the medial end of the clavicles and thus serves as the superior articulation between the axial and appendicular skeletons. As described previously, it also articulates directly with the costal cartilages of the first seven pairs of ribs, and indirectly through the cartilage of the seventh rib with ribs 8 through 10.

The sternum has three distinct parts, as shown in Figure 6–4. The superior part, or **manubrium,** possesses a superior **jugular notch,** or **suprasternal notch,** located at approximately the level of the body of the third thoracic vertebra (T3), lateral **clavicular notches** for the articulation with the clavicles, and **costal notches** for the articulation with the costal cartilage of the first pair of ribs and the upper part of the costal cartilage of the second pair of ribs. The **sternal angle (angle of Lewis)** at the level of T4 or T5 is located at the junction of the manubrium and the body of the sternum, and is found about 5 cm below the jugular notch (see Fig. 6–6). This surface landmark lies approximately at the level of the second costal cartilage and is useful as a reference point in counting ribs (Gardner et al, 1967).

The **body** of the sternum contains the remainder of

TABLE 6–1	Naming of Ribs	
Classification	**Posterior Attachment**	**Anterior Attachment**
True Ribs (Ribs 1–7)	Thoracic vertebrae (T1 to T7)	Direct sternal attachment by means of individual costal cartilages that articulate with costal notches of the sternum.
False Ribs (Ribs 8–12)		No direct sternal attachments.
Ribs 8–10	Thoracic vertebrae (T8 to T10)	Costal cartilages of ribs 8, 9, and 10 are attached to each other and attach indirectly to sternum through the costal cartilage of rib 7.
Ribs 11–12 ("Floating ribs")	Thoracic vertebrae (T11 to T12)	No sternal attachments. Distal ends of ribs attach to muscles of anterolateral body wall.

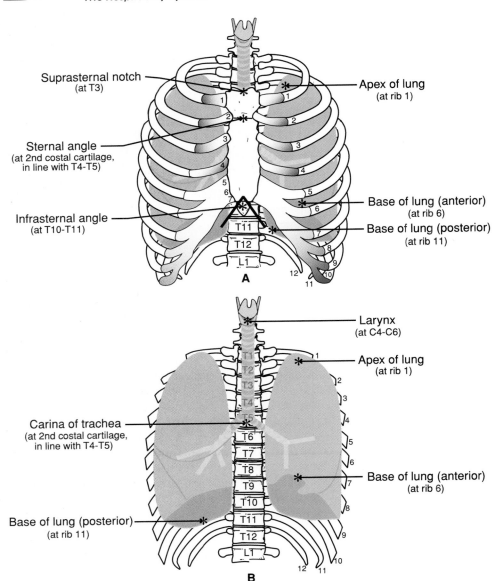

FIGURE 6–6. Surface landmark of the thorax. (A) Anterior view of thorax; (B) anterior part of the chest wall removed to show lungs within thoracic cage. Landmarks indicated on the diagram are approximate. (Considerable variation exists among individuals.)

the lateral costal notches that articulate with the costal cartilages of the second through seventh pairs of ribs (see Fig. 6–4). The posterior surface of the body is slightly concave.

Finally, the **xiphoid** is present as a variable-shaped inferior process on the distal end of the body of the sternum (see Fig. 6–4). The xiphoid process is the smallest of the three parts of the sternum and serves as a muscle attachment point for some of the abdominal muscles. The *epigastric fossa,* or "pit of the stomach," is a small surface depression palpable on the rib cage in front of the xiphoid process. The xiphoid process is situated at the apex of the **infrasternal angle,** or angle formed by the meeting of the right and left costal margins (see Fig. 6–6). This angle lies at approximately the level of the 10th or 11th thoracic vertebrae. Considerable variation among individuals is seen in the size of the infrasternal

angle, ranging from 70 to 110 degrees (Gardner, 1986). *Hyperasthenic* individuals have broad chests and wide infrasternal angles; *asthenic* individuals have characteristic thin chests and narrow infrasternal angles.

Joints of the Thorax

A variety of joints are found in the thorax. **Thoracic joints** impart a remarkable range of movement that permits the bony cage to be changed in both the anteroposterior and transverse directions.

INTERVERTEBRAL JOINTS

The joints of the vertebral column, or **intervertebral joints,** provide both flexibility for the spine and protection for the spinal cord (see Figs. 6–1 and 6–2). Various combinations of extension, flexion, and rotation of the column are made possible by the fibrocartilaginous joints composed of *intervertebral discs*. The resulting joints are classified as slightly movable or amphiarthrotic, based on their range of motion. Intervertebral discs also articulate with the head of a rib at the costovertebral joints.

COSTOVERTEBRAL JOINTS

The two subtypes of joints that make up the **costovertebral joints** of the thorax are (1) joints between the head of the rib and costal facets on the body of thoracic vertebrae and (2) joints between the tubercle of the rib and the transverse facet of thoracic vertebrae (Fig. 6–7).

Joints of the Heads of the Ribs

The articular surface of the head of a typical rib (ribs 2 through 9) articulates with the inferior and superior costal facets of two adjacent vertebrae and the intervertebral disc located between them (see Figs. 6–3 and

6–5). The heads of the 1st, 10th, 11th, and 12th ribs each articulate with only one vertebra, rather than with the costal facets on two adjacent vertebrae.

Costotransverse Joints

The second type of costovertebral joint of a typical rib is the **costotransverse joint.** In this joint, the articular surface on the tubercle of the rib articulates with the costal facet on the transverse process of the corresponding vertebra (see Figs. 6–3 and 6–5). For example, the tubercle of the fourth rib articulates with the transverse process of the fourth thoracic vertebra (T4). Movement of a typical rib about the costovertebral axis that passes through the head and the tubercle is discussed subsequently.

COSTOCHONDRAL JOINTS

Costochondral joints are located between the hyaline cartilage comprising the costal cartilage of the rib and the shallow depression in the distal end of the shaft of the rib. Flexibility at this location adds to the overall elasticity of the bony cage (see Figs. 6–3 and 6–5).

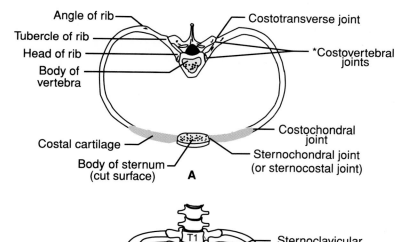

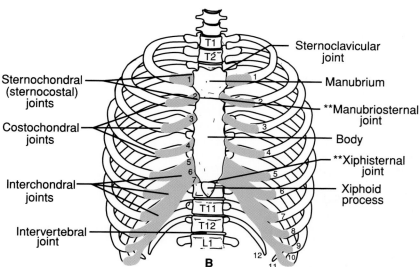

FIGURE 6–7. Joints of the thorax. (A) Superior view; (B) anterior view.

Costovertebral joints consist of (1) the joint between the head of the rib and the body of the vertebra and (2) the costotransverse joint between the tubercle of the rib and the transverse process of the vertebra.

** *Sternal joints* are found in the body of the sternum and consist of (1) the manubriosternal joint (forming the sternal angle) and (2) the xiphisternal joint between the body and the xiphoid process. Individually, the joints of the thorax do not permit a wide range of movement; however, the thoracic cage as a whole can move in several directions as a result of the combined action of the individual thoracic joints.

INTERCHONDRAL JOINTS

Interchondral joints are the joints between the costal cartilages, from the fifth to the eighth or ninth costal cartilage. Each articulates with the costal cartilage below to form a flexible hyaline cartilage framework that can be raised or lowered (see Fig. 6–7).

STERNOCHONDRAL JOINTS

The joints between the costal notches on the lateral side of the sternum and the medial ends of the first seven costal cartilages are called **sternochondral,** or **sternocostal joints** (see Figs. 6–3 and 6–7). Like the interchondral joints of the false ribs, these sternal attachments of the true ribs provide flexibility for thoracic cage movements.

STERNAL JOINTS

The **manubriosternal joint** is the fibrocartilaginous joint between the manubrium and the body of the sternum at the level of the second costal cartilage (see Fig. 6–7). The **xiphisternal joint** is the articulation between the lower margin of the body of the sternum and the xiphoid process at approximately the level of the 10th thoracic vertebra (see Fig. 6–7).

The joints of the thorax are summarized in Table 6–2.

Biomechanics of the Thorax

The thorax is a complex structure consisting of a series of "skeletal arches" formed by the thoracic vertebrae, ribs, costal cartilages, and the sternum. The articular surfaces, cartilages, tendons, and ligaments found at the various joints both stabilize the thorax and limit the ventilatory movements of the bony cage to two basic rotations:

- Pump-handle movement—rotation of the rib about the transverse axis of the costovertebral joint
- Bucket-handle movement—rotation of the rib about the axis passing through the head and the sternal end of the rib.

PUMP-HANDLE MOVEMENT

The ribs of the upper thoracic cage are shaped such that the *plane* of each rib slopes from the back downward to the front but does *not* slope downward toward the side. In other words, the plane of the rib slopes obliquely downward toward the sternum. The plane is defined by

TABLE 6-2	Joints of the Thorax
Joint	**Description**
Intervertebral Joints	Articulations between the bodies of T1 and T12 vertebrae by means of dense fibrocartilage intervertebral discs. Slightly movable (amphiarthrotic) joints provide extension, flexion, and rotation of vertebral column. Vertebrae articulate with the head of rib at costovertebral joint.
Costovertebral Joints	Contribute to pump-handle and bucket-handle movement.
Joints of the heads of the ribs	Heads of ribs 2–9 articulate with the intervertebral disc and the inferior costal facets of the suprajacent vertebra and with the superior costal facets of the subjacent vertebra at the intervertebral joints.
Costotransverse joints	Tubercle of rib articulates with the costal facet of the vertebra.
Costochondral Joints	Articulation between cup-shaped depression on distal end of rib and the corresponding costal cartilage. Hyaline cartilage provides flexibility.
Interchondral Joints	Articulation between adjacent costal cartilages, from approximately the 5th to the 8th costal cartilage. Hyaline cartilage provides flexibility at the sternal attachments.
Sternochondral Joints	Articulation between costal cartilages (ribs 1–7) and corresponding costal notches on the lateral sides of the manubrium and body of the sternum.
Sternal Joints	
Manubriosternal joint	Articulation between manubrium and body to form the sternal angle ("angle of Lewis") at the second costal cartilage.
Xiphisternal joint	Articulation between body and xiphoid process at approximately the level of T10.

three points widely distributed on the arc of the shaft of the rib (De Troyer and Loring, 1995). When such ribs are elevated in inspiration, their sternal (ventral) ends move anteriorly, but their displacement to the side is minimal. This anterior displacement of the sternum produces the characteristic action called **pump-handle movement** (De Troyer and Loring, 1995; Gardner, 1986; Rosse and Gaddum-Rosse, 1997). During maximum inspiration, when the rib cage is elevated in this way, the downward-sloping ribs are raised to a more horizontal position, making the A-P diameter of the chest about 20% greater than it is during maximum expiration (Guyton and Hall, 1996). The axis of rotation is directed laterally along the neck of the rib through the head and tubercle (Fig. 6–8A). Elevation of the rib results in upward and forward movement of the sternum and thus an increase in the A-P diameter of the thorax.

The second through sixth ribs move about the axis described in the next section and exhibit bucket-handle movement in addition to the more obvious pump-handle movement. The costal cartilages of the seventh through tenth ribs turn abruptly upward. Raising the ventral ends of these ribs through the pump-handle effect tends to move the sternum backward slightly by flexing the manubriosternal joint. In general, elevation of the upper ribs results in the sternum being raised and moved forward, whereas eleva-

tion of the lower ribs causes a slight backward movement of the sternum. Bending of both the manubriosternal joint and the costal cartilages occurs in these upward movements of the ribs (Gardner, 1986).

BUCKET-HANDLE MOVEMENT

The planes of the ribs of the lower thorax, like those of the upper thorax, project from the back downward to the front of the thorax. In addition, the planes of the lower ribs slope downward from the midline toward the side. In other words, the ribs appear to "droop" downward at their lateral margins, rather than being oriented in a more horizontal fashion as seen with the upper ribs (see Fig. 6–4). When these lower ribs move upward during inspiration, they exhibit anterior displacement as well as significant lateral displacement (De Troyer and Loring, 1995; Gardner, 1986; Rosse and Gaddum-Rosse, 1997). This action increases the transverse diameter of the thorax and is described as *bucket-handle movement* (Fig. 6–8B). The effect is most noticeable in the lowermost costovertebral joints. The actual plane of the rib passes from the head of the rib to the sternochondral joint. Movement at the costovertebral joint about this axis tends to raise or lower the midpoint of the rib.

In general, the upper ribs and their associated costal cartilages have shorter and more restrictive sternal at-

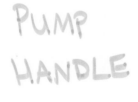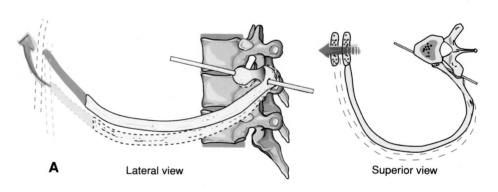

A   Lateral view   Superior view

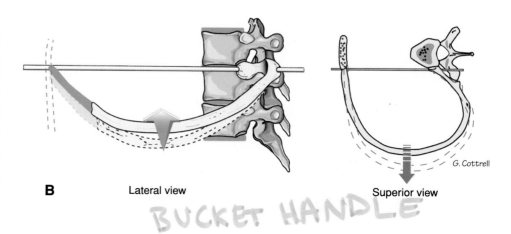

FIGURE 6–8. Biomechanics of the thorax. (A) Pump handle movement. Note the anterior and upward displacement of the sternum when the axis of rotation passes through the tubercle and head of the rib. (B) Bucket handle movement. Lateral and upward displacement of the ribs occurs when the axis of rotation passes through the head of the rib and the sternochondral joint. Axes of rotation are shown by the rigid bars in these movements of the rib.

B   Lateral view   Superior view

tachments; therefore, they tend to move as a unit with the sternum. In contrast, the lower ribs have more flexible cartilaginous attachments at the sternum and, therefore, exhibit more freedom of independent movement (De Troyer and Loring, 1995).

Muscles of Ventilation

Ventilation of the lungs begins with changes in the volume of the thorax. Two groups of ventilatory muscles— the inspiratory and expiratory muscles—provide the necessary changes. Because of the natural elasticity of the thoracic cage and the lung interstitium, the structures tend to recoil once they have been stretched. What this means in terms of ventilation is that under resting conditions, normal breathing (eupnea) requires only that the thorax and lung be expanded through the contraction of inspiratory muscles. Resiliency of the structures will passively return them to their preinspiratory positions once the inspiratory muscles relax. In other words, no expenditure of energy is required by the muscles to initiate expiration under resting conditions.

In the following section, we examine the role of the **diaphragm** and the muscles that assist it in ventilation. Under conditions of eupnea, the diaphragm provides the needed change in thoracic volume and is technically an inspiratory muscle. Under more strenuous conditions the diaphragm is assisted by various muscles of the *accessory inspiratory group* and by those of the *accessory expiratory group*. In effect, the accessory muscles are progressively recruited to assist the diaphragm at higher breathing frequencies.

For simplicity, the following functional descriptions of ventilatory muscles are presented and analyzed separately. However, it should be kept in mind that all these muscles normally work in unison in a coordinated manner to produce the required movements of the thorax (De Troyer and Loring, 1995). Throughout life, the respiratory muscles and the heart muscle must continuously contract. These amazing muscles must be able to respond to sudden metabolic demands and yet be extremely resistant to fatigue (Box 6–1).

PERSPECTIVES

BOX 6–1　　**Fourteen Thousand Contractions per Day**

The muscles that serve as respiratory muscles are classified embryologically, morphologically, and functionally as skeletal muscles. However, the muscle fibers of the principal respiratory muscles—the *diaphragm, intercostals, sternocleidomastoids, scalenes,* and *abdominals*—differ structurally and functionally from those of other skeletal muscles in several important ways. These characteristics include a higher oxidative capacity, higher capillary density, higher maximum blood flow, and greater resistance to fatigue (Edwards and Faulkner, 1995). These unique properties allow the respiratory muscles to meet the metabolic needs associated with both sustained activities and bursts of vigorous activity. For example, during normal quiet respiration, only about 3% to 5% of the total energy used by the body is needed by the muscles of ventilation (Guyton and Hall, 1996). Very heavy exercise can increase the energy consumption of the respiratory muscles by 50-fold, and high duty per rest cycles can ultimately fatigue the muscles. However, under normal workloads the muscles perform admirably well. The respiratory muscles move approximately 10,000 L of air into the lungs per day by moving the associated joints of the thorax some 14,000 times per day, assuming a respiratory rate of around 10 breaths per minute. This frequency of use of joints is one of the highest in the body, with the possible exception of the action of the auditory ossicles of the inner ear.

- De Troyer A and Loring SH: Actions of the Respiratory Muscles. In Roussos C (ed): The Thorax: Part A: Physiology, ed 2. Marcel Dekker, New York, 1995.
- Edwards RHT and Faulkner JA: Structure and Function of the Respiratory Muscles. In Roussos C (ed): The Thorax: Part A: Physiology, ed 2. Marcel Dekker, New York, 1995.
- Guyton AC and Hall JE: Textbook of Medical Physiology, ed 9. WB Saunders, Philadelphia, 1996.
- Thomas CL (ed): Taber's Cyclopedic Medical Dictionary, ed 18. FA Davis, Philadelphia, 1997.

DIAPHRAGM

The diaphragm is one of the most important skeletal muscles in the body because of its primary role in ventilation (Box 6–2). In Chapter 1 we examined how the diaphragm is formed from separate partitions and how it is innervated and invaded with striated muscle fibers to form the dome-shaped muscular separation between the thoracic and abdominopelvic cavities. Recall that the diaphragm is covered with parietal pleura that is continuous with that lining the walls of the thoracic cavity and the outer surface of the mediastinum. The diaphragm consists of radially arranged muscle fibers and a tendinous center called the **central tendon.** The muscular portion and the central tendon of the diaphragm are pierced by several openings for structures such as the esophagus, thoracic duct, aorta, inferior vena cava, and nerves (see Fig. 1–6).

Each half of the diaphragm is called a **hemidiaphragm** and each half of the muscular portion of the diaphragm has three parts: **sternal, costal,** and **lumbar.** All these parts insert into the central tendon. After branches of the phrenic nerve grow into and innervate the diaphragm, motor impulses cause the striated muscle fibers of the hemidiaphragms to contract and increase the tension on the central tendon.

Because the perimeter of the central tendon serves as an insertion for all the muscle fibers of the diaphragm, the dome of the central tendon is pulled toward the periphery of the thoracic cavity as the muscle fibers contract, thus increasing the tension on the central tendon and flattening the dome. This excursion downward of the diaphragm increases the vertical dimension of the thoracic cavity, increases the intrathoracic volume, and decreases the intrathoracic pressure. This action, in turn, causes the lung to expand, increasing the intrapulmonary volume and decreasing the intrapulmonary pressure below atmospheric pressure to result in air being drawn into the conducting passages.

The lumbar part of the diaphragm arises from the lumbar vertebrae to form the *right* and *left crura,* which extend to the central tendon. **Crura** (Latin, *legs;* singular *crus*) are elongated columnlike masses of muscle fibers that resemble legs, or pillars, connecting the vertebral column with the central tendon. The two crura fuse together via a fibrous arch at the aorta and form the opening through which the aorta passes. The right crus is larger than the left and splits to surround the esophagus.

Although some older texts describe innervation of the diaphragm via the phrenic nerve and the thoracic nerve, it has been shown that the *sole* motor control is

P E R S P E C T I V E S

BOX 6–2   Breathing without a Diaphragm

The diaphragm is the principal respiratory muscle in mammals. Although a number of accessory muscles of breathing located in the neck, chest, limbs, and abdomen assist the diaphragm, they cannot support normal activity on their own. They cannot produce the needed changes in thoracic and lung volumes and can only refine, or modify, the diaphragmatic movements that are responsible for the large-scale changes in intrathoracic and intrapulmonic volumes and pressures.

Fish, as well as several groups of air-breathing animals, do not have a diaphragm. Amphibians, reptiles, and birds depend on other combinations of muscles to move air into and out of the lungs. In amphibians and reptiles, muscles in the floor of the mouth, especially the mylohyoid (one of the muscles of the suprahyoid group of laryngeal muscles), move upward as they contract. In this form of *positive pressure ventilation*, air brought in through the nares is forced into the lungs by the muscular action of the floor of the mouth ("frog breathing"). Simultaneously, the action of the trunk muscles moves the trunk outward and results in *negative pressure ventilation* to draw air into the lungs from the outside. Birds evolved from reptiles but, unlike amphibians and reptiles, do not depend on positive pressure ventilation. Instead, birds breathe primarily through the action of intercostal trunk muscles that move the ribs. Unlike human lungs, avian lungs are *attached* to the ribs and are thus moved outward by displacement of the ribs to produce a negative intrathoracic pressure.

• Netter FH: Respiratory System, Vol 7. In Divertie, MB (ed): The CIBA Collection of Medical Illustrations. CIBA Pharmaceutical Co, Division of CIBA-GEIGY Corp, Summit, NJ, 1979.

through the pair of phrenic nerves (De Troyer and Loring, 1995; Moore, 1992). Each hemidiaphragm is innervated separately by the phrenic nerve on the corresponding side' therefore, paralysis of one side of the diaphragm does not affect the other. However, the two halves of the diaphragm normally contract in unison. Each phrenic nerve consists of a variety of nerve fibers that carry (1) motor impulses to the muscle fibers of the diaphragm, (2) sensory impulses from the diaphragm and adjacent pleura and peritoneum, and (3) vasomotor impulses to the arteries of the diaphragm. The peripheral part of the diaphragm is also supplied with sensory and vasoconstrictor fibers through the *thoracoabdominal nerves.*

During normal, quiet breathing the downward excursion of the diaphragm following the arrival of a motor impulse is about 0.5 to 1.5 cm; however, during forced inspiration, this movement can extend from 6 cm to as much as 10 cm. The intrapleural pressures generated as a result of diaphragmatic movement during inspiration range from -3 cm H_2O to -50 cm H_2O, and during expiration may reach $+70$ cm H_2O to as high as $+100$ cm H_2O.

When discussing the attachments and actions of the muscles of breathing, it should be noted that the words "origin" and "insertion" are relative terms that describe the fixed, or anchored attachment of the muscle as the *origin* and the comparatively movable end as the *insertion.* During contraction of a muscle, the insertion is pulled toward the origin by the shortening of the muscle fibers. Although the diaphragm exhibits an unusual movement, the terms regarding its attachments are valid. For most of the other muscles listed in Table 6–3, however, the attachments appear to be "reversed" when compared with similar summary tables presented in other anatomy texts. This apparent discrepancy occurs because Table 6–3 is a summary of the attachments of muscles causing *ventilatory movements,* whereas most summary tables list the origins and insertions for these muscles in relation to their primary role in moving some part of the body, such as a limb.

For example, most anatomy books describe the origin of the *pectoralis major* as the sternum and its insertion as the proximal end of the humerus. Shortening of the muscle fibers causes the arm to be drawn toward the torso, a movement known as adduction. This description of the origin, insertion, and action of the pectoralis major muscle is entirely accurate in the analysis of arm movements at the shoulder joint. However, if the shoulder joint is stabilized, or fixed in position, contraction of the pectoralis major will act upon the sternum and cause it to move forward slightly, thus increasing the intrathoracic volume. Clearly the origin and insertion of the muscle seem to have "reversed" from the description given for adduction of the arm. The description, however, is accurate for movement of

the sternum and the resulting increase in the A-P diameter of the thorax. The origin is relatively stable, and the insertion is moved toward the origin in both of these examples. The reader is cautioned to keep this relationship in mind when studying summary tables of muscle attachments. Some muscles have secondary, or auxiliary, functions such as those described previously for the pectoralis major. In a practical example, the technique of gripping the arms of a chair while inhaling is sometimes practiced by patients suffering from chronic obstructive pulmonary diseases (COPDs) such as emphysema. The pectoralis major and other accessory muscles of ventilation, isolated through such a maneuver, provide additional muscle power for individuals with breathing difficulties.

ACCESSORY INSPIRATORY GROUP

Muscles known as accessory muscles of breathing assist the diaphragm during certain ventilatory actions. The **accessory inspiratory group** of muscles produces changes in the shape of the thorax that increase the volume of the bony cage to decrease the pressure within the container and cause the lungs to expand. In general, these changes increase the A-P diameter of the thorax, the transverse (lateral) diameter of the thorax, or a combination of change in both dimensions. When coupled with an increase in the height, or vertical dimension of the thorax caused by the downward excursion of the diaphragm, the accessory muscles of breathing greatly expand the volume of the chest during forced inspiration. Some of the muscles of the accessory inspiratory group also assist the diaphragm during quiet breathing, although the diaphragm is considered the principal muscle in such activity. Recall that expiration during quiet breathing is primarily a passive process because of the elastic recoil of the lung and thoracic cage. During vigorous breathing, however, virtually all of the muscles of the thoracic wall are active, as well as those of the abdominal group. The progressive recruitment of motor units in each of the muscles of breathing occurs as the rate and depth of ventilation increase (Edwards and Faulkner, 1995).

External Intercostals

The outermost muscle group of the thoracic wall is composed of 11 pairs of **external intercostal muscles** (see Table 6–3). These muscle fibers occupy the outer layer of the intercostal spaces and are attached to the inferior margins of the first through the eleventh rib. The fibers have an oblique orientation, with the fibers passing downward and anteriorly to attach to the superior margin of the rib below. The external intercostals of the lowermost seven spaces blend with the fibers of the external oblique, one of the **abdominal**

TABLE 6-3	Muscles of Ventilation		
Muscle	**Origin**	**Insertion**	**Action**
Diaphragm			
Sternal part	Xiphoid process	Central tendon	Dome of central tendon pulled downward
Costal part	5th–10th costal cartilages; ribs 9–12	Blend with transversus abdominis and insert on central tendon	Same as sternal part
Lumbar part	Fibrous arches in lumbar region	Central tendon	Same as sternal part
	Upper lumbar vertebrae	Form right and left crura, which insert on central tendon	
Accessory Inspiratory Group			
External Intercostals Superficial; 11 pairs of muscles occupy intercostal spaces; fibers of lowermost 7 spaces blend with fibers of external obliques; fibers extend obliquely downward and anteriorly from the tubercles to constochondral junctions.	Inferior margin of ribs 1–11	Superior margin of ribs 2–12	Most of the group raises the ribs. Increased transverse diameter of thorax (bucket-handle movement). Flexion of manubriosternal joint increases the anteroposterior diameter of thorax (pump-handle movement).
Internal Intercostals (Interchondral Parts) Located in upper four or five intercostal spaces	Inferior margin of ribs 1–5	Superior margin of ribs 1–5	Assist external intercostals to elevate ribs.
Subcostals Formed from internal intercostal muscle	Inferior margins of ribs near angle of rib Extend over two or more intercostal spaces	Upper margin of second or third rib below	Elevate ribs.
Levator Costae	Transverse processes of C7–T11	Subjacent rib (the rib below), between the tubercle and angle of rib	Elevate ribs.
Sternocleidomastoids Straplike muscles on either side of neck	Mastoid process of temporal bone	Sternum and clavicle	Elevate sternum to increase anteroposterior diameter of thorax.
Scalenus Group of three muscles; scalenus anterior, scalenus medius, scalenus posterior	C2–C6	Ribs 1–2	Elevate ribs to increasse transverse diameter of thorax
Serratus Anterior "Saw-toothed" appearance; located superior to the external intercostals	Anterior surface and vertebral border of scapula	Ribs 1–8 or 9	Elevate ribs
Pectoralis Major	Proximal end of humerus	Clavicle and sternum	Elevate ribs

(Table continued on following page)

TABLE 6-3	Muscles of Ventilation (*Continued*)		
Muscle	**Origin**	**Insertion**	**Action**
Diaphragm			
Pectoralis Minor	Scapula	Ribs 2–5	Elevate ribs to increase transverse diameter and anteroposterior diameter of thorax
Trapezius	Scapula and clavicle	C7–T12 (dorsal spines)	Elevate ribs to increase anteroposterior diameter of thorax
Accessory Expiratory Group			
Internal Intercostals 11 pairs of muscles located deep to the external intercostals; fibers oriented at right angle to external intercostals and pass obliquely upward and anteriorly; lowermost fibers connect with those of the internal obliques (see below).	Superior margins of ribs and costal cartilages	Inferior margins of ribs and costal cartilages located above origins (suprajacent ribs)	Depress ribs Decrease transverse diameter of thorax Maintain tension on intercostal spaces during forced expiration
Abdominal Group Muscle layers arranged in thin sheets with fibers oriented at right angles to each other; muscle layers function as "postural muscles" in addition to their respiratory role; straplike rectus abdominis layer does not function as a respiratory muscle and is omitted from the table.			
External Oblique	Ribs (lowermost eight pairs)	Ossa coxae (iliac crest and pubis by way of inguinal ligament) Linea alba by way of an aponeurosis	Depresses ribs (ribs moved downward and medially) Upward displacement of diaphragm
Internal Oblique	Ossa coxae (iliac crest and inguinal ligament) Lumbodorsal fascia	Ribs (lowermost three pairs) Linea alba	Same as external oblique
Transversus Abdominis	Ribs (lowermost six pairs) Ossa coxa (iliac crest, inguinal ligament) Lumbodorsal fascia	Ribs (costal cartilages of ribs 5–7 Sternum (xiphoid process)	Same as external oblique

Attachments listed above are based on respiratory actions of the muscles. In the case of arm muscles such as the trapezius and pectoralis major, the respiratory function of the muscle is normally secondary to its limb function. However, during certain forced inspiratory maneuvers, the muscles can assist the diaphragm.

muscles (Fig. 6–9A; see also Color Plate 9). External intercostal muscle fibers extend from the tubercles of the ribs to the costochondral junctions anteriorly (Woodburne and Burkel, 1994). When the intercostal muscles contract, the ribs are raised, which increases the transverse diameter of the thorax (bucket-handle effect) and flexes the sternum at the manubriosternal joint to increase the A-P diameter of the thorax (pump-handle effect). An understanding of the precise action of the intercostal muscles has been uncertain for a considerable length of time. However, the consensus is that the external intercostals, at least in most of the

intercostal spaces, function to *elevate* the ribs (Box 6–3).

Internal Intercostals—Interchondral Parts

The internal intercostals are considered muscles of *expiration,* and will be discussed in a subsequent section as part of the accessory expiratory group (see Table 6–3). However, the **interchondral parts** of the internal intercostal muscles that lie in the upper four or five intercostal spaces function as muscles of *inspiration.* These unique muscle fibers work with the external in-

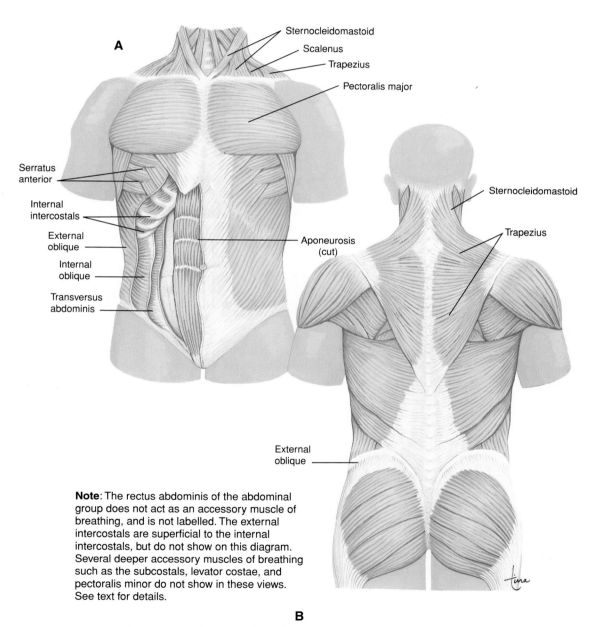

A

Sternocleidomastoid
Scalenus
Trapezius
Pectoralis major
Serratus anterior
Internal intercostals
External oblique
Internal oblique
Transversus abdominis
Aponeurosis (cut)

Sternocleidomastoid
Trapezius
External oblique

Note: The rectus abdominis of the abdominal group does not act as an accessory muscle of breathing, and is not labelled. The external intercostals are superficial to the internal intercostals, but do not show on this diagram. Several deeper accessory muscles of breathing such as the subcostals, levator costae, and pectoralis minor do not show in these views. See text for details.

B

FIGURE 6–9. Accessory muscles of breathing. (A) Anterior view; (B) superior view. (Adapted from Scanlon VC and Sanders T: Essentials of Anatomy and Physiology, ed. 3. FA Davis, Philadelphia, 1999, p 145, with permission.) (See also Color Plate 9.)

P E R S P E C T I V E S

BOX 6-3

Intercostal Muscle Mechanics

The biomechanics of the intercostal spaces have long puzzled and intrigued students and researchers alike. Although it is agreed that the chief function of the intercostal muscles is to *move* the ribs, there has been considerable controversy throughout medical history as to the specific *action* of the various muscles occupying the intercostal (interchondral) spaces. For example, Rosse and Gaddum-Rosse (1997) state that the attachments and fiber orientation of the intercostal muscles suggest that "both the internal and external intercostal muscles could elevate the ribs if their proximal attachment is considered as their point of origin and that both sets of muscles could depress the ribs if the inferior point of attachment is considered the origin." DeTroyer and Loring (1995) point out that controversy exists in this regard as far back as 1749:

The external and internal intercostal muscles have successively been perceived as being (1) all expiratory; (2) all inspiratory; (3) both inspiratory and expiratory, acting simultaneously; (4) either inspiratory or expiratory, depending on the interspace; or (5) only regulating the tension on the intercostal space.

What explanation might shed light on this dilemma?

A biomechanical theory of intercostal muscle movements based on geometrical considerations was postulated by G. E. Hamberger in 1749 and is used today to partially explain the mechanics of the intercostal space. DeTroyer and Loring (1995) summarize this theory in the following manner: The contraction of an intercostal muscle in an intercostal space tends to pull the upper rib down and the lower rib up. However, the fibers of an external intercostal muscle pass obliquely downward and anteriorly. The fibers inserting on the lower rib, therefore, are farther from the center of rotation of the rib at the vertebral articulations than those attaching on the upper rib. As a result, the torque that acts on the lower rib is greater than the torque that acts on the upper rib and the rib is *raised.* The fiber orientation of the internal intercostals is opposite to that of the external intercostals. Therefore, when an internal intercostal muscle contracts, the torque acting on the upper rib is greater than that acting on the lower rib, and the rib is depressed.

The explanations offered in the Hamberger theory are valid for a straight, or planar, model of rib movement where there is equal shortening of all external intercostals, equal lengthening of all internal intercostals, and equal rotation of the ribs around parallel axes. Real ribs, however, are *curved.* The curved shape introduces additional geometric variables that affect muscle fiber length because of the position of the fiber attachment on the curvature of the rib, and the different rotational axes determined by the rotation of ribs of different radii. So, which intercostal muscles *are* responsible for movements of the rib cage?

Electromyographic (EMG) recordings of intercostal muscle activity may provide the best explanation of intercostal space biomechanics. At the present time, such techniques reveal that the *parasternal intercostals, external intercostals,* and the *levator costae* are active during the inspiratory phase of the ventilatory cycle (DeTroyer and Loring, 1995). Electromyographic studies also suggest that, at least in some intercostal spaces, the internal intercostals are active during expiration and that *both* external and internal intercostals are active in forced inspiration and expiration (Rosse and Gaddum-Rosse, 1997). To further confound the situation, other EMG recordings of intercostal muscle activity during costal breathing indicate that the two sets of muscles are not separate in their actions and, instead, function to maintain tension on the intercostal space (Woodburne and Burkel, 1994). This action keeps the spaces at a constant width and minimizes drawing in and bulging out of the intercostal spaces with changes in intrathoracic pressure. Clearly, EMG

(Box continued on following page)

P E R S P E C T I V E S

BOX 6–3   **Intercostal Muscle Mechanics (Continued)**

studies have not provided physiologists with a consistent view of intercostal muscle function. Elucidation of the range of functions of the intercostal muscles continues as new techniques evolve and new equipment such as improved electrodes becomes available. Another few hundred years should bring us a full explanation.

- De Troyer A and Loring SH: Actions of the Respiratory Muscles. In Roussos C (ed): The Thorax: Part A: Physiology, ed 2. Marcel Dekker, New York, 1995.
- Hamberger GE: *De Respirationis Mechanismo et usu Genuino.* Jena, Germany, 1749.
- Rosse C and Gaddum-Rosse P: Hollinshead's Textbook of Anatomy, ed 5. Lippincott-Raven, Philadelphia, 1997.
- Woodburne AM and Burkel WE: Essentials of Human Anatomy, ed 9. Oxford University Press, New York, 1994.

tercostals to elevate the ribs and thus increase the transverse diameter of the thorax.

Subcostals

The **subcostals** arise from the inferior margins of ribs near the angle of the ribs and extend over two or more intercostal spaces to insert onto the upper margin of the second or third rib below (see Table 6–3). Subcostal muscles are formed of fibers of the internal intercostal muscles (Woodburne and Burkel, 1994). Such fibers are better developed in the lowermost part of the thorax where they function to elevate the ribs.

Levator Costae

The transverse processes of the seventh cervical to the eleventh thoracic vertebrae (C7 to T11) serve as the origins of the **levator costae** group of muscles. These spindle-shaped muscles pass at an angle to insert into the rib below (the subjacent rib), between the tubercle and the angle of the rib (De Troyer and Loring, 1995). Contraction of the group raises the ribs (see Table 6–3).

Sternocleidomastoids

The thin straplike **sternocleidomastoid muscles** are located on either side of the neck (Fig. 6–9A and B). These muscles have attachments at the mastoid process of the temporal bone of the skull and at the clavicle and sternum. They are usually described as "muscles that move the neck," responsible for flexion of the neck when there is bilateral contraction ("prayer muscles"), and rotation when there is unilateral contraction. Recall, however, that Table 6–3 lists the attachments and actions of these muscles when they are serving a *respiratory* function. Therefore, with the skull fixed in position, the mastoid process becomes the origin and the sternal

and clavicular end of the muscle serves as the insertion. With such attachments, bilateral contraction elevates the sternum to slightly increase the A-P diameter of the bony cage. Sternocleidomastoids normally contract only during high rates of ventilation or during dyspnea, and can be seen as prominent bulges on the sides of the neck when a subject is breathing strenuously.

Scalenus

Along with the sternocleidomastoids, the **scalenus** muscles are among the most important accessory muscles of inspiration (see Fig. 6–9A). The scalenes, or scalenus muscles, are a group of three small muscles (*scalenus anterior, scalenus medius,* and *scalenus posterior*) that primarily move the neck, but as respiratory muscles they act on the rib cage. Their origins include attachments on the second through sixth cervical vertebrae (C2 to C6) with insertions on the first and second ribs. These muscles elevate the first two ribs and increase the transverse diameter of the thorax during quiet breathing in some individuals and in forced inspiration in most (see Table 6–3).

Serratus Anterior

The **serratus anterior** muscles, located on the anterolateral aspect of the rib cage, have a serrated, or saw-toothed appearance when viewed from the front (see Fig. 6–9A). These muscles primarily depress, abduct, and produce upward rotation of the shoulder (Guyton and Hall, 1996). However, with the shoulder joint in a fixed position, the anterior surface and vertebral border of the scapula serve as the origin and the first eight or nine ribs become the insertion. When acting as accessory muscles of breathing, contraction of the anterior serrati produces a slight elevation of the bony cage (see Table 6–3). The serratus anterior muscles play a relatively minor role as accessory inspiratory muscles compared with the sternocleidomastoids and scalene group discussed above.

> NOTE: In spite of the attachments to the thoracic cage and the relatively large mass of the muscles that normally move the shoulder and arm, the following accessory inspiratory muscles play a negligible role in normal inspiration. They are, however, used by individuals with obstructive breathing disorders to facilitate inspiration, and will be discussed here as inspiratory muscles of breathing.

Pectoralis Major

The fan-shaped **pectoralis major** muscles provide much of the shape and definition of the upper chest (see Fig. 6–9A). These muscles are used in adduction, flexion, and medial rotation of the arm, but as accessory respiratory muscles, they elevate the thorax. With the shoulder joint fixed in position, the proximal humerus becomes the origin, and the clavicle and sternum serve as the insertion for the muscle. Contraction of the pectoralis major muscles, therefore, elevates the thorax and slightly increases the A-P diameter of the chest (see Table 6–3).

Pectoralis Minor

Located beneath the pectoralis major, the **pectoralis minor** muscles connect the scapula (origin) with the second through fifth ribs. With the shoulders fixed, contraction elevates the ribs which slightly increases the transverse (lateral) and A-P diameters of the bony cage (see Table 6–3).

Trapezius

The trapezoid-shaped **trapezius** muscles are located in the upper back (see Fig. 6–9B). Their main actions include retraction, elevation, and depression of the scapulae and extension of the neck. However, with the shoulder joint stabilized, the scapula and clavicle become the origin and the spines of the seventh cervical through the twelfth thoracic vertebrae (C7 to T12) become the insertion. Contraction of the trapezius, therefore, results in elevation of the thorax and an increase in its A-P diameter.

ACCESSORY EXPIRATORY GROUP

As ventilatory rate and depth increase, passive elastic recoil of the lungs and thorax is insufficient to keep pace with demand, and active expiration is required. Most of this assistance is provided by the abdominal group of muscles, functioning as antagonists of the diaphragm. The muscles belonging to the **accessory expiratory group** contribute to expiration by either actively decreasing the volume of the thorax, or by increasing the pressure below the diaphragm and thereby assisting the diaphragm in its upward movement to its preinspiratory position.

Internal Intercostals

Located immediately beneath the external intercostal layer in the intercostal spaces are the fibers of the **internal intercostals** (see Fig. 6–9A). The fibers are oriented at right angles to those of the external intercostals and are separated from them by loose areolar connective tissue. These 11 pairs of muscle arise from the superior margins of the ribs and costal cartilages and pass obliquely upward and anteriorly to insert on the inferior margins of the ribs and costal cartilages above (see Table 6–3). Innervation of the internal intercostals is via the corresponding *intercostal nerves*. Contraction of the **internal obliques** depresses the ribs, decreases the transverse diameter of the thorax, and raises the intrathoracic pressure. Recall, however, that the interchondral parts of the internal intercostals of the upper four or five intercostal spaces function as accessory muscles of *inspiration* (see Box 6–3).

During forced expiration, the function of the internal intercostals may also include the maintenance of tension on the intercostal spaces to prevent them from bulging outward as the intrathoracic pressure rises (Gardner et al, 1967). The lowermost fibers of the internal intercostals blend and connect with those of the internal obliques of the abdominal group.

Abdominal Group

The ventral wall of the abdomen comprises several layers of tough, sheetlike muscle arranged in a unique pattern. The fiber orientation of each layer is different, resulting in a relatively thin but strong structure that resists forces in several directions, much like the distinct wood grain used in each layer of plywood to increase its tensile strength. In general, the abdominals function as postural muscles, compressing the abdomen, pulling the front of the pelvis upward, and flattening the lumbar curvature of the spine. In addition to these functions, the obliques and the **transversus abdominis** located on the anterolateral aspect of the abdomen rotate the trunk laterally and aid in forced expiration. The *rectus abdominis* consists of two longitudinal columns of band-shaped muscle on either side of the midline of the abdomen, rather than the characteristic sheetlike morphology of the other abdominals. This muscle protects the viscera and is a powerful flexor of the vertebral column, but plays no part in expiration as an accessory muscle because of its longitudinal morphology. It is, therefore, not included in the summary given in Table 6–3. By contrast, the remaining three layers—external obliques, internal obliques, and transversus abdominis—contract vigorously during forced expiration and in straining actions such as lifting, coughing, vomiting, defecating, and childbirth. Abdominal muscle fibers originating from lateral pelvic structures insert into a tough, tendinous sheet called an *aponeurosis* (see Fig. 6–9A). Contraction of the fibers increases the tension on this midline structure, moving it inward and compressing the abdomen.

The abdominal compartment contains about 100 to 300 mL of abdominal gas that can be slightly compressed (De Troyer and Loring, 1995). The balance of the compartment, however, is virtually incompressible as a result of nonmovable structures such as the spine dorsally, the pelvis caudally, and the iliac crests of the os coxae laterally. As a result, a localized inward displacement of the container causes outward displacement elsewhere. Such displacement is limited to the ventral abdominal wall and the diaphragm. Contraction of the diaphragm during inspiration causes outward bulging of the ventral abdominal wall; contraction of the abdominal group during expiration causes upward displacement of the diaphragm.

As listed in Table 6–3, the three abdominal layers serving as accessory expiratory muscles all have attachments on the lower rib cage. Therefore, contraction of these muscles pulls the ribs downward and medially, increases the intra-abdominal pressure, and pushes the diaphragm cranially during its relaxation phase. The abdominals and the diaphragm are antagonistic. In other words, when the diaphragm is contracted, the abdominals are relaxed, and vice versa.

In summary, quiet inspiration involves contraction of the diaphragm, assisted in a minor way by contraction of some of the interchondral parts of the internal intercostals. Quiet expiration depends on elastic recoil of the thoracic cage and lungs and does not require any muscle activity. With ventilatory rates up to approximately 50 L/min, the pattern described above is maintained. In the ventilation range of 50 to 100 L/min, however, the sternocleidomastoids are recruited as accessory inspiratory muscles and are joined by the abdominal muscles and internal intercostals functioning as accessory expiratory muscles. Ventilation in excess of 100 L/min requires that the diaphragm and all accessory muscles are active. In addition, the curvature of the thoracic spine is straightened and the back is extended to result in a greater A-P diameter of the thorax (Gardner et al, 1967).

Summary

In this chapter we have examined the anatomy and physiology of the thorax, including a detailed study of the bones, joints, muscles, and movements involved in ventilation of the lungs. The chapter lays important structural and functional groundwork for the study of static and dynamic volume-pressure relationships in the thorax and lungs.

BIBLIOGRAPHY

De Troyer A and Loring SH: Actions of the Respiratory Muscles. In Roussos C (ed): The Thorax: Part A: Physiology, ed 2. Marcel Dekker, New York, 1995.

Edwards RHT and Faulkner JA: Structure and Function of the Respiratory Muscles. In Roussos C (ed): The Thorax: Part A: Physiology, ed 2. Marcel Dekker, New York, 1995.

Gardner E, Gray DJ, and O'Rahilly R: Anatomy: A Regional Study of Human Structure, ed 2. WB Saunders, Philadelphia, 1967.

Guyton AC and Hall JE: Textbook of Medical Physiology, ed 9. WB Saunders, Philadelphia, 1995.

Martini FH: Fundamentals of Anatomy and Physiology, ed 4. Prentice Hall, Upper Saddle River, NJ, 1998.

Moore KL: Clinically Oriented Anatomy, ed 3. Williams & Wilkins, Baltimore, 1992.

O'Rahilly R (with collaboration of Fabiola Müller): Gardner-Gray-O'Rahilly's Anatomy: A Regional Study of Human Structure, ed 5. WB Saunders, Philadelphia, 1986.

Rosse C and Gaddum-Rosse P: Hollinshead's Textbook of Anatomy, ed 5. Lippincott-Raven, Philadelphia, 1997.

Roussos C: Prologue: The Thorax through History into Medicine. In Roussos C (ed): The Thorax: Part A: Physiology, ed 2. Marcel Dekker, New York, 1995.

Thomas CL (ed): Taber's Cyclopedic Medical Dictionary, ed 18. FA Davis, Philadelphia, 1997.

Scanlon VC and Sanders T: Essentials of Anatomy and Physiology, ed 3. FA Davis, Philadelphia, 1999.

Thibodeau GA and Patton KT: Anatomy and Physiology, ed 3. Mosby–Year Book, St Louis, 1996.

Woodburne AM and Burkel WE: Essentials of Human Anatomy, ed 9. Oxford University Press, New York, 1994.

CHAPTER 7

Statics of Breathing

chapter objectives

After studying this chapter the reader should be able to:

☐ Define spirometry

☐ Define the following lung volumes and state a typical value obtained by spirometry in an average person:
    Tidal volume (V_T), inspiratory reserve volume (IRV), expiratory reserve volume (ERV), residual volume (RV).

☐ Define the following lung capacities and state a typical value obtained through spirometry in an average person:
    Vital capacity (VC), inspiratory capacity (IC), functional residual capacity (FRC), total lung capacity (TLC).

☐ Explain the difference between the statics and the dynamics of the mechanics of breathing.

☐ Explain the concept of the pleural space as a potential space.

☐ Describe the source, function, pressure, and recovery of pleural fluid from the pleural space.

☐ Explain how the intrapleural pressure is maintained at a subatmospheric value.

☐ Describe the sequence of events that occur during inspiration and expiration in terms of intra-alveolar and intrapleural pressure changes.

☐ Define transpulmonary pressure in terms of static lung conditions.

☐ Describe the concept of static lung compliance and how this characteristic affects the expansion and deflation of the lungs.

☐ Explain hysteresis and describe why the inspiratory compliance curve is not the same as the expiratory compliance curve.

☐ Describe the concept of specific lung compliance.

☐ Explain how static lung compliance is affected by the elastin network of lung interstitium.

☐ Describe how the elastase-antielastase system of the lung functions to maintain patency of airways and alveoli.

☐ Discuss the contribution to static lung forces made by the following factors: Elastic forces of the lung interstitium, elastic forces caused by surface tension effects, elastic forces of the chest wall.

☐ Define transthoracic pressure.

☐ Describe the interaction of the chest wall and lung as a system of compliances.

☐ Explain why the static compliance of the combined lung-thorax system is less than that of the lungs alone.

☐ Define elastance.

☐ Describe the effect of body position on the statics of the lung and thorax by explaining the changes produced in perfusion and in ventilation of the lung.

☐ Explain how the vertical gradient of pleural pressure and thorax biomechanics affect regional ventilation in the lung.

key terms

α_1-antitrypsin (α_1-AT); α_1-protease inhibitor (α_1-PI)
elastance
expiratory compliance curve
hysteresis (his″ ter-ē′ sis)
inspiratory compliance curve
intra-alveolar pressure; alveolar pressure; intrapulmonary pressure
intrapleural pressure; pleural pressure
lung capacities
   functional residual capacity (FRC)
   inspiratory capacity (IC)
   total lung capacity (TLC)
   vital capacity (VC)

lung volumes
   expiratory reserve volume (ERV)
   inspiratory reserve volume (IRV)
   residual volume (RV)
   tidal volume (V_T)
neutrophil elastase (NE)
pleural cavity; pleural space
pleural fluid
pulmonary mechanics
specific lung compliance
spirometry
static lung compliance (C_{st}, C_L)
transpulmonary pressure (P_{tp})
transthoracic pressure (P_{tt})

Volume-pressure relationships in the lung under conditions of no flow are the subject of this chapter. The *static* considerations of the mechanics of breathing include a review of pertinent gas laws, and of volumes and pressures in the thorax and lung. The concept of compliance of the lung and chest wall is explored, and the role of the vertical hydrostatic gradient in the distribution of gas and blood in the lung is introduced. The dynamics of lung mechanics is examined in the next chapter.

Lung Volumes and Capacities

Spirometry deals with the recording of the volume of air moved into and out of the lungs during different conditions of breathing. In this chapter covering the statics of lung mechanics, we briefly examine the basic pulmonary volumes and capacities obtained by spirometric means. In the following chapter, the dynamic effect of resistance and flow on these measurements are considered. Together, the coverage of the topic in the two chapters serves as an introduction to pulmonary function testing (PFT) for the respiratory care practitioner. A summary of common abbreviations and symbols used in cardiopulmonary physiology, including those used in the assessment of pulmonary function, is given in Appendix A.

To conveniently describe the events of pulmonary ventilation, the spirogram shown in Figure 7–1 is divided into four different **lung volumes** along the left side and four different **lung capacities** along the right side of the graph. Notice that the sum of all the lung volumes equals the maximum volume to which the lungs can be expanded and that the value of each lung

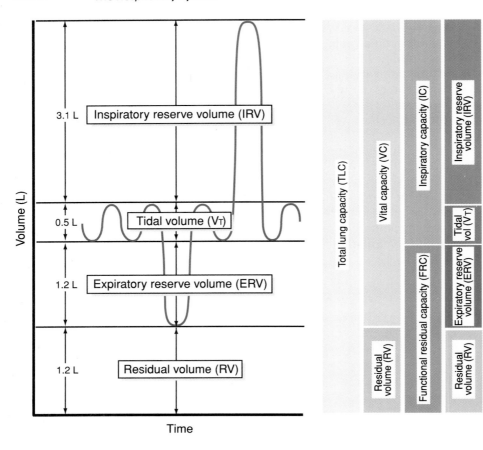

FIGURE 7-1. Spirogram—lung volumes and capacities. Note that lung capacities are composed of two or more lung volumes, and that tidal volume is measured under resting conditions. The values shown are approximate and are affected by variables such as body size.

capacity consists of two or more lung volumes. All lung volumes and capacities are around 20% to 25% less in women compared with men, and all values are correspondingly greater in larger persons (Guyton and Hall, 1996).

LUNG VOLUMES

The various lung volumes depicted in Figure 7–1 are defined as follows.

Tidal Volume

The **tidal volume (V_T)** is that volume of air moved during normal, relaxed, quiet breathing. Shallow diaphragmatic breathing is responsible for tidal volume. The volume inspired and expired is generally about 500 mL in an average young adult man (Guyton and Hall, 1996).

Inspiratory Reserve Volume

The **inspiratory reserve volume (IRV)** is the extra volume of air that can be inhaled beyond the normal tidal volume. Attaining this inspiratory volume of approximately 3.1 L requires the combined effort of the diaphragm and the muscles of the accessory inspiratory group.

Expiratory Reserve Volume

Contraction of the accessory expiratory group of muscles produces a forced expiration. The extra volume of air expelled at the end of a normal tidal breath by such a forced maneuver is usually around 1.2 L and is called the **expiratory reserve volume (ERV).**

Residual Volume

The amount of air remaining in the lungs after the most forceful expiration averages around 1.2 L and is called the **residual volume (RV).**

LUNG CAPACITIES

Various lung capacities are shown in Figure 7–1 and can be described as follows:

Inspiratory Capacity

At the end of a normal expiration, *maximal* inspiratory effort results in inhalation of the **inspiratory capacity (IC),** an amount of air equal to the tidal volume plus the inspiratory reserve volume, usually around 3.6 L in an average-sized adult male.

Functional Residual Capacity

Following the end of a normal expiration, the **functional residual capacity (FRC)** remains in the lungs. This volume of approximately 2.4 L is made up of the expiratory reserve volume and the residual volume. Because part of the FRC is made up of residual volume that cannot be voluntarily exhaled, only a portion of the capacity is "functional" from the physiologic standpoint of gas exchange.

Vital Capacity

The sum of the inspiratory reserve volume, tidal volume, and expiratory reserve volume is around 4.8 L, and is called the **vital capacity (VC).** This is the maximum amount of air that can be expelled from the lungs after first filling the lungs to their maximum extent. The vital capacity represents the total amount of *usable* air that is available in the lungs with both a maximal inspiratory effort and a maximal expiratory effort.

Total Lung Capacity

The maximum amount of air that can be held by the lungs with a maximal inspiratory effort is around 6 L. This **total lung capacity (TLC)** is composed of the vital capacity plus the residual volume, a volume of gas that cannot be expelled.

Volume-Pressure Relationships in the Thorax and Lungs

The study of **pulmonary mechanics** deals with the volume and pressure changes produced in the thorax and lungs by the action of muscles of ventilation. These muscles generate the pressures that overcome the natural elasticity, or static properties, of the respiratory system at times of zero gas flow. In contrast is the study of ventilatory muscle activity in overcoming the flow-resistive pressure losses, or dynamic properties, of the respiratory system during breathing cycles. The *statics* of lung mechanics are covered in the present chapter; the companion topic of the *dynamics* of lung mechanics is dealt with in the following chapter. As a preface to the study of static volume-pressure relationships in the respiratory system, consider the following quotation:

> The lungs do not move naturally of their own motion, but they follow the motion of the thorax and the diaphragm. The lungs are not expanded because they

are filled with air, but they are filled with air because they are expanded.

> Franciscus Sylvius de la Boe—*Opera Medica,* 1681 (Lenfant, 1995). As quoted by Lenfant C: Introduction. In Roussos C (ed): The Thorax—Part A: Physiology, ed 2. Marcel Dekker, New York, 1995.

This concept of thorax and lung movement stated so eloquently over 300 years ago must have been revolutionary at the time. During the preceding era, *movement* of the lung was not considered. Instead, the lung was perceived by medieval physiologists as an internal organ that regulated the heat produced by the heart (Clayton and Philo, 1992). Today we can measure and study the various volumes and pressures generated in both the pleural cavity and the alveoli, and demonstrate that the lungs are indeed "filled with air because they are expanded." However, the relationship between volume and pressure responsible for filling and emptying the lungs is not always easily grasped.

PLEURAL CAVITY, MEMBRANES, AND FLUID

To begin with, the natural elasticity of the lung causes the lung to collapse if no counteracting force keeps it inflated. By contrast, the natural elastic tendency of the thorax is to expand outward unless antagonized by an inward force. These two phenomena—atelectasis, or collapse of the lung, coupled with an outward bulge of the thorax—are visible in a *pneumothorax* when the chest wall is compromised by a penetrating wound and atmospheric air enters the space surrounding the lung. In such a condition, the static forces in the lung and chest wall no longer cancel each other, allowing both structures to exhibit their natural elastic tendencies, resulting in collapse of the lung and expansion of the chest wall. Normally, when the recoil pressure within the lungs equals the outward pressure of chest wall expansion, the lungs are at their FRC, or resting volume. There are no attachments between the lung and the inner walls of the thoracic cage to maintain the resting lung in a state of distention. Instead, the lung is housed in a potential space called the **pleural cavity** or **pleural space** (Fig. 7–2). The "cavity" is so extremely narrow, however, that it is not an obvious physical space at all (Guyton and Hall, 1996). This extremely narrow space is occupied by a monolayer of viscous lubricating fluid called **pleural fluid.** This unique fluid allows the membrane surfaces of the pleural cavity to slide past one another smoothly during chest expansion and contraction. The fluid is derived from interstitial fluid that accumulates in the pleural space. Tissue proteins in the fluid give it a mucoid consistency that reduces friction between the *visceral pleura* that covers the outer surface of the lung and the *parietal pleura* that covers the thoracic wall, diaphragm, medi-

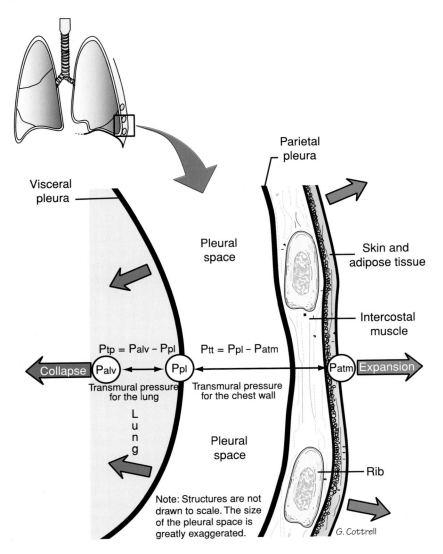

FIGURE 7–2. Transpulmonary and transthoracic pressures. The difference between the intra-alveolar pressure (P_{alv}) and the pleural pressure or intrapleural pressure (P_{pl}) is known as the *transpulmomary pressure* (P_{tp}). This pressure is a measure of the collapse tendency (recoil pressure) of the lung. The difference between the intrapleural pressure (P_{pl}) and the atmospheric pressure at the body surface (P_{atm} or P_{bs}) is the *thoracic pressure* (P_{tt}). This pressure is a measure of the expansion tendency of the chest wall. The difference between the intra-alveolar pressure and the atmospheric pressure ($P_{alv} - P_{atm}$) provides a static measure of the combined lung-thorax system.

astinum, and the region superior to the apex of the lung. Subdivisions of the parietal pleura are named after the structures they cover and are called the *costal, diaphragmatic, mediastinal,* and *pleural cupola* portions, respectively.

INTRAPLEURAL PRESSURE

The normal collapse tendency of the lungs is around −4 mm Hg, therefore, the counteracting pressure in the pleural space must be *at least as negative* as −4 mm Hg to keep the lungs inflated, thus maintaining their FRC. This value is in the range of −5 to −6 cm H_2O (1 mm Hg = 1.36 cm H_2O). Pleural fluid is constantly pumped out of the pleural space by the action of lymphatics draining the region. The lymph is moved into the lymph vessels of the mediastinum, upper surface of the diaphragm, and lateral surfaces of the parietal pleura. This continual lymph flow maintains a *negative* **intrapleural pressure (pleural pressure),** or a

slight suction, of approximately −7 mm Hg, relative to atmospheric pressure (Guyton and Hall, 1996). This negative intrapleural pressure directed outward is *more than* sufficient to counter the collapse tendency of the lung directed inward; therefore, the lungs are kept open and pressed tightly against the inner wall of the rib cage (see Fig. 7–2). Recall that the collapse tendency, or instability, of the lung is due to the combined effect of (1) surface tension forces in the fluid lining of the alveoli, and (2) the elastic recoil of the connective tissue elements of the lung interstitium. In the resting state, these static forces contribute to collapse of the lung, but are balanced by the static forces that cause the chest wall to expand outward.

With expansion of the chest during inspiration, the intrathoracic (intrapleural) volume increases, and the intrapleural pressure is lowered further, from −5 cm H_2O down to about −7.5 cm H_2O. This additional increase in the negativity of the intrapleural pressure is sufficient to increase the lung volume by approximately

0.5 L. During expiration, relaxation of the inspiratory muscles allows the elastic nature of the lungs and thorax to return the structures to their preinspiratory state.

INTRA-ALVEOLAR PRESSURE

The pressure within the alveoli of the lungs is called the **intrapulmonary pressure, intra-alveolar pressure,** or simply, the **alveolar pressure.** At the preinspiratory phase of the respiratory cycle the glottis is open and no gas is flowing. The pressures in all parts of the respiratory system, from the conducting passages down to the alveoli of the respiratory zone, are equal to atmospheric pressure. If the pressures in the respiratory system were anything other than equal to atmospheric pressure, gas would be either flowing into the conducting zone or flowing out of it. Air enters the upper airways during normal inspiration when the intra-alveolar pressure is decreased to about −1 cm H_2O, relative to atmospheric pressure. This drop in intra-alveolar pressure occurs as a result of the increase in lung volume brought about by the decrease in intrapleural pressure. All of these sequential changes occur because of the inverse relationship between volume and pressure ($V \propto 1/P$). The fall in intra-alveolar pressure to −1 cm H_2O relative to atmospheric pressure is sufficient to move about 0.5 L of air into the lungs during normal inspiration—the volume known as the tidal volume. During expiration an increase in intra-alveolar pressure of approximately +1 cm H_2O relative to atmospheric pressure moves about 0.5 L of air out of the lungs.

TRANSPULMONARY PRESSURE

The difference in pressure between the intra-alveolar pressure and the intrapleural pressure is called the **transpulmonary pressure (P_{tp}).** This pressure reflects the difference between the pressure within the alveoli (P_{alv}) and the pleural pressure (P_{pl}), at the outer surface of the lung (see Fig. 7–2). The transpulmonary pressure is also a measure of the collapse tendency, or recoil pressure, of the lung at each point of its expansion:

$$P_{tp} = P_{alv} - P_{pl}$$

Lung Compliance

STATIC LUNG COMPLIANCE

Static lung compliance (C_{st}, C_L) is defined as the change in lung volume (ΔV) per unit change in pressure (ΔP) under conditions of no flow:

$$C_{st} = \frac{\Delta V}{\Delta P}$$

The units used in the measurement of static lung compliance are liters per centimeters of water (L/cm H_2O). Compliance provides us with an assessment of the elastic properties of lung tissue during static conditions. It should be noted that compliance is *not* the same as resistance. Martin and Youtsey (1988) point out that resistance involves a relationship between pressure and flow, such as "centimeters of water per liter per second," and is measured during dynamic conditions. Static lung compliance, on the other hand, involves a relationship between volume and pressure and is measured during conditions of no flow.

In the adult, the normal total compliance of both lungs together is around 0.2 L/cm H_2O (Ganong, 1995; Guyton and Hall, 1996). In other words, the lung is able to expand and accommodate approximately 0.2 L of air each time the transpulmonary pressure increases by 1 cm H_2O (Fig. 7–3). Lungs having increased compliance are very distensible, that is, they expand a large volume for each unit increase in transpulmonary pressure. By contrast, lungs with low compliance are stiff and expand with difficulty (see Fig. 7–3).

When the P_{tp}, or distending pressure, required to maintain lung inflation is plotted against the lung volume generated, the elastic properties of the lung can be determined. Figure 7–4 shows the *compliance diagram of the lung.* The two curves shown in the diagram

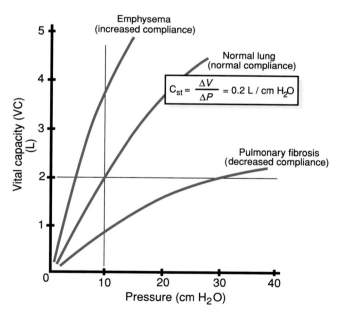

FIGURE 7–3. Static lung compliance. Lungs with substantial fibrotic changes lack elasticity and compliance. Such lungs are stiff and fill with difficulty at any given pressure. By contrast, emphysematous lungs are more complaint than normal lungs. Such lungs tend to become over-distended and thus hyperinflate easily at relatively low pressures. Gas exchange, however, is deficient because of impaired alveolar architecture. Because of the elastic limits of the connective tissue of the lung, compliance tends to decrease as the volume of the lung nears total lung capacity (TLC).

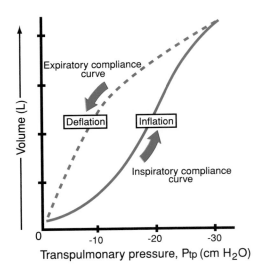

FIGURE 7–4. Compliance diagram of the normal lung. Notice that the shape of the inspiratory and expiratory compliance curves in the static volume-pressure graph is different. Such a disparity is referred to as *hysteresis,* the inability of an effect to keep up to its cause. Changes in the rate of opening of alveoli, and changes in the surface tension of alveoli at different lung volumes, are responsible for the hysteresis effect. Notice also that lung volumes at a given pressure are larger during deflation than those produced during inflation.

are the **inspiratory compliance curve** and the **expiratory compliance curve** (Guyton and Hall, 1996). The shape of the inflation curve differs from that of the deflation curve. Such a disparity in which the appearance of an effect fails to keep up with its cause is referred to as **hysteresis** (Gr., *a coming too late*) (Des Jardins, 1998; Guyton and Hall, 1996; Levitzky, 1995; Taylor et al, 1989). In pulmonary mechanics, hysteresis is the difference between inflation and deflation of the lung, as depicted on a static volume-pressure curve. The lung volume at any given pressure during deflation is larger than the volume attained during inflation (West, 1998). Hysteresis is caused by the gradual opening of alveoli at different volumes and by changes in surface tension that occur as the volume of the lung changes.

SPECIFIC LUNG COMPLIANCE

As described in the preceding section, static lung compliance is dependent upon the volume at which it is measured. Lung compliance progressively decreases as the lungs expand in response to higher volumes. This effect is seen in the plateau region of the compliance curves as TLC is approached (see Fig. 7–3). Larger lungs are more compliant, or distensible, than smaller lungs—whale lungs, for instance, expand with far less effort than mouse lungs. Figure 7–4 shows that there is a greater change in volume for the same change in transpulmonary pressure in the "steeper" part of both the inspiratory and the expiratory compliance curves. Because static lung compliance is volume-dependent, and also varies with lung size (being higher in larger lungs), it must be normalized to the same part of the volume-pressure curve if comparison among different respiratory systems is to be done (Taylor et al, 1989). A value for **specific lung compliance** is obtained when static lung compliance is divided by the functional residual capacity (C_{st}/FRC):

$$\therefore \text{Specific compliance} = \frac{\Delta V}{\Delta P \times V}$$

The units of specific compliance of the lung are liters per cm H_2O per liter (Martin and Youtsey, 1988). Specific compliance eliminates the effect of different lung capacities on lung compliance because the static transpulmonary pressures at TLC and at RV are the same regardless of lung size. Taylor et al (1989) state that specific compliance values are "fairly constant from person to person and from species to species."

LUNG COMPLIANCE AND THE ELASTASE-ANTIELASTASE SYSTEM

In the mid-1960s it was discovered that individuals with a plasma deficiency of α_1-**antitrypsin (α_1-AT),** also known as α_1-**protease inhibitor (α_1-PI),** developed severe, early-onset emphysema and that the deficiency was inherited (Llewellyn-Jones and Stockley, 1993). Of the estimated 2 million people in the United States who have some form of emphysema, it is estimated that only about 1% to 2% have the genetic deficiency for the α_1-AT protein. However, within the group diagnosed with the premature form of the disease, approximately one-half may lack the α_1-antitrypsin gene and develop emphysema before the age of 50.

Emphysema is a debilitating, progressive, and destructive lung disorder grouped with the chronic obstructive pulmonary diseases (COPDs). It is characterized by hyperinflation of the lung, loss of lung compliance, and coalescence of adjacent alveoli in response to destruction of alveolar septa (see Fig. 7–3). As the total number of alveoli decreases, the effective surface area for gas exchange is reduced, resulting in deterioration of arterial blood gas values. The elastic connective tissue of lung interstitium normally contributes to both the elastic recoil of the lung and the patency of small airways. This action occurs because elastin fibers connected to airway walls maintain radial traction, or "mechanical tethering," of the bronchioles (see Fig. 2–8C). Destruction of elastin, therefore, predisposes the lung to collapse and is a major contributing event in the development of emphysema. How is the lung's elastase-antielastase system unbalanced to result in destruction of elastin?

Elastin is prone to enzymatic destruction by proteinases in general, and by **neutrophil elastase (NE)** in particular. Neutrophils play a protective role in the lung but also produce NE, which digests native elastin to destroy the lung's resiliency. NE also damages bronchial epithelium, reduces ciliary beating, and promotes mucous gland hyperplasia (an increase in the number of cells). Clearly, control of such destructive proteases is crucial in the maintenance of healthy, resilient lung tissue. A protective system of protease inhibitors in the lung normally functions to counter the destructive action of NE. The full anti-NE defensive screen is provided by a relatively large volume of α_1-antitrypsin (α_1-AT), augmented by a relatively small volume of other chemicals with antielastase properties. These substances include *secretory leukoprotease inhibitor* (SLPI) and α_2-*macroglobulin* (α_2-M). The most potent inhibitor of neutrophil elastase in the lung is α_1-antitrypsin (Llewellyn-Jones and Stockley, 1993). Therefore, individuals who have an α_1-AT deficiency often develop emphysema as a result of unopposed NE proteolytic activity in the lung interstitium. Without functional elastin, the natural resiliency of the lung is destroyed and overall static lung compliance is decreased (Box 7–1).

The antiproteolytic activity of α_1-AT is theoretically reduced when cigarette smoke activates lung neutrophils and oxidant chemicals. These chemicals, in turn, oxidize and damage a crucial amino acid on an active site of the α_1-AT molecule (Llewellyn-Jones and Stockley, 1993; Witek and Schachter, 1994). The resulting inactivation of α_1-AT tips the elastase-antielastase balance in favor of elastase activity and lung destruction. Clinical and direct studies, however, do not fully support this theory of the pathogenesis, or progression, of COPD in response to inhalation of cigarette smoke (Llewellyn-Jones and Stockley, 1993).

Factors Contributing to Static Lung Forces

The overall characteristics of compliance are determined by the static elastic forces acting in the lungs and contributing to lung instability. The elastic factors that are so crucial in the early days of postnatal life remain as critical factors in lung mechanics throughout our lives. We now briefly review the elastic forces discussed with the neonatal lung, and then add another force capable of influencing the statics of lung mechanics—the force applied by the elasticity of the thoracic wall. The static forces include (1) the elastic force of the lung tissue itself, (2) the elastic force caused by the surface tension of the alveolar lining fluid, and (3) the elastic properties of the chest wall.

ELASTIC FORCES OF THE LUNG INTERSTITIUM

The composition of the lung interstitium includes an interwoven mesh of elastin and collagen protein fibers that are interspersed throughout the lung parenchyma. When the lung is deflated, the fibers are condensed and more or less kinked, but when the lung expands, the fibrous mesh is also stretched. In this distended state, the protein fibers become elongated and exert a static recoil pressure that contributes to the overall elastic force of the lung. Respiratory muscle action generates the pressures required to overcome this elastic force.

ELASTIC FORCES CAUSED BY SURFACE TENSION EFFECTS

About two-thirds of the total elastic force of the lung is produced by the collapse tendency of alveoli lined with fluid. Surface tension in such small-diameter spherical structures is normally very high because of the cohesion between liquid molecules found in the lining fluid (see Fig. 1–12). Recall that the distending pressure, or the pressure required to keep a spherical alveolus open, is proportional to the surface tension of the film of alveolar fluid, but inversely proportional to the radius of the sphere (see Fig. 1–9). Figure 7–5 illustrates the important effect of surface tension on lung elasticity in the statics of breathing.

If the compliance diagrams of two experimental lungs are compared, one filled with saline, and the other with air, striking differences are noted (Fig. 7–6). Both plots produce characteristic hysteresis curves. The compliance diagram of the saline-filled lung, however, is located to the left of that of the air-filled lung, indicating that a relatively low transpulmonary pressure is required to inflate the lung compared with the pressure required to inflate the air-filled lung. The elastin and collagen fibers of the lung interstitium are unchanged, so why is one-third the pressure required to inflate the saline-filled lung? In the air-filled lung there is an interface between the lining fluid and the air in the alveoli, but the saline-filled lung has no air-fluid interface (Guyton and Hall, 1996; Taylor et al, 1989). When the air-fluid interface is replaced by a fluid-fluid interface, the effect of surface tension forces disappears, revealing the elastic forces caused by the recoil tendency of the connective tissue of the lung.

ELASTIC FORCES OF THE CHEST WALL

Another contributing factor in the statics of lung mechanics is the elasticity of the chest wall, a resilient structure that also requires muscular effort to expand. The relevant applied pressure at the chest wall is the **transthoracic pressure (P_{tt}),** which is defined by

P E R S P E C T I V E S

BOX 7-1

Emerging Therapies for the Treatment of α_1-Antitrypsin Deficiency

Elastic connective tissue in lung interstitium can be destroyed by the enzyme *neutrophil elastase* (NE) produced by lung neutrophils. The most potent antielastase substance available to counter the destructive action of NE is α_1-*antitrypsin* (α_1-AT), produced by hepatocytes in the liver, monocytes in the blood, and alveolar macrophages in the lung. Normally, this protein is transported by the bloodstream to the lung where it provides the needed defense against the proteolytic action of NE. However, in an individual lacking the gene for normal production of α_1-AT, the delicate balance of the elastase-antielastase system of the lung is upset, and unrestrained elastase action results in the destruction of the lung's elastic connective tissue.

A variety of therapeutic strategies exist or are being assessed for use in treating α_1-AT deficiency. These therapeutic approaches include *liver transplants, administration of anti-NE agents,* and *gene replacement therapy.* Liver transplantation results in the restoration of the normal concentration of α_1-AT in the serum because liver cells normally synthesize large quantities of the protective protein. Introduction of molecules with anti-NE activity such as the intravenous (IV) administration of the plasma form of α_1-AT (Prolastin), derived from pooled human blood plasma, is currently approved for human use and is effective as an antielastase therapy. The results obtained from animal experiments using aerosol administration of the plasma form of the α_1-AT protein are promising, but the technique is currently not approved for human use (Witek and Schachter, 1994). Aerosol administration of the recombinant form of α_1-AT and of secretory leukoprotease inhibitor (SLPI) also shows promise in the treatment of α_1-AT deficiency in the lung. Finally, gene therapy is a conceptually sound and attractive technique for the treatment of hereditary-based α_1-AT deficiency but is not yet approved for human use.

In several ways, gene therapy exhibits the greatest potential as a future therapeutic strategy in treating α_1-AT deficiency because the hereditary disorder involves a single deficient gene that can be replaced. In simple terms, gene therapy deals with the introduction of functional genetic material to target cells. The recipient cells then incorporate the "new" gene into their genetic code so they can begin synthesis of the deficient substance. A *vector* is required for transfer of the functional α_1-AT gene to the affected cells. Several types of vectors are used in gene therapy, including retroviruses and adenoviruses:

- *Retroviruses* are RNA viruses that can be modified so that they insert a new gene into the target cell. Such vectors are generally used in gene therapy ex vivo, that is, outside the body, to introduce new genetic material (Witek and Schachter, 1994).
- *Adenoviruses* are DNA viruses that can be manipulated so that the functional α_1-AT genetic material can be incorporated into the target cell but the genetic information responsible for the production of infectious adenoviruses is not transferred. Adenoviruses have a natural affinity for the respiratory system, especially the structures of the upper respiratory tract. Use of adenovirus vectors for the transfer of the α_1-AT gene to target cells appears to be the most promising technique for gene therapy intervention in α_1-AT deficiency. Proof of safety and efficacy in humans, however, has not been established (Witek and Schachter, 1994).

- Llewellyn-Jones CG and Stockley RA: The Neutrophil. In Chung KF and Barnes PJ (eds): Pharmacology of the Respiratory Tract: Experimental and Clinical Research. Marcel Dekker, New York, 1993.
- Witek TJ and Schachter EN: Pharmacology and Therapeutics in Respiratory Care. WB Saunders, Philadelphia, 1994.

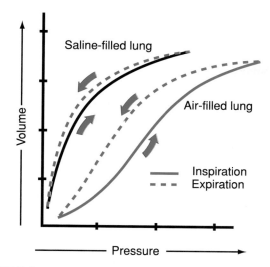

FIGURE 7–5. Comparison of air-filled and saline-filled lungs. The compliance diagram for the air-filled lungs illustrates the typical hysteresis effect. The difference between the inflation and deflation curves disappears, however, when the experimental lungs are filled with a saline solution. The addition of saline solution. The addition of saline creates a fluid-fluid interface in the lung that eliminates the effect of surface tension in the air-fluid interface of the air-filled lung.

Taylor et al (1989) as the difference between the pleural pressure (P_{pl}) and the atmospheric pressure, or pressure at the body surface (P_{atm} or P_{bs}) (see Fig. 7–2).

$$P_{tt} = P_{pl} - P_{atm}$$

Recall that the transmural pressure applied at the lung is known as the transpulmonary pressure, or the difference between alveolar and pleural pressures;

whereas the transmural pressure applied at the chest wall is known as the transthoracic pressure. Therefore, the pressure applied to the combined lung-thorax system is the difference between the alveolar pressure (P_{alv}) and the atmospheric pressure (P_{atm}). Consider what happens to these applied pressures when the chest wall is expanded and contracted.

The walls of the thorax form a flexible container that has a resting volume (0.0 cm H_2O pressure) that is approximately 70% to 78% of the total lung capacity, as shown in Figure 7–6 (Martin and Youtsey, 1988; Taylor et al, 1989; West, 1998). At this volume, the thorax can readily accommodate the expanding lungs as they inflate to their normal V_T. However, if the chest wall is expanded beyond this volume to the TLC, as occurs with forced inspiration, the elastic recoil of the chest wall components such as the ribs, costal cartilages, connective tissue, and muscle, collapse it back to the same resting volume when the expansion force is removed. Conversely, compression of the chest below the resting volume, as occurs when the rib cage is drawn downward and medially during forced expiration, causes the chest wall to recoil outward to its resting volume when the compression force is removed (see Fig. 7–6). Therefore, a subatmospheric pressure must be applied to the inside of the chest wall to decrease the volume of the thorax below its resting volume.

By contrast, the *isolated* lung has a collapse tendency, as a result of the combined effect of connective tissue elasticity and surface tension elasticity, over its *entire* volume range. The recoil pressure causes the isolated lung to collapse all the way to its residual volume at about 20% of TLC (Taylor et al, 1989). During a normal re-

FIGURE 7–6. Pressure-volume curve of the combined lung-chest wall system. TLC = total lung capacity; RV = residual volume; FRC = functional residual capacity; P_{tt} = transthoracic pressure; P_{tp} = transpulmonary pressure. In this relaxation pressure-volume curve note that the lung is minimally distended at RV and that the properties of the combined system at this volume are essentially those of the chest wall alone. At approximately 75%–80% of TLC, the transthoracic pressure is approximately zero; therefore the chest wall contributes relatively little to the elastic nature of the combined system. At this point, the recoil properties of the combined system are determined mainly by the elastic properties of the lung itself. Equilibrium exists at FRC when the transmural pressure for the chest wall (P_{tt}) is equal and opposite to the transmural pressure for the lung (P_{tp}). At this point, the tendency of the chest wall to expand to a larger volume is *balanced* by the tendency of the lung to collapse to a smaller volume. (Adapted from West JB: Respiratory Physiology: The Essentials, ed 5. Williams & Wilkins, Baltimore, 1995, p 102, with permission.)

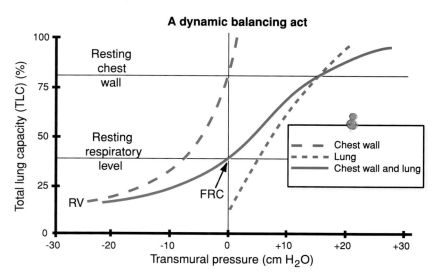

laxed expiration, unlike the events of a forced expiration, deflation of the lung stops at FRC. At this volume, which is approximately 40% of TLC, the collapsing pressure of the lung is balanced by the opposite and equal expanding pressure of the chest wall (see Fig. 7–6). This equilibrium state occurs at the resting *end-expiratory position* (EEP), and it is here that the applied pressure of the *combined* lung-thorax system is at equilibrium, or zero.

Interaction of the Chest Wall and Lung

COMPLIANCE OF THE COMBINED LUNG-THORAX SYSTEM

Ventilation of the combined lung-thorax system requires almost twice as much pressure as needed to ventilate the lungs after their removal from the thoracic cage (Guyton and Hall, 1996). For example, the static compliance of each lung is about 0.1 L/cm H_2O; therefore, the C_{st} of the pair of lungs is approximately 0.2 L/cm H_2O. The combined, or total, compliance of the lung-thorax system (C_T) is much less, measuring only about 0.11 L/cm H_2O. The compliance of a system is made up of individual compliances that act in *parallel;* therefore, the total compliance of a system is determined by adding the *reciprocals* of the individual compliances (Dupuis, 1992; Levitzky, 1995; West, 1998):

$$\frac{1}{C_T} = \frac{1}{C_{st}} + \frac{1}{C_{cw}}$$

where:
C_T = total compliance
C_{st} = static lung compliance
C_{cw} = static chest wall compliance

From this relationship we can calculate the static compliance of the chest wall alone to determine how much of the total compliance is due to the elastic characteristics of thoracic cage structures such as muscle, bone, and cartilage:

$$\frac{1}{C_T} = \frac{1}{C_{st}} + \frac{1}{C_{cw}}$$

$$\frac{1}{C_{cw}} = \frac{1}{C_T} - \frac{1}{C_{st}}$$

$$= \frac{1}{0.11} - \frac{1}{0.2}$$

$$= 9.090909 - 5$$

$$\frac{1}{C_{cw}} = 4.090909$$

$$\therefore C_{cw} = 0.244 \text{ L/cm } H_2O$$

Recall that compliance indicates the degree of distensibility of an elastic structure. The larger the compliance of a distensible structure, the more readily the structure expands to accommodate each incremental increase in pressure. Therefore, over half of the muscular effort required to expand the combined lung-thorax system is needed to overcome the static elasticity, or **elastance,** of the thorax alone. (Elastance is the reciprocal of compliance.) In other words, the lungs have more compliance than the thorax, and the thorax has more elastance than the lungs.

In the normal range of breathing, the elastic characteristics of the lung and chest wall, although somewhat different, generally work in harmony. However, when the lungs are expanded to very high volumes or compressed to very low volumes, the statics of the chest wall become noticeable. Near the extreme upper and lower limits of movement, the compliance of the combined lung-thorax system can decrease to as low as 0.04 L/cm H_2O (40 mL/cm H_2O), or only one-fifth the compliance of the lungs alone (Guyton and Hall, 1996). A lung and thorax overdistended as a result of chronic disease such as emphysema exhibit such elevated compliance that additional expansion of the lung during inspiration is simply not effective. Pathophysiologic conditions such as calcification or ossification of costal cartilages, or arthritic changes in the thoracic spine and rib cage, further reduce the flexibility of these structures and decrease the resiliency and compliance of the thorax. As the thorax becomes more rigid, expansion and contraction of the chest is impaired and breathing becomes progressively more difficult. The effects of aging on the C_{st} and C_{cw} are explored in Chapter 15.

THE EFFECT OF BODY POSITION ON THE STATICS OF THE LUNG AND THORAX

Ventilation and perfusion do not occur uniformly throughout the lung during spontaneous ventilation. The uneven distribution of gas and blood can be partly attributed to static conditions involving the interaction of the chest wall when the body is in different positions. The resulting *vertical gradient* of hydrostatic pressure has an effect on both blood flow and pleural pressure in different regions of the lung.

Perfusion

The vertical hydrostatic (gravitational) effect results in the production of *nondependent* and *dependent* lung regions—classifications based on the degree of reliance of the lung region on gravity for the distribution of blood. In the upright individual, the uppermost region receives the least volume of blood and is considered nondependent. The middle region is a transitional zone between the apex and the base of the lung and is primarily dependent on gravity for its blood supply. The base of the lung is a dependent region, receiving most of its blood flow as a result of the vertical hydrostatic gradient (Dupuis, 1992).

As a general rule, pulmonary vascular flow increases from the least dependent to the most dependent regions of the lung. Much of this regional proportioning of blood occurs as a result of the vertical hydrostatic pressure gradient. The gradient causes progressive dilation of pulmonary capillaries from superior to inferior regions, and facilitates increased blood flow to those areas supplied by larger-diameter, low-resistance blood vessels. Consequently, postural changes affect overall flow of blood in the pulmonary vessels with the lowermost region of the lung becoming the most dependent on gravity for blood distribution. This dependent region of pooled blood is the *base* of the lung in an individual standing upright, but becomes the *posterior surface* of the lungs in a supine individual, and the *lowermost part of each lung* when an individual is lying on his or her side, as occurs in the lateral recumbent position. The relative pressures of pulmonary arteries, veins, and alveoli are also discussed in the *pulmonary perfusion zone model* (see Chap. 11).

Ventilation

Ventilation, like pulmonary perfusion, is also uneven throughout the lung and is affected by body position and the chest wall. The interregional disparity in the distribution of gas to the lung is due to factors such as (1) the vertical gradient of pleural pressure, and (2) thorax biomechanics.

Vertical Gradient of Pleural Pressure

For a subject standing in the upright position, the pleural pressure acting in the upper region of the lung is more subatmospheric than that acting in the lower region. Typically, these intrapleural pressures are around −14 to −10 cm H_2O at the apex, but only about −2 cm H_2O at the base of the upright lung (Dupuis, 1992; Taylor et al, 1989). The change in pleural pressure along the vertical axis of the lung averages approximately 0.4 cm H_2O/cm of lung height, causing the regional lung volume to decrease gradually from superior to inferior regions (Taylor et al, 1989). However, when the pressure-volume curve of each *region* is expressed as a percentage of the VC of each region, the values obtained are identical. What is responsible for this finding?

As a result of the vertical gradient of pleural pres-

sure, the alveoli in the upper, or nondependent, regions of the lung are more distended than those in the dependent regions. Consequently, in the upright position with the entire lung at FRC, the nondependent portion of the lung (apex) is more inflated and, therefore, less compliant, whereas the dependent basal region is less inflated and more compliant.

If a subject in the upright position inhales and increases the transpulmonary pressure equally at all regions of the lung, the following changes occur in the apex and base, respectively:

- The volume of the nondependent region increases by a relatively small percentage of its regional VC. This limited expansion occurs because the low-compliance alveoli of the apex are already inflated (as a result of the greater subatmospheric pleural pressure) and do not easily accommodate a further increase in volume. As a result, relatively little inspired gas is distributed to the nondependent regions of the lung. (Recall, however, that the regional vital capacity of the apex is also correspondingly large due to the distended alveoli.)
- The volume of the dependent basal region of the lung increases by a relatively large percentage of its regional vital capacity. (The regional VC, however, is comparatively small because of underinflated alveoli.) At FRC, inhaled gas tends to be distributed to the dependent regions of the lung because the alveoli are less distended, more compliant, and expand readily for a given pressure change.

NOTE: The interregional differences in ventilation have an important bearing on the matching of ventilation to perfusion in the lung. In the upright position, the dependent base of the lung is better perfused and ventilated than the nondependent apex; therefore, excellent matching of ventilation and perfusion of blood occurs in the base. Similarly, decreased ventilation of the apex of the lung matches the lower blood flow in the region to again result in an optimal relationship between ventilation and perfusion. The ratio and matching of ventilation and perfusion are examined further in Chapters 11 and 14.

Thorax Biomechanics

In addition to the effects of a pleural pressure difference along the vertical axis of the lung, interregional variation in ventilation is also affected by the movement of the ribs affecting the chest wall. In the previous chapter we examined the axes and planes of movement of the various ribs in producing bucket-handle movement of the thorax (see Fig. 6–8B). Recall that the upper ribs have shorter and more restrictive sternal attachments and move as a unit with the sternum, whereas the lower ribs have more flexible attachments and more freedom of movement (De Troyer and Loring, 1995). As a result of these sternal attachments, movement of the more mobile lower ribs displaces more volume, thereby favoring ventilation of the lower regions of the upright lung (Dupuis, 1992).

Summary

Static considerations of volume-pressure relationships were discussed in this chapter through the examination of various pressures in the thorax and the lungs, and through a study of the effect of compliance of the lung, chest wall, and the combined lung-thorax system on the statics of breathing. The interaction between the chest wall and the lung was also explored as a prelude to the study of dynamic factors affecting the mechanics of breathing.

BIBLIOGRAPHY

Beachey W: Respiratory Care Anatomy and Physiology: Foundations for Clinical Practice. Mosby–Year Book, St. Louis, 1998.

Clayton M and Philo R: Leonardo da Vinci: The Anatomy of Man. Museum of Fine Arts, Bullfinch Press/Little, Brown & Co., Houston, 1992.

D'Angelo E and Agostini E: Statistics of the Chest Wall. In Roussos C (ed): The Thorax: Part A: Physiology, ed 2. Marcel Dekker, New York, 1995.

Des Jardins T: Cardiopulmonary Anatomy and Physiology: Essentials for Respiratory Care, ed 3. Delmar Publishers, Albany, NY, 1998.

Dupuis YG: Ventilators: Theory and Clinical Application, ed 2. Mosby–Year Book, St. Louis, 1992.

Ganong WF: Review of Medical Physiology, ed 17. Appleton & Lange, Norwalk, CT, 1995.

Leff AR and Schumacker PT: Respiratory Physiology: Basics and Applications. WB Saunders, Philadelphia, 1993.

Lenfant C: In Roussos C (ed): The Thorax: Part A: Physiology, ed 2. Marcel Dekker, New York, 1995.

Levitzky MG: Pulmonary Physiology, ed 4. McGraw-Hill, New York, 1995.

Llewellyn-Jones CG and Stockley RA: The Neutrophil. In Chung KF and Barnes PJ (eds): Pharmacology of the Respiratory Tract: Experimental and Clinical Research. Marcel Dekker, New York, 1993.

Martin DE and Youtsey JW: Respiratory Anatomy and Physiology. CV Mosby, St. Louis, 1988.

Martini FH: Fundamentals of Anatomy and Physiology, ed 4. Prentice Hall, Upper Saddle River, NJ, 1998.

Taylor AE et al: Clinical Respiratory Physiology. WB Saunders, Philadelphia, 1989.

Thibodeau GA and Patton KT: Anatomy and Physiology, ed 3. Mosby–Year Book, St Louis, 1996.

Vogelmeier C et al: Comparative loss of activity of recombinant secretory leukoprotease inhibitor and alpha 1-protease inhibitor caused by different forms of oxidative stress. Eur Resp J. 10(9):2114–2119.

West JB: Respiratory Physiology: The Essentials, ed 6. Williams & Wilkins, Baltimore, 1998.

West JB: Respiratory Physiology: The Essentials, ed 5, Williams & Wilkins, Baltimore, 1995.

Witek TJ and Schachter EN: Pharmacology and Therapeutics in Respiratory Care. WB Saunders, Philadelphia, 1994.

CHAPTER 8

Dynamics of Breathing

chapter objectives

After studying this chapter the reader should be able to:

☐ Name two factors that cause flow-resistive pressure losses of a fluid moving through a tube.

☐ Define fluid dynamics.

☐ Describe the flow characteristics of laminar flow.

☐ Discuss laminar flow as applied to gas moving in a tube by describing the effect that the pressure gradient, tube radius, tube length, and viscosity have on the flowrate of gas.

☐ Name the types of airways where laminar flow is common.

☐ Define the critical flowrate and describe the flow characteristics of turbulent flow.

☐ Name the types of airways where turbulent flow is common.

☐ Describe the flow characteristics of transitional, or disturbed, flow.

☐ Name the locations in airways where transitional flow is common.

☐ Describe the two types of energy exhibited by gas flowing through a tube.

☐ Describe the phenomenon of convective acceleration that occurs as gas flows from tubes having a large total cross-sectional area to tubes having a small total cross-sectional area.

☐ Explain how a constant flowrate of gas is maintained by dynamic changes in pressure and velocity.

☐ Explain the concept of Reynolds' numbers in the prediction of patterns of flow in the proximal and distal airways.

☐ Define transairway pressure and airway resistance.

☐ Compare the total resistance of a system of pipes connected in series with a system of pipes connected in parallel.

☐ Discuss the airway resistance encountered by air flowing through proximal structures such as the nose, nasopharynx, and larynx.

☐ Describe the change in cross-sectional area and airway resistance observed as gas flows from central airways to peripheral airways.

- ☐ Explain why the impairment of small airways in the "silent zone" of the lung is difficult to detect.
- ☐ Describe the factors that contribute to short time constants and to long time constants.
- ☐ Explain the concept of dynamic lung compliance and the effect of uneven time constants in different lung regions.
- ☐ Explain why the ratio of dynamic lung compliance to static lung compliance decreases at higher breathing frequencies when obstructive disease is present.
- ☐ Compare and contrast frequency-independent compliance with frequency-dependent compliance.
- ☐ Describe the effect that the following resistances have on overall lung resistance during dynamic conditions:
  Airway resistance, tissue viscous resistance, elastic resistance.
- ☐ Differentiate between nonelastic and elastic resistance in the dynamics of breathing.
- ☐ Discuss the concept of work of breathing by comparing elastic work and nonelastic work.

key terms

airway resistance (R_{aw})
alveolar pressure ($P_{a,alv}$)
convective acceleration (Bernoulli effect)
critical flowrate
dynamic lung compliance (C_{dyn})
dynamics
elastic resistance
elastic work; compliance work
flow-resistive pressure loss
fluid dynamics
laminar flow

lung resistance
mouth pressure (P_m)
nonelastic resistance
nonelastic work
Reynolds' number (Re)
time constant (T_C)
tissue viscous resistance
transairway pressure (P_{ta})
transitional flow
turbulent flow
work of breathing (WOB)

The pressures generated in the pleural space during inspiration and expiration must overcome both the *elasticity* of the combined lung-thorax system and the *flow-resistive properties* of the airways. The elastic properties of lung interstitium, airway fluid linings, and the chest wall were analyzed under static conditions of zero flow in the previous chapter. In this chapter we briefly explore the dynamic properties of gases flowing in tubes and discuss the pressures necessary to overcome resistance to flow. A brief review of Poiseuille's law as it relates to gas flow is presented and is followed by a discussion of airway resistance and different types of flow patterns in the airways. The chapter also compares and contrasts dynamic lung compliance with static lung compliance. Measurements of lung mechanics affected by conditions of expiratory flow are considered in the following chapter.

Flow-Resistive Pressure Losses in the Airways

A portion of ventilatory effort is expended to overcome pressure losses in the airways caused by moving gas. **Dynamics** refers to factors such as the type of flow pattern exhibited by a gas in motion or the effect that friction has on the moving gas molecules. Such factors cause **flow-resistive pressure losses.** Clearly, such dynamic factors can only be measured during the actual ventilatory cycle, when gas flow is occurring. The pressures that overcome such resistance to flow depend more on the *rate of change of volume* than on *static lung volume* measured under conditions of zero gas flow.

FLUID DYNAMICS

Although the field of **fluid dynamics**—the study of the behavior of fluids in motion—is well beyond the requirements and scope of this text, certain principles pertaining to fluid motion are applicable to the study of the dynamics of breathing. The term *fluid* refers to both liquids and gases. The properties of these two states of matter, at least in regard to their characteristics when in motion, are surprisingly similar. For instance, when a gas or liquid flows continuously through a tube of fixed diameter, there is a fall in pressure from the proximal to the distal end of the tube as energy is lost to frictional forces. The decrease in pressure is a reflection of the resistance that must be overcome to move a fluid through the tube (Dupuis, 1992). The friction inherent in such a closed system is due, in part, to the type of flow exhibited by the moving molecules of gas or liquid. We now examine the characteristics of the two main types of flow as they relate to the movement of gases in closed tubes: *laminar flow* and *turbulent flow*. A third type, *transitional flow,* is also discussed briefly.

FLOW PATTERNS

Laminar Flow

The primary flow pattern exhibited by gas in motion in the conducting passages of the lung is **laminar flow.** In this efficient type of flow the molecules of gas move in an orderly fashion parallel to the walls of the conducting tube (Fig. 8–1A). The resulting flow pattern is perfectly uniform, with the velocity profile, or leading edge of the flow, assuming a parabolic shape. The moving gas advances as concentric telescoping "rings" of flow along the tube. The layer of gas molecules in contact with the tube walls has zero velocity, but the gas molecules farther from the walls of the tube travel at successively higher velocities. The fastest-moving stream of gas in this axial flow pattern is at the center, hence the three-dimensional shape of a cone is evident at the leading edge of the mass (see Fig. 8–1A).

The layer of gas molecules adjacent to the walls of the tube is essentially at rest. Therefore, frictional forces between the gas molecules and the walls of the tube do not account for the pressure gradient along the tube. In fact, during laminar flow, the pressure drop of a gas from the proximal to the distal end of a tube is due to the *viscosity* of the gas, and different gases exhibit different viscosities.

NOTE: The viscosity of a gas is not the same as the density of a gas. Density is defined as the mass per volume of a substance.

Viscosity has been discussed in relation to the viscoelastic properties of bronchial mucus (see Chap. 5). Viscosity is a measure of the tendency of a fluid to flow and is caused by internal frictional and attractive forces between molecules of the fluid itself.

The relationship between flowrate and viscosity of a fluid, pressure difference along a tube, and the length and radius of the tube is given by the equation known as the Hagen-Poiseuille law, a relationship that describes the unique behavior of fluids during laminar flow:

$$\dot{V} = \frac{\pi\,\Delta P\,r^4}{8\eta l} \quad \text{or} \quad \Delta P = \frac{\dot{V}\,8\eta l}{\pi r^4}$$

where:
$\dot{V}$ = flowrate of the gas
π = mathematical constant (*pi*)
ΔP = pressure gradient (driving pressure)
r = radius of the tube
η = viscosity (*eta*) of the gas
l = length of the tube

From the previous equation, it can be seen that if the viscosity and flowrate are kept constant, the pressure gradient along the tube varies directly with the length of the tube and inversely with the fourth power of the tube radius. Decreasing the *length* of the tube by one-half reduces the pressure gradient across the length of the tube by one-half; however, decreasing the tube *radius* by one-half increases the pressure gradient across the tube by an impressive 16-fold. Consider the two tubes in Figure 8–2. Both are equal in length and are conducting identical gas having the same viscosity and the same flowrate. These variables, therefore, can be represented by a constant (*K*). Tube A has a radius of 1 centimeter, whereas the radius of tube B is 0.5 centimeter:

$$\Delta P = K \times l \times \frac{1}{r^4}$$

where:
ΔP = pressure gradient along the tube ($P_1 - P_2$)
K = constant (flowrate and viscosity of the gas)
l = length of the tube
r = radius of the tube

Therefore,

Tube A:
$$\Delta P = K \times \frac{1}{1^4}$$
$$= K \times \frac{1}{1}$$
$$\Delta P = K \times 1$$

Tube B:
$$\Delta P = K \times \frac{1}{(0.5)^4}$$

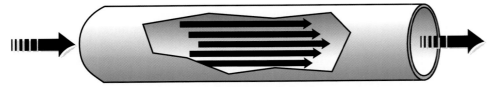

A. Laminar flow

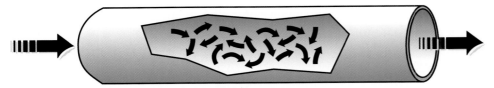

B. Turbulent flow

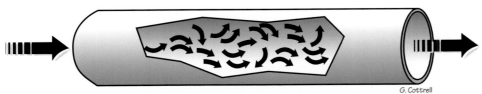

C. Transitional (disturbed) flow

G. Cottrell

FIGURE 8–1. Flow patterns. Note that in conditions of *laminar flow* (A), all flow is parallel to the walls of the tube, and that flow is greatest in the center of the tube. Fluid velocity decreases with the square of the radius; therefore, laminar flow patterns exhibit a conical, or parabolic, velocity profile. In conditions of *turbulent flow* (B), radial as well as axial flow patterns are seen and the velocity of the fluid is uniform, resulting in a more blunt velocity profile. Marginally laminar, disturbed, or *transitional flow* (C) exhibits features of both fully laminar and fully turbulent flow.

$$= K \times \frac{1}{0.0625}$$

$$\Delta P = K \times 16$$

As can be seen by this comparison, decreasing the radius of a tube by one-half causes the pressure drop along the tube to *increase* by a factor of 16. Stated another way, to attain the same flowrate in such a narrowed tube will require a *driving pressure* that is 16 times higher than that required to move gas at the same flowrate in the larger caliber tube.

Finally, if the Poiseuille equation is rearranged so that the viscosity of the gas, as well as the length and radius of the tube is kept constant, it will be seen that the pressure gradient along the tube is directly proportional to the flowrate of the gas (Dupuis, 1992). Therefore:

$$\Delta P = K_1 \dot{V}$$

where:
ΔP = pressure gradient (driving pressure)
K_1 = constant (includes the length and radius of the tube, and the viscosity of the gas)
$\dot{V}$ = flowrate of the gas

True laminar flow patterns in the respiratory system tend to occur at low flowrates. Such conditions are generally found only in the small airways where minimal resistance is encountered.

Turbulent Flow

As the flowrate of a gas increases, the pattern of the flow becomes less uniform. At the **critical flowrate** of the gas, the laminar flow pattern breaks up and becomes uneven and chaotic. Such a pattern is common at high flowrates in structures such as the trachea and large central bronchi. These structures exhibit considerable airflow resistance. All the gas molecules no longer travel in straight lines parallel to the walls of the tube. Instead, some molecules continue in the straight-line *axial* direction, but others move in the *radial* direction, at right angles to the main direction of flow (Leff and Schumacker, 1993). This chaotic pattern forms vortices and results in considerable noise as fluid moving in the radial direction impacts the walls of the tube. This swirling, countercurrent type of flow is called **turbulent flow** (see Fig. 8–1B). The velocity profile of gas traveling through a conducting tube during periods of turbulent flow has a characteristic blunt shape, instead of the parabolic (conical) shape typical of laminar flow. The flat profile is due to the uniform nature of the velocity of the gas. Because of the eddies that thoroughly mix the gas, the velocity of gas along the wall of the tube is the same as that of gas at the center of the flow.

The pressure drop along the tube in cases of turbulent flow is due to the same factors discussed above with laminar flow—geometry of the tube, viscosity, and flowrate of the gas—but is also influenced by the *density* of the gas. Recall that laminar flow exhibits zero

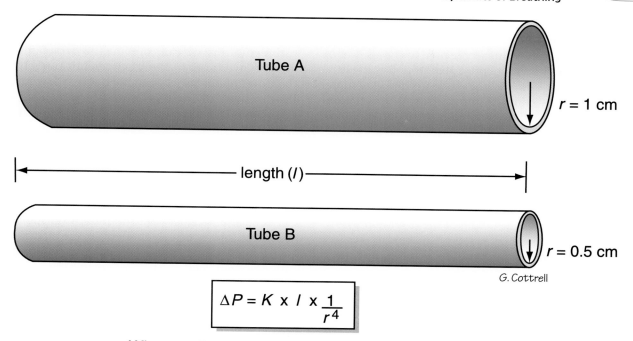

$$\Delta P = K \times l \times \frac{1}{r^4}$$

Where ΔP = pressure gradient
K = constant (flowrate and viscosity of gas)
r = radius of the tube
l = length of the tube

(Assume that both tubes are of equal length)

Tube A: $\Delta P = K \times l \times \dfrac{1}{r^4}$

$= K \times \dfrac{1}{1^4}$

$= K \times \dfrac{1}{1}$

$\Delta P = K \times 1$

Tube B: $\Delta P = K \times l \times \dfrac{1}{r^4}$

$= K \times \dfrac{1}{(0.5)^4}$

$= K \times \dfrac{1}{0.0625}$

$\Delta P = K \times 16$

FIGURE 8–2. Pressure gradient in two tubes of different radius. Note that the pressure gradient along the tube ($P_1 - P_2$, ΔP) is directly proportional to the length of the tube but inversely proportional to the fourth power of the tube radius. To attain the same flowrate of gas in two tubes of different radius requires a higher driving pressure for the gas in the narrower tube (see text for derivation of the formula from the Poiseuille equation).

velocity and, therefore, no frictional resistance at the periphery of the gas flow. In contrast, turbulent flow has a uniform velocity across the diameter of the tube and is prone to a further pressure drop because of friction with the walls of the tube (Dupuis, 1992). In addition to the effect of gas density on the pressure gradient along the tube during conditions of turbulent flow, the pressure drop is also directly proportional to the *square of the flowrate* and can be approximated by:

$$\Delta P \approx K_2 \dot{V}^2$$

where:
ΔP = pressure gradient (driving pressure)
K_2 = constant (includes the length and radius of the tube, and the viscosity and density of the gas)
$\dot{V}$ = flowrate of the gas

Energy is consumed in the production of chaotic fluid movement; therefore, a higher driving pressure is required to maintain the same flowrate under turbulent conditions, as opposed to laminar flow conditions

(Leff and Schumacker, 1993). Laminar pressure-flow relationships are *linear*, meaning that changes in the flowrate of the gas are linearly related to changes in the pressure along the conducting tube. Doubling the driving pressure will double the flowrate of a gas under laminar flow. By contrast, the pressure-flow relationship in turbulent flow is *nonlinear*. In other words, changes in flowrate are not linearly related to changes in the pressure gradient along the conducting tube, but are related to the square of the flowrate (Taylor et al, 1989). Since the pressure difference between two points along a tube increases with the square of the flowrate when the flow is turbulent, doubling the flow requires *more* than a doubling of the driving pressure. This increase in driving pressure is necessary because some of the fluid in turbulent flow exhibits movement in the radial direction.

Figure 8–3 shows the changes in pressure along a tube at different flowrates for both laminar flow and turbulent flow. We can combine the two relationships given above for the pressure gradient caused by laminar flow and the pressure gradient caused by turbulent flow to show the total pressure decrease along a tube (Box 8–1). This value is the total pressure loss in an airway due to the dynamic effect of the flow patterns of a moving gas:

$$\therefore \Delta P_{total} \approx K_1 \dot{V} + K_2 \dot{V}^2$$

The relationship represents the total pressure gradient between the alveolus and the mouth during inspiration. The total pressure gradient in the airways is approximately equal to the sum of the pressure drop in laminar flow regions such as small airways and the

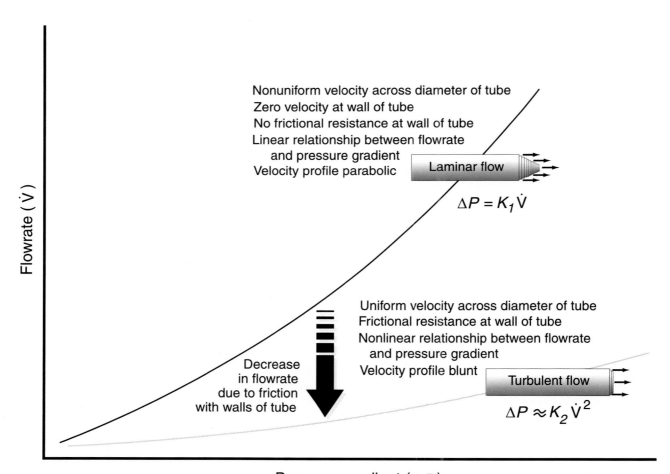

FIGURE 8–3. Relationship between flowrate and pressure gradient in laminar flow and turbulent flow patterns. Where ΔP = pressure gradient; $\dot{V}$ = flowrate of the gas; K_1 = constant (length and radius of tube and viscosity of gas); K_2 = constant (length and radius of tube and viscosity and density of gas).

P E R S P E C T I V E S

BOX 8–1

Corpses and the Measurement of Airway Resistance

Accurate determination of **airway resistance (R_{aw})** has always presented a formidable challenge, partly because of its dynamic nature. The first estimates of airway resistance were made in 1915 by F. Rohrer. Eighty years ago there were no experimental methods to directly assess the resistance encountered by gas flowing through an airway. Therefore, Rohrer estimated it by first performing postmortem measurements of the length and radius of airways and applying the measurements to the laws of fluid dynamics that govern the flow of liquids and gases through tubes. From these calculations the relationships known as the *Rohrer equations* were developed:

$$\Delta P_{total} = K_1 \dot{V} + K_2 \dot{V}^2$$

and

$$R_{aw} = K_1 + K_2 \dot{V}$$

where:

ΔP_{total} = total pressure difference in the airways due to gas flow
$\dot{V}$ = flowrate of the gas
K_1 = constant related to the viscosity of the gas and the radius and length of the airways
K_2 = constant related to the viscosity and density of the gas and the radius and length of the airways
R_{aw} = airway resistance

- D'Angelo E and Milic-Emil J: Dynamics of the Respiratory System. In Roussos C (ed): The Thorax: Part A: Physiology, ed 2. Marcel Dekker, New York, 1995.

pressure drop in turbulent flow regions such as larger airways.

Transitional Flow

At lower flowrates a mixed pattern of laminar and turbulent flow occurs in the larger-diameter airways (see Fig. 8–1C). This uneven pattern of parallel flow lines and eddies is known as **transitional flow.** It is also known as *marginally laminar,* or *disturbed flow,* and is common at locations where larger passages branch, converge, or narrow because of an obstruction (Leff and Schumacker, 1993).

CONVECTIVE ACCELERATION

Up to this point we have considered pressure decreases caused by different types of flow patterns in tubes. At a fixed viscosity of gas, and a constant tube length and radius, we have seen that the pressure changes in a tube are due to flowrate and to gas density. But what hap-

pens to pressure when the tube radii and the total number of tubes change from one region of the respiratory system to another? Since both the conducting and respiratory zones are composed of intricate systems of branched tubes having different diameters, we need to explore what changes occur to pressure when gas moves from a system having a large *total* cross-sectional area to one having a small *total* cross-sectional area.

The flow of gas through a tube possesses energy in two different forms: kinetic energy and potential energy. *Kinetic energy* is associated with *flow velocity,* or the actual movement of the gas, and is determined by the density of the gas and the square of its average velocity:

$$\therefore \text{kinetic energy} = \frac{1}{2} \rho \mu^2$$

where:

ρ = density (*rho*) of the gas (in g/mL)
μ^2 = square of the average velocity

Potential energy in the airways is associated with the *hy-*

drostatic pressure exhibited by the gas. The *total energy* of the system is the sum of the kinetic energy and the potential energy components of the moving gas (Leff and Schumacker, 1993). Fluids such as liquids and gases moving through a tube lose some of their total energy to the frictional loss of potential pressure energy. If the velocity of the flow changes along the tube, some of the potential pressure energy must be converted to kinetic energy.

When a fluid flows from a large-diameter tube into a small-diameter tube, the velocity of the fluid must increase to maintain the same flowrate. This conversion of pressure energy to kinetic energy is shown in Figure 8–4. As fluid enters the narrowed part of a tube, a greater proportion of the total energy is made up of kinetic energy, as compared with the proportions when fluid is traveling in the wider parts of the tube. The change in velocity, or *acceleration,* of the fluid thus causes a decreased pressure in the tube (see Fig. 8–4). This **convective acceleration** effect is named for Bernoulli, the physiologist-physicist who first studied the phenomenon (Taylor et al, 1989).

Consider the following example described by Leff and Schumacker (1993):

EXAMPLE

The flowrate of gas is 1 liter/s as the gas travels through a large-bore passageway having a diameter of 3 cm (see Fig. 8–4). Such a tube has a cross-sectional area of approximately 7.07 cm². The tube tapers abruptly to a diameter of 2.1 cm; therefore, the area of the constricted tube is approximately one-half that of the original tube (3.46 cm²). The average velocity of the gas is calculated by dividing the flowrate (in cm³/s) by the cross-sectional area (cm²) of the tube.

Velocity of gas in large-diameter tube:

$$V_{avg} = \frac{\dot{V}}{A}$$

$$= \frac{1000 \text{ cm}^3/\text{s}}{7.07 \text{ cm}^2}$$

$$= 141.44 \text{ cm/s}$$

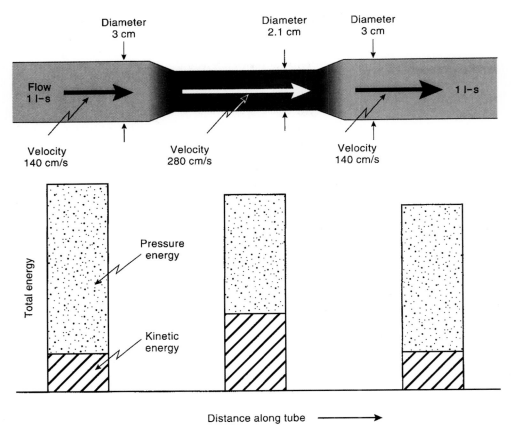

FIGURE 8–4. Convective acceleration (Bernoulli effect) through tubes of different diameter. The Bernoulli principle: When a fluid moves through a tube at a constant flowrate, the total energy of the fluid (potential energy + kinetic energy) decreases because frictional losses convert some of the energy into heat. Increases in fluid velocity occur where the tube narrows, causing an increase in the kinetic energy component ($\frac{1}{2} \rho \mu^2$) at the expense of potential energy (pressure decreases). When the tube widens again, the fluid decelerates and kinetic energy is converted into pressure energy. (From Leff AR and Schumacker PT: Respiratory Physiology: Basics and Applications. WB Saunders, Philadelphia, 1993, p 28, with permission.)

Velocity of gas in small-diameter tube:

$$V_{avg} = \frac{\dot{V}}{A}$$

$$= \frac{1000 \text{ cm}^3/\text{s}}{3.46 \text{ cm}^2}$$

$$= 289.01 \text{ cm/s}$$

From this example it is clear that the fluid must accelerate from a velocity of approximately 141 cm/s to 289 cm/s as it enters the constricted part of the tube to maintain the same flowrate. The hydrostatic pressure falls accordingly within the narrowed part of the tube. The kinetic energy (flow velocity) has increased at the expense of the potential energy (hydrostatic pressure). As the fluid leaves the narrowed part of the tube and enters the larger-diameter portion downstream, it decelerates and the velocity slows considerably. The loss in kinetic energy is converted back to potential (pressure) energy; therefore, the hydrostatic pressure of the system rises. These changes in the proportions of kinetic and potential energy are shown in the graph section of Figure 8–4. Notice that the flowrate is maintained but that the total energy of the system decreases from the proximal to the distal end of the tube. The constant flowrate, as we have seen, is maintained as a result of dynamic changes in pressure and velocity— the Bernoulli effect—as gas flows through passageways of differing diameters. The progressive loss of energy along the passageways occurs as a result of frictional forces and the conversion of some of the energy to heat (Leff and Schumacker, 1993).

According to Taylor et al (1989), the drop in pressure as gas flows from a large-diameter to a smaller-diameter tube is shown by the following relationship:

$$\Delta P \approx \frac{\rho \dot{V}^2}{A}$$

where:
ΔP = pressure gradient (driving pressure)
ρ = density (*rho*) of the gas
$\dot{V}$ = flowrate of the gas
A = area of the tube

The resistance (R) of a fluid to flow is affected by variables such as density, flowrate, and cross-sectional area, and since

$$R = \Delta P / \dot{V}$$

$$R \approx \frac{\rho \dot{V}}{A}$$

The resistance, therefore, is directly proportional to the density and flowrate of the gas, but inversely proportional to the cross-sectional area of the tube.

Now consider what occurs during expiration. As gas leaves the peripheral airways and flows toward the mouth, it enters progressively larger-diameter conducting passageways that are fewer in number. As a result of the declining number of airways, the total cross-sectional area of the proximal (tracheal) end of the conducting system is only about 1/1000 that of the peripheral airways (Taylor et al, 1989). For the same volume of gas to be delivered, a significant increase in gas velocity must occur. The resulting convective acceleration effect causes a dramatic drop in pressure at high flow through these regions of decreased total cross-sectional area. This effect is represented in Figure 8–4 at the point where gas enters the narrowed portion of the tube.

REYNOLDS' NUMBER

Calculation of the **Reynolds' number (Re)** gives an indication of whether the gas flow in a system will exhibit laminar or turbulent characteristics. Reynolds' numbers in excess of 2000 generally indicate that gas flow will be turbulent. The number itself is dimensionless (see following example). As can be seen in the following relationship, the Reynolds' number is directly proportional to three variables: the *diameter* (*D*) of the passageway, the *average velocity* of the gas (*μ*), and the *density* (ρ) of the gas. It is inversely proportional to the *viscosity* (η) of the gas:

$$Re = \frac{D \times \mu \times \rho}{\eta}$$

where:
Re = Reynolds' number (dimensionless)
D = diameter of the airway (cm)
μ = average velocity (*mu*) of the gas (cm/s)
ρ = density (*rho*) of the gas (g/mL)
η = viscosity (*eta*) of the gas (g/s · cm)
       (grams per second per centimeter)

With these factors in mind, it is clear that gas flowing through the larger-diameter passages of the upper airways, such as the nasal cavity, larynx, trachea, and bronchi, will have a larger Reynolds' number indicative of turbulent flow. In addition, as gas flows into the upper airways, which have a small total cross-sectional area, the average velocity of the gas increases. This change in velocity and decrease in pressure is the Bernoulli effect, or convective acceleration. In accordance with the linear (direct) relationship of the Reynolds' equation, as the velocity increases, the Reynolds' number increases. As pointed out above, Reynolds' numbers in excess of 2000 are good predictors of turbulent flow. These findings are in line with observations of actual airflow in the conducting passages: (1) airflow tends to be *laminar* (Re less than 2000) in the peripheral, or distal, airways (toward the alveoli) where the passages have small-diameters and the average airflow velocity is low because of the enormous total cross-sectional area of the system; and (2) airflow tends to be *turbulent* (Re greater than 2000) in the central, or proximal, airways (toward the mouth) where the larger-diameter passages and small total cross-sectional area cause higher velocities to develop. Recall that a higher driving pressure is required to move gas through these high-velocity, low-pressure regions, and that turbulent flow, in general, requires more driving pressure to maintain the same flowrate of gas.

Leff and Schumacker (1993) provide the following data regarding velocity of airflow, density of air, and the viscosity of air. With it we can calculate the Reynolds' number for airflow in the trachea under conditions of normal tidal breathing.

With a flowrate of 1 L/s at the mouth, airflow velocity in a 3-cm-diameter trachea will be approximately 150 cm/s. Air has a density of 0.0012 g/mL and a viscosity of 0.000183 g/s · cm. Therefore, the Reynolds' number (Re) for airflow in the trachea is calculated as follows:

$$Re = \frac{D \times \mu \times \rho}{\eta}$$

$$= \left[3 \text{ cm} \times \frac{150 \text{ cm}}{1 \text{s}} \times \frac{0.0012 \text{ g}}{1 \text{ mL}} \right] \times \frac{1 \text{s} \cdot \text{cm}}{0.000183 \text{ g}}$$

$$= \frac{0.54 \text{ cm}^2 \cdot \cancel{g}}{1 \cancel{s} \cdot \text{mL}} \times \frac{1 \cancel{s} \cdot \text{cm}}{0.000183 \cancel{g}}$$

$$= 2950.8 \frac{\cancel{cm}^3}{\cancel{mL}}$$

$$\therefore Re = 2950.8$$

The calculated value of Reynolds' number is greater than 2000; therefore, the predicted airflow pattern in the trachea will be chaotic and turbulent.

NOTE: The value for Reynolds' number is dimensionless because of the equivalent volume units (1 mL = 1 cm³) used in the calculation. And because 1 L (1000 mL) occupies a cube measuring 10 cm on each side, the volume of such a cube is 10 cm × 10 cm × 10 cm, or 10³ cm³ (1000 cm³). Therefore, 1000 mL = 1000 cm³, and 1 mL = 1 cm³.

Airway Resistance

DETERMINATION OF AIRWAY RESISTANCE

We have examined some of the pressure losses in airways caused by the dynamic effect of moving gas. Recall that the pressure drop along a tube is actually a measure of the *resistance* that must be overcome when a gas is moved through the tube. The factors that contribute to resistance—length and radius of the tube and the viscosity and density of the gas—have been conveniently grouped together as different *constants of proportionality* (K) in the above equations dealing with laminar and turbulent flow. From this we can construct a simplified relationship and conclude that the pressure drop along a tube (ΔP) is determined by the simple product of the resistance (R) and the flowrate ($\dot{V}$):

$$\Delta P = \dot{V} \times R$$

Therefore,

$$R = \frac{\Delta P}{\dot{V}}$$

To analyze the resistance in the tubular components of the conducting and respiratory zone, we need to consider the pressure at the proximal end of the tube (P_1) and the pressure at the distal end of the tube (P_2). From these individual pressures, we can calculate the pressure difference ($P_1 - P_2$, or ΔP) along the tube. The pressure at the proximal end of the tube is called the **mouth pressure (P_m)**, whereas that at the distal end of the conducting tube is the **alveolar pressure (P_a)**. This difference is termed the **transairway pressure (P_{ta})**:

$$P_{ta} = P_m - P_a$$

The **airway resistance (R_{aw})** in a conducting passage is determined by the pressure difference from the proximal end to the distal end of the tube (transairway pressure) divided by the flowrate of the gas:

$$R_{aw} = \frac{P_m - P_a}{\dot{V}}$$

where:
R_{aw} = airway resistance in cm H_2O/L per second
P_m = mouth pressure in cm H_2O
P_a = alveolar pressure in cm H_2O
$\dot{V}$ = flowrate of the gas in L/s

Total airway resistance in a spontaneously breathing adult is normally around 2 cm H_2O/L per second (Des Jardins, 1998; Dupuis, 1992). This value, however, can increase dramatically in obstructive lung disorders such as bronchial asthma, emphysema, or chronic bronchitis.

DISTRIBUTION OF AIRWAY RESISTANCE

Total resistance to the flow of gas through a tubular system is dependent on factors such as the impedance, or resistance, of the individual pipes in the system, and the way in which the pipes are connected together. Assume the pipes in Figure 8–5 all have a resistance of unity. If four of these pipe segments are connected in *series* as shown in Figure 8–5A, the total resistance of the pathway is equal to the sum of the individual resistances of the pipe segments:

$$R_{total} = R_1 + R_2 + R_3 + R_4$$

$$= 1 + 1 + 1 + 1 = 4$$

However, if the pipe segments are connected in *parallel,* the total resistance of the resulting network is *less* than the resistance of any single pipe segment. In Figure 8–5B, the total resistance of the network is one-quarter that of any single segment, as shown in the following relationship:

$$\frac{1}{R_{total}} = \frac{1}{R_1} + \frac{1}{R_2} + \frac{1}{R_3} + \frac{1}{R_4}$$

$$= \frac{1}{4}$$

In a branched system of parallel airways, incoming air has multiple paths to take as it travels toward the peripheral airways. As air enters the tracheobronchial system, it successively passes into smaller-diameter passageways that offer greater and greater resistance to flow. This resistance reaches a peak in the segmental bronchi, between generation 3 and 6 (Leff and Schumacker, 1993). Beyond this point, however, the number of airways increases dramatically, thus increasing the total cross-sectional area of the respiratory tree and lowering the total resistance to flow (Taylor et al, 1989; West, 1998). The system of airways can be viewed as a network of resistances that are arranged in parallel fashion. Because of this unique branching arrangement, most of the airflow resistance occurs in proximal airways whose diameters are greater than 2 mm (Leff and Schumacker, 1993). Substantial airway resistance due to both transitional and turbulent flow is also encountered in the nose, nasal conchae, nasopharynx, and larynx. In fact, it has been estimated that between 25% and 40% of the total airway resistance occurs in the upper airways (Levitzky, 1995; Taylor et al, 1989). Nose breathing, therefore, offers substantially more re-

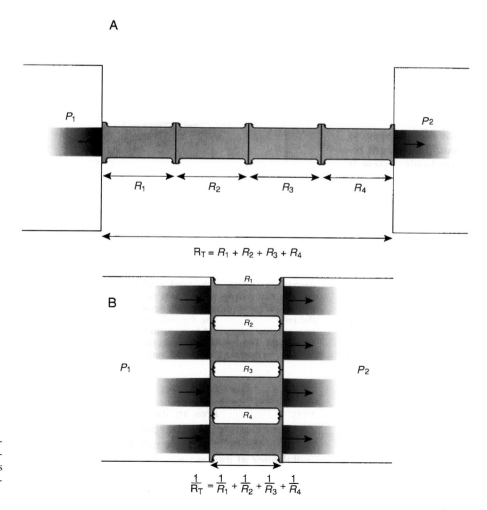

FIGURE 8–5. Flow through pipes. (A) Series; (B) parallel. (From Leff AR and Schumacker PT: Respiratory Physiology: Basics and Applications. WB Saunders, Philadelphia, 1993, p 32, with permission.)

sistance to airflow than does mouth breathing (Taylor et al, 1989). This difference in distribution of resistance in the upper airways is seen with strenuous exercise when breathing automatically shifts to lower-resistance mouth breathing in order to increase the flowrate of air to and from the lungs. Mouth breathing is also seen when viral infections, allergic rhinitis, or occlusions such as nasal polyps substantially increase airway resistance in the nose.

AIRWAY RESISTANCE IN THE "SILENT ZONE"

Figure 8–6 shows the substantial increase in airway resistance found in the intermediate-sized bronchi (generations 5 through 8), and the relatively small amount of resistance present in the smaller-diameter distal airways. Recall that the total cross-sectional area of the distal airways is enormous compared with that of the central airways such as the bronchi and trachea (see Fig. 3–3). As a result of the large total cross-sectional area, the pressure drop in the distal airways is substantial, and the resistance to flow is extremely small. In fact, the forward motion of inspired gas comes to a virtual standstill as the gas reaches this vast system of small airways. Random molecular motion is responsible for the final transfer of gas from the conducting airways to the functional units of the lung. Fortunately, the distance the gas molecules must travel from terminal bronchioles to lung acini is quite short and is completed quickly.

Because of the extremely low resistance of the distal airways, pulmonary clinicians are faced with a formidable diagnostic challenge when it comes to the detection of early airway disease in these structures. The dilemma occurs because the extensively branched system is made up of small-diameter distal airways that comprise a "silent zone" in the lung. Recall that the resistances of the numerous passages are arranged in parallel; therefore, impairment of small airways can be extensive before airway disease is detected through normal measurements of resistance. The large number of parallel pathways effectively masks adverse changes in the total airway resistance of the system. In fact, the entire network of small-diameter airways contributes only around 20% of the total resistance (West, 1998). We now examine how pathophysiologic changes in this "silent zone" can be detected through the measurement of *time constants* and *dynamic compliance*.

Detection of Early Airway Disease in Small Airways

TIME CONSTANTS

A measurement known as the **time constant (T_C)** is the time (in seconds) required to inflate a lung region. This value is the product of airway resistance (R_{aw}) and static lung compliance (C_{st}):

$$T_C = R_{aw} \times C_{st}$$

$$T_C = \frac{\Delta P}{\dot{V}} \times \frac{\Delta V}{\Delta P} = \frac{\Delta V}{\dot{V}}$$

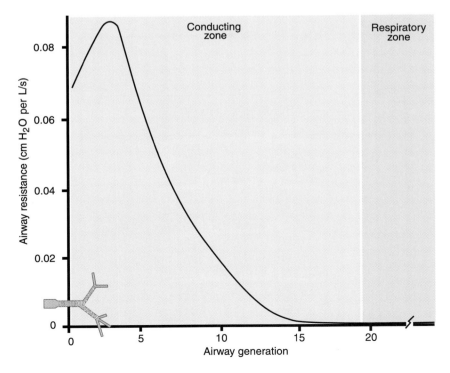

FIGURE 8–6. Airway resistance and airway generations. Note that the intermediate-sized airways (e.g., generations 1–5) are responsible for most of the airway resistance in the system. By contrast, very little resistance is caused by the small-diameter distal airways, beginning with the terminal bronchioles (e.g., generations 16–19). (Adapted from West JB: Respiratory Physiology: The Essentials, ed 5. Williams & Wilkins, Baltimore, 1995, p 107, with permission.)

where:

T_C = time constant (in seconds)
ΔP = pressure gradient (driving pressure)
V = flowrate of the gas
ΔV = volume gradient

As can be seen from this relationship, if the airway resistance or compliance is increased, the alveoli in the lung unit supplied by the restricted passageways will take longer to fill. Such lung units are said to have a *long time constant*. By contrast, if airway resistance is lowered or static lung compliance is decreased, the affected alveoli fill faster and, therefore, exhibit a *short time constant*. Recall, however, that a lung with reduced compliance is stiff and difficult to expand. The overall capacity of such a lung, therefore, is less than that of a lung having more compliance, even though the less-compliant lung can fill at a faster rate. At higher breathing frequencies, a lung region having a long time constant does not have adequate time to fill completely (Laszlo, 1994).

DYNAMIC LUNG COMPLIANCE

Dynamic lung compliance (C_{dyn}) reflects how readily a lung region fills during a period of gas flow. Such a value is profoundly affected by the time constant of the alveoli in the region being inflated. Uneven time constants cause a change in dynamic compliance that is related to the breathing frequency. If respiratory frequency is rapid, alveoli having long time constants do not fill completely. Therefore, pressure is not equalized throughout the lung, and a small lung volume results for a given inspiratory effort compared with that obtained through breathing at lower frequencies (Laszlo, 1994).

Although direct measurement of dynamic compliance was commonly performed in the past, it has been found that for a normal, healthy lung, the ratio of dynamic compliance to static compliance is about the same (1:1) throughout all breathing frequencies (Laszlo, 1994). In patients with partially obstructed airways, however, the ratio of dynamic compliance to static compliance decreases as the rate of breathing increases. Alveoli in such an obstructed lung exhibit a long time constant and, therefore, have insufficient time to fill. The compliance of such obstructed units is described as *frequency dependent*. By contrast, compliance is termed *frequency independent* in lung units having equal time constants. Dynamic compliance is measured in liters per centimeters of water (L/cm H_2O) at a series of frequencies from about 10 up to 120 breaths per minute (West, 1998).

As we have seen in lungs with airway disease of the "silent zone," the measurement of compliance during periods of quiet breathing does not provide a satisfactory means of assessing airway status because of the uneven time constants in different regions of the lungs.

Dynamic compliance, on the other hand, can be viewed as "apparent compliance," or the relative ability of the lung to expand under dynamic conditions of gas flow—expansion that is evident during periods of heavy breathing. At higher breathing frequencies the time for inspiration becomes less and less and the dynamic compliance decreases. This decrease in the apparent compliance of the lung occurs because regions of the lungs that have long time constants are slow to fill; consequently, they receive less and less of the tidal volume. Viewed another way, as dynamic compliance decreases, a smaller and smaller volume of the lung participates in each breath (West, 1998).

To illustrate these relationships, we will compare the dynamic compliance of two respiratory systems—one system with equal time constants, the other having uneven time constants (Fig. 8–7). The systems are composed of lungs each having static compliance (C_{st}) equal to 0.15 L/cm H_2O. Therefore, the total static lung compliance of each system is 0.3 L/cm H_2O, which is the sum of the two individual lung compliances. Static lung compliance and dynamic lung compliance are assumed to be equal. System A is composed of two normal, healthy lungs that are unobstructed and have identical time constants. As breathing frequency increases in System A, the "apparent," or dynamic compliance, does not change from its static value (see Fig. 8–7). Dynamic compliance, therefore, is frequency in-

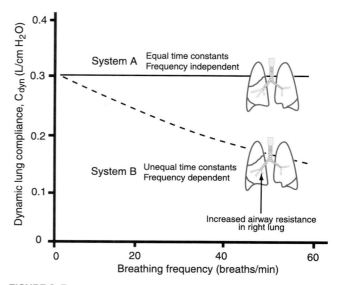

FIGURE 8–7. Dynamic compliance and breathing frequency. System A consists of two lungs having equal time constants. System B consists of two lungs having unequal time constants because of marked airway resistance in one lung. Note that the dynamic lung compliance of the lung units in System A is independent of the breathing frequency, whereas the dynamic lung compliance of the lung units in System B is frequency dependent. At higher frequencies, there is insufficient time for air to enter the obstructed lung, an indication of early airway disease. (Adapted from Taylor AE et al: Clinical Respiratory Physiology. WB Saunders, Philadelphia, 1989, p 124, with permission.)

dependent for lung units having equal time constants. By contrast, when one of the lungs is supplied by a narrowed airway, as shown in System B, differences in static and dynamic compliance become apparent. At low frequencies, the values are the same as those obtained with System A. However, as the breathing rate increases, the dynamic lung compliance decreases as less and less air enters the lung supplied by the obstructed airway. As pointed out previously, such compliance is said to be frequency dependent. Therefore, at higher ventilation rates, gas is only able to ventilate the normal lung in System B. There is simply not enough time in a shortened ventilatory cycle to move air into and out of a lung that has a long time constant. As a result of this time limitation, the *total* dynamic compliance of System B decreases to that of a single, unobstructed lung (0.1 L/cm H_2O). Frequency-dependent dynamic compliance, therefore, may be indicative of early airway disease. Such a measurement offers clinicians a means of detection that static measurements of lung compliance cannot provide.

Work of Breathing

FACTORS CONTRIBUTING TO LUNG RESISTANCE

A lung that is changing volume over time offers more resistance to airflow than a lung that is inflated and deflated under static conditions. The impedance encountered when lung volume changes is called **lung resistance.** The additional pleural pressure required to overcome lung resistance during dynamic conditions depends on the rate at which the lung volume is changing. A rapid change in lung volume requires a greater pleural pressure gradient than that required to change the lung volume slowly. Why would this relationship between driving pressure and the rate of volume change under dynamic conditions be fundamentally different from the conditions that exist during a static lung inflation or deflation to a given volume?

Dynamic conditions involving changes in lung volume over time differ wo basic ways from static inflation or deflation that does not change over time. To start with, the effect of airway resistance on moving air has an important bearing on overall lung resistance because of the pressure decrease that occurs when air enters passageways having a small total cross-sectional area. Recall that this convective acceleration (Bernoulli) effect is responsible for a decrease in hydrostatic pressure in conducting passages.

Second, when lung volume changes rapidly, **tissue viscous resistance** contributes to total lung resistance. Such impedance to air flow is caused by slippage of various lung structures such as pleural membranes,

lung parenchyma, and lung interstitium as they slide past one another during inflation and deflation. By contrast, when the lung is inflated or deflated *slowly*, this viscous effect in the tissues is minimal and contributes little to overall lung resistance. Collectively, lung resistance produced by airway resistance and tissue viscous resistance is referred to as **nonelastic resistance.** This type of resistance is distinct from **elastic resistance** produced by the static elastic recoil of the lung and thorax (Fig. 8–8).

An analogy to help illustrate these different components of resistance is presented by the bellows model shown in Figure 8–9. When the bellows is pumped to move air into and out of the device, much of the resistance to air movement is related to the size of the nozzle where air enters and exits. Changes in the nozzle size affect the airflow of the bellows much like changes in airway resistance affect lung resistance. If the bellows is operated rapidly, the airflow resistance of the nozzle adds considerable resistance to the overall system and more force has to be applied to the handles of the bellows to increase the frequency of operation. Internal moving parts of the bellows such as the accordion folds have intrinsic resistance to changing volume that also adds to the impedance (see Fig. 8–9). If the bellows is gently squeezed and slowly deflated, and then slowly expanded and inflated again, the volume change produced is very gradual and gentle. Under these conditions, internal resistance—the viscous resistance of the device—is relatively low. However, if the bellows is operated rapidly to produce large volume changes over time, the added viscous resistance of the internal moving parts of the bellows must be overcome by the application of additional force to the handles of the bellows. (In the respiratory system, additional lung resistance is overcome by the application of a higher pleural pressure.) Finally, the bellows analogy is useful for illustrating the elastic resistance of the lung. The spring shown in Figure 8–9 represents the elastic resistance in the lung and thorax that must be overcome whenever the handles are pulled apart to inflate the bellows.

OVERCOMING LUNG RESISTANCE

The **work of breathing (WOB)** is the amount of work that must be performed by the muscles of ventilation to overcome the combined effect of airway resistance, tiss viscous resistance, and elastic resistance factorie lung.call that normal quiet breathing requires contraction of respiratory muscles during inspiration only and that elastic recoil of the lung and chest wall occurs during passive expiration. Therefore, ventilatory muscle "work" under quiet conditions is performed only during inspiration.

Static resistance factors such as elasticity of the lung

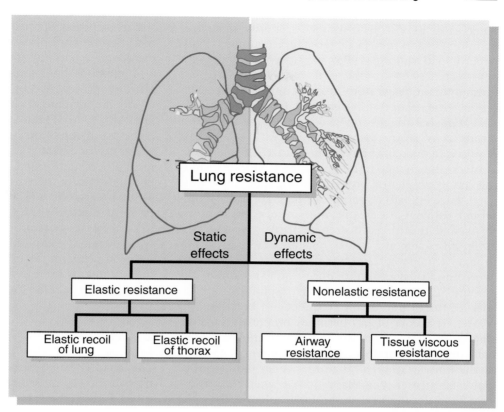

FIGURE 8–8. Elastic and nonelastic resistance.

interstitium, the elasticity imparted by the surface tension effects of alveolar fluid, and the elasticity of the chest wall collectively make up a component of total resistance that must be overcome by **elastic work,** also known as **compliance work.** The elastic work required to inflate the entire respiratory system is less than that required to inflate the lungs alone if they are removed from the chest. This finding is consistent with the compliance values already discussed, namely that the compliance of the *combined* lung-thorax system (C_T = 0.11 L/cm H_2O) is slightly over half that of the lungs alone and is *less than* the sum of the compliance of the lung (C_{st} = 0.2 L/cm H_2O) added to that of the chest wall (C_{cw} = 0.244 L/cm H_2O). Recall that compliance of the lung is in parallel with that of the chest wall and that the compliance values are added reciprocally (see Chap. 7). Stated another way, a portion of the work required to inflate the lungs comes from the elastic energy stored in the thorax. The energy lost from the thorax is gained by the lungs (Ganong, 1995).

The balance of the total resistance in the respiratory system is due to dynamic factors that are overcome by **nonelastic work.** Nonelastic factors include *airway resistance* due to the flow of gas through a tube, and *tissue viscous resistance* caused by slippage of tissue surfaces past one another as they are displaced during the movements of breathing. Airway resistance contributes approximately 80% of the total nonelastic resistance,

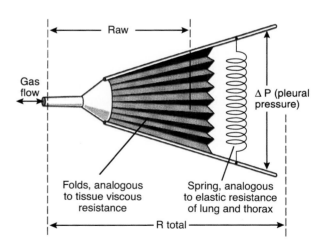

FIGURE 8–9. Bellows analogy and lung resistance. By analogy, respiratory system resistance is similar to the resistance encountered in operating a fireplace bellows (with spring attached). Part of the resistance encountered is due to the work of driving flow through airways that narrow in total area from the alveolus toward the mouth (airways resistance). Another component relates to the resistance in moving the bellows itself, as would be encountered if operated in a vacuum (tissue viscous resistance). The spring represents the force that would be required to operate the bellows very slowly (static lung recoil). R_{aw} = airway resistance; R_{total} = total lung resistance; ΔP = pleural pressure. (From Leff AR and Schumacker PT: Respiratory Physiology: Basics and Applications. WB Saunders, Philadelphia, 1993, p 31, with permission.)

whereas tissue viscous resistance accounts for the remaining 20% of nonelastic resistance (Dupuis, 1992). According to Ganong (1995), elastic work accounts for approximately 65% of the total work of breathing performed by the respiratory muscles during quiet inspiration. Nonelastic work accounts for the remaining 35%, which is roughly divided between the work necessary to overcome viscous resistance (7%) and that required to overcome airway resistance (28%).

When the change in lung volume is plotted against the change in pleural pressure during quiet breathing, the total work of breathing can be graphically represented, showing the relative amount of work required to expand the lungs, overcome tissue viscous resistance, and overcome airway resistance (Fig. 8–10). Although a moderate amount of work is expended to overcome airway resistance during quiet breathing, the amount increases dramatically as respiratory rate increases. Recall that as the frequency of breathing increases, the flow of gas becomes progressively more chaotic, changing from laminar to transitional, and finally to a turbulent flow pattern. The energy expended by the muscles of breathing to move air that is turbulent is far greater than that required when the airflow is laminar. Recall also that during turbulent airflow, the pressure drop in the tube is proportional to the *square* of the flowrate. Hence, higher flowrates cause a profound increase in the pressure gradient across the tube, and the pressure gradient across a tube represents the resistance that must be overcome in the conducting system. Therefore, at higher rates of breathing, the *proportion* of the total work normally expended to overcome airway resistance must increase further to overcome even greater airway resistance. This increased airway resistance is encountered at higher airflow velocities that accompany higher breathing frequencies.

The *total* work of breathing increases dramatically in many pulmonary diseases. For example, in restrictive disorders such as pulmonary fibrosis there is generally an increase in both compliance work and tissue resistance work, whereas in obstructive disorders, there is usually an increase in airway resistance work (Guyton and Hall, 1996). Finally, in activities such as heavy exercise, or in conditions where there is elevated airway resistance or elevated tissue resistance, *expiratory work* must also be performed. In fact, expiratory work often becomes greater than inspiratory work in patients with asthma (Guyton and Hall, 1996). This situation occurs because of greatly increased airway resistance caused, in part, by the dynamic compression of collapsible airways during the expiration phase of breathing. In the following chapter we explore some of the spirometric measurements used to assess expiratory volumes and flows during spontaneous breathing.

Summary

This chapter has explored the factors contributing to pressure losses caused by the effect of moving gas in tubes. In it we have focused on a comparison of laminar and turbulent flow and examined the phenomenon of convective acceleration to help explain the pressure changes observed as gas flows from one part of the respiratory system to another. A brief discussion of the distribution, significance, and measurement of airway resistance was presented in conjunction with an explanation of time constants and dynamic lung compliance. Finally, the elastic and inelastic resistance factors that contribute to the work of breathing were explored. The chapter points out that the forces necessary to overcome airway resistance increase as the fre-

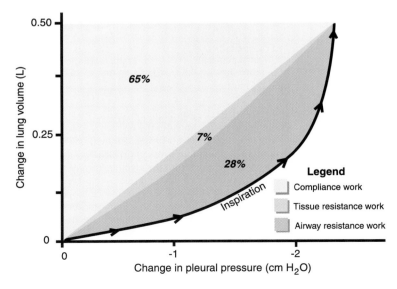

FIGURE 8–10. Work of breathing—change in lung volume as a function of the change in pleural pressure. The *total* work of breathing overcomes the combined resistance of the respiratory system and consists of three different types of work performed during inspiration: (1) compliance of work, (2) tissue resistance work, and (3) airway resistance work. Most of the change in lung volume is due to the performance of compliance work, also known as *elastic work*. Note that the percentages in the art refer to percentage of total work performed. (Adapted from Guyton AC: Textbook of Medical Physiology, ed 8. WB Saunders, Philadelphia, 1991, p 406, with permission.)

quency of breathing increases. It is emphasized that these dynamic factors occur during actual ventilatory cycles, and are not considered during assessment of the statics of breathing when there is zero gas flow.

BIBLIOGRAPHY

D'Angelo E and Milic-Emil J: Dynamics of the Respiratory System. In Roussos C (ed): The Thorax: Part A: Physiology, ed 2. Marcel Dekker, New York, 1995.

Des Jardins T: Cardiopulmonary Anatomy and Physiology: Essentials for Respiratory Care, ed 3. Delmar Publishers, Albany, NY, 1998.

Dupuis YG: Ventilators: Theory and Clinical Application, ed 2. Mosby–Year Book, St. Louis, 1992.

Ganong WF: Review of Medical Physiology, ed 17. Appleton & Lange, Norwalk, CT, 1995.

Guyton, AC: Textbook of Medical Physiology, ed 8. WB Saunders, Philadelphia, 1991.

Guyton AC and Hall JE: Textbook of Medical Physiology, ed 9. WB Saunders, Philadelphia, 1996.

Laszlo G: Pulmonary Function: A Guide For Clinicians. Cambridge University Press, 1994.

Leff AR and Schumacker PT: Respiratory Physiology: Basics and Applications. WB Saunders, Philadelphia, 1993.

Levitzky MG: Pulmonary Physiology, ed 4. McGraw-Hill, New York, 1995.

Taylor AE et al: Clinical Respiratory Physiology. WB Saunders, Philadelphia, 1989.

West JB: Respiratory Physiology: The Essentials, ed 5. Williams & Wilkins, Baltimore, 1995.

West JB: Respiratory Physiology: The Essentials, ed 6. Williams & Wilkins, Baltimore, 1998.

CHAPTER 9

Pulmonary Mechanics

chapter objectives

After studying this chapter the reader should be able to:

☐ Name three practical uses for pulmonary function tests.

☐ Explain why determination of arterial blood gases may not always reveal the extent of functional impairment in the lung.

☐ Define the following terms:
Minute ventilation, maximal voluntary ventilation (ventilatory capacity).

☐ Describe the general shape of a flow-volume loop by analyzing the shape of the forced inspiratory curve and the shape of the forced expiratory curve.

☐ Compare and contrast effort-dependent and effort-independent flowrates.

☐ Define the following terms:
Choke point, transmural pressure, dynamic compression.

☐ Explain the mechanism of expiratory flow limitation by describing the action of choke points in the collapsible airways.

☐ Explain why a slow and gentle expiration does not cause dynamic compression of airways.

☐ Define equal pressure point and describe why the equal pressure point moves toward the alveoli as the lung volume decreases during forced expiration.

☐ Define closing volume and explain why the closing volume increases in obstructive lung diseases such as emphysema.

☐ Define the following terms:
Forced vital capacity (FVC), forced expiratory flow between 25% and 75% of FVC
($FEF_{25\%-75\%}$), forced expiratory volume in 1 second (FEV_1).

☐ List three pathophysiologic factors in the lung that can modify the expiratory flow-volume value.

☐ Compare and contrast the mechanisms of obstructive disease (e.g., emphysema) and restrictive disease (e.g., pulmonary fibrosis) by discussing the significance of spirometric values obtained for total lung capacity (TLC), residual volume (RV), FVC, $FEF_{25\%-75\%}$, and FEV_1.

key terms

choke points
closing volume
dynamic compression
effort-dependent flowrate
effort-independent flowrate
equal pressure point
flow-volume curve
flow-volume loop
forced expiratory flow between 25% and 75% of
 FVC (FEF$_{25\%-75\%}$)

forced expiratory volume in 1 second (FEV$_1$)
forced vital capacity (FVC)
maximal voluntary ventilation (MVV); ventilatory
 capacity
minute ventilation
obstructive disease
restrictive disease
transmural pressure (P$_{tm}$)

In this chapter we introduce the fundamental measurements performed in spirometric studies of forced ventilation. The brief chapter is not designed to be a comprehensive resource covering the techniques and technical aspects of pulmonary function testing (PFT), nor is it meant to be a definitive guide for the interpretation of PFT data. Rather, it introduces some of the basic measurements in lung dynamics that are commonly encountered by the respiratory care practitioner. Performance of proper PFT procedures is generally stressed in practical courses in respiratory care, whereas the interpretation and significance of PFT findings is usually reinforced in diagnostic testing and pulmonary pathophysiology courses.

Early Detection of Pulmonary Impairment

The application of theoretical principles to applied function is seen with *pulmonary function tests* (PFTs). The dynamics of the mechanics of breathing are measured in these objective diagnostic tests which are employed in the following:

- Evaluation of patients with chronic dyspnea
- Determination of severity of impairment of the respiratory system
- Assessment of patient response to therapeutic measures
- Bronchoprovocation testing and evaluation of pulmonary drugs

This list is by no means exhaustive. In fact, spirometric tests of lung function to measure lung volumes, lung capacities, and forced ventilatory maneuvers only tell part of the story. In general, pulmonary function studies also include determination of oxygen uptake, evaluation of oxygen and carbon dioxide transport, measurement of the diffusing capacity of the lung for carbon monoxide, determination of acid-base distur-

bances in the bloodstream, and exercise testing. Several of these determinants of pulmonary function such as arterial blood gases, diffusing capacity of the lung, and pH disturbances are described in subsequent chapters.

Because of the importance of the cardiopulmonary system in maintaining normal blood levels of oxygen and carbon dioxide, determination of arterial blood gases may appear to be one of the most important diagnostic and assessment measures available to the clinician. However, the respiratory system has such a vast functional reserve capacity that considerable disease or damage of the lungs can occur and the arterial blood gas values remain near normal. For example, a portion of the lung can be surgically removed and still have no significant effect on the arterial blood oxygen or carbon dioxide levels if the unaffected lung maintains adequate alveolar ventilation and perfusion to support gas exchange (Farzan and Farzan, 1997). Abnormal blood gas values often indicate functional respiratory impairment, whereas normal values do not necessarily indicate normal lungs. Assessment of lung mechanics, however, often reveals early impairment of the respiratory system and is thus useful in the determination of the severity and progression of the disease, and in the response of the disease to therapeutic measures (Farzan and Farzan, 1997).

Pulmonary Mechanics and Forced Expiratory Flow Measurements

As pointed out previously, the reserve capacity of the respiratory system is substantial. To put this statement in perspective, consider that an adult breathing at rest moves approximately 7 to 10 liters of air per minute. This value is called the **minute ventilation** and is the product of the depth and rate of breathing. During strenuous exercise the minute ventilation can exceed 100 L/min, and in a young healthy subject breathing as hard as possible for 15 seconds, the **maximal voluntary ventilation (MVV)** or **ventilatory capacity** can reach 200 L/min (Leff and Schumacker, 1993). Such a wide range of values illustrates the impressive reserve capacity of normal lungs. It is not surprising that the respiratory system can be considerably stressed by lung diseases with little or no impairment of its ability to meet the metabolic needs of the body *at rest*. However, during pulmonary function tests that measure airflow during *maximal expiration,* early detection of respiratory impairment is possible.

Recall that spirometric tests are used in studies of static lung function to measure changes in lung volume during quiet breathing and during maximal inspiration and expiration (see Fig. 7–1). Spirograms show changes in volume on the *y*-axis (ΔV) as a function of time on the *x*-axis (Δt). Therefore, the slope of any line on a spirogram has units of $\Delta V/\Delta t$, and this relationship (in liters per second) is equivalent to flowrate. The PFT subject is instructed to inhale to TLC and then exhale as forcefully as possible to residual volume (RV). Figure 9–1 shows the type of tracing obtained from this forced expiratory maneuver. It can be seen that the expiratory flowrate is higher (steeper slope) at the beginning of the exhalation compared with that toward the end of expiration.

FLOW-VOLUME MEASUREMENTS

The Flow-Volume Curve

The instantaneous flowrate (in L/s) can be plotted as a function of volume to produce a **flow-volume curve** (Fig. 9–2). As can be seen by the scale on the graph, flows above the horizontal line are expiratory, flows below the line are inspiratory, lung volumes are lowest toward the right, and lung volumes are highest toward the left. The combined inspiratory and expiratory flow-volume curves make up the **flow-volume loop.** Notice that the *exhaled* lung volume is plotted on the *x-axis;* therefore, volumes are lowest at the right side of the graph. In addition, maximal inspiratory flow is about the same or slightly higher than the maximal expiratory flow (see Fig. 9–2). During inspiration the inspiratory flow decreases as the lung volume increases. This decrease in flowrate occurs because the static recoil pressure of the lung increases as the lung expands, thus opposing the force being generated by the contraction of the inspiratory muscles.

Under normal conditions, the peak inspiratory flow occurs about midway between the TLC and RV. The situation is fundamentally different, however, for the expiratory part of the curve. During forced expiration the expiratory flowrate rises rapidly in the first part of the

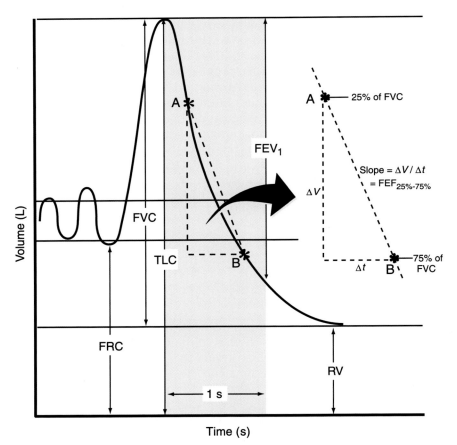

FIGURE 9–1. Spirogram—forced expiratory maneuvers. FVC = forced vital capacity; TLC = total lung capacity; FRC = functional residual capacity; RV = residual volume; FEV_1 = forced expiratory volume in 1 second; $FEF_{25\%-75\%}$ = forced expiratory flow between 25% and 75% of FVC. Note that the slope of any line represents the change in volume as a function of time ($\Delta V/\Delta t$), and is a measurement of flowrate in liters per second (L/s). (Adapted from Leff AR and Schumacker PT: Respiratory Physiology: Basics and Applications. WB Saunders, Philadelphia, 1993, p 37, with permission.)

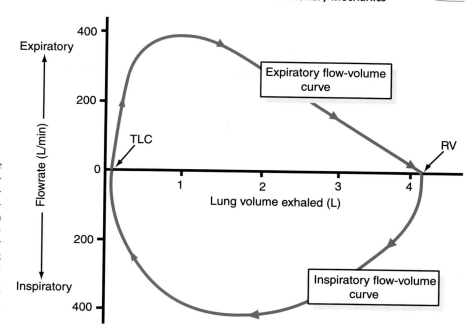

FIGURE 9–2. Flow-volume loop—single expiratory effort. TLC = total lung capacity; RV = residual volume. The instantaneous exhaled flowrate is plotted as a function of exhaled volume to produce a flow-volume loop consisting of an inspiratory flow-volume curve and an expiratory flow-volume curve. Notice that the lung volumes are lowest toward the right and highest toward the left and that the maximal inspiratory flow is the same as or slightly higher than the maximal expiratory flow.

maneuver and reaches its peak early as evidenced by the steep slope of the line representing forced exhalation beginning at TLC (see Fig. 9–2). However, the expiratory flowrate decreases progressively in the latter two-thirds of the expiration, and the slope of the line becomes less steep. Pathologic conditions in the lung may be reflected by changes in the shape of this part of the forced expiratory flow-volume curve. Consequently, the test has become a reliable, sensitive, and reproducible indicator of pulmonary function (Leff and Schumacker, 1993). We now examine why this test is such a useful component of pulmonary function testing.

Effort-Dependent and Effort-Independent Flowrates

Quiet tidal breathing produces characteristic small nested loops in the middle of the flow-volume tracing (Fig. 9–3). However, when a subject performs several forced expirations using differing degrees of effort, interesting features of the flow-volume loop are noted. Figure 9–3 shows three flow-volume loops obtained when a subject forcefully exhales from TLC using progressively greater effort to force air out of the lungs. Notice that both the peak inspiratory flow and peak expiratory flow are **effort-dependent flowrates.** That is, as more ventilatory *effort* is expended with each trial, a higher inspiratory and expiratory flowrate is obtained. Although the peak flowrates occur at different parts of the two maneuvers, the magnitude of the flowrate achieved is related to the respiratory effort of the subject.

Notice also that as the exertion increases, the flowrate in the latter phase of the expiration becomes the same for all expiration trials, and the three curves converge (see Fig. 9–3). In other words, even when the

subject forcefully exhales with maximal effort, the flowrate achieved will be the same as when the subject quietly exhales expending minimal effort. This latter phase of expiration is characterized by an **effort-independent flowrate** because the flowrate achieved is *independent* of the force being generated by the expiratory muscles. In the range that begins after lung volume has fallen by about 20%, the expiratory rate is said to be *flow-limited* by the characteristics of the lung itself (Leff and Schumacker, 1993). Therefore, during most of forced expiration, maximum flow is determined by factors other than effort. According to West (1998), a person cannot breathe "outside" this flow-limited part of the forced expiratory flow curve, no matter how strenuous the exhalation (see Fig. 9–3). What structural and dynamic characteristics in the lung account for such a remarkable finding and, more important, how are these findings derived from forced expiratory flow studies used in the detection and diagnosis of early airway disease?

Mechanism of Expiratory Flow Limitation

The flow-limited phase of forced expiration is due to several factors that include the creation of **choke points** within the airways during exhalation. A choke point is a specific site in the airway where the airway collapses as a result of a negative **transmural pressure (P_{tm}).** This pressure is the difference between the inside and the outside of the airway and is determined by the opposing effects of intrapleural pressure pressing inward on the airway and the outward elastic recoil pressure of the airway (Leff and Schumacker, 1993; Levitzky, 1995). In the alveolus this relationship can be shown by:

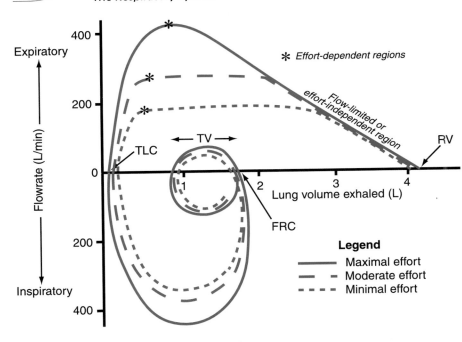

FIGURE 9–3. Effort-independent and effort-dependent regions of forced expiratory flow. TLC = total lung capacity; RV = residual volume; FRC = functional residual capacity; TV = tidal volume. Notice the small nested loops characteristic of quiet tidal breathing (TV). Peak inspiratory and expiratory flowrates are proportional to the ventilatory effort expended (*effort-dependent regions*). During forced expiration, the maximal flow achieved is determined by factors other than the effort expended (*flow-limited* or *effort-independent region*). (Adapted from Leff AR and Schumacker PT: Respiratory Physiology: Basics and Applications. WB Saunders, Philadelphia, 1993, p 39, with permission.)

$$P_{tp} = P_{alv} - P_{pl}$$

where:

P_{tp} = transpulmonary pressure (the transmural pressure, P_{tm}, acting across the airway)

P_{alv} = alveolar pressure

P_{pl} = pleural pressure

NOTE: The concept of a *transmural* pressure gradient can be applied to the pressure difference across any wall, including the chest wall or a blood vessel wall.)

If the distal airways are visualized as floppy, distensible tubes embedded in an air pump, it can be seen that as the pump pressure increases, the tubes are prone to collapse at some critical pressure, an effect known as **dynamic compression.** A useful analogy to help understand what occurs when the transmural pressure in an airway becomes negative is to consider what happens when one attempts to draw water through a floppy, "water-logged" paper soda straw (Fig. 9–4). We will consider the transmural pressure simply as the pressure difference across the wall of the drinking straw (pressure inside the drinking straw minus the pressure outside the drinking straw). If one attempts to forcefully draw water up a soda straw that is soggy and saturated with water, the pressure inside the straw (small arrows) becomes negative with respect to barometric pressure (large arrows), and the straw collapses, preventing fluid from rising up the straw (see Fig. 9–4). On the other hand, if water is drawn up the straw very slowly and gently, dynamic compression does not occur because the distending pressure inside the straw is just sufficient to counter the collapse pressure outside the straw.

Dynamic compression occurs during forced expiration to create a choke point or a critical narrowing of the airway when the pressure within the airway no longer opposes the pressure surrounding the airway (Box 9–1). If expiration occurs slowly and gently, the intrapleural pressure is low enough to not cause collapse of the floppy tubes in the pump. However, in a forced expiration, the high pressure generated outside the tubes causes their collapse, much as the soggy paper straw is collapsed in a forceful attempt to draw water up the straw (see Fig. 9–4). To achieve a low lung volume during forced expiration, contraction of the abdominals and internal intercostal muscles generates a positive intrapleural pressure which can be as high as +120 cm H_2O. Maximal inspiratory intrapleural pressures, on the other hand, may fall as low as −80 cm H_2O during forced ventilatory maneuvers (Levitzky, 1995).

The pressure in an airway immediately before critical closure occurs is called the **equal pressure point.** The transmural pressure at this point is equal to zero. The location of the equal pressure point progressively moves distally toward the alveoli as the lung volume decreases during forced expiration. The change in the location is caused by (1) the intrapleural pressure increases as the muscular effort of expiration increases (thus increasing the *collapse* pressure outside the airway); and (2) the progressive decrease in lung volume causes the elastic recoil pressure of the airway to diminish (thus decreasing the *distending* pressure inside the airway). Let us look briefly at these two effects.

First, recall that noncartilaginous airways have minimal external support and are, therefore, easily collapsed. They are exquisitely sensitive to the degree of bronchomotor tone in their walls and to the pressures

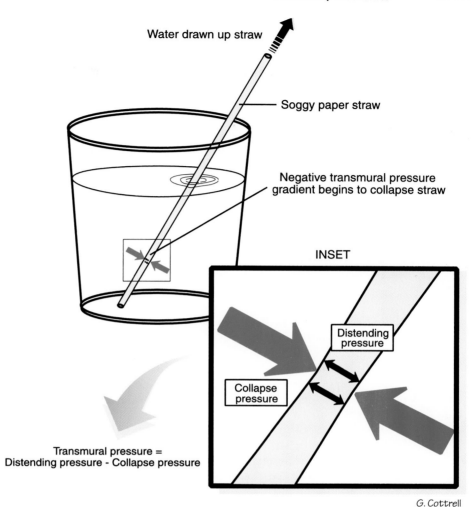

Water drawn up straw

Soggy paper straw

Negative transmural pressure
gradient begins to collapse straw

INSET

Distending
pressure

Collapse
pressure

Transmural pressure =
Distending pressure - Collapse pressure

FIGURE 9–4. Floppy tubes and choke points. In this analogy, when one attempts to forcefully draw water up a soda straw that is soggy and saturated with water, the pressure inside the straw (small arrows) becomes negative with respect to barometric pressure (large arrows), causing the straw to collapse. The critical pressure point occurs as a result of dynamic compression of the collapsible tube to create a choke point. If water is drawn up slowly and gently, the critical narrowing of the tube is not reached.

G. Cottrell

that surround them in the lung. Therefore, an increase in intrapleural pressure tends to decrease the transmural pressure in the small airways, thus increasing airway resistance as the airways begin to constrict. Such a change in airway resistance contributes tremendously to flow-limited forced expiration and helps explain the effort-independent portion of the curve (see Fig. 9–3). The increase in intrapleural pressure in a forced expiration increases the driving pressure for expiratory flow, but the effect is largely canceled out by the development of a choke point.

Second, recall that stabilization of the alveoli and small airways of the lung includes a meshwork of elastin fibers in the lung interstitium. These fibers connect small airways to each other and to surrounding alveolar units (see Fig. 2–8). The resulting *radial traction*, or *mechanical tethering*, of airways helps maintain their patency. However, as lung volume decreases, this elastic recoil effect becomes less pronounced. Consequently, the equal pressure point moves distally toward smaller airways and dynamic compression increases. At a critical point during forced expiration the transmural pressure becomes negative and a choke point develops (Leff

and Schumacker, 1993; Levitzky, 1995). The increase in airway resistance caused by reduced radial traction, like that caused by elevated intrapleural pressure, contributes to the effort-independent portion of forced expiration. The lung volume at which this critical collapse of airways *begins* to occur is called the **closing volume.** Such airway closure generally occurs in healthy subjects only at very low lung volumes, but in patients with chronic obstructive pulmonary diseases (COPDs) such as emphysema, where there is profound loss of radial traction, the closing volume typically occurs at higher lung volumes, causing severe breathing difficulties (Levitzky, 1995).

In summary, the delicate balance that maintains transmural pressure in the noncartilaginous airways is affected by a variety of opposing factors. The most important factor responsible for maintaining a *positive* airway transmural pressure is a high lung static recoil pressure (high lung volume) that keeps the airway pressure higher than the surrounding pleural pressure. Antagonistic factors that cause a *negative* airway transmural pressure and thus contribute to expiratory flow-limitation include (1) flow-resistive pressure losses

BOX 9-1

Wave Speed Theory—The Physics of Expiratory Flow Limitation

Choke points develop in airways when the transmural pressure becomes negative, causing the wall of the airway to collapse inward. This critical closure of an airway depends on the rigidity, or stiffness, of the tube. The rigidity is determined by structural and functional factors such as the amount of supporting cartilage in the wall, the degree of bronchomotor tone of airway smooth muscle, and the radial traction provided by elastic connective tissue tethered to the outside of the airways. Clearly, the development of choke points will occur at much lower transmural pressures in collapsible, noncartilaginous airways.

The *tube wave speed flow,* or theoretical maximum flow that can occur in floppy tubes, is determined by the product of the velocity of propagation of a pressure wave along the tube (the *tube wave speed*), and the *cross-sectional area* of the tube at that point. As the transmural pressure across an airway becomes negative, the cross-sectional area decreases to a minimum. At higher transmural pressures, airway diameter and cross-sectional area increase, but as the elastic elements of the lung parenchyma become stretched to their maximum, further gains in cross-sectional area become minimal.

The tube wave speed flow that an airway can support is thus increased by mechanical factors such as parenchymal tethering at high lung volumes and by supporting cartilage that increases airway rigidity. These factors either increase the cross-sectional area of a tube at a particular point or prevent its collapse. As the actual flow in an airway increases, it reaches a point where it equals the tube wave speed flow. Above this maximum flow a choke point forms and expiratory flow is limited. This limitation is the basis of the effort-independent phase of expiration. The physics of airflow in floppy tubes thus provides insight into the phenomenon of expiratory flow limitation. The theoretical maximum flow, or tube wave speed flow ($\dot{V}_{ws}$), is given by the following equation:

$$\dot{V}_{ws} = \left[\frac{1}{\rho} \times \frac{dP_{tm}}{dA} \right]^{1/2} \times A^{3/2}$$

where:

$\dot{V}_{ws}$	= tube wave speed flow
ρ	= density of the gas
A	= tube cross-sectional area
P_{tm}	= transmural pressure
dP_{tm}/dA	= elasticity of the tube

- Leff AR and Schumacker PT: Respiratory Physiology: Basics and Applications. WB Saunders, Philadelphia, 1993.

(caused by frictional pressure loss) associated with the flow of gas from the alveoli toward the mouth (see Fig. 8–3); (2) convective acceleration pressure losses within airways as gas flows toward the mouth into fewer parallel airways having a smaller total cross-sectional area (see Fig. 8–4); and (3) loss of the radial traction effect exerted on larger noncartilaginous airways as they emerge from the lung parenchyma (Leff and Schumacker, 1993; Levitzky, 1995).

Measurements of Expiratory Flow Limitation in Pulmonary Diseases

Recall that vital capacity (VC) is defined as the total lung capacity (TLC) less the residual volume (RV). Because RV cannot be voluntarily exhaled, the *static* spirometric measurement of TLC represents the total usable portion of air in the lung (see Chap. 7). In this chapter, which focuses on the *dynamics* of breathing, we define the **forced vital capacity (FVC)** as the change in volume from TLC to RV *during a forced expiration*. From the discussion of lung dynamics up to this point the reader should immediately recognize that exhaling forcefully is fundamentally different from exhaling gently. The difference is attributable to the combined effects of dynamic compression of airways, flow-resistive pressure losses, flow-limited (effort-independent) expiration, and other factors. Consider Figure 9–1, which shows the spirometric trace obtained during a single forced expiratory maneuver. The FVC curve has a segment (A–B) showing the average slope ($\Delta V/\Delta t$) in L/s that occurs in the middle half of the forced expiratory maneuver. This region is called the **forced expiratory flow between 25% and 75% of FVC (FEF$_{25\%-75\%}$).** The measurement provides an assessment of FEF in the region where expiration is flow-limited, or effort-independent. Considerable variation exists in the FEF$_{25\%-75\%}$ value; therefore, another measurement of forced expiration is commonly performed to assess pulmonary function—the **forced expiratory volume in 1 second, or FEV$_1$.** (Leff and Schumacker, 1993). The FEV$_1$ value is more reproducible and reliable than the FEF$_{25\%-75\%}$ measurement, and is defined as the volume of air (in liters) exhaled in the first second of the forced expiration. To assess and compare the forced expiratory component of pulmonary function in the same patient or between patients, the FEV$_1$ is normally divided by the FVC, and

the dimensionless answer expressed as a percentage. The resulting FEV$_1$/FVC value is normally between 75% and 85% for normal healthy persons between the ages of 25 and 50 (Leff and Schumacker, 1993).

Measurement of forced expiratory flow maneuvers has applications in pulmonary diagnostics because various types of lung disease change the expiratory flow-volume curve in characteristic ways. The relationship between expiratory flow and volume can be altered by the following:

- Changes in the static lung recoil pressures
- Variation in the degree of airways resistance
- Loss of radial traction (mechanical tethering) of intraparenchymal airways
- Regional differences among lung regions

OBSTRUCTIVE DISEASES

Diverse pulmonary diseases such as bronchial asthma, emphysema, chronic bronchitis, and cystic fibrosis (CF) have distinctive causes, mechanisms of disease, symptoms, clinical presentations, and treatments. For our purposes, we can note that all of these **obstructive diseases** are characterized by *expiratory flow that is limited at relatively low flowrates.* Consequently, a patient with an obstructive lung disorder can usually inspire rapidly at near-normal flows and volumes but is unable to exhale normally (Fig. 9–5). Therefore, expiration tends to be a slow, prolonged process. Spirometric assessment of the pulmonary mechanics of these patients reveals abnormally low values for FEV$_1$, FEF$_{25\%-75\%}$, and FEV$_1$/FVC.

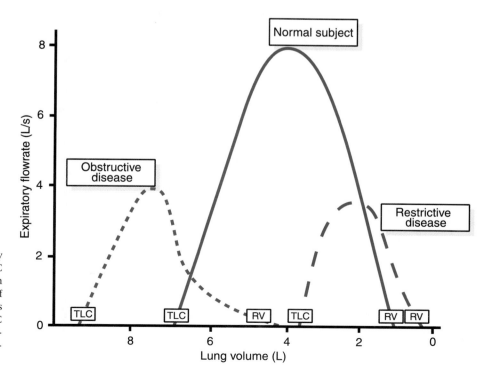

FIGURE 9–5. Spirograms—expiratory flow-volume curves. Notice that the TLC and the RV in obstructive disorders such as emphysema are greater than that of the normal lung. In restrictive disorders such as interstitial fibrosis, both the TLC and the RV are less than that of the normal lung. Other patterns exist for restrictive diseases.

We now look briefly at the mechanical features of these obstructive diseases to find out what mechanisms are responsible for the expiratory flow limitation.

Bronchial asthma is characterized by hypersecretion of tracheobronchial glands, which causes exudate to accumulate in the airways. The disease is also associated with an increase in bronchomotor tone, which reduces airway diameter, and by edema of the wall of the airways (see Fig. 5–5). All of these pathologic changes severely reduce the airway caliber, especially that of the smaller-diameter, collapsible airways within the lung parenchyma. The gas flow within these intra-parenchymal airways is dramatically reduced.

In a similar manner, airflow is reduced as a result of excessive output of high-viscosity secretions that accumulate in the airways of patients with *chronic bronchitis* and *cystic fibrosis*. In addition, clearance mechanisms such as mucociliary transport and cough are often impaired in disorders such as cystic fibrosis, thus worsening the airway obstruction.

Finally, patients with *emphysema* suffer from severely reduced expiratory flows because of the loss of radial traction of small airways. In addition, the destruction of alveolar septa results in greatly decreased static lung recoil, and a corresponding increase in static lung compliance (see Fig. 7–3). Collectively, these structural and functional defects in an emphysematous lung contribute to expiratory flow-limitation and promote the development of choke points in small airways as the transmural pressure becomes negative. In a patient with emphysema, both the total lung capacity (TLC) and the functional residual capacity (FRC) are elevated as a result of the loss of static lung recoil. These volumes in turn, generally cause the patient with emphysema to breathe at higher lung volumes compared with a normal, healthy person.

RESTRICTIVE DISEASES

Pulmonary diseases such as interstitial fibrosis, as well as musculoskeletal abnormalities that cause rigidity of the thorax and neuromuscular diseases that cause weakness of the muscles of breathing, all produce characteristic changes in pulmonary mechanics. Because these disorders restrict the amount of lung inflation, they are grouped together as **restrictive diseases.** TLC is usually decreased in such restrictive diseases (see Fig. 9–5).

In cases of *pulmonary interstitial fibrosis,* increased static lung recoil severely limits both TLC and RV. A typical spirometric finding includes an elevated FEV_1/FVC ratio. This value appears to indicate that the expiratory flow is increased in patients diagnosed with interstitial fibrosis. In fact, FEV_1 may be normal or reduced, while FVC is significantly reduced (Leff and Schumacker, 1993).

Abnormalities of the thorax such as *kyphoscoliosis,* which is an exaggeration of the anterior concave thoracic curve accompanied by a rotation of the thoracic vertebra, cause rigidity of the rib cage and limit chest expansion. The resulting decrease in chest wall compliance reduces FRC because the lung static recoil is unchanged, but the chest wall static recoil is increased. This increase in the outward recoil of the chest wall also decreases TLC because the maximum intrapleural pressure that can be generated by the inspiratory muscles is not sufficient to inflate the lungs to a normal TLC.

Neuromuscular diseases such as *myasthenia gravis,* which is characterized by faulty neurochemical transmission at the neuromuscular junctions of skeletal muscle, may affect the muscles of breathing (see Fig. 4–3). The resulting muscle weakness causes TLC to be low because the muscle strength is insufficient to overcome the combined static recoil of the lungs and chest wall. These static forces must be overcome to reach a normal TLC (see Fig. 7–6). With reduced strength of the expiratory group of muscles, normal residual volume is not reached during exhalation, and an elevated RV results. Expiratory flows in cases of restrictive lung disease are not elevated above normal because static lung recoil is near normal limits and, therefore, does not further impede flow (Leff and Schumacker, 1993).

Summary

The focus of this chapter is the measurement and significance of a select number of spirometric tests of forced expiration (FVC, $FEF_{25\%-75\%}$, and FEV_1). An overview of the flow-volume loop is presented and the significance of the flow-limited part of expiration is discussed. Concepts such as transmural pressure, dynamic compression of airways, equal pressure points, and the closing volume of the lung are examined as mechanisms responsible for the effort-independent part of forced expiration. The chapter concludes with a brief comparison of the spirometric findings and the pathophysiologic mechanisms involved in obstructive and restrictive pulmonary diseases.

BIBLIOGRAPHY

Beachey W: Respiratory Care Anatomy and Physiology: Foundations for Clinical Practice. Mosby–Year Book, St. Louis, 1998.

Farzan S and Farzan D: A Concise Handbook of Respiratory Diseases, ed 4. Appleton & Lange, Norwalk, CT, 1997.

Laszlo G: Pulmonary Function: A Guide For Clinicians. Cambridge University Press, 1994.

Leff AR and Schumacker PT: Respiratory Physiology: Basics and Applications. WB Saunders, Philadelphia, 1993.

Levitzky MG: Pulmonary Physiology, ed 4. McGraw-Hill, New York, 1995.

West JB: Respiratory Physiology: The Essentials, ed 6. Williams & Wilkins, Baltimore, 1998.

CHAPTER 10

Control of Breathing

chapter objectives

After studying this chapter the reader should be able to:

☐ Describe the concept of neural nets in the control of respiratory muscles.

☐ Explain how an intrinsic oscillator functions to generate nerve impulses.

☐ Define the following terms:
   Central pattern generator (CPG), respiratory center.

☐ Describe the structure and function of the following components of the respiratory CPG:
   Dorsal respiratory group (DRG), ventral respiratory group (VRG), pontine respiratory group (PRG), spinal respiratory group (SRG).

☐ Explain the operation of the triphasic model of breathing by describing the following phases of the pattern:
   Early inspiration, postinspiratory inhibition, expiration.

☐ Describe how the medullary CPG is modified by the following neuronal influences:
   Nonrespiratory central pattern generators, cerebrum, cerebellum, hypothalamus.

☐ Describe the structure and function of the carotid and aortic bodies, including the role of the type I and type II cells.

☐ Describe the function of peripheral chemoreceptors and the hypoxic drive mechanism in the chemical control of breathing.

☐ Explain how alveolar P_{O_2} affects ventilation at different P_{ACO_2} levels.

☐ Discuss the stimulation of carotid and aortic bodies by arterial P_{CO_2}/H^+.

☐ Describe the function of central chemoreceptors and the hypercapnic drive mechanism in the chemical control of breathing.

☐ Explain how alveolar P_{CO_2} affects ventilation at different P_{AO_2} levels.

☐ Discuss the ventilation response to acidosis and alkalosis.

☐ Discuss the effect that nonchemical receptors and respiratory reflexes have on the neural control of breathing by discussing the operation of the following: Slowly adapting receptors (SARs), Hering-Breuer reflexes, rapidly adapting receptors (RARs), bronchoconstriction (irritant) reflex, C-fiber afferents, pulmonary chemoreflex, diving reflex, pain reflex, baroreceptor reflex.

key terms

aortic body
baroreceptor reflex
bronchoconstriction reflex; irritant reflex
carotid body
central pattern generator (CPG)
chemoreceptor
chemosensitive area
diving reflex
dorsal respiratory group (DRG)
Hering-Breuer deflation reflex
Hering-Breuer inflation reflex
hypercapnic drive
hypoxic drive
intrinsic oscillator
myelinated fibers
neural net
pain reflex
pontine respiratory group (PRG)
pulmonary chemoreflex
rapidly adapting receptor (RAR); irritant receptor

respiratory center
rhythmogenesis
slowly adapting receptor (SAR)
spinal respiratory group (SRG)
triphasic pattern
   early inspiration
   expiration; stage II expiration; active expiration
   postinspiratory inhibition; stage I expiratory inhibition
type I cells; glomus cells; chief cells; principal cells
type II cells; capsule cells; sheath cells; sustentacular cells
unmyelinated fibers (C-fiber afferents)
   bronchial C fibers
   pulmonary C fibers
ventral respiratory group (VRG)
   caudal VRG (cVRG)
   intermediate VRG (iVRG)
   rostral VRG (rVRG)

We have seen how the contractions of respiratory pump muscles such as the diaphragm, intercostals, and abdominals bring about changes in pleural pressure. We have also examined how inflation and deflation of the lung is affected by the static and dynamic properties of pulmonary mechanics. These contractions continue from birth until death, with only the briefest of interruptions. Now we consider the *control* of such muscles and examine how breathing adapts to accommodate changes in metabolic demand, posture, disease, and cardiopulmonary function. The basic neural control of ventilation resides in the brain, embedded in an intricate network of nerve cells. It is here that we focus our attention, but we also examine several peripheral mechanisms that modify the central control of breathing. Exploration of the various ventilatory control systems and their effect on ventilation is the subject of this chapter.

Overview of Ventilatory Control

Ventilatory control systems must respond to both *short-term conditions* of the stimulus-response variety; and to *long-term conditions* related to adaptation where the changed condition is prolonged. Strenuous exercise is an example of a short-term condition that temporarily decreases oxygen levels in the bloodstream and acts as an acute stimulus to trigger an increase in breathing. On the other hand, the low partial pressure of inspired oxygen that exists at high elevation is an example of a long-term condition that evokes adaptation changes in the body's cardiopulmonary system that permit a person to live comfortably and permanently at such altitudes. We now examine the neural and chemical control systems of ventilation that respond to both short-term and long-term conditions.

Neural Control

NEURAL NETS AND CENTRAL PATTERN GENERATORS

Many parts of the brain are composed of elaborate networks of interconnected neurons. These **neural nets** provide complex pathways for high-speed nerve impulse distribution among nerve cells and between nerve cells and effectors. In respiratory control systems, neural nets link various parts of the brain, spinal cord, and muscles of the thorax and ventral abdominal wall into a highly coordinated and integrated neuromuscular system capable of responding rapidly to changes in ventilatory needs. The focal point of respiratory control is an **intrinsic oscillator** located in the brainstem (Feldman and Smith, 1995). This functional area receives afferent impulses related to sensations such as temperature and movement, and integrates them with the functional state of the controlling neurons, as well as with the sensory impulses sent into the brain from peripheral mechanoreceptors and chemoreceptors (Fig. 10–1).

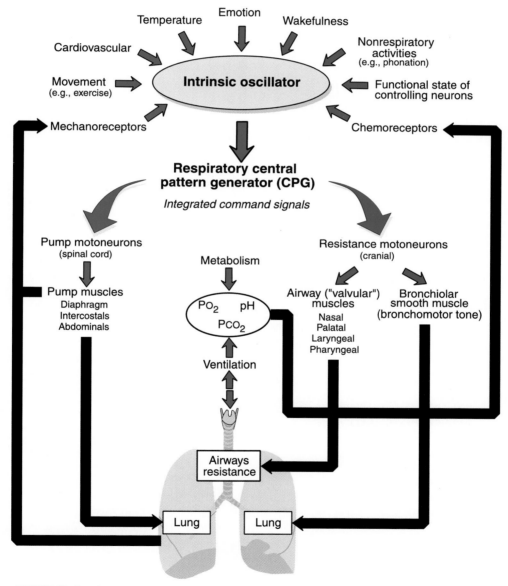

FIGURE 10–1. Schematic—respiratory central pattern generator (CPG). In the respiratory control system, neural nets link various parts of the brain, spinal cord, and muscles of the thorax and ventral abdominal wall into a highly in-tegrated neuromuscular system. The respiratory central pattern generator drives and coordinates the activities of motoneurons that control breathing. (Adapted from Feldman, JL and Smith JC: Neural control of respiratory patterns in mammals: An overview. In Dempsey JA and Pack AI (eds): Regulation of Breathing, Marcel Dekker, New York, 1995, p 40, with permission.)

This central neural structure then converts the various incoming signals into integrated command signals sent to the respiratory muscles. *Oscillation* refers to a system whereby control alternates between different functional groups of neurons. Such functional groups are mutually antagonistic. That is, while one group of nerve cells is sending excitatory motor impulses to a particular group of muscles, it is simultaneously sending inhibitory signals to the opposing group of nerve cells to suppress motor activity to antagonistic muscles. Following this phase of the cycle, control alternates to the opposing group of nerve cells and the process repeats.

Through the reciprocal mechanism described above, the intrinsic oscillator generates output signals that influence the respiratory rhythm. Such networks of cells having patterned motor outputs that result in rhythmic, repetitive behaviors such as respiration or locomotion, are called **central pattern generators** (CPGs). The respiratory CPG in the brainstem is responsible for driving and coordinating motor nerve cells, or *motoneurons*, that control breathing (Box 10–1). Motoneurons are nerve cells with their cell body located in the central nervous system (CNS), and their axons extending peripherally to muscle cells. In addition to controlling respiratory activ-

---

P E R S P E C T I V E S

BOX 10–1   ### Control of Respiration: Network or Pacemaker?

Details of the operation of the respiratory **central pattern generator (CPG)** are far from clear, in spite of decades of study. Investigations into the structure and function of the neural substrate of the pattern generator have focused on two distinct animal models: an in vivo model based on the adult cat, and an in vitro model based on neonatal rat brainstem and spinal cord tissue. The results of the studies have yielded two different hypothetical models to help explain the control of respiration; however, in both models the interconnections among neurons and the functional state of the neuronal membranes are responsible for the *rhythmogenesis,* or the generation of the intrinsic firing pattern, that drives the muscles of breathing. The main difference between the hypothetical models is in the *degree* to which the synaptic connections and membrane properties generate the rhythm.

In vivo studies of the phenobarbital-anesthetized, paralyzed, vagotomized adult cat have led to a *network model* to explain the function of the respiratory CPG. In this hypothesis, synaptic inhibition of networked cells is carried out via membrane hyperpolarization brought about through the opening of chloride channels in the neuronal membrane. This inhibitory action, in turn, helps determine phase duration. By contrast, the in vitro animal model involves the study of the complete brainstem or 400-μm–thick slices of medulla from the neonatal rat. In this experimental method, chloride channels in the neuronal membrane are selectively blocked and the discharge patterns of the "pacemaker" cells are studied. Rhythmogenesis (and thus phase duration) in this *pacemaker model* is determined by the endogenous firing properties of the neurons involved.

It is now known that control of respiration is an extremely complex mechanism affected by multiple factors. The overall process is probably governed by "pacemaker" cells in the immature brainstem, followed by the development of elaborate synaptic interconnections that lead to a "network" model in the mature brainstem. Because of this chronological shift in the structural and functional makeup of the brainstem, researchers have found that study of the respiratory CPG in the developing newborn often leads to valuable insights into the nature of the neural control of respiration.

- Dick TE, Van Lunteren E, and Kelsen SG: Control of respiratory motor activity. In Roussos C (ed): The Thorax—Part A: Physiology, ed 2. Marcel Dekker, New York, 1995.
- Lawson EE, Czyzyk-Krzeska MF, Dean JB, and Milhorn DE: Developmental aspects of the neural control of breathing. In Beckerman RC, Brouillette RT, and Hunt CE (eds): Respiratory Control Disorders in Infants and Children. Williams & Wilkins, Baltimore, 1992.
- Richter DW, Ballanyi K, and Ramirez J: Respiratory rhythm generation. In Miller AD, Bianchi AL, and Bishop BP (eds): Neural Control of the Respiratory Muscles. CRC Press, Boca Raton, FL, 1997.

ity, the respiratory CPG coordinates respiratory movements with nonrespiratory activities such as swallowing. The motor output from the respiratory CPG is sent to muscles of the respiratory system through two groups of motoneurons, the *spinal motoneurons* and *cranial motoneurons*. Spinal motoneurons innervate the muscles of the respiratory pump, such as the diaphragm, intercostal, and abdominal muscles. Cranial motoneurons innervate the muscles that control airways resistance, such as bronchiolar, laryngeal, and pharyngeal muscles. The pump muscles produce changes in pleural pressure that bring about lung inflation and deflation, whereas valvular muscles of the laryngeal, pharyngeal, palatal, and nasal regions change airway resistance, thus affecting airflow. Such muscles consist of both abductors that decrease airway resistance and adductors that increase airway resistance (Dick, Van Lunteren, and Kelsen, 1995).

RESPIRATORY CENTERS

A *center* is a functional collection of nerve cells. These cells work together to perform the same function but are not necessarily concentrated in one location. Such nerve cells are typically distributed throughout a section of brain tissue and are linked together to form a neural network that includes the relatively long efferent nerve fibers that control the muscles of breathing. Three different **respiratory centers** are organized as major neuronal complexes in the brainstem: the *dorsal respiratory group* and *ventral respiratory group* of the medulla, and the *pontine respiratory group* located in the pons.

> **NOTE:** The *brain stem* is a loosely defined term referring to the medulla oblongata and pons, plus several associated structures. Full agreement regarding the structures, in addition to the medulla and pons, that constitute the brainstem, has not been reached.

Dorsal Respiratory Group

The medullary center known as the **dorsal respiratory group (DRG)** is located in the region of the *nucleus of the solitary tract* (NST) (Fig. 10–2). Most of the DRG neurons exhibit discharge patterns that provide the main excitatory input to phrenic motoneurons. These motoneurons, in turn, bring about contraction of the diaphragm to initiate inspiratory airflow. The neurons of the DRG, therefore, are characterized as inspiratory (I) neurons (Berger and Bellingham, 1995; Bianchi and Pásaro, 1997).

Ventral Respiratory Group

The **ventral respiratory group (VRG)** of the medulla is roughly divided into three anatomic regions: a *caudal*

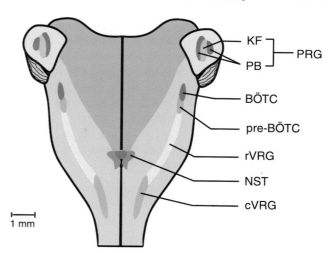

FIGURE 10–2. Respiratory centers of the brainstem. Dorsal view of the brainstem region. The cerebellum has been removed to show the major respiratory centers. KF = Kölliker-Fuse nucleus; PB = parabrachial nuclei; PRG = pontine respiratory group; BÖTC = Bötzinger complex; pre-BÖTC = pre-Bötzinger complex; rVRG = rostral ventral respiratory group; cVRG = caudal ventral respiratory group; NST = nucleus of the solitary tract. (Adapted from Feldman, JL and Smith JC: Neural control of respiratory patterns in mammals: An overview. In Dempsey JA and Pack AI (eds): Regulation of Breathing, Marcel Dekker, New York, 1995, p 50, with permission.)

VRG at the inferior end of the group; an *intermediate VRG* located in the middle region; and a *rostral VRG* at the superior end of the grouping (see Fig. 10–2).

The **caudal VRG (cVRG)** begins at the border between the spinal cord and the medulla and is composed of the *nucleus retroambigualis* (NRA). It contains a high concentration of expiratory (E) neurons intermingled with a few I neurons (Berger and Bellingham, 1995; Bianchi and Pásaro, 1997).

The **intermediate VRG (iVRG)** is located in the ventrolateral medulla, anterior to the DRG. The iVRG includes the *nucleus ambiguus* (NA) and *para-ambigual* regions. The NA includes laryngeal motoneurons that drive intrinsic and extrinsic laryngeal and pharyngeal muscles to modify airway resistance. The nerve cells of the iVRG include both E and I neurons with outputs to the spinal motoneurons that innervate thoracic respiratory muscles. In addition, the cells of the iVRG coordinate activities of the pump muscles with those of the valvular muscles controlling upper airway resistance, thus playing a key role in the respiratory CPG (Bianchi and Pásaro, 1997).

The **rostral VRG (rVRG)** includes the rostral, or cranial, portion of the nucleus ambiguus and contains pharyngeal motoneurons that exhibit both I and E discharge patterns. The rVRG also contains interneurons that project to the caudal medulla and spinal cord and exhibit E discharge patterns. These neurons are collectively referred to as the *Bötzinger complex* (BÖTC). Located in the ventral medulla, caudal to the BÖTC, is a region that contains neurons essential in **rhythmo-genesis,** or the generation of rhythmic impulses (Ganong, 1995). This key medullary area exhibits intrinsic discharge pattern activity and has been identified as the *pre-Bötzinger complex* (pre-BÖTC) (see Fig. 10–2). Bianchi and Pásaro (1997) report that even *isolated* slices of this tissue exhibit respiratory-like rhythm. Both in vitro and in vivo studies suggest that the pre-BÖTC is *the* kernel of the respiratory CPG, "containing all types of respiratory neurons that are assumed to be necessary for the generation of a normal respiratory rhythm" (Richter, Ballayni, and Ramirez, 1997).

Pontine Respiratory Group

Several groups of respiratory-related neurons in the dorsolateral pons are located in the *parabrachial nuclei* (PB) and the *Kölliker-Fuse* (*KF*) *nucleus* (see Fig. 10–2). These regions are referred to collectively as the **pontine respiratory group (PRG).** PRG neurons do not appear to be essential for respiratory rhythm generation, but they may act to stabilize the respiratory pattern, slow the rhythm, and influence the timing of respiratory phases (Bianchi and Pásaro, 1997). Relatively little is known about this group of cells; however, electrical recordings have shown that the respiratory activity of the PRG appears less phasic (rhythmic) than that of the medulla (Dick, Van Lunteren, and Kelsen, 1995). On the basis of animal studies, it has been proposed that the PRG interacts with vagal afferents to determine the duration of respiratory phases.

> **NOTE:** In older texts, the pons is often described as the site of the "pneumotaxic center," a conceptual area controlling the duration of inspiration.

Animal studies also suggest that the PRG assists in the stabilization of the medullary respiratory rhythm. For example, when the pons is lesioned in a *vagotimized* animal (that is, in an animal in which vagus nerve connections have been blocked), the phase duration of respiration is dramatically lengthened, resulting in a breathing pattern characterized by prolonged inspiration. Such a pattern is called *apneusis.* Similarly, pontine lesions reduce the stability of the medullary rhythm so that the breathing pattern becomes more erratic. Interactions between the respiratory groups in the pons and those in the medulla as well as between pontine and spinal respiratory groups have been illustrated by electrophysiologic and neuroanatomic studies; however, the precise nature of the interactions remains unclear (Dick, Van Lunteren, and Kelsen, 1995). PRG neurons may also function to relay information from the hypothalamus to the respiratory centers of the medulla (Bianchi and Pásaro, 1997).

Spinal Respiratory Group

Prior to the 1980s it was believed that the respiratory pattern generated in the medulla was transmitted directly to motoneurons which, in turn, functioned solely to relay the impulses to the respiratory muscles. Electrophysiologic and neuroanatomic evidence now suggests that interneuronal pools making up the **spinal respiratory group (SRG)** are found in the cervical and thoracic spinal cord (see Fig. 10–2). Such neuronal pools shape the respiratory pattern in some way, probably through inhibitory synaptic connections to respiratory motoneurons (Dick, Van Lunteren, and Kelsen, 1995). Details of the function of the SRG await further study.

Table 10–1 summarizes the function of important regions of the respiratory centers in the brainstem, including the presumed distribution of I and E motor neurons in the various respiratory groups.

TRIPHASIC PATTERN OF BREATHING

Through the use of sophisticated electrophysiologic techniques and the study of animal models (both neonatal and adult), researchers have shown that respiration in higher mammals is controlled through a *three-phase sequence* of synaptic activity occurring in the respiratory neurons of the brainstem (Feldman and Smith, 1995; Lawson et al, 1992). Such a model depends on reciprocal inhibitory interactions between phase-specific groups of neurons. Each group exhibits depolarization and rapid firing of action potentials during a particular phase of the respiratory cycle (Fig. 10–3):

- *Inspiratory neurons* depolarize during inspiration.
- *Postinspiratory neurons* depolarize immediately after inspiration.
- *Expiratory neurons* begin to depolarize in a ramplike fashion immediately following the postinspiratory period. This period of ramp depolarization, whereby the resting membrane potential gradually creeps upward, is followed by a plateau period of repetitive firing.

The **triphasic pattern** of breathing involves the following network interactions among respiratory interneurons and is summarized in Table 10–2.

Early Inspiration

The initiation of a cycle of breathing begins with brainstem inspiratory interneurons that bring about **early inspiration.** Such neurons exhibit ramplike depolarization after being released from expiratory inhibition. This ramplike pattern of activity drives the phrenic mo-

TABLE 10-1	Function of Respiratory Centers		
Respiratory Center	**Classification of Neurons**	**Location**	**Function**
Dorsal respiratory group (DRG)	I	Medulla Nucleus of the solitary tract (NST)	Excitatory impulses to phrenic motoneurons which innervate diaphragm
Ventral respiratory group (VRG)			
Caudal VRG (cVRG)	Mostly E Few I	Between spinal cord and medulla Nucleus retroambigualis (NRA)	Expiratory motor impulses to thoracic muscles
Intermediate VRG (iVRG)	I and E	Ventrolateral medulla, anterior to the DRG Nucleus ambiguus (NA) Para-ambigual region	Excitatory to laryngeal and pharyngeal muscles to control upper airway resistance Output to spinal motoneurons which innervate thoracic respiratory muscles Coordination of "valvular muscles" (airway resistance) with "pump muscles" (lung volume changes)
Rostral VRG (rVRG)	I and E	Cranial portion of NA Pharyngeal motoneurons	Motor output to pharyngeal muscles
	E	BÖTC Interneurons to caudal medulla and spinal cord	Expiratory motor
	I and E	Pre-BÖTC Ventral medulla, caudal to BÖTC	Intrinsic discharge pattern responsible for rhythm of respiratory CPG (rhythmogenesis)
Pontine respiratory group (PRG)	n/a	Parabrachial nuclei (PB) Kölliker-Fuse nucleus (KF)	Stabilize respiratory pattern, slow rhythm, modify timing of respiratory phases ("pneumotaxic center"); relay information from hypothalamus to medullary respiratory center
Spinal respiratory group (SRG)	n/a	Interneuronal pools in the cervical and thoracic spinal cord	Modification of output to respiratory motoneurons

I = inspiratory discharge pattern; E = expiratory discharge pattern; CPG = central pattern generator; n/a = not applicable.

toneurons resulting in diaphragmatic contraction and inspiratory airflow (see Fig. 10-3).

Postinspiratory Inhibition (Stage I Expiratory Inhibition)

The early neuronal activity of the inspiratory neurons is immediately followed by **postinspiratory inhibition,** or **stage I expiratory inhibition.** Such activity prevents reactivation of the inspiratory neurons until expiration has been completed (see Fig. 10-3). Simultaneously, vagal motoneurons in the rostral ventral respiratory group (rVRG) are activated by the ramplike activity pattern, resulting in contraction of laryngeal adductors. Contraction of these intrinsic laryngeal muscles increases upper airway resistance to passive expiratory airflow. Nonvagal motoneurons such as postinspiratory interneurons in the BÖTC also depolarize during this postinspiratory phase, thus preventing additional inspiratory activity and prolonging the onset of expiration.

Expiration (Stage II Expiration, Active Expiration)

Once the respiratory network is released from postinspiratory inhibition, it enters the third phase of the respiratory cycle. This phase is called **active expiration, stage II expiration,** or simply **expiration,** and occurs during the period of relative phrenic nerve "silence" (see Fig. 10-3). Elastic recoil of the lungs and thorax follows, initiating passive expiration. During periods of increased respiratory activity, expiratory neurons activate spinal expiratory motoneurons, which innervate expiratory intercostal and abdominal muscle groups (Feldman and Smith, 1995; Lawson et al, 1992).

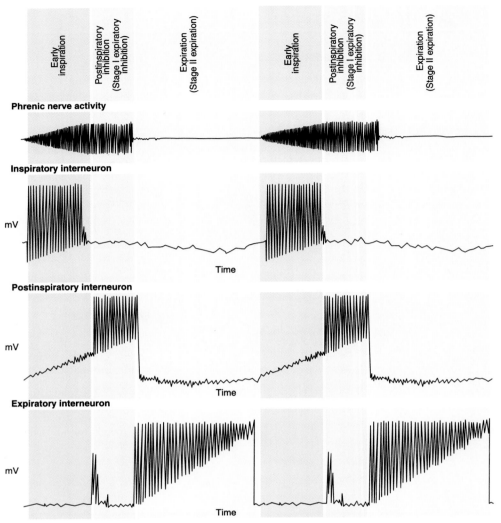

FIGURE 10–3. Neural activity in triphasic breathing (mammalian model). Note the height of the action potential curves are not drawn to scale (mV = millivolt). The tops of the curves have been truncated (cut off) in order to show the distinctive action potentials of the three types of respiratory interneurons on the same graph. See text for an explanation of the discharge patterns. (Adapted from Lawson EE, Czyzk-Krezeska MF, Dean JB, and Milhorn DE: Developmental aspects of the neural control of breathing. In Beckman RC, Brouillette RT, and Hunt CE (eds): Respiratory Control Disorders in Infants and Children, Williams & Wilkins, Baltimore, 1992, p 11, with permission.)

MODIFICATION OF RESPIRATORY CENTERS

Nonrespiratory Central Pattern Generators

As explained previously, CPGs are responsible for several kinds of rhythmic, repetitive actions in addition to respiration. Chewing (mastication) and swallowing (deglutition) are examples of nonrespiratory activities controlled by CPGs. These activities must be coordinated with those of the respiratory CPG in the brainstem to prevent aspiration of food or liquid. In chewing, both the respiratory rate and the activity of muscles of mastication *increase*. For example, the mas-

seter, a powerful muscle that elevates the lower jaw, is activated at the phase transitions occurring at the onset of both inspiration and expiration. As a result of this coordination, the action of chewing is smoothly coupled with that of breathing in a 2:1 or 3:1 ratio (Fontana et al, 1992). In contrast to chewing, respiratory rate *decreases* during swallowing, and tends to be initiated in late inspiration (Dick, Van Lunteren, and Kelsen, 1995).

Cerebrum

Although the neural networks of the brainstem and spinal cord respond exquisitely to minor changes in the

TABLE 10-2	Network Interactions in a Three-Phase Model of Breathing
Phase	**Major Features**
Early Inspiration	Ramplike activation after inspiratory interneurons are released from expiratory inhibition.
	Action potentials occur during same period as phrenic nerve activity.
	Inspiratory interneurons drive phrenic motoneurons resulting in contraction of diaphragm and inspiratory inflow.
Postinspiratory Inhibition (Stage I Expiratory Inhibition)	Expiratory inhibition prevents reactivation of inspiratory interneurons until expiration has occurred.
	Ramp increase of resting membrane potential "baseline" during inspiratory period.
	Decreased frequency of firing during postinspiratory burst.
	Inhibition of inspiratory interneurons during both inspiration and expiration.
	Ramplike activity pattern activates rVRG motoneurons resulting in contraction of laryngeal adductors.
	Postinspiratory interneurons of the BÖTC are presumed to be the source of the postinspiratory inhibition, which prolongs the onset of expiration.
Expiration (Stage II Expiration; Active Expiration)	After release from postinspiratory inhibition, a ramp increase of firing rate occurs during the expiratory period.
	Third phase of the cycle is associated with phrenic nerve silence.
	During high demand states expiratory interneurons activate expiratory muscles (e.g., internal intercostals, abdominals).
	Expiratory interneurons strongly inhibited during inspiration.

rVRG = rostral ventral respiratory group; BÖTC = Bötzinger complex.

internal environment of the body to bring about rapid and precise control of airflow, higher brain areas in the cerebrum have the ability to override the basic rhythm by inhibiting or initiating breathing (Fig. 10–4). We perform these commonplace functions when we adjust our breathing to speak. We also alter diaphragmatic breathing to express emotions such as laughter or sorrow (Harper, 1997). Additionally, humans consciously sense their breathing, an ability that can produce the distressing sensation of dyspnea, or "air hunger," under certain pathologic conditions such as an asthma attack (Davenport and Reep, 1995; Harper, 1997). The precise cortical mechanisms involved in the alteration of the respiratory CPG are not fully understood. It is presumed (Harper, 1997) that the conscious perception of breathing involves sensory cortical elements, whereas the voluntary initiation of breathing or breath-holding involves the cortical action of traditional motor areas (Box 10–2).

Cerebellum

Although the function of the cerebellum in fine-tuning the motor drive to the muscles of locomotion is well established, controversy exists as to the role the cerebellum plays in the regulation of the muscles of breathing (see Fig. 10–4). Recent findings suggest that the cerebellum is primarily involved in integrating and modulating the reflex respiratory responses to chemical and mechanical changes in the respiratory system. In addition, experimental evidence reveals that the cerebellum is most active in the regulation of breathing during high-demand states rather than during normal, quiet breathing (Frazier, Xu, and Lee, 1997).

Hypothalamus

The hypothalamus is a relatively small part of the forebrain located on the cranial floor immediately behind the nasal cavity (see Fig. 10–4). This small mass of tissue is involved with thermoregulation; primitive emotions such as rage, fear, and sex drive; hunger and thirst; central arousal; and hormonal control.

To date, relatively few studies have been conducted to determine the extent of hypothalamic control of cardiopulmonary function. However, recent investigations suggest that neurons in the hypothalamus have connections to regions in the medulla and spinal cord that serve cardiovascular and respiratory functions. It is known that cardiovascular, sympathetic, and respiratory neurons are found in the hypothalamus; however, it is not clear if their neural activity originates in the hypothalamus or is a result of feedback from other brain areas, peripheral receptors, or both. The most important role of the hypothalamus may involve the integration of cardiopulmonary activity with other functions such as temperature regulation and behavior (Waldrop and Porter, 1995).

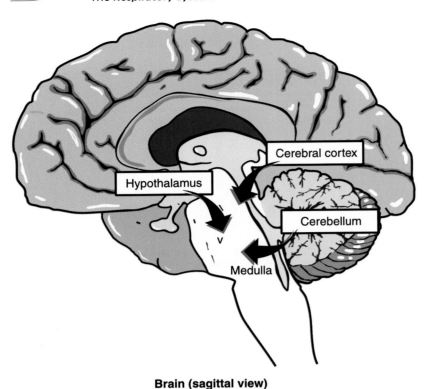

Brain (sagittal view)

FIGURE 10–4. Modification of respiratory centers by higher brain areas. *Cerebral centers* can override the basic rhythm of breathing for a short time (e.g., speaking); the *cerebellum* may function to integrate and modulate the reflex respiratory responses to chemical and mechanical stimuli; the *hypothalamus* may serve to integrate cardiopulmonary activity with other central nervous system functions such as thermo- regulation and behavior.

Chemical Control

CHEMORECEPTORS AND HYPOXIC DRIVE

An increase in the activity of the neurons found in the respiratory CPG in the medulla can be triggered by an increase in the P_{CO_2} or hydrogen ion (H^+) concentration of arterial blood, or by a decrease in the P_{O_2} of arterial blood (Fig. 10–5). A decrease in the activity of the respiratory neurons in the medulla results from a decrease in arterial P_{CO_2} or arterial hydrogen ion (H^+) concentration, or by an increase in arterial P_{O_2}. These variations in blood chemistry are detected by **chemoreceptors,** which are unique sensory structures composed of groups of specialized neuroepithelial cells (see Fig. 10–1). Respiratory chemoreceptors are found in the *carotid bodies* and *aortic bodies*, as well as in groupings of cells located within the *medulla*. These peripheral and central chemoreceptors are sensitive to changes in blood chemistry; however, the degree of sensitivity to oxygen and carbon dioxide tension, and to hydrogen ion concentration, is quite different in the various monitoring locations.

Carotid and Aortic Bodies

A **carotid body** is associated with the common carotid artery on each side of the neck, close to the bifurcation where the external and internal carotid arteries branch from the common carotid artery. Several **aortic bodies** are located near the arch of the aorta (Fig. 10–6). The chemoreceptors at these different locations are organized as groupings of two types of cells—*type I cells* and *type II cells*. The carotid and aortic bodies are surrounded and penetrated by numerous fenestrated sinusoidal capillaries (Ganong, 1995). Such capillaries have relatively large endothelial pore spaces (fenestrations, or "windows"), and many small outpouchings (sinusoids). This unique structural arrangement brings the arterial blood supply very close to the functional cells of the carotid and aortic bodies.

In fact, the perfusion of these small groupings of chemically sensitive cells is quite remarkable. For example, each 2-mg carotid body receives blood flow of about 0.04 mL/min. This minuscule blood flow is not impressive when compared with the 1000 to 1200 mL/min that flows through the kidney or brain. However, when the *mass* of the tissues are considered, the true perfusion rates are revealed. The tiny carotid body is perfused at a rate of about 2000 mL of blood per 100 g of tissue per minute. This rate compares with a blood flow of 420 mL per 100 g of tissue per minute in the kidney, and only about 54 mL per 100 g of tissue per minute in the brain; large organs are generally considered to be highly perfused (Ganong, 1995). How is the chemical composition of this blood sensed by the chemoreceptors of the carotid and aortic bodies?

The parenchymal cells of the carotid and aortic body are separated by interstitial connective tissue contain-

PERSPECTIVES

BOX 10–2

Remembering to Breathe—Ondine's Curse

According to ancient German legends, a mortal lover was once unfaithful to a water nymph named Ondine. To exact revenge, the king of the water nymphs placed a curse on the mortal that removed all of the man's automatic functions, including the basic rhythm of breathing. As a result of the curse, the man was no longer able to sleep because he had to stay awake and remember to breathe. Ultimately, he fell asleep from sheer exhaustion and promptly died of respiratory failure. The moral standards of water nymphs are not to be taken lightly.

Certain neuromuscular or lung diseases such as viral encephalitis caused by polio may cause alveolar hypoventilation, but the condition is rare in the *absence* of these diseases. In the early 1950s, however, several patients were diagnosed with an alveolar hypoventilation syndrome characterized by sleep and wake apnea, reduced hypercapnic drive, insufficient ventilation during sleeping, but adequate voluntary ventilation while awake. These patients did not exhibit neuromuscular or lung disease to account for their symptoms. The syndrome was named *Ondine's curse.* Comroe (1993) has reviewed the literary references to Ondine's doomed lover and concluded that they have not been accurately applied. Instead, the syndrome *at best* describes a patient in whom alveolar hypoventilation is congenital and idiopathic (a disease without recognizable cause).

Alveolar hypoventilation syndromes in children are classified as *congenital, acquired,* or *transient.* The most common and severe congenital forms include *central hypoventilation syndrome (CHS)* and malformation of the hindbrain causing compression and direct damage to the respiratory centers in the medulla. Acquired forms of alveolar hypoventilation may result from asphyxia associated with traumatic birth, encephalitis resulting from infections, trauma of the brainstem, tumor, or infarction. Transient forms of alveolar hypoventilation may be associated with cases of severe obstructive sleep apnea (OSA). In infants and children with CHS, the following symptoms are recognized:

- Hypoventilation during quiet sleep, with progressive hypercapnia and hypoxemia
- Absent or negligible ventilatory and arousal sensitivity to hypercapnia and hypoxia during sleep
- Unresponsiveness to respiratory stimulants
- Absence of autoresuscitation and perception of asphyxia
- Absent or negligible ventilatory sensitivity to hypoxia and hypercapnia while awake
- Normal ventilation during wakefulness

Because these patients exhibit no arousal response from sleep, and have no perception of asphyxia, they do not experience the sensation of dyspnea, which is a conscious awareness of shortness of breath, or "air hunger."

Clinical management of CHS presents a formidable challenge. Pharmacologic treatment includes the use of respiratory stimulants such as theophylline, caffeine, progesterone, or methylphenidate. In spite of the short duration of effect, the ventilatory response to these CNS stimulants has been satisfactory in some patients. Other types of management include (1) mechanical ventilatory support with positive pressure ventilator and tracheostomy, (2) positive pressure ventilator and nasal mask, and (3) diaphragm pacing. Again, the patient response has been satisfactory in some cases. However, CHS remains a rare, difficult-to-treat neural disorder of breathing.

- Comroe JH: Frankenstein, Pickwick, and Ondine (Retrospective Redux). Respiratory Care. 38:940–943, 1993.
- Weese-Mayer DE, Hunt CE, and Brouilette RT: Alveolar hypoventilation syndromes. In Beckerman RC, Brouillette RT, and Hunt CE (eds): Respiratory Control Disorders in Infants and Children. Williams & Wilkins, Baltimore, 1992.

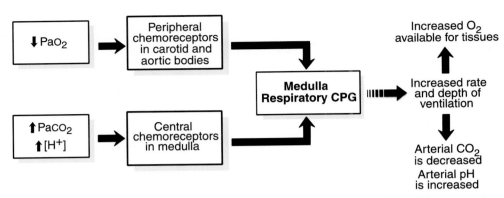

FIGURE 10–5. Chemical regulation of the respiratory CPG. The example in this figure illustrates an increase in respiratory minute volume caused by either: (1) a decrease in arterial oxygen tension or (2) an increase in arterial carbon dioxide tension or in hydrogen ion concentration (a decrease in pH). A decrease in respiratory minute volume is triggered by blood chemistry conditions such as increased arterial oxygen tension, decreased arterial carbon dioxide tension, or decreased hydrogen ion concentration.

ing nerve fiber bundles and the special blood vessels described above. Each carotid and aortic body is enclosed by a capsule and is composed of clusters of **type I,** or **glomus, cells** closely associated with afferent nerve fibers belonging to the *carotid sinus nerve* (Fig. 10–7). Glomus cells are also known as **chief,** or **principal cells.** These cells are similar to the secretory cells of the adrenal medulla and contain granules of stored catecholamines that are released when the glomus

cells are exposed to hypoxemia. The precise mechanism responsible for the release of catecholamines is not fully understood (Ganong, 1995; Gonzalez, Dinger, and Fidone, 1995).

The catecholamines stimulate the nerve endings of the carotid sinus nerve which, in turn, transmits sensory impulses to the medullary respiratory area. As the PO_2 of arterial blood decreases or the PCO_2 increases, the frequency of impulse transmission of the carotid si-

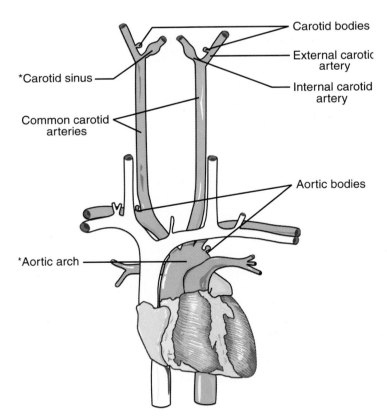

Anterior view

FIGURE 10–6. Location of carotid and aortic bodies. The carotid and aortic bodies are composed of groupings of specialized neuroepithelial cells, called *chemoreceptors,* that function to monitor changes in blood chemistry. Because of their location, the carotid bodies have been studied in more detail than the aortic bodies.

*Specialized mechanoreceptors, called *baroreceptors* or *pressoreceptors,* are located in the aortic arch and carotid sinuses. These sensory cells monitor systemic blood pressure by detecting changes in the stretch of major arterial walls.

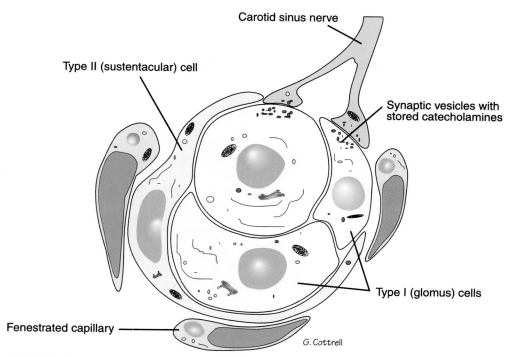

FIGURE 10–7. Structure of the carotid body. The parenchymal (functional) cells of the carotid body are the chemoreceptor cells known as type I (*glomus*) cells. Capillaries bring a large volume of blood into close proximity to the chemoreceptor cells. When stimulated by hypoxemic conditions, the highly perfused glomus cells released stored catecholamines near the cuplike nerve endings of the carotid sinus nerve. Sensory impulses are then transmitted to the medulla. The type II cells are known as *sustentacular cells,* and function in a support role for the glomus cells.

nus nerve increases. **Type II cells,** also known as **sustentacular, capsule,** or **sheath cells,** are located within the aortic and carotid bodies, supporting clusters of type I cells (see Fig. 10–7). The ratio of chemoreceptor to sustentacular cells in the lobule of the carotid body is approximately 5:1. The type II cells resemble the supporting glial cells of nervous tissue (Ganong, 1995; Gonzalez, Dinger, and Fidone, 1995).

Hypoxic Drive and Ventilatory Response to Oxygen Deficiency

In humans, the carotid bodies have been studied in more detail than the aortic bodies. The location of the aortic bodies makes their investigation difficult; however, on the basis of animal and human studies it is believed that the aortic body responses are similar, but of lesser magnitude, than those of the carotid bodies (Ganong, 1995).

Carotid body chemoreceptors are activated when arterial oxygen tension (Pao_2) drops below the normal homeostatic range of 80 to 100 mm Hg (Fig. 10–8). Through this response to arterial hypoxia, or *hypoxemia,* the peripheral chemoreceptors provide the main afferent stimulus, or **hypoxic drive,** to the respiratory centers of the brain stem. Surprisingly, this control system is relatively insensitive to falling Pao_2 values, which must decrease to low levels before the carotid and aortic bodies trigger an increase in breathing. As can be seen in Figure 10–8, carotid body chemoreceptors are maximally driven at a relatively low Pao_2 value of about 26 mm Hg (Gonzalez, Dinger, and Fidone, 1995).

When the partial pressure of oxygen in the alveoli (PAO_2) is greater than 60 mm Hg, the effect on respiratory minute volume is slight. However, as PAO_2 falls below 60 mm Hg, marked stimulation of respiration occurs. It should be noted that a normal alveolar-capillary membrane allows oxygen molecules to quickly diffuse from the alveolus to the pulmonary blood. As a result of this efficient transfer of gas, the Po_2 of the mixed venous blood entering the lung is raised to the Po_2 of the alveolus. In other words, equilibrium is reached so rapidly in this dynamic system that an alveolar Po_2 of 100 mm Hg quickly translates into an arterial Po_2 of 100 mm Hg in the blood leaving the lung and being pumped to the rest of the body. Carotid and aortic body chemoreceptors monitor *arterial* blood levels of Po_2. However, the reader is reminded that these blood levels usually mirror the *alveolar* Po_2. Therefore, graphs that depict alveolar partial pressure values are often used to describe the activity of arterial chemoreceptors. We examine details of the alveolar-capillary gas-

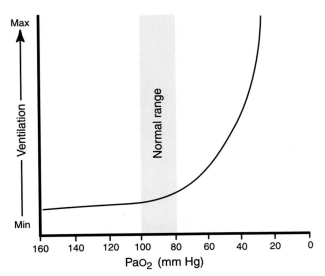

FIGURE 10–8. Ventilation response at different PaO$_2$ values. The curve illustrates the effect of different arterial PO$_2$ values on alveolar ventilation. Ventilation is not affected dramatically until the PaO$_2$ falls below 100 mm Hg, with maximal effect occurring at approximately PaO$_2$ = 26 mm Hg. Arterial PCO$_2$ and pH are kept constant.

exchange mechanism in a later chapter. In the meantime, it is useful to consider why the peripheral chemoreceptors are relatively unresponsive to a decrease in arterial (and alveolar) PO$_2$ values from a normal level of about 100 mm Hg to a hypoxemic level of about 60 mm Hg:

1. As arterial PO$_2$ decreases, hemoglobin (Hb) becomes less saturated, causing the amount of unbound Hb to increase. Unbound Hb is a weaker acid than bound Hb, also known as oxyhemoglobin (HbO$_2$). Therefore, the increase in Hb causes a decrease in the H$^+$ concentration in arterial blood, resulting in metabolic alkalosis and depressed ventilation.
2. Any increase in ventilation causes a reduction in alveolar PCO$_2$ and arterial PCO$_2$, which further inhibits ventilation.

As a result of these changes, the stimulatory effects of hypoxemia are not evident until the condition becomes severe enough to override the effects of the decrease in arterial hydrogen ion concentration and the decrease in PaCO$_2$. Normally, this threshold level for detection occurs at an arterial PO$_2$ of approximately 60 mm Hg (Ganong, 1995).

If carotid body chemoreceptors are not stimulated until the PaO$_2$ drops to low levels, why is the hypoxic drive mechanism not activated by conditions such as anemia or carbon monoxide poisoning, conditions that are certainly accompanied by arterial hypoxia? The answer lies in the fact that the O$_2$ needs of the glomus cells are easily met by *dissolved* oxygen in the high volume of blood perfusing the carotid body. Dissolved

oxygen normally makes up a comparatively small fraction of the total oxygen transported in a given volume of blood, but in the case of glomus cells in intimate contact with this blood, the amount of dissolved oxygen is sufficient to prevent the chemoreceptors from being stimulated. In cases of anemia and carbon monoxide poisoning, the saturation of hemoglobin, or the amount of O$_2$ *combined* with Hb, is severely depressed. This particular oxygen deficiency, in which the amount of HbO$_2$ is decreased, does not activate the carotid bodies because the dissolved amount of O$_2$ in the bloodstream remains above the threshold for detection by the glomus cells. Peripheral chemoreceptors are stimulated when (1) the PaO$_2$ is extremely low; (2) the total amount of O$_2$ delivered to the carotid body per unit time is severely depressed; or (3) drugs such as cyanide are given which prevent the utilization of O$_2$ at a cellular level, including the utilization of O$_2$ by the glomus cells themselves (Ganong, 1995).

Effect of Alveolar PO$_2$ on Ventilation at Different PACO$_2$ Levels

As we have seen, a significant ventilatory response is lacking at PAO$_2$ values above 60 mm Hg (see Fig. 10–8). This observation should be qualified somewhat by stating that the detection threshold of hypoxia (PAO$_2$ ≈ 60 mm Hg) normally occurs when the alveolar PCO$_2$ is fixed at a level near normal or slightly below normal (Fig. 10–9). However, when the PACO$_2$ is stabilized at a level a few mm Hg above normal, the minute volume of ventilation increases, even at a considerably higher

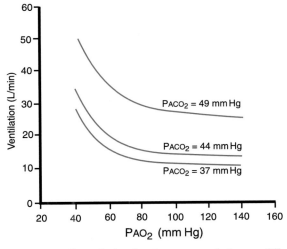

FIGURE 10–9. Effect of alveolar PO$_2$ on ventilation at different PACO$_2$ levels. The hypoxic response curves illustrate the effect of different alveolar PO$_2$ values on alveolar ventilation when the alveolar PCO$_2$ is held constant at values of 37, 44, and 49 mm Hg. As the PACO$_2$ increases, the ventilation response at a given PAO$_2$ is increased, as shown by the shift of the hypoxic response curves to the right and upward.

PaO$_2$ range of 90 to 110 mm Hg (see Fig. 10–9). Put another way, the threshold for detection of hypoxia "improves," indicating that the peripheral chemoreceptors are more sensitive to hypoxia when the PaCO$_2$ is increased. The graph in Figure 10–9 shows this trend with the higher PaCO$_2$ curves displaced to the right and higher than the curve corresponding to the subnormal values (PaCO$_2$ less than 40 mm Hg).

Such a change in the sensitivity threshold of the peripheral chemoreceptors represents a compensatory mechanism seen in patients with severe chronic obstructive pulmonary disease (COPD), such as the end-stage of emphysema. In these patients, a low PaO$_2$ is accompanied by a chronically elevated PaCO$_2$ attributable to severely impaired gas diffusion at damaged alveolar-capillary membranes. The abnormally high PaCO$_2$ levels that result from the impaired gas exchange ultimately reduce the sensitivity of the *central* chemoreception mechanism. (This mechanism is the main chemical control of breathing and is discussed subsequently.) As a result of the reduced sensitivity of the central mechanism, the patient with severe emphysema becomes increasingly dependent on the hypoxic drive mechanism of the peripheral chemoreceptors. Fortunately, the elevated PaCO$_2$ increases the O$_2$-sensitivity of the carotid and aortic body chemoreceptors, so that hypoxic drive becomes the primary chemical control of breathing in these individuals.

In addition to the primary O$_2$-sensing activity of the peripheral chemoreceptors, the cells of the carotid and aortic bodies monitor blood chemistry via detection of CO$_2$/pH levels. An increase in the PaCO$_2$ causes a decrease in intracellular pH when CO$_2$ diffuses into the glomus cells and becomes hydrated, thus liberating H$^+$, as shown by the following equation:

$$CO_2 + H_2O \rightarrow H_2CO_3 \rightarrow H^+ + HCO_3^-$$

The acidification process is enhanced by the enzyme, carbonic anhydrase, present in the chemoreceptor cells. As the pH within the cells decreases, an ion exchange mechanism is activated, which results in the release of catecholamine neurotransmitters that stimulate the afferent nerves (Gonzalez, Dinger, and Fidone, 1995).

In animal studies in which both the carotid and aortic bodies have been denervated, and in humans in whom the carotid bodies have been removed but the aortic bodies are intact, the respiratory responses to blood gases are essentially the same. Namely, there is little change in ventilation at rest, but the response to hypoxia is lost. In addition, there is a 30% reduction in the ventilatory response to CO$_2$ (Ganong, 1995). This loss of hypoxic drive implies that the aortic and carotid bodies are the primary chemoreceptors for detection of falling PaO$_2$ values, and that they play a minor role in the detection of rising PaCO$_2$ values. However, since the response to PaCO$_2$ is not *completely* abolished by the blockade of carotid and aortic bodies, some other chemoreceptor mechanism must be assisting these peripheral receptors in the detection of rising PCO$_2$ levels in the bloodstream. We now consider a central control mechanism responsible for detecting high PaCO$_2$ and low pH values.

CHEMORECEPTORS AND HYPERCAPNIC DRIVE

Medullary Chemosensitive Area

The hyperventilation response to an increase in PaCO$_2$ is mediated by medullary chemoreceptors located at or within a few hundred μm of the ventrolateral surface of the medulla oblongata (Fig. 10–10) (Nattie, 1995). These central chemoreceptors making up the **chemosensitive area** are found near the medullary respiratory center but are distinct from it. Central chemoreceptors exhibit a remarkable sensitivity to arterial PCO$_2$ but, as we shall see, the detection is accomplished in a very indirect manner. It should be noted that medullary chemoreceptors do not detect arterial PO$_2$ levels.

Hypercapnic Drive and Ventilatory Response to Carbon Dioxide Excess

In conditions of *hypercapnia* the arterial PCO$_2$ is elevated. Central chemoreceptors indirectly detect this blood gas abnormality and send afferent signals to the medullary respiratory center which, in turn, increases the minute volume of ventilation to correct the imbalance (see Fig. 10–1). For this reason, the central mechanism is referred to as the **hypercapnic drive.** In actual fact, medullary chemoreceptors do not directly detect the partial pressure of CO$_2$. Instead, they monitor the H$^+$ concentration of both the cerebrospinal fluid (CSF) and the interstitial fluid of brain cells located on the ventrolateral surface of the medulla. Brain cells are bathed by interstitial fluid that is in contact with CSF; therefore, they are affected by the ionic composition and pH of CSF. The composition of CSF is determined, in part, by membrane transporters that move substances from the bloodstream through the blood-brain barrier into the CSF (Leff and Schumacker, 1993). When blood levels of PCO$_2$ are elevated, CO$_2$ rapidly crosses cell membranes, including those of the blood-brain barrier (Fig. 10–11). By contrast, H$^+$ and bicarbonate (HCO$_3^-$) penetrate the blood-brain barrier very slowly. As CO$_2$ enters the interstitial fluid and CSF, it combines with H$_2$O to form carbonic acid (H$_2$CO$_3$), which immediately dissociates to H$^+$ and HCO$_3^-$:

$$CO_2 + H_2O \rightarrow H_2CO_3 \rightarrow H^+ + HCO_3^-$$

The Respiratory System

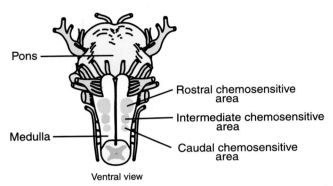

FIGURE 10–10. Chemosensitive areas of the medulla. Central chemoreceptors are located in the chemosensitive areas on the ventral surface of the medulla, in close contact with the CSF that bathes the surface.

As the hydration of CO_2 continues, the concentration of H^+ in the CSF increases, proportionately activating the medullary chemoreceptors. Stimulation of the respiratory center follows. The central chemoreceptors are unusually sensitive to $PaCO_2$ levels, providing minute-to-minute adjustments in the depth and rate of breathing to maintain homeostasis of blood gases. What accounts for this exquisite sensitivity of the hypercapnic drive mechanism?

HCO_3^- is a common ion found in the bloodstream and is the most important plasma buffer for neutralizing H^+. However, it is not normally found in the CSF in large amounts. Additionally, HCO_3^- does not readily cross the blood-brain barrier to enter the CSF. As a result of this nearly total absence of buffering capability, any accumulation of H^+ within the CSF results in an immediate fall in the pH of the CSF from its normal value of about 7.33. As the hydrogen ion concentration increases, the respiratory center is activated to increase ventilation and offset the hypercapnia. Under conditions in which the arterial PCO_2 is abnormally changed, the blood-brain barrier regulates the pH of the CSF by slowly adjusting the HCO_3^- concentration of the CSF over a period of several hours (Leff and Schumacker, 1993).

Recall that COPDs such as emphysema are characterized by elevated $PaCO_2$, and decreased sensitivity of the central chemoreceptor mechanism. This impairment accompanies a chronic state of hypercapnia because there is sufficient time for HCO_3^- to transfer from the plasma into the CSF. As a result of this movement of HCO_3^-, the cerebrospinal fluid gains buffering capacity and is able to neutralize H^+ before medullary chemoreceptors are activated. In short, the hypercapnic drive becomes unreliable in individuals with COPD. Instead, they become almost totally dependent on a compensated hypoxic drive mechanism that exhibits increased sensitivity to changes in arterial PO_2, even in the homeostatic range of 90 to 110 mm Hg (see Fig. 10–9).

In a similar way, drug overdoses involving CNS depressants such as barbiturates or narcotics reduce the effectiveness of the hypercapnic drive. Because medullary respiratory centers are progressively depressed in such toxicities, HCO_3^- has adequate time to enter the CSF and buffer H^+ generated through the hydration of CO_2. The main chemical control of breathing, therefore, switches to the hypoxic drive mechanism, just as in the end-stages of emphysema. If a CNS overdose victim is given supplemental oxygen without supported ventilation, there is risk of suppressing hypoxic drive as the PaO_2 increases in response to O_2 therapy. Consequently, the patient is deprived of his or her remaining chemical control of breathing. For this reason, assisted ventilation is normally provided. (Cottrell and Surkin, 1995).

Effect of Alveolar PCO_2 on Ventilation at Different PAO_2 Levels

Figure 10–12 shows the ventilation response to alveolar PCO_2 at a normal alveolar PO_2 of 100 mm Hg, and to

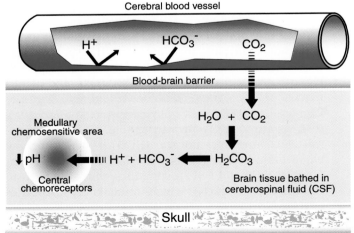

FIGURE 10–11. Hypercapnic drive. The blood-brain barrier is relatively impermeable to hydrogen ions and bicarbonate ions. Carbon dioxide, however, passes from the bloodstream into the ECF with relative ease and is rapidly hydrated to form carbonic acid. Dissociation of carbonic acid generates hydrogen ions, which stimulate the central chemoreceptors. Buffers in the ECF and CSF are normally not present in large quantities; therefore, the pH falls rapidly, stimulating the chemosensitive area of the medulla.

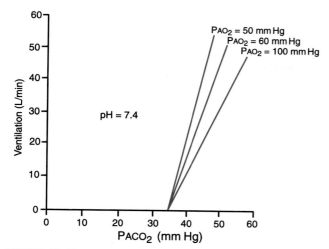

FIGURE 10–12. Effect of alveolar P_{CO_2} on ventilation at different P_{AO_2} levels. The curves illustrate the effects of different alveolar P_{CO_2} values on alveolar ventilation when the alveolar P_{O_2} is held constant at 100, 60, and 50 mm Hg. As the P_{AO_2} decreases, the ventilation response at a given P_{ACO_2} is increased, as shown by the shift of the response curves to the left and upward. At a constant pH, hypoxia increases the sensitivity of the central control system to arterial P_{CO_2} levels.

varying degrees of hypoxia. It can be seen that the slope of the response curve becomes steeper at increasing levels of hypoxia. In other words, hypoxia increases the sensitivity of the control system to an increase in arterial P_{CO_2}. As a result of this change in sensitivity, the respiratory minute volume increases and the blood level of CO_2 is restored to a normal range.

Effect of Acid-Base Levels on Ventilation

A decrease in the pH of the bloodstream may be caused by the accumulation of acidic substances in the tissues, or by the inability of the body to buffer H^+. Either way, a condition of *acidosis* develops as the blood pH falls below its homeostatic range. Acidosis triggers an increase in ventilation, which allows larger quantities of CO_2 to be expelled from the body. As alveolar P_{CO_2} decreases, there is a compensatory fall in H^+ concentration to return the blood pH to the normal range of 7.35 to 7.45, as shown by the following equation:

$$CO_2 + H_2O \leftarrow H_2CO_3 \leftarrow H^+ + HCO_3^-$$

An increase in the pH of the bloodstream may be caused by the accumulation of alkaline substances in the tissues, or by the addition of excess buffer that reduces H^+ concentration. In these examples, a condition of *alkalosis* develops as the blood pH rises above the normal range. Alkalosis brings about a decrease in ventilation, which causes retained CO_2 to be hydrated to carbonic acid. This acid dissociates into H^+, which

lowers the blood pH toward normal, as shown by the following equation:

$$CO_2 + H_2O \rightarrow H_2CO_3 \rightarrow H^+ + HCO_3^-$$

Comparison of different types of acidosis and alkalosis, and a detailed discussion of respiratory system involvement in the maintenance of acid-base levels, is found in Chapter 24.

Nonchemical Receptors and Respiratory Reflexes

Up to this point we have focused on the role of peripheral and central chemoreceptors in providing afferent impulses that modify the basic neural rhythm of breathing. We now consider how respiratory drive is further regulated by sensory receptors in the airways and lungs. These receptors send afferent information that is superimposed on the basic neural control of breathing.

The various receptors of the airways and lungs providing nonchemical reflex modulation of ventilation are innervated by two types of nerve fibers—*myelinated fibers* and *unmyelinated fibers* (also known as *C fibers*). Impulses from nonchemical receptors travel to the medulla through the vagus nerve.

MYELINATED FIBERS

The receptors innervated by **myelinated fibers** are classified as *slowly adapting receptors* or *rapidly adapting receptors* on the basis of the duration of discharge of their afferent nerves following sustained stimulation. Slowly adapting receptors transmit afferent information related to the volume state of the lung, whereas rapidly adapting receptors are involved in augmented breaths or sighs (Leff and Schumacker, 1993).

Slowly Adapting Receptors

The rate of firing of **slowly adapting receptors (SARs)** accommodates (adapts) *slowly* to a stimulus. SARs reside among airway smooth muscle cells and are responsible for mediating an *inspiratory time-shortening response* in the lung as well as the *Hering-Breuer reflexes*. These reflexes are mediated by *pulmonary stretch receptors* (PSRs), which are mechanoreceptors that detect the degree of stretch in the lung parenchyma. The **Hering-Breuer inflation reflex** provides inspiratory inhibition and is triggered following steady lung inflation. This reflex results in an increase in the duration of expiration to limit excessive lung expansion. The **Hering-Breuer deflation reflex** provides expiratory facilitation by reducing the period of expiration following marked defla-

The Respiratory System

tion of the lung (Table 10–3). Recall that parasympathetic output via the vagus nerve is the primary neural control responsible for maintaining smooth muscle tone in airways (see Chap. 4). SARs in the airways are mechanically stimulated during inspiration, resulting in inhibition of parasympathetic bronchomotor tone and a reflex increase in airway diameter. Such stimulation occurs with each inspiration (Leff and Schumacker, 1993).

Rapidly Adapting Receptors

Rapidly adapting receptors (RARs) are also known as **irritant receptors** because they are readily stimulated by exogenous and endogenous chemical substances. Application of stimuli causes the RARs to fire rapidly, and then quickly accommodate to slow firing of impulses. Subepithelial irritant receptors are found

TABLE 10–3	Nonchemical Receptors and Respiratory Reflexes		
Type of Receptor or Reflex	**Location**	**Stimulus**	**Response**
Myelinated Fibers			
Slowly adapting receptors (SARs)	Scattered among airway smooth muscle	Mechanically stimulated during lung inflation	Inhibition of bronchomotor tone, resulting in bronchodilation Inspiratory time-shortening response *Hering-Breuer inflation reflex (increases duration of expiration to limit lung expansion; i.e inspiratory inhibition)
		Mechanically stimulated during lung deflation	*Hering-Breuer deflation reflex (reduces period of expiration following marked deflation of lung; i.e., expiratory facilitation)
Rapidly adapting receptors (RARs) (subepithelial irritant receptors)	Scattered among epithelial cells of large airways	Endogenous and exogenous irritants and particulate matter (e.g., dusts, histamine, noxious chemicals)	Bronchoconstriction reflex Cough Mucus production
Unmyelinated fibers (C-Fiber Afferents; Also Known As J Receptors) Pulmonary C fibers	Located near blood vessels in the lung	Endogenous and exogenous chemicals Lung hyperinflation	Pulmonary chemoreflex (apnea, bronchoconstriction, bradycardia, hypotension) Vasodilation
Bronchial C fibers	Located near blood vessels in the bronchi	Endogenous and exogenous chemicals Lung hyperinflation	Pulmonary chemoreflex (apnea, bronchoconstriction, bradycardia, hypotension)
Diving reflex	Nasal and facial receptors	Cold water	Apnea and bradycardia
Irritant receptors	Irritant receptors in nose and upper airways	Inhalation of irritating chemicals (e.g., ammonia)	Apnea
Pain reflex	Pain receptors (generalized location throughout the body)	Pain	Apnea
Baroreceptor reflex	Aortic arch and carotid sinus baroreceptors	Elevated blood pressure	Bradycardia Decreased force of contraction Decreased ventilation
		Depressed blood pressure	Tachycardia Increased force of contraction Increased ventilation

Hering-Breuer reflexes are mediated by mechanoreceptors known as pulmonary stretch receptors (PSRs).
Source: Ganong, 1995; Kubin & Davies, 1995.

among epithelial cells of large airways and are stimulated by irritants and inflammatory mediators such as histamine. Stimulation of RARs by particulate matter, noxious chemicals, or cold air provides the sensory component of the **bronchoconstriction (irritant) reflex** in the trachea (see Table 10–3). Recall that this protective reflex prevents the entry of potentially damaging substances to distal parts of the lung (see Fig. 5–5). The motor response of the reflex includes coughing, bronchoconstriction, and mucus production. Some patients with asthma exhibit a hyperreactive irritant receptor response that accounts, in part, for the dramatic reaction seen in these individuals when noxious substances are inhaled.

UNMYELINATED FIBERS (C-FIBER AFFERENTS)

The terminal endings of **unmyelinated fibers** or **C-fiber afferents** are found close to pulmonary capillaries. Because of this proximity to capillaries and airways, over the years these fibers have been variously referred to as *juxtacapillary receptors, juxtapulmonary capillary receptors, juxta-alveolar receptors,* or simply, *J receptors.* **Pulmonary C fibers** and **bronchial C fibers** are both found near blood vessels in the lung and bronchi, respectively, and both are stimulated by lung hyperinflation and by chemicals (see Table 10–3). The respiratory response produced by stimulation of C-fiber afferents is called the **pulmonary chemoreflex.** This reflex is characterized by apnea, followed by rapid breathing, bronchoconstriction, bradycardia, and hypotension. The precise role of this reflex in altering breathing patterns is unclear; however, it probably occurs in association with pathophysiologic conditions such as interstitial lung edema, pulmonary congestion, and pulmonary embolism (Ganong, 1995; Leff and Schumacker, 1993).

Mild bronchoconstriction is often observed following cold air hyperpnea, especially in individuals with asthma. Operation of this cold air–induced asthma response is not fully understood; however, the bronchoconstriction response is similar to that seen with respiratory system heat loss and water loss associated with exercise-induced bronchoconstriction (EIB) (Leff and Schumacker, 1993). It is believed that cold air hyperpnea stimulates C fibers to release *tachykinins* such as *substance P.* These mediators cause edema of the airways and bronchoconstriction of airway smooth muscle (Leff and Schumacker, 1993).

OTHER REFLEXES

Extrapulmonary airways and other sites contain several types of receptors that contribute to the reflex control of respiration (see Table 10–3). These reflexes and receptors include:

- **Diving reflex:** Stimulation of nasal or facial receptors with cold water causes apnea and bradycardia
- **Irritant receptors:** Inhalation of irritating chemicals such as ammonia stimulates irritant receptors in the nose and upper airways to result in reflex apnea
- **Pain reflex:** Sudden pain causes apnea
- **Baroreceptor reflex:** Elevated systemic blood pressure stimulates aortic arch and carotid sinus baroreceptors to reduce the heart rate, force of contraction, and the rate of ventilation. Depressed systemic blood pressure produces an increase in heart rate, force of contraction, and rate of ventilation. (Details of the baroreceptor reflex are studied in the cardiovascular unit.)

Table 10–3 summarizes the location, stimulation, and responses associated with some of the nonchemical receptors of the airway and lung.

Summary

We have seen that the muscles of breathing are controlled by a central pattern generator that consists of networked cells in the brain and spinal cord. This basic neural mechanism is responsible for the rhythmic generation of motor impulses. The repetitive neural pattern is modified by a variety of chemoreceptors and mechanoreceptors located both peripherally and centrally. The basic chemical modification of breathing depends on the operation of a peripheral hypoxic drive mechanism as well as a central hypercapnic drive mechanism. We have also seen that the basic neural control of breathing can be further modified by nonchemical receptors and reflexes of the airways and lungs.

BIBLIOGRAPHY

Berger AJ and Bellingham MC: Mechanisms of respiratory motor output. In Dempsey JA and Pack AI (eds): Regulation of Breathing. Marcel Dekker, New York, 1995.

Bianchi AL and Pásaro R: Organization of central respiratory neurons. In Miller AD, Bianchi AL, and Bishop BP (eds): Neural Control of the Respiratory Muscles. CRC Press, Boca Raton, FL, 1997.

Bisgard GE and Neubauer JA: Peripheral and central effects of hypoxia. In Dempsey JA and Pack AI (eds): Regulation of Breathing. Marcel Dekker, New York, 1995.

Cottrell GP and Surkin HB: Pharmacology for Respiratory Care Practitioners. FA Davis, Philadelphia, 1995.

Davenport PW and Reep RL: Cerebral cortex and respiration. In Dempsey JA and Pack AI (eds): Regulation of Breathing. Marcel Dekker, New York, 1995.

Dick TE, Van Lunteren E, and Kelsen SG: Control of respiratory motor activity. In Roussos C (ed): The Thorax—Part A Physiology, ed 2. Marcel Dekker, New York, 1995.

Feldman JL and Smith JC: Neural control of respiratory pattern in mammals: An overview. In Dempsey JA and Pack AI (eds): Regulation of Breathing. Marcel Dekker, New York, 1995.

Fontana GA, et al (1992). Changes in respiratory activity induced by mastication in humans. J Appl Physiol. 72:779–86.

Frazier DT, Xu F, and Lee L: Respiratory-related reflexes and the cerebellum. In Miller AD, Bianchi AL, and Bishop BP (eds): Neural Control of the Respiratory Muscles. CRC Press, Boca Raton, FL, 1997.

Ganong WF: Review of Medical Physiology, ed 17. Appleton & Lange, Norwalk, CT, 1995.

Gonzalez C, Dinger BG, and Fidone SJ: Mechanisms of carotid body chemoreception. In Dempsey JA and Pack AI (eds): Regulation of Breathing. Marcel Dekker, New York, 1995.

Haddad GG, Donnelly DF, and Bazzy-Asaad AR: Developmental control of respiration: Neurobiological basis. In Dempsey JA and Pack AI (eds): Regulation of Breathing. Marcel Dekker, New York, 1995.

Harper RM: Higher brain areas involved in respiratory control. In Miller AD, Bianchi AL, and Bishop BP (eds): Neural Control of the Respiratory Muscles. CRC Press, Boca Raton, FL, 1997.

Jean A, Car A, and Kessler JP: Brainstem organization of swallowing and its interaction with respiration. In Miller AD, Bianchi AL, and Bishop BP (eds): Neural Control of the Respiratory Muscles. CRC Press, Boca Raton, FL, 1997.

Kubin L and Davies RO: Control pathways of pulmonary and airway vagal afferents. In Dempsey JA and Pack AI (eds): Regulation of Breathing. Marcel Dekker, New York, 1995.

Lawson EE, Czyzyk-Krzeska MF, Dean JB, and Milhorn DE: Developmental aspects of the neural control of breathing. In Beckerman RC, Brouillette RT, and Hunt CE (eds): Respiratory Control Disorders in Infants and Children. Williams & Wilkins, Baltimore, 1992.

Leevers AM and Road JD: Reflex influences acting on the respiratory muscles of the chest wall. In Roussos C (ed): The Thorax—Part A Physiology, ed 2. Marcel Dekker, New York, 1995.

Leff AR and Schumacker PT: Respiratory Physiology: Basics and Applications. WB Saunders, Philadelphia, 1993.

Mathew OP and Ghosh TK: Role of airway afferents on upper airway muscle activity. In Dempsey JA and Pack AI (eds): Regulation of Breathing. Marcel Dekker, New York, 1995.

Mines AH: Respiratory Physiology, ed 3. Raven Press, New York, 1993.

Nattie EE: Central chemoreception. In Dempsey JA and Pack AI (eds): Regulation of Breathing. Marcel Dekker, New York, 1995.

Nunn JF: Nunn's Applied Respiratory Physiology, ed 4. Butterworth-Heinemann, Oxford, 1993.

Richter DW, Ballanyi K, and Ramirez J: Respiratory rhythm generation. In Miller AD, Bianchi AL, and Bishop BP (eds): Neural Control of the Respiratory Muscles. CRC Press, Boca Raton, FL, 1997.

Waldrop TG and Porter JP: Hypothalamic involvement in respiratory and cardiovascular regulation. In Dempsey JA and Pack AI (eds): Regulation of Breathing. Marcel Dekker, New York, 1995.

West JB: Respiratory Physiology: The Essentials, ed 6. Williams & Wilkins, Baltimore, 1998.

CHAPTER 11

Ventilation, Perfusion, and Metabolic Function of the Lung

chapter objectives

After studying this chapter the reader should be able to:

☐ Describe the depth and frequency of breathing seen with the following ventilatory patterns and maneuvers:
  Eupnea, apnea, orthopnea, hyperpnea, tachypnea, dyspnea.

☐ Compare and contrast the following types of breathing:
  Hyperventilation, hypoventilation, Kussmaul's breathing, Biot's breathing, Cheyne-Stokes breathing.

☐ Explain why the entire tidal volume with each breath does not reach the alveoli by describing the following volumes:
  Anatomical dead space volume, alveolar volume.

☐ Compare and contrast the following:
  Minute or total ventilation, alveolar ventilation, anatomical dead space ventilation.

☐ Calculate the minute ventilation, alveolar ventilation, and anatomical dead space ventilation given the tidal volume, anatomical dead space volume, and respiratory frequency.

☐ Calculate the anatomical dead space ventilation given the total ventilation and the dead space to tidal volume ratio.

☐ Define physiologic dead space ventilation.

☐ Compare and contrast physiologic dead space ventilation and anatomical dead space ventilation.

☐ Calculate the physiologic dead space volume (Bohr dead space) given the mixed expired partial pressure of carbon dioxide ($P_{E}CO_2$) and the arterial partial pressure of carbon dioxide ($P_{a}CO_2$).

☐ Explain why alveolar ventilation is made more effective by an increase in the depth of breathing than by an increase in the rate of breathing.

☐ Define hydrostatic pressure gradient as it applies to regional ventilation in the lung.

☐ Explain why the alveoli in the apex of the upright lung are less compliant than those in the base by discussing intrapleural pressure differences in the lung.

☐ Briefly describe the parallel flow of blood through the systemic and pulmonary circuits.

☐ Describe pulmonary vascular resistance (PVR) in terms of pressure gradients and cardiac output.

☐ Describe the effect that differences in transmural pressure have on the diameter, resistance, and flow characteristics of pulmonary capillaries.

☐ Discuss the effect the following factors have on the active control of pulmonary vascular resistance and flow:

   Autonomic vasomotor tone, cardiovascular drugs with vascular effects.
   Discuss the effect the following vasoactive substances have on the active control of pulmonary vascular resistance and flow:
   Nitric oxide, angiotensin-converting enzyme (ACE), norepinephrine, epinephrine, histamine, bradykinin, prostaglandins, serotonin.

☐ Describe the mechanism of hypoxic pulmonary vasoconstriction and its effect on pulmonary vascular resistance and flow.

☐ Describe the effect lung inflation and deflation have on the diameter, resistance, and flow characteristics of the following pulmonary blood vessels by comparing the response at high and low lung volumes:

   Alveolar septal capillaries, extra-alveolar capillaries.

☐ Describe how flow in the pulmonary blood vessels is affected by the vertical hydrostatic pressure gradient of the lung.

☐ Explain the zone model of perfusion in the lung and describe the relationships among arterial, venous, and alveolar pressures in the various zones of the upright lung.

☐ Explain why the lung is at continual risk of accumulating fluid that has leaked out of pulmonary capillaries.

☐ Describe the Starling forces acting at the capillary wall by discussing the factors that generate the force and describing the direction of flow of fluid into or out of capillaries.

☐ Describe how the lymphatic capillaries scavenge fluid from interstitial tissue in the lung.

☐ Briefly describe the metabolic function of the lung.

☐ Explain how the lung activates angiotensin I as the substance passes through pulmonary circulation.

☐ Name three substances synthesized by the lung and three substances inactivated by the lung.

key terms

alveolar dead space	Bohr dead space
alveolar septal capillaries	capillary pressure (P_c); capillary hydrostatic
alveolar ventilation ($\dot{V}_A$)	pressure
anatomical dead space ventilation ($\dot{V}_D$)	Cheyne-Stokes breathing (chān′ stōks′)
angiotensin-converting enzyme (ACE)	dead space to tidal volume ratio (V_D/V_T)
apnea (ap-nē′ a)	dyspnea (disp-nē′ a; disp′ nē-a)
Biot's breathing (bē-oz′)	eupnea (ūp-nē′ a)

extra-alveolar capillaries
hydrostatic pressure gradient
hyperpnea (hī''perp-nē' a)
hyperventilation
hypoventilation
hypoxic pulmonary vasoconstriction
interstitial fluid colloid osmotic pressure (π_i);
   interstitial fluid colloid oncotic pressure
interstitial fluid pressure (P_i); interstitial fluid
   hydrostatic pressure
Kussmaul's breathing (koos' mowl)
minute ventilation; minute volume; total ventilation
   ($\dot{V}_E$)

orthopnea (or'' thop' nē-a)
physiologic dead space ventilation
plasma colloid osmotic pressure (π_c); plasma
   colloid oncotic pressure
pulmonary vascular resistance (PVR)
Starling forces
tachypnea (tak'' ip-nē' a)
zone model of perfusion
   zone 1
   zone 2
   zone 3
   zone 4

This chapter introduces the reader to the different ventilatory patterns and the effect that dead space has on overall ventilation of the lung. Factors that contribute to regulation and modification of both ventilation and perfusion are also introduced. In addition, the chapter examines the regional differences in the lung that contribute to the zone model of ventilation and perfusion. These topics provide valuable background information for an understanding of ventilation-perfusion relationships to be discussed later. The chapter continues with an introduction to lung fluid balance and clearance, and concludes with a brief discussion of the metabolic function of the lung that allows it to synthesize, activate, and inactivate substances found in pulmonary circulation.

Ventilation of the Lung

TYPES OF BREATHING AND VENTILATORY MANEUVERS

A variety of breathing patterns is seen in response to both normal and abnormal physiologic conditions. Following is a brief description of common ventilatory patterns and maneuvers.

Eupnea

Normal, spontaneous breathing is known as **eupnea** (Fig. 11–1A). The rhythmic pattern is produced by the central pattern generator of the medulla. Efferent activity transmitted to the diaphragm results in *diaphragmatic breathing,* a gentle downward and upward excursion of the diaphragm that moves the tidal volume (VT) of air into and out of the lung, a volume approximately 500 mL in a normal, healthy adult. *Costal breathing* refers to the rib cage movements that occur as the depth of ventilation increases.

Apnea

A temporary cessation in ventilatory activity is called **apnea.** This breathing pattern is characterized by sustained deep inspirations separated by short periods of expiration (Fig. 11–1B). Clearly, this interruption of breathing can only be tolerated for a brief period of time. Typically, apnea occurs only during voluntary breath-holding and during nonrespiratory activities such as speaking, singing, coughing, and sneezing. Apnea is occasionally seen in patients with central nervous system (CNS) injury in which inspiratory inhibition is reduced, and is also a component in several types of *sleep apnea syndromes,* including obstructive sleep apnea and central sleep apnea. In these disorders, the duration of apnea extends long enough to cause hypercapnia (elevated P_{aCO_2}), hypoxemia (depressed P_{aO_2}), and reduced quality of sleep.

Orthopnea

In a ventilatory condition known as **orthopnea,** a subject feels discomfort and anxiety breathing in any but the erect sitting or standing position. In orthopnea, muscles of breathing are used forcefully to ventilate the lungs. Patients often brace themselves to stabilize joints such as the shoulder joint, allowing the accessory muscles of breathing to assist the diaphragm. This condition may be observed in cases of bronchial asthma, pulmonary edema, severe emphysema, or pneumonia.

Hyperpnea

An increase in the depth of breathing, with or without an increase in the rate of breathing, is called **hyperpnea** (Fig. 11–1C). Such a pattern occurs in response to increased metabolism that raises the arterial P_{CO_2}, activating the hypercapnic drive to the medullary respiratory center.

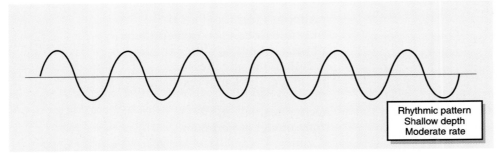

Rhythmic pattern
Shallow depth
Moderate rate

A - Eupnea

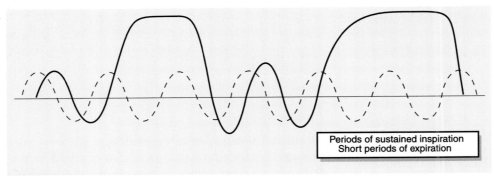

Periods of sustained inspiration
Short periods of expiration

B - Apnea

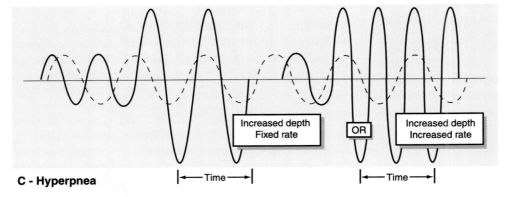

Increased depth
Fixed rate

OR

Increased depth
Increased rate

C - Hyperpnea |← Time →| |← Time →|

FIGURE 11–1. Basic breathing patterns. For comparison purposes, breathing patterns are shown superimposed on a graph of normal tidal breathing. (Eupnea is represented by the dotted line in B and C.)

Tachypnea

An abnormally rapid respiratory rate is known as **tachypnea.** If the rate is prolonged, it can lead to excessive loss of carbon dioxide and acid-base imbalance.

Hyperventilation

An increase in ventilation that reaches the alveoli can result from an increase in the depth of breathing, rate of breathing, or both, and is termed **hyperventilation.** Such a pattern causes carbon dioxide to be exhaled to the atmosphere, thus decreasing the partial pressure of carbon dioxide (alveolar carbon dioxide tension) (P_{ACO_2}) and Pa_{CO_2}.

Hypoventilation

A decrease in the ventilation reaching the alveoli can be caused by a decrease in the depth of breathing, rate

of breathing, or both, and is termed **hypoventilation.** With this type of breathing pattern, carbon dioxide is retained in the body, thus increasing both the P_{ACO_2} and Pa_{CO_2}.

Dyspnea

The sensation of shortness of breath is termed **dyspnea.** This respiratory system response is a symptom, not an actual breathing maneuver. Dyspnea results when the work of breathing increases in response to an increase in airway resistance. Patients suffering an acute asthma attack experience severe dyspnea that causes them to hyperventilate, producing a Pa_{CO_2} that is less than the normal value of approximately 40 mm Hg.

Kussmaul's Breathing

An increase in both the rate and depth of breathing is seen in a ventilatory pattern called **Kussmaul's**

breathing (Fig. 11–2A). This very deep gasping type of breathing increases both P_{AO_2} and Pa_{O_2}, and decreases both P_{ACO_2} and Pa_{CO_2}. Kussmaul's breathing is occasionally seen in patients with severe nonrespiratory, or metabolic, acidosis. This condition is associated with early stages of acetylsalicylic acid (ASA) toxicity and with diabetic ketoacidosis.

Biot's Breathing

Short periods of rapid breathing at uniform depth, followed by periods of apnea, characterize the ventilatory pattern known as **Biot's breathing** (Fig. 11-2B). The pattern is occasionally seen in patients with increased intracranial pressure.

Cheyne-Stokes Breathing

Both the tidal volume and frequency are variable in the common and bizarre ventilatory pattern known as **Cheyne-Stokes breathing** (Fig. 11–2C). In this breathing pattern, a period of apnea lasting 10 to 60 seconds is followed by a period of increasing depth and frequency of respirations. This activity is then followed by decreasing depth and frequency until another period of apnea develops. Although the mechanisms underlying Cheyne-Stokes ventilation are not fully understood, the pattern is sometimes observed with head trauma as well as with CNS dysfunctions associated with CNS depressant drug overdoses, or reduced cerebral blood flow.

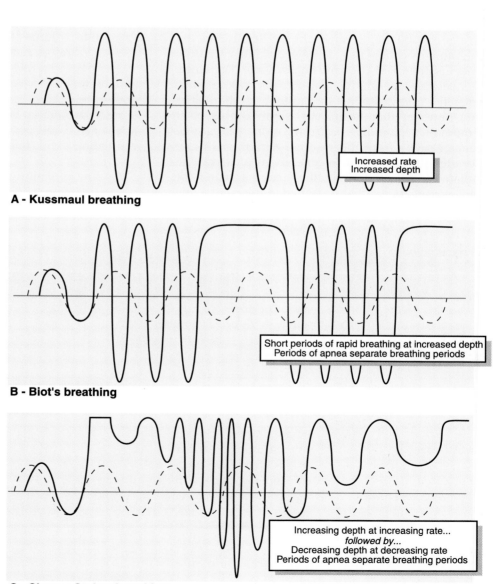

A - Kussmaul breathing

Increased rate
Increased depth

B - Biot's breathing

Short periods of rapid breathing at increased depth
Periods of apnea separate breathing periods

C - Cheyne-Stokes breathing

Increasing depth at increasing rate...
followed by...
Decreasing depth at decreasing rate
Periods of apnea separate breathing periods

FIGURE 11–2. Types of breathing. For comparison purposes, types of breathing are shown superimposed on a graph of normal tidal breathing. (Eupnea is represented by the dotted line in A, B, and C.)

Table 11–1 summarizes different types of breathing and ventilatory maneuvers.

ALVEOLAR AND DEAD SPACE VENTILATION

General Remarks

Recall from our study of the conducting and respiratory zones of the lung that most of the total cross-sectional area (and volume) of the respiratory system is contained in the alveoli. At functional residual capacity (FRC), an average adult lung contains about 3000 mL of gas in the alveoli, whereas the conducting passages contain only about 150 mL of gas. As a rough estimate of this conducting zone volume, the dead space in the conducting passages, in milliliters, has been found to be approximately equal to the weight, in pounds, of an adult subject (Ganong, 1995; West, 1995). Recall also that during a normal inspiration, the lung volume increases by a tidal volume (V_T) of approximately 500 mL. Because of their rigidity, the extrapulmonary conducting airways expand very little during inspiration of a 500 mL tidal volume. Therefore, the *alveolar volume* will be approximately 500 mL immediately following this inspiration. It should be noted, however, that the first gas to enter the alveoli at the onset of inspiration is *not* fresh gas that has entered the nasal cavity from the external environment and descended through 15 or so generations of airways to ventilate the alveoli. Instead, the first gas to enter the alveoli is *nonfresh* gas that remained in the conducting passages at the end of the previous breath. In other words, if the volume of nonfresh gas in the conducting passages is 150 mL, and the tidal volume is 500 mL, only 350 mL of *fresh* gas will enter the alveoli with each breath. In effect, the nonfresh gas that re-enters the alveoli, after being exhaled as the final 150 mL of gas in the previous breath, "dilutes" the concentration of atmospheric gas entering with the next breath.

Minute Ventilation and Alveolar Ventilation

The product of the tidal volume and the respiratory frequency (in breaths per minute) is called the **minute ventilation** or **minute volume.** This ventilation flowrate is also known as the **total ventilation ($\dot{V}E$),** and is shown by the following equation:

$$\dot{V}_E = V_T \times RR$$

where:
$\dot{V}_E$ = minute ventilation
V_T = tidal volume
RR = respiratory rate

EXAMPLE 1

If the V_T is equal to 500 mL and the respiratory rate is 12 breaths per minute, what is the minute ventilation in mL/min?

$$\text{Minute ventilation} = \frac{500 \text{ mL}}{1 \text{ breath}} \times \frac{12 \text{ breaths}}{1 \text{ min}}$$

$$= 6000 \text{ mL/min}$$

TABLE 11–1	Types of Breathing and Ventilatory Maneuvers
Breathing Pattern	**Description**
Eupnea	Rhythmic pattern
	Shallow depth (V_T approximately 500 mL)
	Moderate rate (RR approximately 8/min)
Apnea	Periods of sustained inspiration
	Short periods of expiration
	Commonly occurs during nonrespiratory activities such as speaking, swallowing, or coughing
Hyperpnea	Increased depth at the same rate, or increased depth with increased rate
*Kussmaul's breathing	Increased rate
	Increased depth
Biot's breathing	Short periods of rapid breathing
	Uniform pattern with increased depth
	Periods of apnea separate the breathing periods
Cheyne-Stokes breathing	Increasing depth at increasing frequency, followed by decreasing depth at decreasing frequency
	Periods of apnea separate the breathing periods

V_T = tidal volume; RR = respiratory rate.
Note: Comparisons such as "increased" or "decreased" are relative to the normal, quiet breathing pattern of eupnea.
*Kussmaul's breathing is a sustained type of hyperpnea, lasting for a period of time. The unusual pattern is sometimes seen in cases of acute toxicity due to aspirin (salicylate) overdose.

Recall that the entire gas flow of minute ventilation does not reach the alveoli as fresh gas. The portion of minute ventilation reaching those alveoli involved in gas exchange is called the **alveolar ventilation ($\dot{V}A$)**.

EXAMPLE 2

If the tidal volume of the lung is 500 mL and the volume of the conducting passages is 150 mL, what is the alveolar ventilation in mL/min when the respiratory rate is 12 breaths per minute?

$$\text{Alveolar volume} = \text{tidal volume} - \text{dead space volume}$$
$$= 500 \text{ mL} - 150 \text{ mL} = 350 \text{ mL}$$

$$\therefore \text{Alveolar ventilation} = \frac{350 \text{ mL}}{1 \text{ breath}} \times \frac{12 \text{ breaths}}{1 \text{ min}}$$
$$= 4200 \text{ mL/min}$$

Anatomical Dead Space Ventilation

The portion of minute ventilation that does not contribute to alveolar ventilation is called **anatomical dead space ventilation ($\dot{V}D$)**. This ventilation is the product of dead space volume and respiratory frequency. Using the data given in the previous example, the anatomical dead space ventilation is calculated as follows:

EXAMPLE 3

$$\text{Anatomical dead space ventilation} = \frac{150 \text{ mL}}{1 \text{ breaths}}$$

$$\times \frac{12 \text{ breaths}}{1 \text{ min}} = 1800 \text{ mL/min}$$

The volume of gas that does not contribute to ventilation of the alveoli occupies *dead space* in the conducting passages. Clearly, the portion of total ventilation used to ventilate this space is wasted. The **dead space to tidal volume ratio (VD/VT)** provides a measure of how much of the minute ventilation is wasted ventilating the conducting zone of the lung. $\dot{V}D$, therefore, can be calculated as the product of the total ventilation and the dead space to tidal volume ratio:

$$\dot{V}D = \dot{V}E \times \frac{VD}{VT}$$

Using the same data from the above examples, the anatomical dead space ventilation ($\dot{V}D$) can be calculated using the dead space to tidal volume ratio (VD/VT):

EXAMPLE 4

$$\text{Anatomical dead space ventilation} = \frac{6000 \text{ mL}}{1 \text{ min}}$$
$$\times \frac{150 \text{ mL}}{500 \text{ mL}} = 1800 \text{ mL/min}$$

Note that the calculated value for the anatomical dead space ventilation ($\dot{V}D = 1800$ mL/min), is the same in both Examples 3 and 4.

Physiologic Dead Space Ventilation

At any given time, even in healthy lungs, some of the gas entering the respiratory zone may reach alveoli that are unperfused or underperfused. These alveoli represent the **alveolar dead space.** The volume of gas that ventilates these nonfunctional alveoli is essentially wasted. In a functional sense, this portion of total ventilation is just as ineffective as the portion of gas ventilating the conducting zone. **Physiologic dead space ventilation,** therefore, refers to the *total* amount of wasted ventilation—both the ventilation of the anatomical dead space and the excessive ventilation of alveoli that are not adequately perfused. Physiologic dead space ventilation will always be at least as large as the anatomical dead space ventilation, typically comprising about 25% to 35% of the total ventilation in healthy individuals (Leff and Schumacker, 1993). However, in lungs with severely underperfused regions, the physiologic dead space ventilation may be substantially greater than the anatomical dead space ventilation.

In the *two-compartment lung model* shown in Figure 11–3, one group of alveoli is both ventilated and perfused; the other group is ventilated but does not receive blood flow. A sample of alveolar gas from the perfused compartment has a $PACO_2$ of approximately 40 mm Hg, roughly the same as the arterial carbon dioxide tension ($PaCO_2 = 40$ mm Hg). The alveoli which are unperfused, however, have a $PACO_2$ equal to zero, because no carbon dioxide is able to leave the bloodstream to enter the alveoli. Exhaled gas from this two-compartment model has a PCO_2 that is less than that of the perfused alveoli but greater than that of the unperfused alveoli. In effect, the exhaled carbon dioxide from the perfused respiratory units is "diluted" by the gas from the units that did not participate in gas exchange. This *mixed expired PCO_2* or $PECO_2$ can be used to calculate the physiologic dead space volume when the $PACO_2$ is known. This volume is also known as the **Bohr dead space,** named after the Danish physiologist Christian Bohr (1856–1923) (Leff and Schumacker, 1993):

$$\frac{\dot{V}D}{\dot{V}T} = 1 - \frac{PECO_2}{PACO_2}$$

The Respiratory System

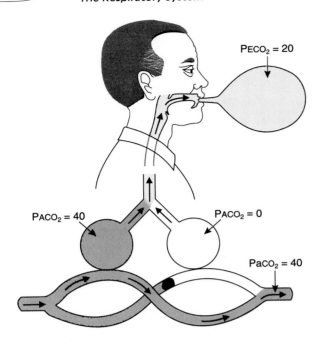

FIGURE 11–3. Physiologic dead space ventilation. Physiologic dead space can be determined by measuring the P_{CO_2} in alveolar gas and in mixed expired gas. The dilution of carbon dioxide in mixed expired gas, relative to alveolar gas, provides a functional measure of the amount of wasted ventilation relative to the minute ventilation. Dead space is 50% (0.5) in this example. (From Leff AR and Schumacker PT: Respiratory Physiology: Basics and Applications. WB Saunders, Philadelphia, 1993, p 55, with permission.)

It has been found that arterial and alveolar values of P_{CO_2} are nearly identical; therefore, Pa_{CO_2} values can be substituted for PA_{CO_2} values. This finding is especially useful because the tension of arterial blood gases can be determined more easily than the tension of alveolar gases. Therefore,

$$\frac{\dot{V}_D}{\dot{V}_T} = 1 - \frac{P_{ECO_2}}{Pa_{CO_2}}$$

EXAMPLE 5

If the P_{ECO_2} value of an expired sample of gas from a subject is found to be 27 mm Hg, and the arterial P_{CO_2} is 40 mm Hg, calculate the physiologic dead space as a percentage of total ventilation.

$$\frac{\dot{V}_D}{\dot{V}_T} = 1 - \frac{27 \text{ mm Hg}}{40 \text{ mm Hg}} = 0.325 \times 100\% = 32.5\%$$

In other words, 32.5% of the total ventilation did not contribute to effective ventilation in this subject.

From these relationships it can be seen that anatomical dead space ventilation varies inversely with tidal volume. The *volume* of the rigid conducting airways is essentially fixed, changing relatively little during a breath. Therefore, this fixed volume of the conducting zone airways (approximately 150 to 200 mL) represents a larger *proportion* of a small tidal volume. At a fixed breathing rate, an increase in the depth of breathing decreases the proportional ventilation of anatomical dead space, thus increasing alveolar ventilation. The delivery of more gas to those alveoli which participate in gas exchange is thus accomplished. For this reason, total alveolar ventilation is made more effective by an increase in the *depth* of breathing than by an increase in the *rate* of breathing.

REGIONAL DIFFERENCES IN VENTILATION

Although we explore the relationships between ventilation and perfusion in a later chapter, it should be noted here that ventilation of the lung is *nonuniform*. In other words, some alveoli are better ventilated than others, even at the same depth and frequency of breathing. This nonuniform ventilation is due to differences in lung compliance related to regional differences in intrapleural pressure. In a subject standing erect, the intrapleural pressure at the apex of the lung is approximately −10 cm H_2O, whereas the intrapleural pressure at the base of the lung is about −2 cm H_2O (Dupuis, 1992; West, 1998). This regional difference in intrapleural pressure is caused by the weight of lung tissue (see Fig. 7–7). Figure 11–4 shows the vertical **hydrostatic pressure gradient** that exists in the upright lung. The effects of gravity, therefore, are progressively greater going down through the mass of lung tissue. West (1998) points out that the sup-

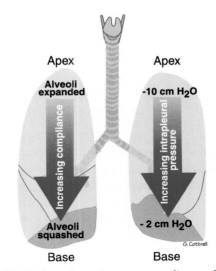

FIGURE 11–4. Hydrostatic pressure gradient and regional ventilation. The regional difference in intrapleural pressure is due to the weight of lung tissue, which requires a higher pressure at the base of the lung in order to support the mass. The more negative conditions at the apex cause alveoli in the region to expand, thus becoming less compliant than those in the base.

port of a structure requires a greater pressure below it than above it. This pressure is required to counteract the downward-acting weight forces on an object. In the respiratory system, the lung is supported by the diaphragm and thorax; furthermore, the pressure at the base is higher, or *less negative*, than the pressure at the apex (-2 cm H_2O compared with -10 cm H_2O).

Perfusion of the Lung

THE PULMONARY CIRCUIT

To understand the role of blood flow through the lung in the exchange of gases, it is necessary to briefly review the basics of general circulation. The reader is encouraged to consult general anatomy and physiology textbooks for a more detailed treatment of the subject. Suitable anatomy and physiology textbooks are included in the chapter bibliography.

The cardiovascular system operates as two parallel circuits, each driven by a ventricle of the heart. Working in tandem, the physiologic left heart pushes blood through the systemic circuit to all parts of the body except the lungs, while the physiologic right heart supplies the lungs via the pulmonary circuit. Blood leaving the left ventricle (LV) exits under high pressure through the aortic valve into the large-diameter aorta, reaching the various organs of the body through progressively smaller arteries that supply numerous arterioles. Arterioles are the body's principal resistance vessels, functioning to regulate the flow of blood into the vast capillary beds that perfuse the tissues. Here, at the site of internal respiration, oxygen and carbon dioxide are exchanged, along with wastes and nutrients to support cellular metabolism. Blood leaves the tissues through venules that drain into small veins. These vessels are collected into progressively larger-diameter veins that return blood to the right atrium (RA) through the vena cavae. The right atrium forces blood into the right ventricle (RV) through the tricuspid valve, working in unison with the left atrium (LA), which pumps blood through the mitral valve to the LV at the same time.

Contraction of the RV propels blood into the pulmonary circuit. Deoxygenated blood leaves the RV through the pulmonary valve and enters the pulmonary trunk, which bifurcates into the right and left pulmonary arteries. These arteries branch into the lobar arteries, which supply the major lobes of the lung. Within the lung, lobar arteries branch successively into the sublobar, segmental, subsegmental, and lobular arteries (Leff and Schumacker, 1993). The pulmonary alveolar septal capillaries branch from the lobular arteries and penetrate the alveolar septa. This intimate association between septal capillaries and the thin-walled squamous epithelial cells (type I pneumocytes) of the alveolar walls provides a large surface area for efficient gas exchange, similar to a continuously moving thin sheet of blood in close contact with the air contained in the alveoli. Equilibration of gas occurs between the alveoli and capillaries. Blood leaves the pulmonary capillaries through venules that are collected into progressively larger-diameter veins. After leaving the lung at the hilum, the pulmonary veins enter the left atrium, returning oxygenated blood to the heart.

As previously described, the two vascular systems operate in parallel. Therefore, the entire cardiac output must pass through both the systemic and pulmonary circuits each minute. In other words, the average blood volume pumped through the pulmonary and systemic circulatory loops over time must be equal in order to prevent excessive damming of blood in either the systemic or the pulmonary veins.

PULMONARY VASCULAR PRESSURE AND RESISTANCE

The pulmonary vascular bed has low resistance compared with that of systemic vascular beds. For this reason the average pressure in the pulmonary arteries is about 18 mm Hg, compared with about 100 mm Hg in typical systemic arteries (Leff and Schumacker, 1993; West, 1998). The **pulmonary vascular resistance (PVR)** is calculated as the pressure difference between proximal and distal pressures divided by the cardiac output:

$$PVR = \frac{P1 - P2}{\dot{Q}}$$

where:
PVR = pulmonary vascular resistance
$P1$ = proximal (upstream) vessel pressure or pulmonary artery pressure
$P2$ = distal (downstream) vessel pressure or left atrial pressure
$\dot{Q}$ = cardiac output

Pulmonary circulation involves blood flow through a low-resistance, low-pressure vascular bed. These hemodynamic conditions are ideal for efficient gas exchange because they provide optimal time for slow-moving pulmonary blood in the alveolar septal capillaries to be exposed to gas in the alveoli.

The right ventricle only has about one-third the muscle mass of the left ventricle. The LV requires a large muscle mass to eject blood under high pressure into the systemic circulation. By contrast, the low pressure generated by contraction of the RV is sufficient to perfuse all regions of the lung. The efficient distribution of blood in the pulmonary circuit is also assisted by the lower hydrostatic pressures in the lung, compared with that in the systemic circuit. For example, the hydrostatic effect acting upon blood in the legs must be overcome in order to pump blood upward toward the heart. This requirement adds greatly to the workload of the physiologic left heart. By contrast, the physiologic right heart does not have to pump blood uphill toward the lungs.

FACTORS AFFECTING PULMONARY VASCULAR RESISTANCE AND FLOW

Active Factors

Active changes in blood vessel diameter are brought about by *neural impulses, cardiovascular drugs* such as digitalis (a vasodilator) or adrenaline (a vasoconstrictor), and by *vasoactive substances* that produce localized effects in the pulmonary vasculature. These influences are examples of *active factors* that modify PVR by altering the tone of vascular smooth muscle.

Sympathetic innervation provides the dominant autonomic nervous system (ANS) control of blood vessels in the lung; parasympathetic control is less common (Nunn, 1993). Sympathetic control of pulmonary blood vessels is mediated through both α_1-adrenergic receptors, which bring about vasoconstriction, and β_2-adrenergic receptors, which cause vasodilation (see Chap. 4). The influence of sympathetic nerves on pulmonary blood vessels is not as great as on systemic blood vessels. Additionally, sympathetic influences on lung vasculature are relatively minor under resting conditions, but increase dramatically under the stress conditions of the fight-or-flight response (Nunn, 1993). Parasympathetic stimulation (M_3-muscarinic cholinergic) results in pulmonary vasodilation via release of acetylcholine, which causes the release of nitric oxide (NO) from pulmonary endothelial cells.

Vasoactive substances acting as tissue hormones to produce local effects include *nitric oxide* and **angiotensin-converting enzyme (ACE),** both produced by pulmonary endothelial cells. Nitric oxide is a potent vasodilator that exhibits selective vasodilation of the pulmonary blood vessels (see Box 14–1), whereas ACE catalyzes the production of a powerful vasoconstrictor called angiotensin II. (This mechanism is discussed later in the chapter with metabolic functions of the lung.) *Norepinephrine* (NE) and *epinephrine* are naturally occurring catecholamine hormones that produce constriction of blood vessels, including those of pulmonary circulation. NE is an especially powerful vasoconstrictor, whereas epinephrine produces less intense vasoconstriction (West, 1998). *Histamine, bradykinin,* and *prostaglandin E_2* (PDE$_2$) are powerful vasodilators produced and released by lung tissue during inflammatory responses, whereas *prostaglandin $F_{2\alpha}$* (PGF$_{2\alpha}$) is a vasocon-

strictor released during such inflammatory reactions. *Serotonin* (5-hydroxytryptamine, 5-HT) is a vasoactive mediator released from platelets in the circulatory system, producing either vasodilation or vasoconstriction, depending on the circulatory region targeted. The functions of serotonin in the control of circulation are not fully understood (Guyton and Hall, 1996).

Decreased oxygen tension of alveolar gas (PAO$_2$) causes contraction of vascular smooth muscle in precapillary pulmonary vessels proximal to alveoli that are operating under hypoxic conditions. In other words, blood vessels that are upstream from capillaries supplying alveoli having decreased PAO$_2$ undergo intense vasoconstriction, thus shutting down blood flow to poorly ventilated alveoli. Capillaries lack smooth muscle in their walls and, therefore, cannot actively change diameter. Arterioles, on the other hand, are located proximal to pulmonary capillaries, possess a large proportion of smooth muscle in their walls, and are equipped with precapillary sphincters which function as "gateways" to regulate blood flow into capillary beds. The response to depressed PAO$_2$ is called **hypoxic pulmonary vasoconstriction,** but the precise mechanism of action is not known (Ganong, 1995; Leff and Schumacker, 1993). This response to alveolar hypoxia is a self-regulating reaction that reduces perfusion to those areas of the lung that are underventilated. Such diversion of local alveolar blood flow to better ventilated lung regions helps regulate ventilation-perfusion ($\dot{V}/\dot{Q}$) ratios in the normal lung (see Chap. 14).

Passive Factors

Changes in the diameter of **alveolar septal capillaries** are not caused by changes in vascular tone. Instead, they are caused by changes in the *transmural pressure* acting across the wall of the vessels. Any decrease in the pressure inside the vessel, or increase in pressure outside the vessel, tends to occlude the small-caliber blood vessels, much as the "floppy tubes" discussed in Chapter 9 (see Fig. 9–4). These special capillaries have a large surface area relative to their volume, thus providing an efficient air-blood exchange surface (Leff and Schumacker, 1993). Their delicate shape, however, can be easily changed by different lung volumes (Fig. 11–5). Because pulmonary alveolar septal capillaries pass through the alveolar septa, they are stretched and constricted as the alveoli inflate. This distortion in the thin-walled capillaries increases the pressure acting on the *outside* of the vessel, decreases capillary diameter, increases PVR, and reduces pulmonary perfusion. The change in vessel diameter reduces the ratio between the total surface area of the bloodstream delivered to the alveoli and the surface area of the air contained in the alveoli. Transmural pressure is also increased when the pressure on the *inside* of the capillary is decreased,

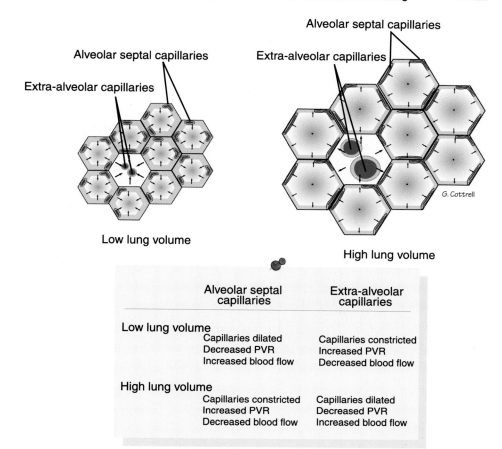

FIGURE 11–5. Pulmonary capillaries. *Alveolar septal capillaries* are located within alveolar septa, which lack significant structural support. Volume changes directly affect the transmural pressure of the septal capillaries. An increase in lung volume above FRC stretches the septa, thins the walls, and compresses the capillaries. *Extra-alveolar capillaries* are located between alveoli and are not directly affected by changes in the wall thickness of alveolar septa. Mechanical tethering to lung parenchyma causes capillary diameters to increase at lung volumes up to FRC. (PVR = pulmonary vascular resistance; FRC = functional residual capacity.)

as occurs in cases of falling blood pressure. Such a condition may accompany hemorrhage. In this condition, the fall in capillary hydrostatic pressure results in collapse of pulmonary blood vessels and reduced PVR, even when alveolar inflation is within normal limits.

Such changes in transmural pressure are examples of *passive factors* that modify pulmonary vascular resistance. Interestingly, the blood vessels that make up pulmonary *microcirculation*, that is, blood vessels without smooth muscle in their walls, make up more than half of the total resistance in the pulmonary circuit (Nunn, 1993). These vessels, lacking the power of active vasoconstriction, are primarily responsible for determining PVR and the distribution of blood flow in the lung. Consider what happens to pulmonary vascular resistance and flow when the shape of these passive vessels is changed.

Changes in transmural pressure also affect the diameter of the numerous thin-walled pulmonary blood vessels that course through lung parenchyma, but lie *outside* alveoli (see Fig. 11–5). These **extra-alveolar capillaries** are tethered to surrounding connective tissue elements of the parenchyma, much like the distal airways of the conducting zone (see Fig. 2–8). During inflation of the alveoli, the diameter of extra-alveolar blood vessels *increases* at higher lung volumes, unlike that of the alveolar septal capillaries. The increase in

vessel diameter occurs because the outward traction exerted by the parenchymal fibers increases the transmural pressure by pulling the vessel wall outward. This change reduces PVR and increases blood flow through the pulmonary vessels. At lower lung volumes, the outward traction on the walls of the extra-alveolar blood vessels is less, resulting in decreased vessel diameter and an increase in PVR.

At higher driving pressures, the flowrate in the pulmonary blood vessels increases more for a given increment in pressure than occurs at lower driving pressures. In other words, the relationship between blood pressure and flow in the pulmonary circuit is *nonlinear*. Furthermore, the vascular resistance of the pulmonary vessels changes at different rates of flow. Decreased PVR can be caused by (1) *increased distention* of thin-walled pulmonary arteries and veins at higher vascular pressures, thus decreasing overall vascular resistance; and (2) *vascular recruitment* of additional pulmonary vessels as higher intravascular pressures cause previously collapsed blood vessels to dilate.

In summary, it can be said that changes in lung volume cause changes in the transmural pressure acting on the pulmonary blood vessels. This change, in turn, modifies PVR and affects pulmonary blood flow. Pulmonary vascular resistance is at its lowest at functional residual capacity because the diameter of pulmonary vessels is optimal (Fig. 11–6). At FRC the two types of pulmonary capillaries are both *dilated:* alveolar septal capillaries are dilated because low lung volumes do not stretch and thin the alveolar walls that contain them; extra-alveolar capillaries are dilated because of the traction applied to them by mechanical tethering to the lung parenchyma. As lung volume increases above FRC, however, the resistance to pulmonary blood flow increases, reaching a peak at total lung capacity (TLC) (see Fig. 11–6). At these higher lung volumes, the increase in PVR is primarily due to alveolar inflation that stretches and narrows alveolar septal vessels, thus restricting flow (see Fig. 11–5). At lung volumes below FRC there is also an increase in pulmonary vascular resistance, caused primarily by loss of mechanical tethering of extra-alveolar vessels to the surrounding lung parenchyma (see Fig. 11–6). This change results in a decrease in the diameter of extra-alveolar vessels (see Fig. 11–5). Although the diameter of alveolar septal vessels is increased at lung volumes below FRC, the decrease in the diameter of extra-alveolar vessels counteracts this change to result in a *net increase* in PVR and a decrease in overall pulmonary perfusion.

Table 11–2 provides a summary of active and passive

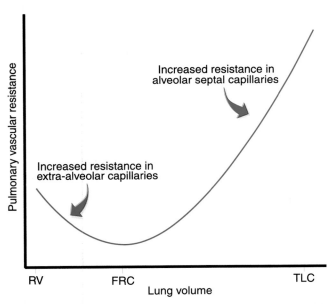

FIGURE 11–6. Pulmonary vascular resistances at different lung volumes. At lung volumes below FRC, loss of radial traction on the extra-alveolar capillaries results in vasoconstriction and an increase in pulmonary vascular resistance. At lung volumes above FRC, the thinning of alveolar walls causes vasoconstriction of alveolar septal capillaries and an increase in pulmonary vascular resistance. Pulmonary vascular resistance is lowest at FRC. (FRC = functional residual capacity; RV = residual volume; TLC = total lung capacity.) (Adapted from Leff AR and Schumacker PT: Respiratory Physiology: Basics and Applications. WB Saunders, Philadelphia, 1993, p 65, with permission.)

factors that modify pulmonary vascular resistance and blood flow.

REGIONAL BLOOD FLOW IN THE LUNG AND THE ZONE MODEL OF PERFUSION

Hydrostatic Effects

The distribution of blood in the pulmonary circuit is nonuniform. Instead, it is affected by gravity and increases almost linearly from the apex to the base of the upright lung. The uppermost regions are the *least dependent* on gravity for their supply of blood, whereas the middle and lowest regions of the lung are considered gravity *dependent.* Hydrostatic (gravitational) forces alter both the driving pressure in pulmonary blood vessels and their diameter. Specifically, perfusion is reduced in the superior part of the lung but is enhanced in the inferior region of the lung in a person standing upright (Fig. 11–7). These relationships are changed when a person is in a different position. In the supine position the vertical distance from the "top" to the "bottom" of the lung is reduced. This postural change causes the perfusion of apical regions to increase while the perfusion of basal regions remains the same, thus redistributing blood flow so that it becomes almost uniform from apex to base (West, 1998).

An adult lung is approximately 30 cm in height. If the pulmonary arterial system is represented as a continuous "column" of blood, stretching from the apex to the base of the upright lung, the pressure difference from top to bottom is about 30 cm H_2O. West (1998) points out that such a pressure differential is remarkable in a low-pressure vascular system, and that regional blood flow is dramatically affected by the pressure difference. In a subject standing upright, the vertical pressure gradient from superior to inferior regions of the lung occurs because hydrostatic pressure is changed by approximately 1 cm H_2O for each cm change in vertical height (Leff and Schumacker, 1993). Consider the following: blood leaving the right ventricle must travel upward in the pulmonary circuit within the lung in order to reach the apical region. The pressure of this blood is the mean pulmonary artery pressure and is normally around 12 to 18 mm Hg (1 mm Hg = 1.36 cm H_2O) (Ganong, 1995; Leff and Schumacker, 1993; West, 1998). However, the upward movement of blood in branches of the pulmonary artery is immediately affected by a fall in arterial pressure of −1 cm H_2O per cm of height (−1 cm H_2O/cm), resulting in decreased perfusion of the uppermost regions of the lung. Conversely, the flow of blood pumped from the right ventricle to the middle and lowest regions of the lung is aided by gravitational effects that increase arterial pressure (+1 cm H_2O/cm), thereby improving perfusion of these regions.

| TABLE 11–2 | Factors Modifying Pulmonary Vascular Resistance and Blood Flow in the Lung |

Factors	Vascular Effect		PVR	Flow
	Vasoconstriction	Vasodilation		
Active factors—changes in vascular tone affect the diameters of pulmonary blood vessels:				
Neural impulses				
α_1-Adrenergic stimulation	✓		↑	↓
β_2-Adrenergic stimulation		✓	↓	↑
*M_3-Muscarinic stimulation		✓	↓	↑
†Cardiovascular drugs				
Epinephrine or adrenalin (catecholamine)	✓		↑	↓
Nitroglycerin (nitrate)		✓	↓	↑
Verapamil (calcium channel blocker)		✓	↓	↑
Propranolol (β-blocker)		✓	↓	↑
Nitric oxide (inhaled pulmonary vasodilator)		✓	↓	↑
Vasoactive substances				
Nitric oxide (NO)		✓	↓	↑
Angiotensin II (catalyzed by ACE)	✓		↑	↓
Epinephrine	✓		↑	↓
Norepinephrine	✓		↑	↓
Histamine		✓	↓	↑
Bradykinin		✓	↓	↑
Prostaglandin E_2 (PGE$_2$)		✓	↓	↑
Prostaglandin I_2 (PGI$_2$, prostacyclin)		✓	↓	↑
Prostaglandin $F_{2\alpha}$ (PGF$_{2\alpha}$)	✓		↑	↓
Prostaglandin D_2 (PGD$_2$)	✓		↑	↓
Serotonin (5-hydroxytryptamine, 5-HT)	✓	✓	↑,↓	↓,↑
Passive factors—changes in lung volume change the transmural pressures acting on pulmonary blood vessels (Their diameters are not affected by changes in vascular tone.):				
Alveolar septal capillaries				
Low lung volume		✓	↓	↑
High lung volume	✓		↑	↓
Extra-alveolar capillaries				
Low lung volume	✓		↑	↓
High lung volume		✓	↓	↑

PVR = pulmonary vascular resistance; NO = nitric oxide; ACE = angiotensin-converting enzyme.
*Stimulation causes nitric oxide to be released from pulmonary endothelial cells which brings about vasodilation.
†Representative sample only. Cardiovascular drugs having vascular effects are too numerous to list here. Consult a suitable cardiopulmonary pharmacology text such as Cottrell and Surkin (1995).

Venous drainage from pulmonary capillary beds is also affected by gravitational effects that operate along the vertical axis of the lung in the upright position. For instance, the venous pressure of blood leaving pulmonary capillaries located in the apical regions of the lung is less than left atrial pressure, which is normally around 5 to 7 mm Hg (Ganong, 1995; Leff and Schumacker, 1993). Therefore, venous return from these upper regions is sluggish. By contrast, the venous pressure of blood exiting from capillaries in the base of the lung is greater than left atrial pressure, thus the flow of blood back to the heart is enhanced.

The Zone Model of Perfusion

Regional differences in pulmonary blood flow are determined by relative pressures in the pulmonary arterial system, pulmonary venous system, and alveoli.

The Respiratory System

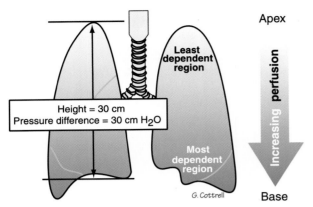

FIGURE 11–7. Regional blood flow in the lung. The vertical pressure gradient in the upright lung changes by approximately 1 cm H_2O/cm of height. Pulmonary arterial pressure is affected by this hydrostatic gradient, resulting in decreased perfusion of the apical regions of the lung and increased perfusion of the gravity-dependent basal regions.

These differences have led to the **zone model of perfusion.** Figure 11–8 shows that alveolar diameters are greatest in the apex of the upright lung, and progressively decrease in diameter toward the base, finally assuming a "squashed" look in the lowest regions. Because the majority of alveoli near the top of the lung are expanded (because of the larger intrapleural pressure at the apex), most of the FRC of the lung is distributed in the apex. These alveoli of the upper regions, therefore, are less compliant than those in the lower regions.

Recall that a distensible structure having low compliance is "stiff" and does not expand readily per unit change in pressure. At FRC, alveoli of the apical region in the upright lung already contain a proportionally large volume of gas and, therefore, resist further expansion. Put another way, the change in lung volume per unit resting volume (effective alveolar

ventilation) is *least* near the apex of the lung, becoming progressively *greater* near the base. (Leff and Schumacker, 1993; West, 1998). The alveoli at the base of the lung have a smaller resting volume but a larger change in volume than their counterparts in the apex of the lung. Consequently, the base of the upright lung is better ventilated than the apex in spite of being poorly expanded at FRC. In the supine position, the regional differences disappear so that apical ventilation is approximately equal to basal ventilation (West, 1998).

Zone 1

The apical regions comprise **zone 1** of the upright lung. In this zone, pulmonary arterial pressure is less than alveolar pressure because of the substantial vertical distance of the apex above the heart (approximately 12 cm). Alveolar pressure in this region of the lung is normally close to atmospheric pressure, collapsing the low-pressure pulmonary capillaries and severely restricting blood flow. Under normal circumstances, zone 1 conditions do not occur in the lung because pulmonary arterial pressure (12 to 18 mm Hg) is just sufficient to raise blood to the top of the lung (West, 1998). However, any compromise in right-side heart function leading to pulmonary hypotension, or any condition such as hemorrhage that leads to hypovolemia and a fall in blood pressure, causes a negative transmural pressure to develop across the pulmonary capillary wall (Dupuis, 1992; West, 1998). Such a change collapses pulmonary capillaries and halts blood flow. Similarly, if alveolar pressure is raised during positive pressure ventilation, pulmonary capillaries may be compressed (Leff and Schumacker, 1993). These changes result in ventilated but unperfused lung tissue and contribute to *alveolar dead space*. When local

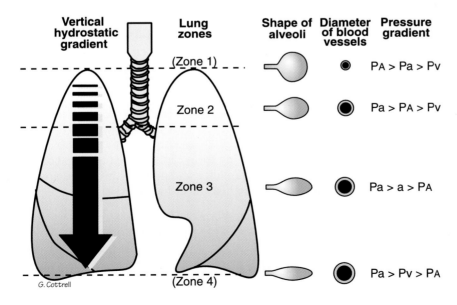

FIGURE 11–8. Zone model of perfusion (upright lung). Different regions of the lung operate under different flow conditions caused by gravitational effects that alter alveolar pressure (PA), pulmonary artery pressure (Pa), and pulmonary vein pressure (Pv). See text for description of perfusion in the different zones. (Note: Blood vessels and alveoli are not drawn to scale.)

venous pressure is *less than* alveolar pressure, as occurs in the upper regions, the effective pressure influencing pulmonary blood flow becomes the *alveolar-arterial* pressure gradient (see Fig. 11–8). The low pressure at the venous end of the capillaries causes them to collapse as a result of negative transmural pressure, thus restricting flow. As the pressure builds in the capillaries, they reopen and flow is restored.

Zone 2

Because of the proximity of **zone 2** to the heart, most of the alveoli are normally perfused. In other words, the vertical hydrostatic gradient does not impede blood flow because the pulmonary arterial pressure is sufficient to deliver blood to the alveoli. Perfusion in the upper portion of zone 2 is sporadic because the region is slightly above the heart, but perfusion in the middle and lower portions of the zone is normal (Dupuis, 1992). Optimal perfusion occurs as a result of the vertical hydrostatic effect that increases pulmonary artery pressure downward through zone 2. The elevated pulmonary artery pressure exceeds alveolar pressure (see Fig. 11–8). Blood flow in zone 2 is determined by this *arterial-alveolar* pressure difference, rather than the arterial-venous pressure gradient that normally drives blood flow in vascular systems (Leff and Schumacker, 1993).

Zone 3

Blood flow increases further down the vertical hydrostatic gradient in the lung, reaching peak flow in **zone 3.** In zone 3, pulmonary artery pressure is higher than pulmonary venous pressure. Furthermore, pulmonary venous pressure exceeds alveolar pressure (see Fig. 11–8). Therefore, blood flow through this zone is determined by the driving pressure provided by the *arterial-venous* pressure gradient (Leff and Schumacker, 1993). Since local venous pressure is greater than alveolar pressure in zone 3, the pulmonary capillaries tend to remain open so that blood flow continues. In fact, distention of the capillaries in this zone, as well as recruitment of previously closed capillaries, contribute dramatically to the enhanced perfusion of alveoli in zone 3 (West, 1998).

Zone 4

Recall that pulmonary blood flow is also affected by the diameter of both alveolar and extra-alveolar vessels. At low lung volumes (below FRC), poorly inflated alveoli at the base of the lung cause the parenchyma to collapse inward on the extra-alveolar vessels, reducing their diameter and increasing vascular resistance (see Fig. 11–5). This region of reduced blood flow in the base of the lung is known as **zone 4** (West, 1998) (see Fig. 11–8).

LUNG FLUID BALANCE AND THE PULMONARY LYMPHATIC SYSTEM

Capillary Membrane Fluid Dynamics—The Starling Forces

Several forces act on each side of the capillary wall to influence the transfer of fluid into and out of the capillary (Fig. 11–9). These pressures are known as the four primary **Starling forces,** named after Ernest H. Starling (1866–1927), the English physiologist who first described them a century ago (Guyton and Hall, 1996).

Two fluid dynamic forces act on the *luminal* side of the capillary wall:

- **Capillary pressure (P_c),** also known as **capillary hydrostatic pressure,** is generated by contraction of the ventricles of the heart. This pressure, although relatively low, is sufficient to force fluid and dissolved substances through capillary pores into the surrounding tissue spaces. This outward movement of fluid through the capillary wall illustrates the permeable nature of these small vessels.
- **Plasma colloid osmotic pressure (π_c)** is also known as **plasma colloid oncotic pressure.** Colloid osmotic pressure (COP) is produced by the presence of proteins such as albumin in the plasma. These proteins exert an osmotic force that causes fluid to move from the interstitial spaces back into the capillaries. Through this mechanism, excessive depletion of plasma volume is prevented.

Two fluid dynamic forces also operate on the *tissue* side of the capillary wall:

- **Interstitial fluid pressure (P_i)** or **interstitial fluid hydrostatic pressure,** generally imposes an outward force on fluids in the capillaries. This pressure results from the "pumping" action of the lymph capillaries that remove fluid from tissue spaces and propel it into general circulation.
- **Interstitial fluid colloid osmotic pressure (π_i),** also known as **interstitial fluid colloid oncotic pressure,** exerts an outward force on the fluid in capillaries. This osmotic effect is produced by the proteins found in tissue spaces.

Fluid Scavenging by the Pulmonary Lymphatic System

As shown by the Starling forces, a variety of dynamic forces interact at the capillary membrane (see Fig. 11–9). *Net inward forces* are created by plasma colloid osmotic pressure, whereas *net outward forces* are generated by capillary hydrostatic pressure, interstitial fluid os-

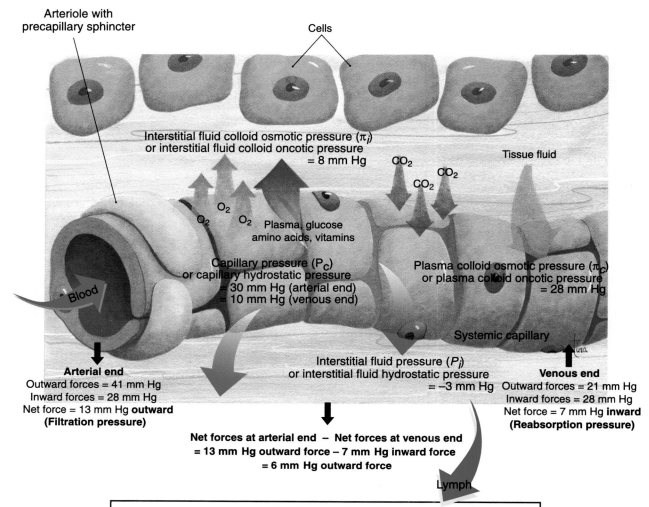

FIGURE 11–9. Starling forces acting at the capillary wall. Exchanges between blood and the surrounding tissue fluid. Filtration takes place at the arterial end of the capillary. Osmosis takes place at the venous end. Gases are exchanged by diffusion. Although pressure values shown are typical for a systemic capillary, the *processes* are the same for a pulmonary capillary. Arrows depict the direction of movement of fluid between the vascular and tissue fluid compartments. (Adapted from Scanlon VC and Sanders T: Essentials of Anatomy and Physiology, ed. 3. FA Davis, Philadelphia, 1999, p 279, with permission.) (See also Color Plate 10.)

motic pressure, and interstitial fluid hydrostatic pressure (Box 11–1). These opposing forces are not balanced; therefore, the small volume of fluid (approximately 10%) that escapes from the permeable capillaries must be recovered by other means.

Fortunately, tissues are well equipped with an extensive branched system of thin-walled *lymphatic capillaries*. These unique vessels are closed-ended, porous, and equipped with numerous valves (Fig. 11–10). Any external compression of tissues containing lymphatics,

such as occurs during rhythmic inflation and deflation of the lung, squeezes these thin-walled vessels, causing them to passively "pump" fluid out of the tissue spaces. The fluid (now called *lymphatic fluid,* or *lymph*) is slowly transported toward the superior vena cava where it is returned to general circulation.

This mechanism of fluid recovery continues at all times and is normally able to keep up with net fluid loss out of the capillaries. The lymphatic system essentially functions as a scavenger system to remove excess fluid,

P E R S P E C T I V E S

BOX 11–1

The Starling Equation and the Flow of Fluid Through Tissue Spaces

Fluid movement across the capillary membrane is dictated by fluid dynamic pressures known as the four primary **Starling forces,** named after Ernest H. Starling (1866–1927). The interaction of forces can be summarized by the following relationship known as the **Starling equation:**

$$Q = K[(P_c - P_i) - \sigma(\pi_c - \pi_i)]$$

where:

Q = *filtration rate,* or *flux* (net fluid out)

K = *capillary filtration coefficient,* an expression of the net imbalance of forces at the capillary membrane

σ = *protein reflection coefficient,* an expression of the resistance of the capillary membrane to protein leakage. When protein molecules are unable to pass through the pores between endothelial cells of capillaries, they are "reflected" from the pore and cause osmotic pressure. When all of the protein molecules are reflected, $\sigma = 1.0$ and a maximum osmotic effect is created; when all of the proteins pass through the pores, $\sigma = 0.0$ and no osmotic effect is produced.

P_c = *capillary (hydrostatic) pressure,* which forces fluid outward through the capillary membrane. Capillary, or microvascular, pressure is created by systemic or pulmonary blood pressure.

P_i = *interstitial fluid (hydrostatic) pressure,* which forces fluid inward when P_i is positive but outward when P_i is negative. In loose connective tissue, the pumping action of the lymphatic vessels scavenges fluid from the tissue spaces to create a *negative,* or subatmospheric, interstitial fluid pressure.

π_c = *plasma colloid osmotic (oncotic) pressure,* which causes inward movement of fluid from the interstitial spaces to the vascular compartment. Only those substances unable to pass through membrane pores exert osmotic pressure, and since proteins are normally "reflected" from the capillary membrane pores, it is the plasma proteins in the vascular compartment that generate an inward osmotic force at the capillaries.

π_i = *interstitial fluid colloid osmotic (oncotic) pressure,* caused by the presence of plasma proteins in the tissue spaces. Proteins slowly leak into the interstitial spaces through larger capillary membrane pores and generate an outward osmotic force at the capillaries.

Because the four Starling forces dramatically affect capillary membrane dynamics, a relatively large volume of fluid is filtered out of the arterial ends of capillaries and reabsorbed at the venous ends of capillaries. The net outward force at the arterial ends of capillaries is called the net *filtration pressure* and is created by the interaction of the forces discussed above. (*Diffusion* refers to the movement of fluid in both directions across the capillary membrane, whereas *filtration* refers to the net flow of fluid out of the proximal ends of capillaries.) Filtered fluid leaving the arterial end of capillaries enters the loose connective tissue of interstitial spaces and "flows" toward the venous ends of capillaries. Here, the summation of Starling forces produces a net inward force called the *reabsorption pressure.* This mechanism is responsible for recovery of approximately 90% of the filtered fluid while lymphatic vessels recover the remaining filtered fluids and dissolved substances and return them to general circulation.

• Guyton AC and Hall JE: Textbook of Medical Physiology, ed 9. WB Saunders, Philadelphia, 1996.
• Leff AR and Schumacker PT: Respiratory Physiology: Basics and Applications. WB Saunders, Philadelphia, 1993.

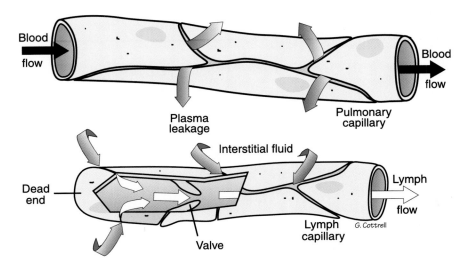

FIGURE 11–10. Fluid scavenging by pulmonary lymphatics. Approximately 90% of the fluid that leaks into the tissue spaces is recovered as a result of the inward force generated by plasma colloid osmotic pressure. The remaining 10% is recovered by the pumping action of the pulmonary lymphatic system. Approximately 50 mL of lymph is transported per hour out of the lung and returned to general circulation. (Note: For simplicity, the basement membranes around the vessels are not shown.)

cellular debris, and other material from tissue spaces. The loose tissue spaces serve as a sump, or storage area, from which the fluid is removed. When the amount of fluid entering the spaces is very slight, the pumping action of the lymphatics propels lymph forward and creates a slight *negative* interstitial fluid pressure. As a result of the pumping action of the lymph capillaries, the average pressure in loose connective tissue such as the interstitium of the lung is about −3 mm Hg (Guyton and Hall, 1996). This semivacuum, or suction, helps propel interstitial fluid out of the tissue spaces. In tight fibrous connective tissues, the interstitial fluid hydrostatic pressure is usually more positive (Guyton and Hall, 1996). Lymph carried by the pulmonary lymphatic system leaves the adult lung at the hilum at a rate of approximately 10 to 50 mL/h and is returned to systemic circulation (Leff and Schumacker, 1993).

If the rate of lymph production increases slightly, the rate of lymphatic fluid clearance increases to keep pace; however, a significant increase in lymph formation may surpass the scavenging ability of the pulmonary lymphatic system. The risk in this type of arrangement is the development of pulmonary edema, a condition that may begin with accumulated fluid in the tissue spaces (interstitial edema) but leads to a far more serious condition if this fluid transfers through the alveolar wall and fills the alveoli (alveolar edema). Such an accumulation of fluid in the alveoli may lead to impaired gas exchange, intrapulmonary shunting, ventilation-perfusion inequalities, and hypoxemia (Box 11–2). These topics are examined in Chapter 14.

Metabolic Function of the Lung

Although the primary role of the lung is to provide an extensive surface area for gas exchange, other important functions such as *elimination* and *metabolism* are routinely carried out by the organ. For example, the removal of anesthetic gas from the bloodstream occurs when the drug leaves the pulmonary blood and enters the alveoli prior to being exhaled. The lung also functions as an organ of *biotransformation*, or chemical change. The lung participates in important metabolic reactions made possible by the action of pulmonary enzymes or mechanisms operating in the organ. In general, metabolic functions of the lung include *activation* of precursor substances found in the blood, *synthesis* of substances such as proteins, and *inactivation* of substances that either pass through the lung or are produced by it. Several of the following chemicals were discussed previously in relation to the active control of blood flow through the lung. It should be noted that the lung is the only organ, other than the heart, that receives the entire cardiac output. This exposure to the entire circulation provides ample opportunity for the lung to modify substances in the blood, add substances to it, or remove substances from it.

ACTIVATION OF SUBSTANCES

In response to hypotension, kidney cells secrete the hormone renin, which converts angiotensinogen to angiotensin I (Fig. 11–11). (Angiotensinogen is an inactive precursor synthesized by the liver.) As angiotensin I passes through the pulmonary microcirculation, pulmonary endothelial cells secrete ACE, which converts angiotensin I into a powerful vasoconstrictor called angiotensin II (see Fig. 11–11). This vasoactive substance is up to 50 times more potent than its immediate precursor (West, 1998). In fact, angiotensin II is one of the most powerful vasoactive substances known. Guyton and Hall (1996) note that as little as 1 µg of angiotensin II is capable of increasing arterial

P E R S P E C T I V E S

BOX 11-2

Pulmonary Edema

In conditions of cardiac failure caused by left-side failure as a result of chronic systemic hypertension or aortic valve stenosis (narrowing), increased left atrial pressure causes the pulmonary venous and capillary pressures to increase. The rise in capillary hydrostatic pressure forces additional fluid out of the capillaries into the interstitial spaces causing a type of *pulmonary edema* known as *cardiac pulmonary edema*. This condition is also known as *hydrostatic* or *high pressure edema*. The interstitial edema may lead to alveolar edema. The combined effect of the accumulated fluid in the interstitium and alveoli of the lung causes a reduction in lung compliance, lung volumes, and lung capacities. In addition, an increase in airway resistance occurs as fluid accumulates within the lumen of airways and within their walls. Unequal changes in compliance and airway resistance throughout the lung result in ventilation-perfusion mismatching, intrapulmonary shunting, and arterial hypoxemia. Hydrostatic edema often resolves within hours once the pressures return to normal and the lymphatic system catches up to the rate of fluid outflow from the pulmonary capillaries.

Noncardiac pulmonary edema occurs when capillary membrane permeability increases dramatically, allowing the movement of proteins from pulmonary capillaries to interstitial spaces. This type of pulmonary edema is also known as *low-pressure* or *high-permeability edema*. Cardiac dysfunction is not the cause of the edematous condition. Hydrostatic pressures are normal but the permeability of the capillaries to proteins is increased. This protein transfer reduces the plasma colloid osmotic pressure while increasing the interstitial fluid osmotic pressure. Because the presence of proteins within the vascular compartment normally opposes the capillary hydrostatic pressure, the leakage of proteins outward results in diminished inward forces, thus allowing fluid to accumulate in the interstitial spaces and, ultimately, flood the alveoli to produce the changes noted above with cardiac pulmonary edema. Noncardiac pulmonary edema is often seen with conditions such as the adult respiratory distress syndrome (ARDS).

Differentiation between the two types of pulmonary edema is normally performed with a combination of heart catheterization procedures (see Chap. 20), and laboratory analysis of the protein content of alveolar fluid.

- Guyton AC and Hall JE: Textbook of Medical Physiology, ed 9. WB Saunders, Philadelphia, 1996.
- Leff AR and Schumacker PT: Respiratory Physiology: Basics and Applications. WB Saunders, Philadelphia, 1993.
- West JB: Pulmonary Pathophysiology: The Essentials, ed 5. Williams & Wilkins, Baltimore, 1997.
- West JB: Respiratory Physiology: The Essentials, ed 6. Williams & Wilkins, Baltimore, 1998.

pressure by more than 50 mm Hg. Fortunately, pulmonary blood vessels are unaffected by angiotensin II as the substance passes through pulmonary circulation. Angiotensin II causes widespread vasoconstriction and stimulates the release of aldosterone, a hormone that promotes plasma expansion and a further increase in blood pressure.

SYNTHESIS OF SUBSTANCES

Type II pneumocytes in the lung are active in the synthesis of the phospholipid, *pulmonary surfactant*. This complex substance is critical in the maintenance of alveolar stability because it effectively lowers surface tension to minimize alveolar collapse (see Chap. 1). The lung is also active in the synthesis of structural proteins such as *collagen* and *elastin*, both of which contribute to the interstitium of lung tissue. The resulting meshwork of fibers is responsible for the radial traction exerted on airways and blood vessels in the lung as well as the elastic recoil and compliance characteristics of healthy lung tissue. *Mucopolysaccharides* are essential carbohydrates synthesized by the lung and incorporated into the structure of bronchial mucus. This im-

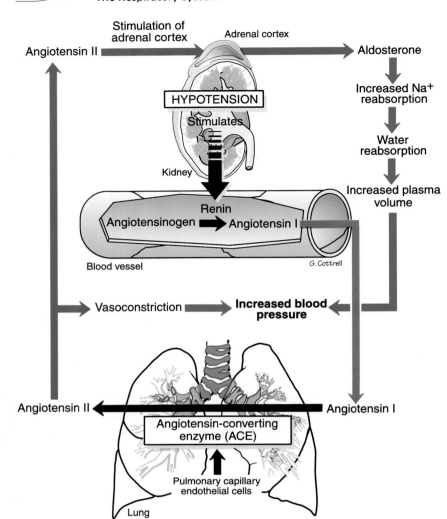

FIGURE 11–11. Renin-angiotensin-aldosterone mechanism. Angiotensin I is changed into angiotensin II within the pulmonary circulation by ACE, secreted by pulmonary endothelial cells. Angiotensin II elevates blood pressure by promoting vasoconstriction and stimulating the release of aldosterone, which expands plasma volume. (Adapted from Cottrell GP and Surkin HB: Pharmacology for Respiratory Care Practitioners. FA Davis, Philadelphia, 1995, p 290, with permission.)

portant chemical complex is involved with humidification of inspired air (see Chap. 2) and defense of the lung (see Chap. 5).

The lung is also involved in the metabolism of several vasoactive and bronchoactive substances. Several of these inflammatory mediators are released into pulmonary circulation or into small airways during inflammatory reactions in the lung. Many of the symptoms of bronchial asthma can be attributed to the actions of these potent chemicals. In response to antigen challenge or tissue insult, *histamine* is released from sensitized mast cells that line the small airways and blood vessels of the lung. This powerful mediator causes bronchoconstriction and vasodilation (see Table 5–3). Inflammatory reactions in lung tissue also involve activation of the enzyme phospholipase A_2, which catalyzes the conversion of cell membrane phospholipids to an intermediate compound. This intermediate compound serves as the starting point for synthesis of a variety of potent inflammatory mediators such as *leukotrienes, prostaglandins,* and *thromboxane A_2* (see Fig. 5–9).

INACTIVATION OF SUBSTANCES

A variety of vasoactive substances are neutralized as they pass through the lung, largely because the lung is equipped with the catabolic enzymes necessary for the inactivation of mediators such as the *leukotrienes, bradykinin, serotonin, norepinephrine,* and certain *prostaglandins,* namely PGE_2 and $PGF_{2\alpha}$. In general, vasoactive substances having local effects tend to be removed or inactivated by pulmonary circulation. In contrast, vasoactive substances such as *angiotensin II, epinephrine, histamine,* and *vasopressin* (also known as *antidiuretic hormone, ADH*), exhibit generalized actions in the body and pass through pulmonary circulation unchanged.

TABLE 11–3	Metabolic Function of the Lung	
Process	**Substance**	**Comments**
Activation		
	Angiotensin I	Converted to angiotensin II by ACE
Synthesis		
	Angiotensin-converting enzyme (ACE)	Produced by pulmonary endothelial cells; converts angiotensin I to angiotensin II, a powerful vasoconstrictor
	Nitric oxide (NO)	Produced by pulmonary endothelial cells; NO originally called endothelium-derived relaxing factor (EDRF) because of its vasodilating effect on pulmonary vasculature
	Pulmonary surfactant	Produced by type II pneumocytes lining the alveoli
	Collagen; elastin	Structural proteins responsible for support, radial traction, elastic recoil, and compliance characteristics of lung interstitium
	Mucopolysaccharides	Protein-carbohydrate complexes incorporated into the structural matrix of bronchial mucus
	Inflammatory mediators (histamine and arachidonic acid metabolites such as the leukotrienes, prostaglandins, and thromboxanes)	Inflammatory mediators are released or produced following antigenic challenge or tissue injury
Inactivation*		
	Bradykinin	Up to 80% inactivated by ACE
	Serotonin (5-hydroxytryptamine, 5-HT)	Almost completely removed via uptake and storage in pulmonary tissue
	Norepinephrine	Up to 30% removed via uptake and storage in pulmonary tissue
	PGE_2, $PGF_{2\alpha}$	Almost completely inactivated
	Leukotrienes	Almost completely inactivated

ACE = angiotensin-converting enzyme; EDRF = endothelium-derived relaxing factor; NO = nitric oxide; PGE_2 = prostaglandin E_2; $PGF_{2\alpha}$ = prostaglandin $F_{2\alpha}$.
*Vasoactive substances with generalized effects tend to pass through pulmonary circulation unchanged (e.g., angiotensin II, epinephrine, histamine, vasopressin or antidiuretic hormone)
Source: Adapted from West (1998).

Table 11–3 summarizes the metabolic functions of the lung.

Summary

In this chapter a variety of ventilatory patterns was discussed as well as the effect that dead space, rate of breathing, and depth of breathing, have on alveolar ventilation. Basic physiologic calculations were introduced that allow the reader to determine total ventilation, alveolar ventilation, anatomical dead space ventilation, and physiologic dead space ventilation. The theoretical differences among the various types of ventilation were also examined.

The various mechanisms that operate in the lung to prevent fluid accumulation in the interstitial spaces and alveoli were briefly explored in this chapter. The chapter continued with a discussion of the regional effect of hydrostatic pressure gradients and different lung volumes on both ventilation and perfusion, and concluded with a discussion of the nonrespiratory metabolic functions of the lung.

BIBLIOGRAPHY

Cottrell GP and Surkin HB: Pharmacology for Respiratory Care Practitioners. FA Davis, Philadelphia, 1995.

Dupuis YG: Ventilators: Theory and Clinical Application, ed 2. Mosby–Year Book, St. Louis, 1992.

Ganong WF: Review of Medical Physiology, ed 17. Appleton & Lange, Norwalk, CT, 1995.

Guyton AC and Hall JE: Textbook of Medical Physiology, ed 9. WB Saunders, Philadelphia, 1996.

Leff AR and Schumacker PT: Respiratory Physiology: Basics and Applications. WB Saunders, Philadelphia, 1993.

Levitzky MG: Pulmonary Physiology, ed 4. McGraw-Hill, New York, 1995.

Martini FH: Fundamentals of Anatomy and Physiology, ed 4. Prentice Hall, Upper Saddle River, NJ, 1998.

Mines AH: Respiratory Physiology, ed 3. Raven Press, New York, 1993.

Nunn JF: Nunn's Applied Respiratory Physiology, ed 4. Butterworth-Heinemann, Oxford, 1993.

Shier D, Butler J, and Lewis R: Hole's Human Anatomy and Physiology, ed 7. Wm C Brown, Dubuque, IA, 1996.

West JB: Pulmonary Pathophysiology: The Essentials, ed 5. Williams & Wilkins, Baltimore, 1997.

West JB: Respiratory Physiology: The Essentials, ed 6. Williams & Wilkins, Baltimore, 1998.

CHAPTER 12

Gas Exchange

chapter objectives

After studying this chapter the reader should be able to:

☐ Describe how the partial pressure of a gas is calculated by explaining the terms dry gas fraction and barometric (ambient) pressure.

☐ Explain Dalton's law of partial pressures.

☐ Explain the concept of water vapor partial pressure (P_{H_2O}) and describe how the partial pressures of gases in a mixture are affected by the P_{H_2O}.

☐ Define the term diffusivity.

☐ Explain Fick's law of diffusion by describing the role played by the following factors:

Area of the membrane, thickness of the membrane, partial pressure gradient, diffusion coefficient.

☐ Explain Graham's law and Henry's law by describing how the diffusion coefficient of a gas is affected by the solubility of the gas and the molecular weight of the gas.

☐ Explain the concept of transit time in the pulmonary capillary as it applies to gas diffusion in the lung.

☐ Describe how equilibration of gases occurs in the dynamic pulmonary circuit by explaining partial pressure gradients and the role played by the continuous perfusion of blood in pulmonary capillaries.

☐ Describe gas solubility by explaining the relationship between the volume of gas entering a fluid and the partial pressure of gas in the fluid.

☐ Explain why the volume-pressure relationship of some gases is linear while that of others is nonlinear.

☐ Discuss effective solubility of a gas by comparing the solubilities of oxygen, carbon dioxide, and carbon monoxide.

☐ Compare and contrast perfusion limited and diffusion limited characteristics of gas exchange in the lung by describing the transfer of nitrous oxide and carbon monoxide into the pulmonary blood.

☐ Explain the concept of diffusing capacity of the lung for carbon monoxide (DLCO).

☐ Describe how the transfer of oxygen gas can be perfusion limited or diffusion limited.

☐ Explain how diffusion of gas occurs between systemic capillaries and the tissues of the body.

key terms

Dalton's law of partial pressures
diffusing capacity of the lung for carbon monoxide (DLCO)
diffusion-limited gas exchange
diffusivity (di-fū-siv′-i-tē)
dry gas fraction (FGAS)
effective solubility
equilibration of gases

Fick's law of diffusion
Graham's law
Henry's law
partial pressure; tension (PGAS)
perfusion-limited gas exchange
transit time
water vapor partial pressure (PH₂O)

In preceding chapters we discussed different types of dead space ventilation and saw that only the portion of air reaching the alveoli is useful in a functional sense. But how much *oxygen* is actually delivered to the alveoli by this inspired air? More importantly, what determines whether or not oxygen leaves the alveoli to enter the blood perfusing the lung? Since only the amount of oxygen entering the pulmonary bloodstream will be available to support cellular metabolism, the answers to these questions are critical, especially in view of the fact that several pulmonary pathophysiologic conditions impair the exchange of respiratory gases in the lung.

As a prelude to the study of gas exchange, gas transport, and ventilation-perfusion relationships, we begin this chapter with a brief review of the composition of ambient, inspired, and alveolar gas mixtures. The chapter then examines applicable gas laws, gas solubilities, and equilibration of gas along a pulmonary capillary, and concludes with a discussion of perfusion and diffusion factors that limit gas exchange in the lung and tissues.

Composition of Gas Mixtures

BAROMETRIC PRESSURE AND DRY GAS FRACTIONS

A sample of air taken from the external environment contains a mixture of gases that includes oxygen, car-

bon dioxide, nitrogen, water, and trace gases such as argon. In addition, atmospheric pollutants such as ozone, methane, sulfur, and carbon monoxide may be present in some ambient air samples. The gases of respiratory importance found in a mixed sample of dry ambient air are present as **dry gas fractions** totaling 100%. This gas mixture can be described in terms of either the percentage composition of the gas fractions or the **partial pressure (tension)** of the gases comprising the total pressure (Table 12–1). The *partial pressure (PGAS)* of a gas, therefore, is the product of the *dry gas fraction (FGAS)* and the total ambient pressure, or *barometric pressure (PBAR)* of the mixture:

$$\therefore \text{PGAS} = \text{FGAS} \times \text{PBAR}$$

EXAMPLE 1

At a barometric pressure of 760 mm Hg (sea level), calculate the partial pressure of oxygen (PO_2) in the air sample when the dry gas fraction of oxygen is 20.93%.

$$\text{PO}_2 = 0.2093 \times 760 \text{ mm Hg}$$

$$= 159 \text{ mm Hg (159 torr)}$$

NOTE: The pressure unit, *torr*, was named in honor of Evangelista Torricelli (1608–1647), the Italian mathematician credited with inventing the

TABLE 12–1	Partial Pressures of Respiratory Gases (mm Hg)				
Percentage Composition (dry)	PO_2	PCO_2	PN_2	PH_2O	Total
	20.93%	0.04%	79.03%	0%	100.00%
Atmospheric gas (dry)	159	0	601	0	760
Inspired gas (saturated)	149	0	564	47	760
Expired gas (saturated)	116	28	569	47	760
Alveolar gas (saturated)	100	40	573	47	760

barometer and proving that a column of air extending into the atmosphere has weight and, therefore, exerts a pressure at the Earth's surface (1 torr = 1 mm Hg) (Box 12–1).

DALTON'S LAW OF PARTIAL PRESSURES

Because each of the gases in an ambient air sample contributes a portion of the total barometric pressure, the sum of all the partial pressures must equal the total barometric pressure of the mixture. This relationship is known as **Dalton's law of partial pressures,** and can be shown as:

$$P_{TOTAL} = P_1 + P_2 + P_3 + \cdots + P_n$$

where P_1, P_2, P_3, and P_n are the partial pressures of the individual gases.

Barometric pressure is inversely proportional to altitude. Therefore, at higher elevations, the total pressure exerted by atmospheric air decreases. The composition of air, however, is remarkably uniform at various altitudes, meaning that the gas fractions essentially remain the same as those found at sea level. Therefore, the *partial pressures* of ambient gases decrease at high altitude because they are fractions of a smaller and smaller *total* pressure (see Table 12–1).

WATER VAPOR PARTIAL PRESSURE

Recall that one of the functions of the upper airways is to *condition* incoming air so that it is filtered, warmed, and humidified before reaching the lower respiratory passages. Inhaled particulate matter that impacts the mucus blanket lining the passages is entrapped and effectively removed from the airstream. In addition, dry inspired gas that comes into contact with the warm, moist mucous lining of the nasopharynx is *warmed* by blood perfusing the rich vascular beds and *humidified* by mucus produced by glands in the nasal and sinus cavities. As a result of this contact, inspired air is quickly warmed to about 33°C by passage through the pharynx, reaching body temperature (approximately

37°C) by the time it gets to the carina of the trachea. Inspired air also becomes saturated with water vapor picked up from moist mucosal surfaces. The total amount of water added to the incoming airstream is about 120 mL per day (Taylor et al, 1989).

The degree of saturation, however, depends on the temperature. At 37°C, saturated inspired gas has a constant **water vapor partial pressure (PH_2O)** of approximately 47 mm Hg. Water vapor partial pressure reduces the partial pressures of other inspired gases before they reach the alveoli. This reduction is attributable to the fact that the total pressure of inspired air is unchanged, but the mixture now includes an additional gas—water vapor. The partial pressure of water vapor causes a *relative* decrease in the partial pressures of other gases such as nitrogen, oxygen, carbon dioxide, and inert gases. *Inspired air* is described as ambient air that has entered the conducting zone of the lung but has not yet reached the alveoli. Note in Table 12–1 that the oxygen tension of dry ambient air at sea level is approximately 159 mm Hg, whereas inspired oxygen tension is reduced to approximately 149 mm Hg by the addition of water vapor to the incoming airstream. To correctly calculate the partial pressure of a gas in a humidified mixture, the water vapor partial pressure must first be subtracted from the total pressure of the mixture.

Understandably, it is important to know the temperature, pressure, and water vapor pressure of the gas mixture being analyzed when calculating the partial pressures of the individual gases in the mixture, as shown by the following example:

EXAMPLE 2

Mt. Everest, in the Himalayan range, is the tallest mountain peak on Earth (elevation ≈ 8000 m). The barometric pressure at the summit of Mt. Everest is approximately 247 mm Hg. Calculate the ambient and inspired partial pressure of oxygen at this altitude. (Assume that the ambient air is *dry* at the top of Mt. Everest.)

$$F_{O_2} = 20.93\%; P_{BAR}$$
$$= 247 \text{ mm Hg}; P_{H_2O}$$

P E R S P E C T I V E S

BOX 12–1

Living at the Bottom of a Sea of Air

Evangelista Torricelli was a brilliant mathematician of the Renaissance. His contemporaries included Descartes, Huygen, Pascal, Hooke, Newton, Halley, Boyle, Wren, and dozens more—a stellar company of thinkers and tinkerers who revolutionized philosophy and shaped scientific thought for centuries to come. In 1641, Torricelli became assistant to Galileo, the most illustrious scientist of the age. When Galileo died in 1642, Torricelli was appointed to succeed him as Mathematician to Grand Duke Ferdinando II of Tuscany. Torricelli held the Chair in Mathematics until his own death in 1647. Torricelli was a typical Renaissance man, accomplished in a variety of disciplines, including mathematics, mechanics, hydrodynamics, and meteorology. He was a gifted lens grinder and instrument maker, producing several high-quality telescopes and microscopes. He also worked on a mathematical value for gravity, the theory of projectiles, fluid motion, and even dabbled in the practical field of military fortifications.

One of the most important events in physics in the seventeenth century was the *Torricellian experiment,* which marked the introduction of the barometer and provided convincing arguments regarding the characteristics of atmospheric pressure and the nature of vacuums.

We live immersed at the bottom of a sea of elemental air, which by experiment undoubtedly has weight, and so much weight that the densest air in the neighborhood of the surface of the earth weighs about one four-hundredth part of the weight of water.

(FROM A LETTER TO MICHELANGELO RICCI CONCERNING THE BAROMETER—JUNE 11, 1644)
MAGIE, 1935

Torricelli also correctly observed:

. . . on the peaks of high mountains the air begins to be more pure and to weigh much less than the four-hundredth part of the weight of water.

MAGIE, 1935

The Torricellian experiment demonstrated that barometric pressure determines the height to which a column of fluid will rise in a tube that has been inverted over a reservoir of the same fluid. The contemporary (Aristotelian) thinking denied the possibility of a vacuum—Torricelli's experiment not only produced a sustained vacuum above the column of fluid but also introduced the principle of the barometer. In this elegant experiment a glass tube open on one end and "two cubits long" (approximately 115 cm), was filled with quicksilver and turned upside down, with the open end closed by a finger placed over it. We now know quicksilver as mercury (Hg). (We also now know to not put our fingers in the shimmering but toxic liquid!) Torricelli found that when the mercury-filled glass tube was placed in a bowl of mercury, and the finger was removed, the column of mercury always fell to a height a little more than a "cubit and a quarter" (approximately 70 cm), and created a vacuum above the surface of mercury.

Later, he noticed that the height of mercury fluctuated slightly from day to day and seemed to be influenced by temperature. By employing glass tubes and vessels of differing diameters and shapes, Torricelli's experiments in 1644 provided evidence that resistance to the descent of the column of mercury was caused exclusively by the weight of the atmosphere pressing down externally on the reservoir of mercury and

continued

BOX 12-1

Living at the Bottom of a Sea of Air (Continued)

countering the mass of the liquid—not by the presence of an "exceedingly rarefied substance" acting within the space in the tube above the surface of mercury to reduce its descent.

On the surface of the liquid which is in the bowl there rests the weight of a height of fifty miles of air. . . . [Quicksilver enters the tube and rises] . . . in a column high enough to make equilibrium with the weight of the external air which forces it up.

Water also in a similar tube, though a much longer one, will rise to about 18 cubits, that is, as much more than quicksilver does as quicksilver is heavier than water, so as to be in equilibrium with the same cause which acts on the one and the other.

MAGIE, 1935

Through this simple observation of the relative heights of two liquids in glass tubes, Torricelli showed that mercury is about 14 times denser than water (18 cubits/1.25 cubits = 14.4). The density of mercury has been accurately calculated as $d = 13.6$. Through these insightful experiments, Torricelli laid the groundwork for much of the subsequent work concerning gases and pressures. When we record the barometric pressure at sea level as 760 mm Hg, or 760 torr, we recognize the invaluable contributions of a true Renaissance thinker.

- Magie WF: A Source Book in Physics: Collected Works Vol III (1919) [Reprinted letter posted on the World Wide Web]. McGraw-Hill, New York, 1935. Retrieved March 23, 1998 from the World Wide Web: URL http://maple.lemoyne.edu/~guinta/torr.htm.
- Westfall RS: Evangelista Torricelli: The Galileo Project Development Team [Biography posted on the World Wide Web]. Indiana University, n.d./1998. Retrieved March 23, 1998 from the World Wide Web: URL http:es.rice.edu/ES/humsoc/Galileo/Catalog/Files/torriceli.html.

$$= 47 \text{ mm Hg}$$

$$\therefore \text{Ambient P}_{O_2} \text{ (dry)}$$

$$= 247 \text{ mm Hg} \times 0.2093$$

$$= 51.7 \text{ mm Hg}$$

$$\therefore \text{Inspired P}_{O_2} \text{ (saturated)} = (247 \text{ mm Hg}$$

$$- 47 \text{ mm Hg}) \times 0.2093 = 41.9 \text{ mm Hg}$$

PARTIAL PRESSURE GRADIENTS IN THE LUNG

Recall from the discussion of the conducting zone that a substantial proportion of the total cross-sectional area of the airways is contained in the distal passageways. Recall also that in systems where laminar flow occurs, gas velocity varies inversely with tube radius. Therefore, as gas enters a tube of small radius, its velocity increases because of the convective acceleration effect. Remember that this energy conversion is accompanied by a fall in pressure. Overall, as gas enters a branched network

of small airways, the driving pressure drops appreciably until the forward velocity of the gas reaches zero. This dramatic reduction in gas velocity in the distal airways occurs at a point *upstream* from the alveoli. The final movement of gas into the alveoli is brought about by the random molecular motion of the gas, a type of movement known as *Brownian motion* (West, 1998).

As the gas molecules begin to impact the alveolar epithelial surface, their rate of movement through the membrane is dictated, in part, by the partial pressure *gradient* that exists between the partial pressure of alveolar gas and that of the mixed venous blood perfusing the alveolus. *Gases always diffuse from an area of high partial pressure to an area of low partial pressure.* For example, if a gas sample from an alveolus has an oxygen tension of $\text{P}_{AO_2} = 100$ mm Hg, and a mixed venous sample of blood from pulmonary capillaries perfusing the alveolus has an oxygen tension of $\text{P}\bar{v}_{O_2} = 40$ mm Hg, a *net diffusion* of oxygen out of the alveolus and into the pulmonary capillaries occurs because of the partial pressure gradient ($\Delta\text{P}_{O_2} = 60$ mm Hg). This transfer of gas continues until *equilibration* occurs, that is, until the partial pressure of gas in the pulmonary capillary equals that of gas in the alveolus. (Equilibration is discussed further in a subsequent section).

Gas Diffusion

FICK'S LAW OF DIFFUSION

What factors dictate the *rate* at which gas molecules move through a membrane along a partial pressure gradient? If we consider a model in which two regions having differing partial pressures (P_1 and P_2) are separated by a membrane, or a layer of fluid in which they briefly dissolve during transit, we can predict some of the factors influencing the rate of gas diffusion through the membrane. For instance, common sense tells us that a *thin membrane* with a *very large surface area* would presumably contribute to efficient gas transfer. This is precisely the structural arrangement found in the lung—an alveolar-capillary membrane 0.35 μm thick coupled with an alveolar surface area of roughly 80 m². But what of other, less obvious factors such as the behavior of the diffusing gas within the membrane itself? The behavior of the gas is related to its *solubility* in the membrane and the *molecular weight* of the gas. Fortunately there is a mathematical relationship that links all of these variables so that we can calculate the **diffusivity** of a gas, that is, the rate of diffusion of a gas through a membrane along a partial pressure gradient. **Fick's law of diffusion** combines the various factors described above in the following equation (Fig. 12–1):

$$\dot{V} = \frac{Ad}{T} \times \Delta P$$

where:

$\dot{V}$ = volume of gas diffusing across the membrane or liquid film per unit time (mL/min)
A = area of the membrane (cm²)
d = diffusion coefficient (cm²/mm Hg per minute), or diffusivity of a particular gas
T = thickness of the membrane (cm)
ΔP = gas partial pressure gradient across the membrane (mm Hg)

From this relationship we can see that the transfer of gas is directly proportional to the area of the membrane and inversely proportional to its thickness, when all other factors are held constant. Doubling the area of the membrane doubles the flow rate of gas across the membrane, whereas doubling the thickness of the membrane reduces the rate of diffusion by one-half. Fick's law also shows us that the rate of diffusion is directly proportional to the magnitude of the partial pressure gradient (ΔP) across the membrane. Finally, gas transfer through a membrane is influenced by the *diffusion coefficient* (d) of the gas. The diffusion coefficient is directly proportional to the *solubility* of gas in the barrier material, but inversely proportional to the square root of the *molecular weight* (*mw*) of the gas, as shown by the following relationship:

$$d \propto \frac{\text{Solubility}}{\sqrt{\text{mw}}}$$

From our example of ambient and inspired gas pressures at the summit of Mt. Everest, it is clear that high altitude effectively reduces the rate of transfer of oxygen in the lung by reducing the partial pressure gradient across the alveolar-capillary membrane, as revealed by the Fick equation.

GRAHAM'S LAW

The diffusion rate of a gas is inversely proportional to the square root of its gram molecular weight, a relationship known as **Graham's law:**

$$\text{Gas diffusion rate} \propto \frac{1}{\sqrt{\text{gmw gas}}}$$

NOTE: The gram molecular weight of O_2 is 32 g; the gram molecular weight of CO_2 is 44 g.

Because oxygen is a lighter molecule, it diffuses through a gaseous medium 1.17 times faster than carbon dioxide, as shown by a comparison of the relative rates of diffusion of the two gases:

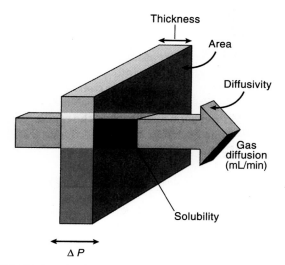

FIGURE 12–1. Fick's law and the diffusivity of gas through a membrane. Diffusion of a gas from one region to another through a barrier. Fick's law of diffusion describes the factors influencing the rate of gas diffusion from a region of high partial pressure to a region of lower partial pressure. (From Leff AR and Schumacker PT: Respiratory Physiology: Basics and Applications. WB Saunders, Philadelphia, 1993, p 83, with permission.)

$$\frac{O_2 \text{ diffusion rate}}{CO_2 \text{ diffusion rate}} \quad \frac{\sqrt{\text{gmw } CO_2}}{\sqrt{\text{gmw } O_2}} = \frac{\sqrt{44\text{ g}}}{\sqrt{32\text{ g}}}$$

$$= \frac{6.63}{5.66} = \frac{1.17}{1} = 1.17$$

HENRY'S LAW

Carbon dioxide is more soluble in water than is oxygen. For example, at a body temperature of 37°C and a pressure of 760 mm Hg, 0.592 mL of CO_2 dissolves in 1 mL of water. Under the same conditions, however, only 0.0244 mL of O_2 dissolves in 1 mL of water (Beachey, 1998; Des Jardins, 1998). This difference in solubility has an important bearing on gas transport and is examined in Chapter 13. At a given temperature, the volume of gas that dissolves in a liquid is directly proportional to the partial pressure of the gas. This relationship is known as **Henry's law.** Comparing the solubilities of CO_2 and O_2, it is seen that CO_2 is approximately 24 times more soluble in water than O_2, as shown by the following calculation:

$$\frac{CO_2 \text{ Solubility}}{O_2 \text{ Solubility}} = \frac{0.592 \text{ mL/mL } H_2O}{0.0244 \text{ mL/mL } H_2O}$$

$$= \frac{24.3}{1.0} = 24.3$$

Because the overall rate of diffusion of gas in the lung is inversely proportional to the gram molecular weight of the gas and directly proportional to the solubility of the gas, we can combine Graham's and Henry's laws to calculate the overall diffusion rate of a gas through a membrane. CO_2 diffuses through the alveolar-capillary membrane approximately 20 times faster than O_2, as shown by the following calculation:

Combined Graham's and Henry's laws:

$$\frac{\text{Overall } CO_2 \text{ diffusion rate}}{\text{Overall } O_2 \text{ diffusion rate}} = \frac{\sqrt{32}}{\sqrt{44}} \times \frac{0.592}{0.0244}$$

$$= \frac{3.35}{0.16} = 20.7$$

From the above comparison it is clear that a defect in the alveolar-capillary membrane will affect the diffusion of oxygen more than the diffusion of carbon dioxide.

Gases impacting the membrane surface must ultimately dissolve in the membrane material to pass through to the other side. Gases that readily dissolve in the barrier will diffuse through it at a faster rate than those that are relatively insoluble in the barrier. Solubility is defined as the volume of gas (in mL) that must be dissolved in 100 mL of the barrier liquid to raise the partial pressure by 1 mm Hg (Leff and Schumacker, 1993). Interestingly, synthetic fluids called *perfluorocarbons* (*PFCs*) have been developed that can be in-

stilled into collapsed alveoli and oxygenated with a technique called *partial liquid ventilation* (Box 12–2). Oxygen is very soluble in such fluids; therefore, large volumes of oxygen can be delivered to patients suffering from acute respiratory distress. Because the fluids produce a liquid-liquid gas exchange barrier, the high surface tension typical of the air-blood interface in the lung is dramatically reduced, thus improving lung compliance, decreasing atelectasis, and providing a valuable adjunct to conventional positive-pressure ventilator therapy.

MOLECULAR VELOCITY AND GAS DIFFUSION

Gases having a high molecular weight have a low molecular velocity that causes them to diffuse slowly through a membrane. By contrast, gases having a lower molecular weight possess a higher molecular velocity and, therefore, diffuse relatively quickly through a membrane. The velocity determines the speed at which gas molecules impact each other and collide with the barrier material in which they dissolve. At a given temperature, gas molecules have the same kinetic energy (KE), as shown by the classic equation, $KE = \frac{1}{2} mv^2$, where m is the mass and v is velocity. Therefore, the velocity of a gas is inversely proportional to the square root of its molecular weight (m), as shown by the following equation (Leff and Schumacker, 1993):

$$KE = \frac{1}{2} mv^2$$

$$2KE = mv^2$$

$$v^2 = \frac{2KE}{m}$$

$$\therefore v = \sqrt{\frac{2KE}{m}}$$

Dissimilar gas molecules having the same kinetic energy illustrate this relationship between the molecular weight and the molecular velocity of a gas:

Assume:

Kinetic energy of gas A = kinetic energy of gas B

$$\frac{1}{2}m_A v_A^2 = \frac{1}{2}m_B v_B^2$$

$$\therefore m_A v_A^2 = m_B v_B^2$$

From this relationship it can be seen that the same kinetic energy can be achieved by a fast-moving, low-molecular-weight gas molecule or by a slow-moving, high-molecular-weight gas molecule. Recall, however, that the rate of passage through a barrier is determined by the *velocity* with which the gas molecules impact the barrier. Stated simply, lighter gas molecules having high velocities impact the barrier at high speed and dif-

PERSPECTIVES

BOX 12–2 ## Liquid Ventilation

Infants and pediatric patients diagnosed with severe respiratory failure serious enough to warrant extracorporeal life support (ECLS) generally require immediate ventilatory treatment. In these cases, inflammatory processes within the lung, and the gas exchange disturbances that accompany them, develop so quickly that aggressive, and often damaging, ventilatory regimens must be employed. Acute respiratory failure is characterized by the rapid loss of surfactant function, development of high surface tension, extensive atelectasis of the lung, and severe impairment of respiratory gas exchange.

Conventional treatment with gas ventilation is potentially damaging because of barotrauma or volutrauma, leading to pulmonary air leaks. Such ventilator-induced lung injury results from the high inflation pressures employed, a problem exaggerated in the lungs of immature patients. For these reasons, new treatment modalities are being investigated to treat acute respiratory failure and reduce the occurrence of additional lung injury. Modern adjuncts to ventilator therapy include high-frequency ventilation, administration of exogenous surfactant (see Box 1–1), inhaled nitric oxide (see Box 14–1), extracorporeal membrane oxygenation (see Box 3–1), and partial liquid ventilation.

Liquid ventilation (LV) is a process involving gas ventilation of liquid-filled lungs. Because the lungs are not completely filled with a liquid serving as a respiratory medium, the term *partial liquid ventilation (PLV)* is more accurate. The technique is also called *perfluorocarbon-associated gas exchange (PAGE)*. The breathable fluids employed in the therapy are known as *perfluorocarbon (PFC) liquids* (e.g., *perflubron*). Originally, a complex liquid ventilator was used to produce tidal liquid breathing in which infusion and active removal of tidal volumes of PFCs was carried out. Today, repetitive doses of PFCs are instilled through the trachea and pushed into collapsed alveoli to keep them open. Conventional positive-pressure gas ventilators are then used to oxygenate the fluid. The PFCs are instilled to tidal volume (V_T) where they fill the dependent zone of the lung. Such compounds have a high binding capacity for oxygen and carbon dioxide. In addition, PFCs are bioinert and nonbiotransformable. These unique respiratory media exhibit characteristics such as high respiratory gas solubility, low surface tension, minimal absorption, and tissue compatibility. Advances in fluorine chemistry promise to deliver PFCs with improved respiratory qualities for future PLV therapies.

Partial liquid ventilation provides significant improvements in the treatment of respiratory failure in neonates and pediatric patients. Advantages of PLV over conventional high insufflation pressure ventilator therapy include more effective gas exchange, improved lung mechanics, increased lung compliance, elimination of the high surface tension of the gas-lung interface, improved acid-base balance, and improved ventilation-perfusion matching.

Potential neonatal applications of PLV therapy include the treatment of surfactant deficiency, persistent pulmonary hypertension of the newborn, meconium aspiration, and pneumonia. The use of PLV to deliver drugs to lung tissues and systemic circulation is also being studied. Complications of PLV therapy include pneumothorax. Liquid ventilation represents a radical departure from the normal mode of ventilator therapy and seems especially bizarre for air-breathing animals. The advantages, however, of reducing the high surface tension of collapsed alveoli and filling them instead with an

continued

P E R S P E C T I V E S

BOX 12–2   Liquid Ventilation (Continued)

oxygen-rich fluid that promotes gas exchange, appear to outweigh the risks associated with the unconventional therapy.

- Cox CA, Wolfson MR, and Shaffer TH: Liquid ventilation: A comprehensive review. Neonatal Netw. 15:31–43, 1996.
- Elixson EM, Myrer ML, and Horn MH: Current trends in ventilation of the pediatric patient. Crit Care Nurs Q. 20:1–13, 1997.
- Gabriel JL et al: Quantitative structure-activity relationships of perfluorinated hetero-hydrocarbons as potential respiratory media: Application to oxygen solubility, partition coefficient, viscosity, vapor pressure, and density. ASAIO-J. 42:968–973, 1996.
- Gauger PG et al: Initial experience with partial liquid ventilation in pediatric patients with the acute respiratory distress syndrome. Crit Care Med. 24:16–22, 1996.
- Leach CL et al: Partial liquid ventilation with perflubron in premature infants with severe respiratory distress syndrome. The LiquiVent Study Group. N Engl J Med. 335:761–767, 1996.
- Norris MK, Fuhrman BP, and Leach CL: Liquid ventilation: It's not science fiction anymore. AACN Clin Issues. 5:246–254, 1994.
- Paulson TE, Spear RM, and Peterson BM: New concepts in the treatment of children with acute respiratory distress syndrome. J Pediatr. 127:163–175, 1995.
- Shaffer TH and Wolfson MR: Liquid ventilation: An alternative ventilation strategy for management of neonatal respiratory distress. Eur J Pediatr. 155 Suppl 2:S30–40, 1996.

fuse rapidly through it. Thus, the molecular weight of a gas and its inherent velocity at the membrane, along with its solubility in the membrane, determine the diffusion coefficient (*d*) in the Fick equation—and the greater the diffusion coefficient, the greater the diffusivity of the gas through the membrane.

Equilibration of Gas at the Alveolar-Capillary Membrane

TRANSIT TIME IN PULMONARY CAPILLARIES

The exchange system between the air and blood is formed by the type I pneumocytes of the alveolar wall and the endothelial cells of pulmonary capillaries. Recall that pulmonary capillaries are so narrow that erythrocytes must nearly fold in half to pass through the vessels in single file. This continuous flow occurs under nearly pulseless conditions because the pulmonary circuit is a low-pressure, low-resistance vascular system. The **transit time** of blood in the pulmonary capillary system is affected by the driving pressure provided by the right ventricle and the vascular resistance of the pulmonary vessels. Perfusion of the lung is affected by different lung volumes because both alveolar septal capillaries and extra-alveolar blood vessels are changed by the degree of lung inflation or deflation. In addition, pulmonary vascular resistance (PVR) and perfusion are influenced by the vertical hydrostatic effect in the lung (see Chap. 11). Under normal conditions, the transit time of an

erythrocyte in a capillary perfusing a single alveolus is approximately 0.75 s (Des Jardins, 1998; Leff and Schumacker, 1993). In this brief period, respiratory gases are exchanged across the alveolar-capillary membrane according to the partial pressure gradient and Fick's law of diffusion. In fact, this exchange normally takes place in the first one-third of the time available for gas diffusion—about 0.25 s. The additional time available provides a buffer against physiologic stress. For example, as cardiac output increases, more of the 0.75-s exposure time is used to complete oxygenation of the red blood cell. During the transit time, equalization of partial pressures occurs on the two sides of the alveolar-capillary membrane, a process called **equilibration of gases** (Fig. 12–2).

Consider what happens when mixed venous blood traveling in a pulmonary capillary passes a ventilated alveolus. A normally ventilated alveolus has a partial pressure of oxygen (P_{AO_2}) of 100 mm Hg and a P_{ACO_2} of 40 mm Hg (see Fig. 12–2). These values are maintained at a more or less constant level because fresh gas continually enters the alveolus. The pulmonary capillary blood has a partial pressure of oxygen ($P\bar{v}_{O_2}$) of 40 mm Hg and a $P\bar{v}_{CO_2}$ of approximately 45 to 47 mm Hg. Notice in Figure 12–2 that the pulmonary *arterial* gas tensions are raised to the alveolar gas tension levels. In other words, as blood leaves the venous end of a pulmonary capillary that has just perfused a normally ventilated alveolus, the partial pressure of arterial gases equals the partial pressure of alveolar gases.

How is this so? In fact, if respiratory gases reach an equilibrium across the alveolar-capillary membrane,

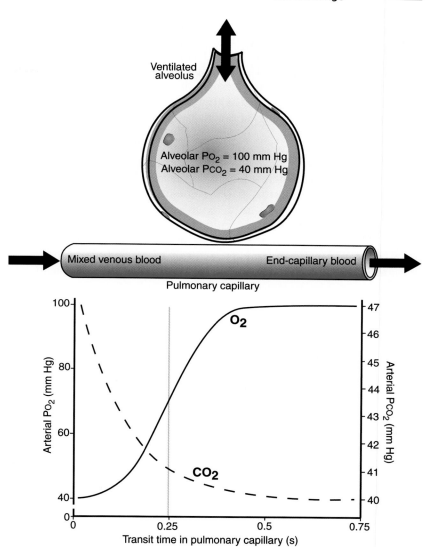

FIGURE 12–2. Equilibration of gases at the alveolar-capillary membrane. Mixed venous blood enters the proximal end of the pulmonary capillary with $PO_2 = 40$ mm Hg and $PCO_2 = 47$ mm Hg. Equilibration with alveolar gas occurs rapidly because of the substantial pressure gradient. Under normal conditions, much of the exchange takes place in the first one-third of the available transit time.

why are the arterial gas tensions not a mean, an *average* of the alveolar and mixed venous values? The answer is that the diffusion of gases and the transit of pulmonary blood through capillaries is part of a *dynamic system*. In this constantly changing system, both the air stream and the bloodstream are continually moving and are continually being replaced. For instance, at the arteriole end of the capillary, "fresh" blood with a relatively low oxygen tension of about 40 mm Hg continually enters the exchange zone next to a single alveolus. If this is a normally ventilated alveolus, "fresh" air will have already entered the respiratory system to maintain an alveolar oxygen tension of approximately 100 mm Hg. Therefore, at the instant erythrocytes begin to stream past this single alveolus, the partial pressure gradient for oxygen will be 60 mm Hg. This partial pressure differential ensures that oxygen diffuses out of the alveolus into the pulmonary capillary. The PAO_2 begins to fall as oxygen leaves the alveolus, but the gas is immediately replaced by fresh gas to restore the alveolar

oxygen tension to 100 mm Hg. Similarly, the entry of oxygen into the pulmonary capillary causes the PaO_2 to rise, but the oxygenated blood is pushed toward the venule end of the capillary and quickly replaced by deoxygenated blood pumped from the right ventricle. This continual flow transports reoxygenated blood ($PaO_2 = 100$ mm Hg) out of the lung and brings in mixed venous blood ($P\bar{v}O_2 = 40$ mm Hg).

The transfer of carbon dioxide in this dynamic system is similar—that is, continual movement of blood with a $P\bar{v}CO_2 = 45$ mm Hg and continual tidal flow of alveolar air with a $PACO_2 = 40$ mm Hg maintains the partial pressure gradient that transfers carbon dioxide out of the bloodstream (see Fig. 12–2). As carbon dioxide begins to leave the pulmonary blood vessel at its arteriole end, the $P\bar{v}O_2$ decreases and the $PACO_2$ begins to rise. However, the bloodstream quickly replaces this blood with mixed venous blood having a high carbon dioxide tension, while alveolar ventilation quickly delivers fresh air having a low carbon dioxide tension, thus maintaining the low carbon dioxide tension of the alveolus. At the venule end of the capillary the $P\bar{v}CO_2$ has been decreased by gas diffusion to approximately 40 mm Hg, the same as that of the alveolus. Through this dynamic mechanism, the carbon dioxide partial pressure gradient is maintained at about 5 mm Hg. Notice that the ΔPCO_2 of 5 mm Hg is considerably smaller than the ΔPO_2 of 60 mm Hg. In spite of this small partial pressure gradient, carbon dioxide achieves equilibration well within the available transit time, a characteristic related to its high solubility in plasma.

Equilibration of respiratory gases in the lung is easy to visualize if one imagines an alveolar-capillary system in which both air and blood suddenly *cease* to flow. In such a stagnant system, the gases already present at the respiratory membrane impact each side of the barrier and move through it at a flow rate determined by the various diffusion factors—solubilities, molecular weights, and partial pressure gradients of the gases, as well as thickness and surface area characteristics of the membrane itself. The gases continue to diffuse in both directions across the respiratory membrane until equilibrium is reached. In this fictitious system, the partial pressures in the alveoli and bloodstream approach the mean of the two values—approximately 70 mm Hg PO_2 and 42 mm Hg PCO_2 on *each side* of the membrane. In the dynamic system, however, the mean is never reached. Instead, the partial pressure of gas on the capillary side of the membrane mirrors that of gas on the alveolar side of the membrane.

GAS SOLUBILITY AND EQUILIBRATION

As we have seen in the Fick's law relationship, gases with high solubility diffuse at faster rates through membranes. This rapid flow rate occurs because high solubility gases quickly dissolve in the liquid matrix of the barrier material and pass from the side of higher partial pressure to the side of the barrier with the lower partial pressure. The transfer of gas results in equilibration. Figure 12–3 shows the direct relationship between the volume of gas dissolved in a liquid and the partial pressure exerted by the gas dissolved in the liquid. Gases that do not combine chemically with the liquid exhibit linear relationships at a given temperature. A straight line on such a volume-pressure graph represents a gas having constant solubility. The steeper the slope, the greater the solubility. In other words, the change in volume of dissolved gas entering the liquid matrix of the membrane is greater for each incremental change in partial pressure of the gas. This characteristic applies to high-solubility gases such as *diethyl ether,* an early general anesthetic no longer used (see Fig. 12–3). By contrast, the solubility of *nitrous oxide* (N_2O), another general anesthetic, is much less than that of diethyl ether, as shown by the lower slope of the N_2O pressure-volume rela-

tionship. As we will see later, gases that combine chemically with the liquid in which they are passing through exhibit nonlinear volume-pressure relationships—that is, their solubility is not constant; therefore, their slope is not a straight line. Only the fraction of gas actually dissolved in liquid is capable of exerting partial pressure in the liquid. Gases chemically combined with the liquid in which they are found do not exert partial pressure.

The equilibration of gases through membranes is also determined by their *relative* solubilities in different media. For instance, if a gas exhibits roughly the same solubility in the alveolar membrane as it does in plasma (which is mostly water), the equilibration rate for the gas will be very rapid. In other words, the gas quickly exerts a tension in the plasma because its solubility in the blood-gas barrier is similar to its solubility in the plasma. Inhalational anesthetics with such characteristics exhibit rapid onset of action because they quickly reach high partial pressures in the bloodstream and begin to depress the central nervous system. By contrast, anesthetic gases having dissimilar solubilities in different media are slow to reach anesthetic levels in the blood; therefore, their onset of action is much slower. If an anesthetic gas slowly leaves the alveolus to enter the pulmonary capillary, the perfusion of the alveolus will effectively "dilute" the gas as it is carried downstream. Consequently, a large partial pressure of gas in the plasma is not achieved, nor is an effective level of anesthesia rapidly attained.

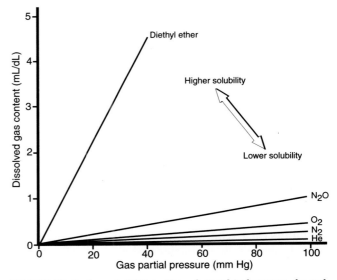

FIGURE 12–3. Gas solubilities. The relationship between the volume of gas dissolved in a liquid and the partial pressure of the gas in the liquid is shown by the graph. The *slope* of the line is the solubility of the gas in the liquid. These linear relationships are characteristic of gases that do not combine chemically with the liquid in which they are dissolved. (Adapted from Leff AR and Schumacker PT: Respiratory Physiology: Basics and Applications. WB Saunders, Philadelphia, 1993, p 83, with permission.)

EFFECTIVE SOLUBILITY

As pointed out previously, gases that combine chemically with blood do not exhibit *linear* partial pressure–volume relationships and do not have straight-line slopes representing constant solubility. Instead, gases of physiologic importance such as oxygen, carbon dioxide, and carbon monoxide combine with blood and exhibit nonlinear partial pressure–volume relationships. Graphs of these relationships reveal relatively complex curves having differing slopes (Fig. 12–4). These slopes represent the **effective solubility** of the gas, or the volume of gas that combines with a given volume of blood at a particular partial pressure. The

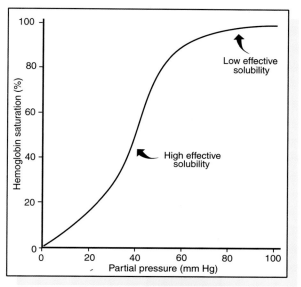

A - Oxygen plus hemoglobin

B - Carbon dioxide

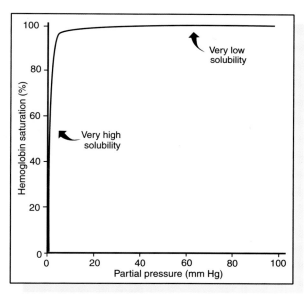

C - Carbon monoxide plus hemoglobin

FIGURE 12–4. Effective solubility. The *effective solubility* of each gas in blood is equivalent to the slope of the line at any given point. (A) Note that oxygen is highly soluble in the partial pressure range of 20–60 mm Hg but relatively insoluble above 100 mm Hg. (B) The solubility of carbon dioxide is relatively constant as a function of partial pressure, but it is still considered a nonlinear relationship. (C) The effective solubility of carbon monoxide is extremely high at partial pressure as low as 1 mm Hg. Above 1 mm Hg, carbon monoxide solubility is small, and additional carbon monoxide content occurs by adding dissolved gas. (Adapted from Leff AR and Schumacker PT: Respiratory Physiology: Basics and Applications. WB Saunders, Philadelphia, 1993, p 86, with permission.)

content of gas is usually expressed as mL of gas per 100 mL of blood, or mL/dL. (The letter "C" is used to denote *content* of gas, as in Ca_{O_2}, meaning "arterial content of oxygen.") Such nonlinear curves graphically show that the solubility and resulting plasma content of these gases vary according to the partial pressure of the gas, and that the change in content is different for each incremental change in tension of the gas.

Consider the sigmoid curve for oxygen shown in Figure 12–4A. The flattened plateau portion of the curve that starts at an oxygen tension of approximately 80 mm Hg illustrates that the effective solubility of oxygen is quite low at P_{O_2} values above 100 mm Hg. (Most of the hemoglobin binding sites are occupied in this partial pressure range.) Clearly, oxygen content is at a maximum level at such elevated partial pressures. The change in oxygen content, however, is minimal for each incremental change in partial pressure; therefore, the *effective* solubility of oxygen is low at higher partial pressures (Leff and Schumacker, 1993). The effective solubility of oxygen increases markedly at P_{O_2} values below 60 mm Hg. This trend is evident in the steep part of the slope, which represents a greater change in oxygen content for each incremental change in partial pressure (see Fig. 12–4A). In the next chapter we examine oxygen transport and the mechanisms responsible for generating both the flat portions and the steep portion of the curve.

Figure 12–4B shows the partial pressure–content curve for carbon dioxide. As can be seen by the nearly straight line of the curve, the effective solubility of carbon dioxide in blood is reasonably high and exhibits a relationship that is nearly constant. In other words, as the carbon dioxide tension of the blood increases, its content in the blood rises at a more or less steady rate.

Carbon monoxide (CO) is a toxic gas produced as a by-product of combustion. The gas has considerable physiologic importance because of its unusually high affinity for hemoglobin in blood. At extremely low partial pressures of carbon monoxide, a large volume of CO rapidly diffuses out of the alveoli and enters the bloodstream, significantly raising the CO content of the blood by chemically combining with hemoglobin (Fig. 12–4C). Put another way, the effective solubility of carbon monoxide is remarkably high. The high solubility of the gas in blood is represented by an extremely steep slope on the graph (see Fig. 12–4C).

Limiting Factors in Gas Exchange

PERFUSION-LIMITED GAS EXCHANGE

Recall that the partial pressure of gas in a fluid medium is produced when gas molecules do not chemically combine with the fluid in which they are found. Their pres-

ence in the plasma is what generates gas tension in the blood. In the case of physiologically inert gases, such as inhaled helium, ether, or nitrous oxide, equilibration of gas in the plasma with gas in the alveoli occurs very rapidly. Once equilibrium occurs, no further net exchange of gas takes place. The transfer of high-solubility gases into the plasma occurs so rapidly that the membrane itself is not the limiting factor in the exchange. Instead, the movement of blood through the pulmonary capillaries determines how much gas is loaded into circulation. For the transfer of high-solubility gases to continue, more blood must enter the alveolar-capillary system. Cardiac output, therefore, limits the diffusion of gases such as nitrous oxide, ether, and helium. The transfer of such gases into the bloodstream is described as **perfusion-limited** (Fig. 12–5A). As a result of the rapid diffusion, the partial pressure of gas in the plasma increases rapidly. This rapid rise to equilibrium implies that the diffusion occurs early in the transit of blood

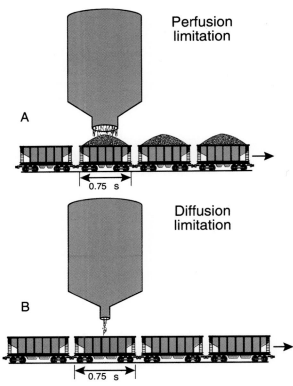

FIGURE 12–5. Gas transfer across the blood-brain barrier. (A) Perfusion-limited gas exchange; (B) diffusion-limited gas exchange. The rate at which alveolar gas and blood equilibrate depends on the solubility of the gas in the blood-gas barrier (diameter of the coal chute) relative to the effective solubility in blood (size of the railroad cars). Each car spends 0.75 second under the chute before moving on. (A) Membrane solubility is well matched to the solubility in blood, so the cars leaving the dock are filled fully (perfusion limitation). (B) Membrane solubility is low while blood solubility is high, and the cars leave without being completely filled (diffusion limitation). (From Leff AR and Schumacker PT: Respiratory Physiology: Basics and Applications. WB Saunders, Philadelphia, 1993, p 88, with permission.)

through the pulmonary capillary (Fig. 12–5). Any further time spent by blood in the capillary will not increase the amount of gas transferred into the bloodstream.

DIFFUSION-LIMITED GAS EXCHANGE

Gas transfer dependent on the integrity of the alveolar-capillary membrane is said to be **diffusion-limited** (Fig. 12–5B). Some gases such as carbon monoxide move through the respiratory membrane with relative ease but take a relatively long time to reach equilibration with the plasma. The slow rise to equilibration is due to the fact that CO combines chemically with hemoglobin in red blood cells to form *carbon monoxide hemoglobin*. Since this binding with hemoglobin effectively "removes" CO from the plasma as quickly as it diffuses out of the alveolus, the gas in the bloodstream fails to reach equilibrium with gas in the alveolus and is, therefore, unable to exert a high partial pressure in the blood. In effect, the capillary transit time of approximately 0.75 s is expired before a substantial volume of CO gas enters the plasma.

Under normal circumstances, mixed venous blood entering the alveolar-capillary system of a single alveolus contains no CO. However, if an individual has breathed carbon monoxide and the gas is present in the alveolus, CO immediately begins to diffuse out of the alveolus and into the plasma because of the carbon monoxide partial pressure gradient. The gas briefly enters the plasma and then rapidly passes through the cell membranes of red blood cells. Here, it chemically combines with hemoglobin because of its unusually high affinity, estimated to be as much as 200 times greater than the affinity exhibited by oxygen toward hemoglobin. As explained above, this rapid transfer of CO out of the plasma and into the red blood cells keeps the carbon monoxide tension of the blood extremely low. Pulmonary perfusion has little effect on the movement of such gases out of the alveolus. In other words, a change in the flow rate of pulmonary blood will not appreciably change the volume of CO entering the plasma. Instead, the movement of such gases is dependent on the *diffusing capacity*, or *conductance* characteristics of the alveolar-capillary membrane itself; such characteristics contribute to the diffusion limited nature of gas transfer.

DIFFUSING CAPACITY OF THE LUNG

As explained previously, the integrity of the alveolar-capillary membrane determines the *diffusing capacity of the lung* (D_L). In Fick's law of diffusion, it was seen that the rate of gas diffusion (diffusivity) through a membrane is directly proportional to the partial pressure gradient:

$$\dot{V} = \frac{Ad}{T} \times \Delta P$$

In this relationship, the term Ad/T represents the *conductance* or the *diffusing capacity* of the lung for the transfer of a particular gas from the alveolus to the bloodstream. (Recall that conductance is the reciprocal of resistance.) Conductance, as applied to the entire lung, is affected by the total area available for diffusion (A), the average thickness of the alveolar-capillary membrane (T), and the diffusion coefficient of the specific gas (d).

Because of the phenomenal ease and speed with which CO diffuses out of the alveoli to chemically combine with hemoglobin, and its extremely slow rate of equilibration along the pulmonary capillary, CO is used as a test gas to assess the overall ability of the lung to diffuse gases. (Recall that the movement of CO into the bloodstream is *not* perfusion limited.) Substituting CO into Fick's law gives us the **diffusing capacity of the lung for carbon monoxide (D_{LCO}):**

$$\dot{V}_{CO} = \frac{Ad}{T} \times \Delta P$$

and

$$D_{LCO} = \frac{Ad}{T}$$

$$\therefore \dot{V}_{CO} = D_{LCO}\, \Delta P$$

Because the bloodstream is normally devoid of CO, capillary blood carbon monoxide partial pressure ($P\bar{v}_{CO}$) is assumed to be zero. Therefore, the difference (ΔP) between alveolar carbon monoxide partial pressure ($P_{A_{CO}}$) and capillary blood carbon monoxide partial pressure can be expressed simply as the alveolar value. Using this value ($P_{A_{CO}}$), the diffusing capacity of the lung for carbon monoxide can be calculated. Note that the units for D_{LCO} are given in milliliters per minute per millimeter of mercury:

$$\therefore \dot{V}_{CO} = D_{LCO} \times P_{A_{CO}}$$

and

$$D_{LCO} = \frac{\dot{V}_{CO}}{P_{A_{CO}}}.$$

By measuring how much CO diffuses out of the lung in a given time, an estimate can be made of alveolar-capillary membrane function. For instance, pathologic conditions such as alveolar fibrosis or edema compromise the structure and function of the alveolar-capillary system, thereby reducing the diffusing capacity of the lung for CO. The D_{LCO} value for normal lungs is approximately 25 mL/min per mm Hg, increasing to two or three times this value in response to exercise (West, 1998). This increase in the diffusing capacity of the lung upon exercising is related to the increase in the total area of lung tissue available for gas exchange. Such an increase occurs as a result of the recruitment and distension of additional pulmonary capillaries (see Chap. 11).

OXYGEN AS A PERFUSION-LIMITED AND DIFFUSION-LIMITED GAS

Oxygen exhibits both perfusion-limited and diffusion-limited characteristics of gas exchange. As we have seen, oxygen diffuses into the bloodstream because of a partial pressure gradient of approximately 60 mm Hg. Although the transfer of oxygen does not occur nearly as rapidly as the transfer of physiologically inert gases such as nitrous oxide, the diffusion of oxygen from the alveolus into the pulmonary capillary occurs in approximately one-third of the transit time available for blood in the pulmonary capillary. This means that the Po_2 of mixed venous blood is substantially raised within 0.25 s as blood perfuses past a single alveolus and equilibration occurs with alveolar gas (see Fig. 12–2).

Most of the oxygen that diffuses into the bloodstream combines chemically with hemoglobin and does not contribute to the partial pressure of the plasma. A small but significant volume of oxygen, however, *does* enter the plasma and exert partial pressure. The alveolar-capillary membrane in a normal lung does not impede the diffusion of oxygen. However, abnormalities in the number of red blood cells or in the amount or function of hemoglobin result in reduced oxygen-binding sites, anemia, and reduced volume of oxygen in the blood. Similarly, impairment of right heart function causes a reduction in pulmonary blood flow and reduced loading of oxygen into the bloodstream. These abnormal conditions cause a reduction in the oxygen content of the blood (Cao_2), illustrating the *perfusion-limited* nature of oxygen transfer in the lung.

Interestingly, the transfer of oxygen across the alveolar-capillary membrane is also described as *diffusion-limited*. Under normal lung conditions, as we have seen, oxygen transfers out of the alveolus in the first one-third of the time available, meaning that the exchange is usually not slowed by the diffusion properties of the alveolar-capillary membrane. However, under abnormal pulmonary conditions such as interstitial or alveolar fibrosis, the movement of oxygen out of the alveoli is slowed by the impaired alveolar-capillary membrane. The flow rate of blood through the pulmonary circuit in such conditions does not appreciably change the transfer of oxygen out of the alveoli.

In summary, the movement of oxygen from the alveolus into the bloodstream normally occurs very rapidly because of the favorable diffusion properties of the exchange membrane and the diffusing properties of the gas itself. Also, the loading of oxygen into the bloodstream is carried out effectively by the adequate

perfusion of the lung. It is under unusual pathophysiologic conditions that the exchange of oxygen is seen as either perfusion-limited or diffusion-limited.

Diffusion in the Tissues

In the systemic capillaries, oxygen and carbon dioxide exchange occurs because of passive diffusion. The exchange is considered diffusion limited under normal conditions (Leff and Schumacker, 1993). This limitation tells us that if blood remained in the systemic capillaries for a longer period of time, more oxygen would be extracted and more carbon dioxide would be loaded. Such a situation is common in tissues in which membrane solubili ty is low and blood solubility is high. In effect, capillary blood leaves the tissues before all of the gases have been exchanged. For example, the oxygen tension of mixed venous blood leaving the systemic capillaries is normally reduced to about 40 mm Hg, indicating that all of the oxygen in the arterial blood (Pao_2 = 100 mm Hg) was *not* given up in transit through systemic capillaries. Similarly, the carbon dioxide tension of tissue fluid in the immediate vicinity of the systemic capillaries is normally 45 mm Hg. The carbon dioxide in the tissues quickly equilibrates with arterial blood ($Paco_2$ = 40 mm Hg) and is lowered to approximately 40 mm Hg—but is *not* reduced to zero.

As occurs at the sites of external respiration, gas exchange at the sites of internal respiration is determined by differences in partial pressures between the capillaries and the tissues. Unlike the structural arrangement in the lung, however, systemic cells may be located at some distance from a capillary. A fall in partial pressure of oxygen in the tissues triggers recruitment of additional capillaries so that blood flow is increased and adequate amounts of oxygen are delivered to metabolically active tissues. This type of vascular adaptation to hypoxia is seen in strenuous exercise where skeletal muscle blood flow increases dramatically. At rest, perfusion of approximately 20% of the available capillaries in skeletal muscle occurs, increasing to nearly 100% during heavy exercise (Leff and Schumacker, 1993). Compare this systemic vascular response to hypoxia with that of pulmonary blood vessels, where *reduced* blood flow occurs as a result of pulmonary vasoconstriction (see Chap. 11).

Summary

In this chapter we examined the classical gas laws of Dalton and Fick as they relate to the diffusion of gas across the alveolar-capillary membrane in the lung. Here we saw that partial pressures are affected both by the percentage composition of gas in a mixture and, in a relative way, by the partial pressures of *other* gases in the mixture. Most importantly, we noted that gases always diffuse from an area of high partial pressure to an area of lower partial pressure. The chapter also discussed the variables that affect the rate of transfer of gas through a membrane along a partial pressure gradient. These variables include the area and thickness of the membrane as well as the partial pressure gradient across the membrane, the solubility of the gas in the membrane matrix, and the molecular weight of the gas transferring through the barrier. The chapter also examined the transit time of blood in pulmonary capillaries, the equilibration of gas along the capillary, and the effective solubility of gas in different media. The chapter concluded with a brief discussion of perfusion and diffusion factors that limit gas exchange across membranes.

BIBLIOGRAPHY

Beachey W: Respiratory Care Anatomy and Physiology: Foundations for Clinical Practice. Mosby–Year Book, St. Louis, 1998.

Des Jardins T: Cardiopulmonary Anatomy and Physiology: Essentials for Respiratory Care, ed 3. Delmar Publishers, Albany, NY, 1998.

Ganong WF: Review of Medical Physiology, ed 17. Appleton & Lange, Norwalk, CT, 1995.

Leff AR and Schumacker PT: Respiratory Physiology: Basics and Applications. WB Saunders, Philadelphia, 1993.

Martini FH: Fundamentals of Anatomy and Physiology, ed 4. Prentice Hall, Upper Saddle River, NJ, 1998.

Taylor AE et al: Clinical Respiratory Physiology. WB Saunders, Philadelphia, 1989.

Thibodeau GA and Patton KT: Anatomy and Physiology, ed 3. Mosby–Year Book, St Louis, 1996.

West JB: Respiratory Physiology: The Essentials, ed 6. Williams & Wilkins, Baltimore, 1998.

CHAPTER 13

Gas Transport

chapter objectives

After studying this chapter the reader should be able to:

☐ Explain the concept of oxygen consumption as the difference between systemic oxygen delivery and systemic oxygen return.

☐ Define Henry's law as it applies to the transport of oxygen in the plasma.

☐ Describe how oxygen is transported in a dissolved form in the plasma.

☐ Define hematocrit.

☐ Discuss the morphology of red blood cells that contributes to their suitability as oxygen carriers.

☐ Describe the structure of the hemoglobin molecule by explaining the arrangement of heme units, iron ions, and the polypeptide chains that make up the globin protein.

☐ Explain the importance of the hydrophobic interior and the hydrophilic exterior of the hemoglobin molecule.

☐ Discuss the elimination of hemoglobin from the body by describing the role of bile pigments.

☐ Differentiate between the theoretical oxygen-binding capacity and the physiologic oxygen-binding capacity of hemoglobin.

☐ Explain why the actual volume of oxygen bound to hemoglobin is less than the theoretical volume of oxygen bound to hemoglobin.

☐ Explain how the total oxygen content of the blood is calculated.

☐ Differentiate between linear and nonlinear chemical relationships and describe the shape of the oxyhemoglobin dissociation curve.

☐ Describe the conformational and kinetic factors responsible for producing the flat and steep parts of the oxyhemoglobin dissociation curve.

☐ Describe carbon monoxide poisoning and explain the effect of carboxyhemoglobin on the oxygen-transporting ability of the hemoglobin molecule.

☐ Describe the standard oxyhemoglobin dissociation curve known as hemoglobin P_{50} and explain how the curve is useful in gas transport studies.

☐ Discuss the significance of a left or a right shift in the oxyhemoglobin dissociation curve in terms of affinity of hemoglobin towards oxygen and the relative ease that oxygen associates with and dissociates from hemoglobin.

☐ Discuss how the following physiologic factors shift the oxyhemoglobin dissociation curve:

Blood temperature, pH, P_{CO_2}, 2,3-DPG, fetal hemoglobin.

☐ Explain how the Bohr effect influences the release of oxygen from oxyhemoglobin.

☐ Discuss the clinical significance of left and right shifts in the oxyhemoglobin dissociation curve in terms of loading of oxygen in the lung and unloading of oxygen in the tissues.

☐ Explain the concept of total carbon dioxide content by explaining the role of the following:

Bicarbonate, carbamino compounds, dissolved form of carbon dioxide.

☐ Explain how bicarbonate is formed in red blood cells, including the role of the chloride shift mechanism.

☐ Describe the role of carbonic anhydrase in carbon dioxide transport.

☐ Explain how carbaminohemoglobin is formed.

☐ Describe how the carbon dioxide dissociation curve is affected by changes in hemoglobin oxygen saturation by explaining the role of the Haldane effect.

key terms

Bohr effect
carbon dioxide transport
  bicarbonate transport
  carbaminohemoglobin
  plasma dissolution
carboxyhemoglobin (COHb)
chloride shift; anion shift
2,3-diphosphoglycerate (2,3-DPG)
erythrocyte; red blood cell (RBC)
Haldane effect
hematocrit (Hct)
hemoglobin (Hb)
hemoglobin P_{50}

oxygen consumption ($\dot{V}O_2$)
oxyhemoglobin dissociation curve; hemoglobin saturation curve
  left shift
  right shift
oxyhemoglobin
physiologic oxygen-binding capacity
systemic oxygen delivery
systemic oxygen return
theoretical oxygen-binding capacity
total carbon dioxide content

This chapter introduces the mechanisms involved in the transport of oxygen and carbon dioxide by the bloodstream, including the factors that influence the loading and unloading of the two gases in the lung and in the systemic tissues. A common theme stressed in this chapter is the interdependency of the simultaneous transport of the two gases by the bloodstream. The uptake and release of the gases represents a unique synergistic arrangement—the uptake of oxygen in pulmonary capillaries is facilitated by the simultaneous release of carbon dioxide from blood; the release of carbon dioxide is facilitated by simultaneous uptake of oxygen. In the tissues the roles reverse so that the loading of carbon dioxide is enhanced by the unloading of oxygen, and the release of oxygen is facilitated by the uptake of carbon dioxide.

Systemic Oxygen Consumption

Although gases always diffuse down a partial pressure gradient, blood does not give up *all* of its oxygen content as it passes through systemic tissues, nor does it completely take up *all* of the carbon dioxide (CO_2) present in the tissues. Similarly, pulmonary capillary blood does not give up *all* of its carbon dioxide content as it passes through the pulmonary circuit, nor does it completely take up *all* of the oxygen available in the alveoli. This lack of complete gas transfer in the tissues is evident in the partial pressure of blood gases sampled proximal and distal to systemic capillaries. For example, arterial oxygen tension is about 100 mm Hg (Pa_{O_2} = 100 mm Hg), yet only falls to approximately 40 mm Hg after blood passes through systemic capillaries to enter the veins ($C\bar{v}_{O_2}$ = 40 mm Hg). Oxygen has clearly left the bloodstream, thus lowering the partial pressure of oxygen—but some oxygen remains in the blood vessels and is returned to the heart and lungs. The difference between oxygen delivery and return is the amount of oxygen *consumed*, or *extracted*, by the tissues per unit time. This volume can be shown by the following relationships:

Systemic oxygen delivery is the product of total cardiac output ($\dot{Q}$) and the arterial oxygen content (Ca_{O_2}):

$$\text{Systemic oxygen delivery} = \dot{Q} \times Ca_{O_2}$$

Systemic oxygen return is the product of total cardiac output ($\dot{Q}$) and the mixed venous blood oxygen content ($C\bar{v}_{O_2}$):

$$\text{Systemic oxygen return} = \dot{Q} \times C\bar{v}_{O_2}$$

Therefore, **oxygen consumption ($\dot{V}_{O_2}$)** in the tissues is the *difference* between systemic oxygen delivery and systemic oxygen return, thus:

$$\dot{V}_{O_2} = \dot{Q} \times (Ca_{O_2} - C\bar{v}_{O_2})$$

Note that oxygen content in blood is usually expressed in units of *milliliters of oxygen per deciliter of blood* (*mL/dL*), or as *volume percent* (*vol%*). The equivalence is based on a volume-volume relationship between the amount of solute contained in a given amount of solution, as in the volume of oxygen (in mL) contained in 100 mL of blood. For example, "15 vol%" is read as "15 mL of oxygen per 100 mL of blood," or as "15 mL of oxygen per deciliter of blood." (1 mL = 1 $\times$ 10^{-3} L; 1 dL = 1 $\times$ 10^{-1} L.)

EXAMPLE

If the resting cardiac output of an individual is 5 L/min, calculate the systemic oxygen consumption in milliliters per minute when the arterial oxygen content is 20 vol% and the mixed venous oxygen content is 14 vol%.

Recall that vol% = mL/dL; therefore, 20 vol% = 20 mL/dL, and 14 vol% = 14 mL/dL

$$\dot{V}_{O_2} = \dot{Q} \times (Ca_{O_2} - C\bar{v}_{O_2})$$

$$= \frac{5 \text{ L}}{1 \text{ min}} \times (20 \text{ mL/dL} - 14 \text{ mL/dL})$$

$$= \frac{5 \text{ L}}{1 \text{ min}} \times \frac{6 \text{ mL}}{1 \text{ dL}} \times \frac{10 \text{ dL}}{1 \text{ L}}$$

$$\therefore \dot{V}_{O_2} = 300 \text{ mL/min}$$

NOTE: Calculations should always be performed using *base units* of the metric system. In this example, liters (L) are converted to other units by applying appropriate *unit conversion factors* such as "10 dL/1 L", or "1 L/10 dL."

Transport of Oxygen

DISSOLVED OXYGEN

Recall that oxygen rapidly diffuses in less than one second from the alveolus into the pulmonary capillary, according to the partial pressure gradient in the lung (ΔP_{O_2} = 60 mm Hg). Oxygen quickly loads the binding sites on hemoglobin within red blood cells (see following discussion) and then enters plasma solution, where it exerts a partial pressure.

In terms of solubility, oxygen is described as sparingly soluble in aqueous solution, including aqueous solutions such as plasma. However, certain chemical solvents can dissolve large amounts of oxygen. Such compounds are promising candidates as artificial blood products (Box 13–1). Recall that the volume of gas that enters solution at a given temperature is proportional to the tension of the gas, a relationship known as Henry's law. Determination of the oxygen content in the plasma is calculated by multiplying the oxygen tension by the solubility of oxygen in plasma. At body temperature (37°C), this solubility is equal to 0.00304 mL of oxygen per 100 mL of blood per mm Hg. The total volume of oxygen transported in **plasma dissolution,** therefore, is stated as 0.00304 mL O_2/100 mL per mm Hg, or 0.00304 mL O_2/ dL per torr (Leff and Schumacker, 1993).

PERSPECTIVES

BOX 13-1

What Goes Best with Surgery—Red or White?

The first successful human blood transfusion was performed in 1667 by Jean-Baptiste Denis. The practice was considered safe for a time but was discontinued when a transfusion patient died unexpectedly. We now know that the death was caused by an incompatibility reaction. The use of natural blood for transfusions was subsequently deemed unsafe, and substitutes such as oil and milk were tried. These blood substitutes were dismal failures and were also abandoned. In the early part of the 20th century, however, the A, B, O, and AB human blood types as well as the Rh factor had been identified by one researcher, an Austrian immunologist and pathologist named Karl Landsteiner (1868–1943). Discovery of the ABO system in 1900 and the Rh factor in the early 1920s led to the Nobel Prize in Medicine or Physiology for Landsteiner in 1930. These discoveries, along with routine cross-matching of blood samples from donor and recipient changed public and medical opinion so that transfusions were once again considered safe. The 1980s and the blood-borne pathogen known as human immunodeficiency virus (HIV), the etiologic agent of acquired immunodeficiency syndrome (AIDS), changed all that.

The threat of HIV and hepatitis infections, ABO incompatibility reactions, short shelf life of the natural product, and the chronic shortage of blood stored in blood banks have led to renewed interest in a reliable, effective, and safe substitute blood product. Although virtually no progress has been made in the creation of a blood substitute that mimics vital functions such as clotting, nutrient transport, or infection control, recent biotechnology advances have resulted in the production of *artificial blood* replacements that function admirably well in gas transport. Research into gas transport via blood substitutes has led to the development of two types of products that are now undergoing clinical trials in humans: *polymerized hemoglobin preparations* ("red blood") and *perfluorocarbon (PFC) emulsions* ("white blood").

Hemoglobin cannot be extracted from red blood cells and used on its own because it is quickly destroyed by enzymes, resulting in the production of breakdown products that are toxic to the kidney. Secondly, hemoglobin requires the red blood cell for stability. Finally, hemoglobin's affinity for oxygen is too high when it is present as a "stroma-free" product, that is, without its protective red blood cell carrier. Therefore, hemoglobin must either be modified in some way so that it gains the needed stability, or it must be produced through alternate means. After it has been stabilized, hemoglobin can be sterilized to remove microorganisms such as HIV.

One method that has been developed to produce "red blood" for human use involves the use of bovine (cattle) hemoglobin molecules. These molecules are considerably smaller than the human variety and must be encapsulated or cross-linked so that they "appear" larger than they really are. In this way, bovine hemoglobin provides gas transporting capability yet still exerts a normal osmotic pressure in the human recipient. Additionally, encapsulated hemoglobin molecules do not stimulate the body's immune system. Several bovine hemoglobin products are available: Hemopure is being tested for human use, while Oxyglobin has received Food and Drug Administration (FDA) approval for use in dogs. Recombinant hemoglobin such as *Somatogen rHb 1.1* has been engineered by splicing the gene responsible for the production of human hemoglobin into *Escherichia coli* bacteria. The bacteria are then cultured and the hemoglobin product is removed and purified. Bioengineered forms of hemoglobin mimic the normal oxyhemoglobin dissociation curve of whole blood.

continued

P E R S P E C T I V E S

What Goes Best with Surgery—Red or White? (Continued)

Some of the most promising blood substitutes for effective gas transport are PFC emulsions. These artificial substances are ideal gas transport media because they are chemically inert and act as solvents for common gases such as oxygen, carbon dioxide, and nitrogen. In fact, the oxygen transporting ability of such fluids is superior to whole blood (e.g., 45 mL oxygen per 100 mL PFC compared with 19.5 mL oxygen per 100 mL whole blood). Perfluorocarbon emulsions are not hemoglobin-based and do not bind iron; therefore, they do not have the reddish color of natural blood. Instead, PFC blood substitutes have a color resembling milk. These "white blood" products are insoluble in other fluids and must be emulsified with surfactant to make them compatible with plasma. In addition, they exert little or no osmotic pressure; therefore, electrolytes and volume expanders must be added. Finally, the insolubility of PFCs means that they cannot be excreted by the kidney, but must be removed by the lung. In spite of these technical and physiologic drawbacks, the ability of perfluorocarbon emulsions to transport large volumes of oxygen and carbon dioxide to and from the lung and tissues is remarkable. *Fluosol DA* and *Oxygent* are PFC emulsion products currently undergoing clinical trials in humans for use as blood substitutes in limited clinical applications (e.g., coronary artery angioplasty).

- Chang TMS and Geyer RP (eds): Blood Substitutes. Marcel Dekker, New York, 1989.
- Gibbs WW: Artificial blood quickens: Several short-term substitutes approach final clinical trials (Biotechnology news). Sci Am. 275: 44, 48, 1996.
- Marieb EN: Human Anatomy and Physiology, ed 4. Benjamin/Cummings, Menlo Park CA, 1998.
- Moreno J et al: Artificial blood [Current research survey article posted on the World Wide Web]. Michigan State University, n.d./1998. Retrieved May 4, 1998 from the World Wide Web: URL http://www.cem.msu.edu/~cem181h/blood/blood.htm.
- Neergaard L: FDA OKs artificial blood for dogs [Associated Press news item posted on the World Wide Web]. Washington, Jan 31, 1998. Retrieved May 4, 1998 from the World Wide Web: URL http://www.techserver.com/newsroom/ntn/health/013198/health11_10074_noframes.htm.
- Saladin KS: Anatomy and Physiology: The Unity of Form and Function. WCB/McGraw-Hill, Boston, 1998.
- Spiess BD and Cochran RP: Perfluorocarbon emulsions and cardiopulmonary bypass: A technique for the future. J Cardiothorac Vasc Anesth. 10:83–89, 1996.
- Winslow RM: Hemoglobin-based Red Cell Substitutes. The Johns Hopkins University Press, Baltimore, 1992.

EXAMPLE

Given an arterial oxygen tension of 100 torr, calculate the volume (content) of oxygen carried in a dissolved form in the plasma.

$$PaO_2 = 100 \text{ torr} = 100 \text{ mm Hg}$$

Plasma dissolution =

$$\frac{0.00304 \text{ mL } O_2/100 \text{ mL}}{1 \text{ mm Hg}} \times 100 \text{ mm Hg}$$

$$= 0.304 \text{ mL } O_2/100 \text{ mL}$$

In other words, at 37°C (body temperature), at a PaO_2 of 100 mm Hg, approximately 0.3 mL of oxygen dissolves in solution for each 100 mL of blood. Arterial oxygen content (CaO_2) in this example is often expressed as 0.3 vol% (mL solute per 100 mL solvent). The "vol%" units are not true SI metric unit, but are used extensively in the clinical setting, along with the metric unit "mL/dL."

This volume of gas (0.3 mL/100 mL) is far too small to support the metabolism of higher life forms. The metabolic oxygen demands of complex organisms easily exceed the capacity of an oxygen supply system based solely on the solubility of oxygen in the aqueous part of plasma. Instead, special *respiratory pigments* such as hemoglobin function to transport large volumes of oxygen to the metabolically active cells of the body. However, in spite of the small volume of oxygen carried in dissolved form in the plasma, the fraction of gas is important for at least two reasons—one physiologic, the other diagnostic. First, the presence of oxygen in the plasma is the factor that generates the actual partial pressure of oxygen. Oxygen bound to hemoglobin does not exert partial pressure. Recall that the partial pressure *gradient* determines the direction of movement of oxygen, either into or out of a capillary. Second, for practical purposes, detection of the partial pressure of oxygen in the plasma is the basis of arterial blood gas (ABG) analysis and interpretation, an important clinical diagnostic tool in cardiopulmonary medicine.

HEMOGLOBIN-BOUND OXYGEN

Erythrocytes

Hemoglobin is an essential molecule needed to meet the oxygen requirements of metabolically active tissue. This complex, pigmented molecule is found only within **erythrocytes (red blood cells [RBCs]).** Therefore, the number and function of red blood cells directly influence the oxygen-transporting ability of the bloodstream because, as we have seen, plasma transport of dissolved oxygen is severely limited. Determination of the number of erythrocytes in the blood is carried out in a hematology laboratory procedure in which a blood sample is spun in an ultracentrifuge at high revolutions per minute until the various components of whole blood settle out. The sedimentation of blood elements is based on differences in their densities. Erythrocytes, because they possess heavy, iron-containing hemoglobin molecules, pack into the bottom of small hematocrit tubes during the centrifugation process. This fraction of blood found in the bottom of the tubes is made up primarily of red blood cells, and is called the **hematocrit (Hct).** Most of the *packed cell volume* (PCV) is made up of erythrocytes. The normal PCV for a person living at sea level is about 45%, with the balance of the whole blood sample made up of plasma containing substances such as electrolytes, wastes, nutrients, gases, and pro-

teins (Fig. 13–1). Such substances are dissolved in, or transported by, the plasma component of blood. As noted in Chapter 14, PCV is affected by conditions such as *hypoxia* associated with living at higher altitudes.

The normal number of erythrocytes in men is about 5 to 6 million cells per microliter (μL) of blood; women have approximately 4 to 5 million cells per microliter (μL) of blood (1 μL = 1×10^{-6} L).

> **NOTE:** Cell concentrations are also commonly stated in terms of *cubic millimeters,* as in "5 million cells/mm³."

Differences in RBC counts generally reflect differences in average body sizes of men and women. Each red blood cell possesses approximately 250 to 280 million hemoglobin molecules, and each hemoglobin molecule is capable of transporting up to four oxygen molecules. Mature erythrocytes have a unique shape consisting of a flattened disk that is slightly concave on each side (Fig. 13–2). These biconcave discs lack a nucleus and are, therefore, incapable of reproducing themselves or repairing routine cellular damage. As a result of these limitations, erythrocytes have a relatively short life span of about 90 to 120 days and must be continually replaced by erythropoietic (blood-producing) tissues such as bone marrow. The biconcave shape of normal erythrocytes increases the cells' total surface area, thus improving their diffusion characteristics. Recall Fick's law of diffusion, which states that the rate of diffusion of a gas through a membrane is directly proportional to the surface area of the membrane. The anucleated arrangement of the mature erythrocyte allows the cytoplasm to contain a larger volume of hemoglobin, the main determinant of the bloodstream's oxygen transport capacity. In a later section, as well as in Chapter 14, we explore the effect of both red blood cell and hemoglobin anomalies on the transport of oxygen.

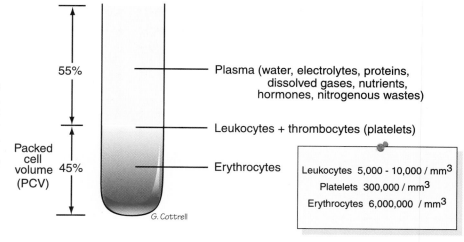

FIGURE 13–1. Hematocrit. Hematocrit is the volume percentage of erythrocytes in whole blood. (Erythrocytes make up most of the packed cell volume.) The term *hematocrit* originally described the apparatus or procedure used in its determination, but it is now used to describe the result of the determination. Values shown are typical for a healthy adult living at sea level (PBAR = 760 mm Hg). The hematocrit is affected by altitude, nutrition, dehydration, body size, anemia, and other factors.

Packed cell volume (PCV)

55%

45%

G. Cottrell

Plasma (water, electrolytes, proteins, dissolved gases, nutrients, hormones, nitrogenous wastes)

Leukocytes + thrombocytes (platelets)

Erythrocytes

Leukocytes 5,000 - 10,000 / mm³
Platelets 300,000 / mm³
Erythrocytes 6,000,000 / mm³

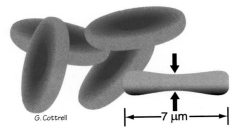

FIGURE 13–2. Mature erythrocytes. Note the unique biconcave surface feature of the flattened, disk-shaped, anucleated cells. Each erythrocyte contains approximately 250 million hemoglobin molecules, providing a total of up to 1 billion oxygen-binding sites.

Hemoglobin Structure

Hemoglobin (Hb) is a large and complex molecule with a molecular weight of approximately 64,500 daltons. (A *dalton* [Da] is an arbitrary unit of mass equal to 1/12 the mass of carbon-12, or 1.657×10^{-24} g [Thomas, 1997].) The hemoglobin molecule is composed of two basic parts:

- *Heme units*—Each hemoglobin molecule is made up of four pigmented heme units, each of which contains an iron ion in the reduced state (Fe^{2+}, iron (II), or ferrous iron). One oxygen molecule can reversibly bind to one heme group. Therefore, a single hemoglobin molecule has the potential to transport four oxygen molecules. Such a hemoglobin molecule carrying four oxygen molecules is considered to be 100% saturated, although lower saturation levels exist (see "Oxyhemoglobin Dissociation Curve" later in this chapter).
- *Globin protein*—Each globin protein associated with hemoglobin is composed of four separate amino acid chains. These polypeptide chains mesh together to form a complex structure with an interior that is *hydrophobic* and an exterior that is strongly *hydrophilic*.

The hydrophilic exterior of the molecule allows hemoglobin to be compatible with the aqueous nature of plasma, whereas the hydrophobic interior promotes oxygen binding. For example, heme groups are located within hydrophobic crevices in the globin molecule, and each contains an iron atom oxidized to the iron II (ferrous) state. This hydrophobic environment repels water and, therefore, protects the ferrous iron ion from being oxidized to the nonfunctional iron III (ferric) state by water molecules. Oxygen, on the other hand, is lipophilic and easily gains access to the hydrophobic environment of the heme groups, where it reversibly binds to form *oxyhemoglobin*. This binding does not change the ferrous state of the iron ion. Unfortunately, carbon monoxide molecules are also lipophilic and can easily gain access to the oxygen-binding sites on heme units (see "Carboxyhemoglobin" section).

Adult hemoglobin (HbA) consists of two α (alpha) polypeptide chains and two β (beta) polypeptide chains ($\alpha_2\beta_2$). Fetal hemoglobin (HbF) differs structurally and functionally from adult hemoglobin and is made up of two α polypeptide chains and two γ (gamma) polypeptide chains ($\alpha_2\gamma_2$). The two γ chains of fetal hemoglobin enhance the attraction of oxygen to facilitate gas transfer at the placenta. This prenatal mechanism compensates for the less efficient exchange structures of the placenta compared with those of the alveolar-capillary membrane of postnatal lungs. Fetal hemoglobin is gradually replaced with adult hemoglobin over the course of the first year of life.

Elimination of Hemoglobin

The total amount of hemoglobin in the bloodstream is proportional to the total number of red blood cells in circulation and is typically measured as grams of hemoglobin per 100 mL of blood, or as "grams%" of hemoglobin (Table 13–1). Adult men, because of higher average body weights, normally possess more erythrocytes and, therefore, more hemoglobin than adult women. The increased amount of hemoglobin is required to support the metabolic needs of a larger body. Surprisingly, fetuses and infants typically have more hemoglobin per volume of blood than adults, a value reflected in the higher packed cell volume of fetuses and neonates. Following birth, with efficient alveolar-capillary structures handling the task of external respiration, the newborn must eliminate excess of red blood cells.

During destruction and recycling of red blood cell components and hemoglobin molecules in the liver,

TABLE 13–1	Hemoglobin—Normal Values
Subject	g of Hemoglobin/100 mL of Blood (g Hb/dL or g% Hb)
Average adult man	14–16
Average adult woman	12–15
Average infant	14–20

Hb = hemoglobin.

the cyclical heme units of hemoglobin are split open to form linear molecules known as *bile pigments.* These toxic substances include *bilirubin* and *biliverdi,* which must be continually excreted via the bile and eliminated with fecal material. Accumulation of bile pigments, as occurs with excessive destruction of red blood cells or with occlusion of the bile duct, results in the clinical condition of *jaundice,* a yellowish discoloration of skin. In especially severe conditions, even the sclera ("whites") of the eyes may be discolored. Jaundice is a normal but temporary condition seen in newborns immediately following birth. It occurs as the liver processes large numbers of excess red blood cells and recycles portions of the hemoglobin molecules.

Hemoglobin Dysfunctions

Alteration in the structure of hemoglobin can result in the deformation of erythrocytes. Such cells lose their flexibility and cannot easily go through blood vessels. The altered structure of hemoglobin can be caused by changes in the number, sequence, or conformation of amino acids comprising the globin protein of hemoglobin. For example, in a congenital disorder of the blood called *sickle cell anemia,* defective β-chains result in the creation of sickle cell hemoglobin (HbS). Abnormal hemoglobin causes the red blood cells in which it is contained to assume a crescentlike shape that lacks flexibility. These abnormal red blood cells are easily damaged as they pass through narrow blood vessels. They are also more likely to form thrombi (clots) within blood vessels. As the extent of the cellular damage increases, the ability of the blood to transport oxygen is impaired, resulting in an anemic condition.

Oxygen transport can also be impaired by *methemoglobin,* a molecule that cannot function as a reversible oxygen carrier. In this abnormality the structure and function of the amino acids in hemoglobin is normal, but the valence state of iron found in the heme units is changed from ferrous iron (Fe II, Fe^{2+}) to ferric iron (Fe III, Fe^{3+}). Iron ions in the Fe III oxidized state exhibit impaired oxygen-transporting ability, resulting in an anemic condition called *methemoglobinemia.*

Oxyhemoglobin

Hemoglobin bound to oxygen is known as **oxyhemoglobin.** Because of the high-affinity oxygen-binding sites on the heme units of hemoglobin, each gram of *fully saturated* hemoglobin ($SaO_2 = 100\%$) can transport 1.39 mL of oxygen. This volume of gas is known as the **theoretical oxygen-binding capacity** of the blood. In actual gas transport studies, however, the volume of oxygen bound to each gram of hemoglobin is found to be approximately 1.34 mL, a volume known as the **physiologic oxygen-binding capacity** (Leff and Schu-

macker, 1993). This reduced value of 1.34 mL O_2 per gram of hemoglobin is used to determine the amount of oxygen transported as oxyhemoglobin (see subsequent calculation). The physiologic oxygen-binding capacity is less than the theoretical oxygen-binding capacity because the oxygen-binding sites on hemoglobin are not *all* available at the same time. According to Leff and Schumacker (1993), approximately 4% of the sites cannot function as oxygen carriers because, at any given time, some of the hemoglobin is present as methemoglobin (1% to 2%), and some of the oxygen-binding sites are occupied by carbon monoxide (1% to 2%). The effect of carbon monoxide on oxygen transport is discussed in a later section.

With hemoglobin levels of 15 g%, and hemoglobin saturation of 100%, the *theoretical* volume of oxygen transported per 100 mL of blood is calculated as follows:

Theoretical volume of O_2 bound to hemoglobin

$$= \frac{1.34 \text{ mL } O_2}{1 \text{ g\% Hb}} \times 15 \text{ g\% Hb} = 20.1 \text{ mL}$$

This calculation assumes that the hemoglobin saturation is 100% ($SaO_2 = 100\%$). However, at a normal PaO_2 of 100 mm Hg, hemoglobin saturation is normally about $SaO_2 = 97\%$. Therefore, the amount of oxyhemoglobin transported by the blood must be corrected to account for hemoglobin saturation that is less than 100%:

$$\therefore \text{ At } PaO_2 = 100 \text{ mm Hg:}$$

Actual volume of oxygen bound to hemoglobin = 20.1 mL $O_2 \times 0.97 = 19.5$ mL O_2 (or 19.5 vol%, since 19.5 mL oxygen is contained in 100 mL of blood)

Why is hemoglobin saturation less than 100% when multiple oxygen-binding sites are present on each hemoglobin molecule, as many as 250 million hemoglobin molecules are found in each red blood cell, and as many as 6 million red blood cells are found in each microliter of blood? With such impressive numbers, why is hemoglobin saturation only 97% when the PaO_2 is 100 mm Hg?

Hemoglobin saturation is generally less than 100% in most circulatory routes in the body because of various *physiologic shunts* that prevent the entire blood volume from reaching the lung, and thus being oxygenated. For instance, bronchial venous drainage returns deoxygenated blood from lung tissue not involved in the alveolar-capillary system, directly to the pulmonary arteries and left atrium. This volume of blood effectively bypasses the gas exchange units of the lung and thus contributes to the reduction in hemoglobin saturation of arterial blood. Similarly, ventilation-perfusion inequalities involving alveoli that are underventilated relative to pulmonary blood flow represent another type of shunt and, therefore, contribute to reduced arterial hemoglobin saturation. Anatomic and physiologic shunt mechanisms are discussed in Chapter 14.

Note that in spite of the reduced value for the physiologic oxygen-binding capacity of the blood *and* the correction factor for the effect of physiologic shunts on oxygen transport, the volume of hemoglobin-bound oxygen is more than 60 times greater than the very small volume of oxygen that dissolves in plasma at an oxygen tension of 100 mm Hg (19.5 mL O_2/100 mL versus 0.304 mL O_2/100 mL). Thus oxyhemoglobin is primarily responsible for supplying the large volumes of oxygen required by metabolically active tissues.

We can calculate the *total* oxygen content of the blood by adding the volume of oxygen bound to hemoglobin to the volume of oxygen dissolved in plasma. Oxygen is found at the following three "locations", or circulatory sites:

- Arterial blood (CaO_2)
- Mixed venous blood ($C\bar{v}O_2$)
- Pulmonary capillary blood ($Cc'O_2$)

The total oxygen content of the blood can be calculated when the amount of hemoglobin is known, along with the percent saturation of hemoglobin in the arterial and mixed venous blood. In addition, the alveolar, arterial, and mixed venous blood oxygen tensions must be known. The sum of the following three oxygen contents will give the total oxygen transported by 100 mL of blood:

- Arterial blood:

$$CaO_2 = \frac{(1.34 \text{ mL } O_2 \times x \text{ g\% Hb} \times SaO_2)}{1 \text{ g\% Hb}}$$
$$+ \frac{(0.003 \text{ vol\% } O_2 \times x \text{ mm Hg } PaO_2)}{1 \text{ mm Hg } PaO_2}$$

- Mixed venous blood:

$$C\bar{v}O_2 = \frac{(1.34 \text{ mL } O_2 \times x \text{ g\% Hb} \times S\bar{v}O_2)}{1 \text{ g\% Hb}}$$
$$+ \frac{(0.003 \text{ vol\% } O_2 \times x \text{ mm Hg } P\bar{v}O_2)}{1 \text{ mm Hg } P\bar{v}O_2}$$

- Pulmonary capillary blood:

$$Cc'O_2 = \frac{(1.34 \text{ mL } O_2 \times x \text{ g\% Hb} \times 1^*)}{1 \text{ g\% Hb}}$$
$$+ \frac{(0.003 \text{ vol\% } O_2 \times x \text{ mm Hg } PAO_2)}{1 \text{ mm Hg } PAO_2}$$

NOTE: *The saturation of hemoglobin in pulmonary capillary blood is assumed to be 100%.

Also, the "prime" notation used with the symbol $Cc'O_2$ refers to the oxygen content of capillary blood coming from normally ventilated alveoli, the end-capillary ideal oxygen content (see Chap. 14). The symbol should not be confused with CcO_2, the symbol for carbon dioxide content.

Oxyhemoglobin Dissociation Curve

REACTION KINETICS

Linear relationships between two variables result in a straight-line graph when the data is plotted. The plot of some chemical reactions takes this form when the kinetics of the reaction are uniform (Fig. 13–3). That is, when the interaction between two substances is more or less constant, a linear relationship exists. In these relationships, an incremental change in one variable produces a constant incremental change in the other (see Fig. 13–3). Recall that small amounts of oxygen are carried in a dissolved form in the plasma. However, as shown by Figure 13–3, relatively little change in the arterial hemoglobin saturation (SaO_2) or the arterial oxygen content (CaO_2) occurs in the oxygen tension range up to 100 mm Hg as a result of plasma dissolution. In fact, the amount of oxygen dissolved in plasma produces relatively little change in hemoglobin saturation, even at partial pressures as high as 600 mm Hg (Leff and Schumacker, 1993).

Nonlinear relationships, on the other hand, generate complex curves when the data is plotted. Chemical interactions in which the kinetic rate is constantly changing fall into this category and are typical of the interactions between oxygen and hemoglobin to form oxyhemoglobin (Fig. 13–4). The *association,* or binding, between oxygen and hemoglobin produces oxyhemoglobin; *dissociation* of oxygen refers to the release of oxygen from such binding sites. As can be seen in Figure 13–4, a sigmoid-shaped curve is generated when oxygen interacts with hemoglobin. The *steep part* of the curve occurs in the oxygen tension range of 10 mm Hg to 60 mm Hg. In this range, oxygen rapidly binds with hemoglobin at a particular partial pressure, producing a large change in hemoglobin saturation and oxygen content for each incremental change in oxygen tension. However, in the range between 60 mm Hg and 100 mm Hg, large-scale changes in hemoglobin saturation and oxygen content do not occur. Notice in Figure 13–4 that when the $PO_2 = 60$ mm Hg the arterial oxygen saturation is approximately 90%, but that a large increase in the oxygen tension to $PO_2 = 100$ mm Hg only results in a relatively small increase in arterial oxygen saturation, to about 97%. What factors affect

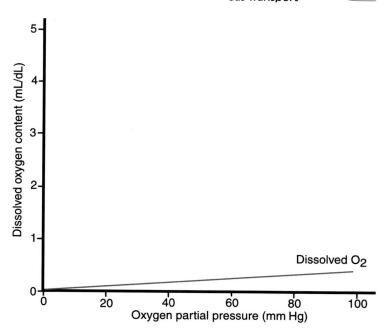

FIGURE 13–3. Linear relationship—oxygen dissolved in the plasma. The relationship between the volume of oxygen dissolved in the plasma (mL/dL) and the partial pressure of oxygen in the blood (mm Hg) is *linear*. That is, the amount of oxygen that dissolves in plasma increases at a constant rate as the oxygen tension increases. Doubling the partial pressure will double the dissolved oxygen content in the plasma. Such a linear relationship is typical of low-solubility gases.

the kinetics of the reaction between oxygen and hemoglobin to account for such differences in saturation over a fairly broad range of partial pressures?

CONFORMATIONAL CHANGES IN HEMOGLOBIN

The kinetics of the reaction and the shape of the **oxyhemoglobin dissociation curve** are determined primarily by the unique three-dimensional spatial features of the hemoglobin molecule itself. Although many biologic molecules exhibit differences in activity based on their shape, certain ones have sufficient *flexibility* to alter their shape under different conditions, often by rotating around internal bonds within the molecule. For example, the neurotransmitter molecule *acetylcholine* adapts its shape to match that of different types of receptors on effector cells to control them. Hemoglobin also exhibits the characteristic of flexibility. When hemoglobin combines with the first oxygen molecule, the binding causes oxyhemoglobin to alter its shape slightly. This conformational change "exposes" two additional oxygen-binding sites in the hydrophobic interior of the molecule that were previously not readily accessible. Assuming there is an adequate partial pressure gradient, additional oxygen molecules rapidly move onto the hemoglobin molecule to occupy the two new binding sites, thus producing a steep slope in the **hemoglobin saturation curve** in the partial pressure range of PaO_2 = 10 to 60 mm Hg. The binding of additional oxygen molecules causes a further change in the shape of hemoglobin. However, the fourth oxygen-binding site is not occupied as rapidly as the previous two. Consequently, the slope of the hemoglobin satu-

ration curve decreases, flattening to form a plateau section in the partial pressure range of PaO_2 = 60 to 100 mm Hg (see Fig. 13–4). Through these complex interactions the sigmoid shape of the oxyhemoglobin dissociation curve is generated when the data are plotted.

Analysis of the sigmoid curve reveals subtle features. For example, the relatively small increase in the hemoglobin percentage saturation from 90% to 97%, occurring between 60 mm Hg and 100 mm Hg, points out the "safety margin" that hemoglobin possesses as it passes through the alveolar-capillary system. Recall that the transit time through a pulmonary capillary is approxi-

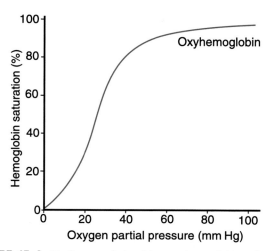

FIGURE 13–4. Nonlinear relationship—oxyhemoglobin. The relationship between the oxygen partial pressure in blood (mm Hg) and the percentage of hemoglobin-binding sites that are occupied by oxygen molecules is a *nonlinear* relationship. In this oxygen dissociation curve, adult hemoglobin is approximately 50% saturated at 27 mm Hg, 90% saturated at 60 mm Hg, and 98% saturated at 100 mm Hg.

mately 0.75 s. Even after most of the oxygen has diffused, a significant oxygen-partial pressure gradient exists because the alveolar oxygen tension is maintained at 100 mm Hg as a result of the partial pressure of inspired gas. An increase in the alveolar partial pressure beyond 100 mm Hg adds relatively little additional oxygen to the blood because hemoglobin is already fully saturated. Some additional oxygen, however, enters the plasma at these elevated PO_2 levels, as discussed previously.

Another observation to make from analysis of the shape of the oxyhemoglobin dissociation curve is that in the steep portion of the curve, a large volume of oxygen is released from hemoglobin for a relatively small decrease in the arterial oxygen tension. Therefore, oxygen dissociation at the tissues—the site of *internal respiration*—is enhanced both by the kinetics of the reaction and the conformational changes of hemoglobin.

Carboxyhemoglobin

Carbon monoxide (CO) is a lipophilic molecule that binds at the same heme sites that normally bind oxygen. The resulting compound is called **carboxyhemoglobin (COHb).** CO is produced as a byproduct of combustion and is commonly found in cigarette smoke, urban environments, and as a component of industrial pollution. CO has an affinity for hemoglobin approximately 200 times greater than that of oxygen for hemoglobin. It is estimated that an increase in the arterial carbon monoxide tension (PaCO) to as little as 0.5 mm Hg results in a nearly total blockade of oxygen-binding sites on hemoglobin (Leff and Schumacker, 1993). This occupation of binding sites functionally reduces the physiologic oxygen-binding capacity of the blood, resulting in severe hypoxemia.

When some of the oxygen-binding sites are occupied by CO, the remaining sites continue to function as oxygen carriers, although the total oxygen transport capability of the blood is reduced proportionately. Interestingly, the affinity of hemoglobin for oxygen is *increased* when carboxyhemoglobin is produced, even though relatively few oxygen-binding sites are available for oxygen transport. Therefore, the few oxygen molecules that manage to combine with hemoglobin in the lung do not readily dissociate from hemoglobin in the tissues, a feature discussed in a later section. To unload sufficient oxygen in the tissues, a lower PO_2 must be maintained outside the systemic capillaries. This factor, in turn, reduces the partial pressure *gradient* critical for diffusion of oxygen away from the capillary into the surrounding tissues. For these reasons, carbon monoxide poisoning effectively deprives the tissues of oxygen. Not only is the total oxygen-carrying capacity of the blood functionally reduced, but increased affinity of hemoglobin for oxygen and a lower oxygen tension outside the capillaries ensures that relatively little oxygen leaves the bloodstream to meet the metabolic demands of the tissues.

COHb is responsible for about 1% to 2% of the total hemoglobin-binding capacity of the bloodstream. This value is typical of a healthy subject living in an urban environment; however, heavy smokers have carboxyhemoglobin levels in excess of 10% (Leff and Schumacker, 1993). In cases of accidental carbon monoxide poisoning, patients are given supplemental oxygen at high concentrations. The higher concentration allows oxygen to compete more effectively for heme binding sites and also hastens the removal of CO from the body. Occasionally a *hyperbaric chamber* is employed in cases of carbon monoxide poisoning to raise barometric pressure artificially. With such a device, PaO_2 values in excess of 1000 mm Hg can be produced. Such a high-pressure environment accelerates the displacement of carbon monoxide molecules from oxygen-binding sites and promotes their elimination from the body.

Hemoglobin P_{50}—The Standard Oxyhemoglobin Dissociation Curve

A common reference point used in gas transport studies is the **hemoglobin P_{50},** which represents the partial pressure at which hemoglobin is 50% saturated (Fig. 13–5). The normal P_{50} is approximately 27 mm Hg in an adult human at rest (Des Jardins, 1998; Leff and Schumacker, 1993). The benefit of such a reference system is seen in blood gas studies that permit comparison of a patient's hemoglobin saturation to the standard. Certain pathophysiologic conditions shift the oxyhemoglobin dissociation curve either to the left or to the right of the standard P_{50} curve (see Fig. 13–5). In the following section we examine the clinical significance of these shifts. In general, conditions that increase the affinity of hemoglobin for oxygen shift the curve to the left. These shifts result in a P_{50} curve with a value less than 27 mm Hg. Conditions that decrease the affinity of hemoglobin for oxygen shift the dissociation curve to the right, producing a P_{50} curve with a value greater than 27 mm Hg. A higher P_{50} value implies that a higher PO_2 is needed to attain a given oxygen saturation. Figure 13–5 shows that a straight line extended horizontally from the 50% hemoglobin saturation point intercepts the left-shifted curve at a PO_2 value of about 20 mm Hg. This same horizontal line intercepts the right-shifted oxyhemoglobin dissociation curve at a PO_2 of approximately 45 mm Hg.

Another way to view the relative degree of hemoglobin saturation is to simply look at the vertical line that passes through the 27 mm Hg point on the *x*-axis.

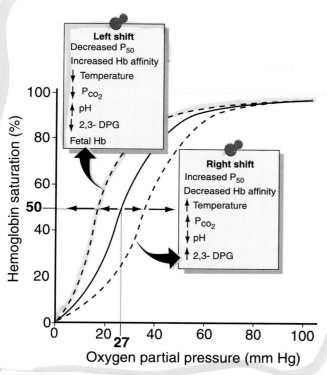

FIGURE 13–5. Hemoglobin P_{50}. At a hemoglobin saturation level of 50%, partial pressure of oxygen is 27 mm Hg, a value referred to as the *hemoglobin P_{50}*. Shifts to the right of this standard oxyhemoglobin dissociation curve are caused by conditions that decrease the affinity of hemoglobin for oxygen. The opposite conditions, as well as fetal hemoglobin, increase the affinity of hemoglobin for oxygen and shift the curve to the left. 2,3-DPG = 2,3-diphosphoglycerate; Hb = hemoglobin. (See text for full explanation.)

As can be seen in Figure 13–5, this line intercepts the normal oxyhemoglobin dissociation curve at the 50% level (the standard P_{50} curve). Notice, however, that the vertical line intercepts the right-shifted curve at a point where the hemoglobin saturation is relatively low but intercepts the left-shifted oxyhemoglobin dissociation curve at a point where the hemoglobin saturation is quite high. These differences in hemoglobin saturation *at the same oxygen tension* clearly illustrate the differences in oxygen affinity exhibited by hemoglobin under conditions that shift the curve either to the right or to the left of the standard P_{50} position. What conditions are capable of altering the affinity of the hemoglobin molecule for oxygen and thus shifting the oxyhemoglobin dissociation curve?

Left and Right Shifts of the Oxyhemoglobin Dissociation Curve

The change in hemoglobin's affinity for oxygen is related to conformational changes that the molecule

goes through in response to different conditions. As discussed previously, the shape of hemoglobin is affected by certain conditions that cause oxygen-binding sites on the molecule to become either more or less accessible. As a result of such three-dimensional changes in the shape of the molecule, oxygen binds to hemoglobin with greater or lesser avidity. Before we examine the factors that shift the oxyhemoglobin dissociation curve away from its standard position, we first need to understand the significance of a left or a right shift in the curve in terms of oxygen-binding sites, the resulting affinity of hemoglobin toward oxygen, and the relative ease with which oxygen associates with and dissociates from hemoglobin.

SIGNIFICANCE OF LEFT SHIFTS

Conformational changes in hemoglobin that enhance the loading, or association, of oxygen to form oxyhemoglobin, *increase* the affinity of the molecule for oxygen. As pointed out previously, this change results in a **left shift** in the oxyhemoglobin dissociation curve and a lower P_{50} value. Such a change enhances the loading of oxygen in the lung but impairs the unloading, or dissociation, of oxygen in the tissues.

Increased loading of oxygen as blood passes through the alveolar-capillary system occurs because oxygen-binding sites in the interior of the hemoglobin molecule are more readily accessible. Therefore, at a given partial pressure gradient, a greater volume of oxygen diffuses from the alveoli to the pulmonary blood, thus increasing the saturation of hemoglobin (Fig. 13–5). Such a change in the conformation of hemoglobin *increases* the efficiency of gas transfer during external respiration but *decreases* the efficiency of gas transfer during internal respiration.

Reduced unloading of oxygen at the sites of internal respiration occurs because of hemoglobin's increased affinity for oxygen. In other words, oxygen is "held" more tightly to the hemoglobin molecule. As a result of this increased affinity, less oxygen is released from hemoglobin for a given change in partial pressure. This reduced unloading of oxygen in the tissues with a left-shifted oxyhemoglobin dissociation curve is evident in Figure 13–5. Notice that a relatively small reduction in hemoglobin saturation occurs for a given change in oxygen tension.

SIGNIFICANCE OF RIGHT SHIFTS

Certain conditions induce conformational changes in hemoglobin that reduce the loading of oxygen in the lung, thus bringing about a *decrease* in the affinity of the molecule for oxygen and an overall reduction in the formation of oxyhemoglobin. (see Fig. 13–5). Such a change causes a **right shift** in the oxyhemoglobin dissociation curve and a higher P_{50} value. Hemoglobin conformational changes that cause a right shift in the oxyhemoglobin dissociation curve result in increased unloading of oxygen in the tissues.

Because of conformational changes in hemoglobin that decrease access to the oxygen-binding sites, a decreased volume of oxygen leaves the alveoli to bind with hemoglobin. This reduced loading of oxygen results in reduced hemoglobin saturation at a given partial pressure of oxygen (see Fig. 13–5). Therefore, the efficiency of external respiration is *decreased* with a right-shifted oxyhemoglobin dissociation curve. The efficiency of gas transfer in the tissues, however, is *increased* under such conditions.

Because of the reduced affinity for oxygen, hemoglobin readily gives up the gas in the tissues. Therefore, for a given change in partial pressure, a relatively large volume of oxygen is unloaded, or dissociated, from hemoglobin as blood passes through the systemic capillaries. This enhanced unloading of oxygen with a right-shifted oxyhemoglobin dissociation curve is shown in Figure 13–5. Note that a large decrease in hemoglobin saturation occurs for a given change in oxygen tension.

Factors that Shift the Oxyhemoglobin Dissociation Curve

BLOOD TEMPERATURE, pH, AND P_{CO_2}

Physiologic factors such as changes in *blood temperature, pH,* and *carbon dioxide tension* cause conformational changes in the hemoglobin molecule that affect its affinity for oxygen (see Fig. 13–5). These changes in hemoglobin's affinity toward oxygen occur rapidly as blood travels through a capillary from arterial to venous end. The rapid change in affinity causes a dynamic shift in the oxyhemoglobin dissociation curve that favors oxygen loading in the lung and oxygen unloading in the systemic tissues. These changes enhance the diffusion of oxygen into or out of the capillary for a given change in oxygen content.

Slight changes in blood temperature alter the conformation of the hemoglobin molecule. Actively metabolizing tissues have relatively higher temperatures compared to other tissues. For example, the temperature in skeletal muscles during strenuous exercise may rise to 40°C or more for short periods of time. This increase in temperature alters the shape of the hemoglobin molecule and shifts the dissociation curve to the right, thus enhancing the unloading of oxygen in hard-working tissues (see Fig. 13–5). Lower blood temperatures, as occur in the alveolar-capillary system of the lung, increase the affinity of hemoglobin for oxygen, shift the dissociation curve to the left and facilitate the loading of oxygen in the lung (see Fig. 13–5). Through these subtle changes in the shape of hemoglobin and shifts in the oxyhemoglobin dissociation curve in response to small changes in blood temperature, the saturation of hemoglobin is maintained within homeostatic limits.

In working muscles acidic conditions predominate. The increase in hydrogen ion (H^+) concentration occurs as a result of the accumulation in the tissues of both carbon dioxide and acidic by-products of metabolism. The buildup of CO_2 results in the production of carbonic acid as CO_2 combines with H_2O in the tissues. In addition, metabolic acids such as lactic acid normally accumulate in the tissues, especially during anaerobic exercise. The ionization of acids such as carbonic acid and lactic acid is responsible for the decrease in pH. The fall in pH, in turn, induces a conformational change in hemoglobin that shifts the oxyhemoglobin dissociation curve to the right, indicating a decrease in oxygen affinity (see Fig. 13–5). As a result of this shift, more oxygen unloads in active tissues to support the elevated metabolism of the cells.

The effect of increased carbon dioxide levels on the affinity of hemoglobin for oxygen is called the **Bohr effect,** named after the physiologist, Christian Bohr. The reduced affinity of hemoglobin for oxygen as a result of the Bohr effect is due to (1) the decrease in pH that occurs as the P_{CO_2} increases and (2) direct effects of carbon dioxide on the hemoglobin molecule (Leff and Schumacker, 1993).

A decrease in the P_{CO_2} and an increase in the pH is common in the lungs where carbon dioxide is being expelled. As a result of the alkaline conditions, the conformation of hemoglobin changes to favor the binding of oxygen, thus increasing the affinity of hemoglobin toward oxygen. Therefore, the oxyhemoglobin dissociation curve is shifted to the left (see Fig. 13–5). As explained above, such a shift indicates that a relatively large volume of oxygen is loaded for a given change in oxygen tension.

RED BLOOD CELL 2,3-DIPHOSPHOGLYCERATE

During the anaerobic conditions that develop during strenuous exercise, erythrocytes form an intermediate product called **2,3-diphosphoglycerate (2,3-DPG).** This intermediate compound accumulates within red blood cells and causes hemoglobin molecules to become less flexible and not bind oxygen as readily. The affinity of hemoglobin for oxygen varies inversely with 2,3-DPG concentration (see Fig. 13–5). Therefore, as 2,3-DPG concentration rises, the affinity of hemoglobin for oxygen decreases. This change in affinity is typical of a right shift in the oxyhemoglobin dissociation curve, indicating that large volumes of oxygen are released from systemic capillaries for a given change in the partial pressure gradient of oxygen. The magnitude of the shift is proportional to the concentration of 2,3-DPG. This type of change is precisely what is needed to deliver additional oxygen to metabolically active tissues.

The effect on hemoglobin affinity for oxygen occurs for two reasons: (1) 2,3-DPG binds directly to hemoglobin and causes a conformational change that decreases the affinity of hemoglobin for oxygen; and (2) the accumulation of 2,3-DPG within red blood cells lowers the pH of red blood cells, which promotes a right shift in the oxyhemoglobin dissociation curve.

The concentration of 2,3-DPG is affected by several factors, including hypoxemia, anemia, hydrogen ion concentration, and stored blood. Conditions such as hypoxemia and anemia cause 2,3-DPG to accumulate in cells. These conditions contribute to an anaerobic environment in metabolically active tissues, but the associated buildup of 2,3-DPG in red blood cells causes oxygen to dissociate from hemoglobin more readily. Factors such as living at high altitude or chronic lung disease decrease the average level of blood hemoglobin saturation and contribute to hypoxemia and a rightward shift in the oxyhemoglobin dissociation curve. Although several factors are known to play a role, the average blood hemoglobin saturation level seems to be the most important factor in the regulation of 2,3-DPG concentration in red blood cells (Leff and Schumacker, 1993).

In blood bank samples that have been stored over a 2-week period in acid-citrate-dextrose anticoagulant solution, there is a gradual depletion of red blood cell levels of 2,3-DPG. This decrease in 2,3-DPG concentration increases the affinity of hemoglobin for oxygen. As a result of the left shift in the oxyhemoglobin dissociation curve when stored blood is given to a patient, more oxygen is loaded in the lungs, but less oxygen is unloaded in the tissues.

Although the effect of red blood cell 2,3-DPG on hemoglobin's affinity for oxygen has been studied and debated for some time, it appears that the physiologic significance of the effect is minor (Leff and Schumacker, 1993).

FETAL HEMOGLOBIN

Fetal hemoglobin (HbF) has a greater affinity for oxygen (P_{50} = 20 to 22 mm Hg) than adult hemoglobin (P_{50} = 27 mm Hg) (Leff and Schumacker, 1993). This characteristic ensures that adequate amounts of oxygen are transferred from maternal blood to fetal blood at the placenta. The left shift in the oxyhemoglobin dissociation curve of fetal hemoglobin compensates for less efficient gas exchange at the placenta, when compared with gas exchange in the fully functioning postnatal lung (see Fig. 13–5). During the first year following birth, fetal hemoglobin is gradually replaced by the adult form of hemoglobin (HbA).

Table 13–2 summarizes the type of shift in the oxyhemoglobin dissociation curve produced by the various factors discussed above.

Clinical Significance of Shifts in the Oxyhemoglobin Dissociation Curve

After discussing the various factors that shift the oxyhemoglobin dissociation curve, it seems ironic that neither right nor left shifts in the curve significantly alter the oxygen-transporting capability of hemoglobin, as long as the arterial oxygen tension is in the normal range of PaO_2 = 80 to 100 mm Hg. This observation is true because the partial pressure range of 80 to 100 mm Hg occurs on the *flat portion* of the oxyhemoglobin dissociation curve. Consequently, shifts of the dissociation curve to either side of the P_{50} standard position do not cause appreciable changes in either the percentage of hemoglobin saturation (SaO_2) or in the oxygen content of arterial blood (CaO_2). What changes, however, occur when arterial blood gas values are *not* in this normal range, as seen in patients with bronchial asthma? In the following section we briefly examine the clinical significance of left and right shifts in the oxyhemoglobin dissociation curve when these shifts occur in patients having *abnormal* values for oxygen tension and hydrogen ion concentration.

LEFT SHIFTS UNDER ABNORMAL CONDITIONS

Loading of Oxygen in the Lung

Recall that hemoglobin's affinity for oxygen is increased as a result of alkaline conditions (e.g., pH = 7.6), shifting the oxyhemoglobin dissociation curve to the left. Such a shift has important consequences for the person with asthma. In acute asthma, alveolar oxygen tension (PAO_2) depressed to 60 mm Hg normally causes hypoxia in a patient. However, with increased affinity for oxygen occurring under alkaline conditions, hemoglobin is saturated in the lung to approximately SaO_2 = 95%, *in spite of* a depressed arterial oxygen tension of only PaO_2 = 60 mm Hg (Fig. 13–6A).

Unloading of Oxygen in the Tissues

Although a left shift in the oxyhemoglobin dissociation curve favors loading and enhances the total delivery of oxygen to the tissues, the increased affinity of hemoglobin for oxygen means that less oxygen dissociates from hemoglobin in the systemic capillaries for a given change in partial pressure. For example, at a depressed arterial oxygen tension of PaO_2 = 60 mm Hg, hemoglobin is

TABLE 13-2	Factors that Shift the Oxyhemoglobin Dissociation Curve	
Factors	**Right Shift**	**Left Shift**
	Decreased O_2 affinity for hemoglobin Reduced O_2 loading in lungs Enhanced O_2 unloading in tissues	Increased O_2 affinity for hemoglobin Enhanced O_2 loading in lungs Reduced O_2 unloading in tissues
Blood Temperature		
Increased temperature	√	
Decreased temperature		√
pH		
*Decreased	√	
Increased		√
Pco$_2$		
*Increased	√	
Decreased		√
2,3-DPG		
Increased concentration caused by:		
hypoxemia	√	
anemia	√	
Decreased concentration caused by:		
stored blood		√
fetal Hb		√

*Oxygen unloading along the capillary is enhanced by (1) a decrease in pH caused by the accumulation of hydrogen ions in metabolically active tissues, and (2) an increase in Pco$_2$, which has a direct effect on the affinity of the hemoglobin molecule for oxygen. The combination of these mechanisms is called the *Bohr effect*. (Carbon dioxide loading in the tissues is enhanced by the simultaneous desaturation of hemoglobin, a mechanism known as the *Haldane effect*.) 2,3-DPG = 2,3-diphosphoglycerate; Hb = hemoglobin.

95% saturated when the dissociation curve is shifted to the left, as we have seen. This compares favorably with $Sao_2 = 90\%$ when the oxyhemoglobin dissociation curve has not undergone a shift of any kind. In order to unload 5 mL of oxygen per 100 mL of blood with an *unshifted* curve, the Pao_2 must decrease from 60 mm Hg to 35 mm Hg ($\Delta Po_2 = 25$ mm Hg). With a left-shifted dissociation curve, however, a greater decrease in arterial partial pressure from 60 mm Hg to 30 mm Hg ($\Delta Po_2 = 30$ mm Hg), is required to unload an equivalent amount (5 vol%) of oxygen in the tissues (Fig. 13–6B). This limitation decreases the efficiency of internal respiration and offsets the enhanced loading of oxygen that occurs in the lung when the dissociation curve is shifted to the left by factors such as alkaline conditions.

RIGHT SHIFTS UNDER ABNORMAL CONDITIONS

Loading of Oxygen in the Lung

At a decreased alveolar oxygen tension of $Pao_2 = 60$ mm Hg, as occurs with acute asthma, hemoglobin saturation is normally about 90% (Fig. 13–7A). A right shift of the oxyhemoglobin dissociation curve, however, re-sults in a decrease in the hemoglobin saturation from a predicted value of about 90% to an actual value of approximately 75%. As discussed previously, a right shift in the curve may be caused by an acidic pH (e.g., pH = 7.2). Because acidosis often accompanies an asthmatic condition, total oxygen delivery may be much less than indicated by a particular arterial oxygen tension. This anomaly is especially important to keep in mind when a patient has clinical signs such as acidosis that produce right shifts of the oxyhemoglobin dissociation curve.

Unloading of Oxygen in the Tissues

Recall that right shifts in the dissociation curve represent conditions that reduce the affinity of hemoglobin for oxygen. Acidic conditions in the tissues promote such a change to enhance the unloading of oxygen. For example, when the dissociation curve is normal, the Pao_2 must decrease by 25 mm Hg, from 60 mm Hg to approximately 35 mm Hg to unload 5 mL of oxygen per 100 mL of blood (Fig. 13–7B). Under acidotic conditions, however, the decreased affinity of hemoglobin for oxygen causes an equivalent amount of oxygen (5 vol%) to be transferred to the tissues for a smaller

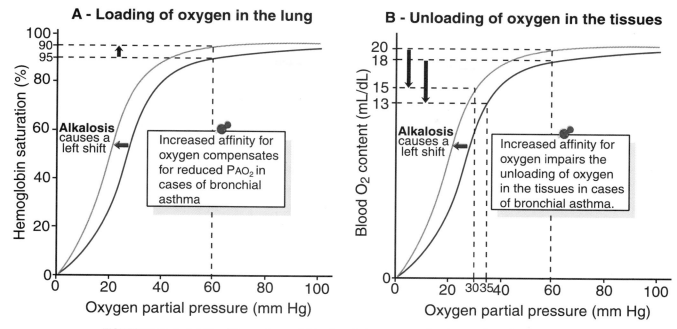

FIGURE 13–6. Left shifts of the oxyhemoglobin dissociation curve under abnormal conditions. In cases of bronchial asthma, alveolar and arterial oxygen tension is typically depressed (e.g., $PO_2 = 60$ mm Hg). A left shift of the oxyhemoglobin dissociation curve causes increased loading of oxygen in the lung, resulting in an increase in hemoglobin saturation from approximately 90% to 95%, thus offsetting the lowered oxygen tension. In the tissues, oxyhemoglobin does not give up its oxygen readily under alkaline conditions. In order to release 5 mL of oxygen per dL of blood, the partial pressure must normally change by approximately 25 mm Hg in a person with asthma (60–35 mm Hg). With a left-shifted curve, however, a greater partial pressure change of 30 mm Hg is required to unload an equivalent amount of oxygen (60–30 mm Hg).

change in partial pressure. Notice with the right-shifted curve in Figure 13–7B that arterial oxygen tension only has to decrease from 60 mm Hg to 40 mm Hg to unload 5 mL oxygen per 100 mL of blood. This lower partial pressure gradient ($\Delta PO_2 = 20$ mm Hg versus $\Delta PO_2 = 25$ mm Hg) may not seem significant, but remember that a relatively short transit time is available for the systemic capillaries to unload oxygen in the tissues. Therefore, a smaller oxygen tension gradient that unloads an equivalent volume of oxygen translates into more efficient internal respiration—a feature especially important to the patient with asthma. Recall that patients with asthma have reduced hemoglobin saturation because of the effects in the lung of a right shift of the oxyhemoglobin dissociation curve.

Carbon Dioxide Transport

An adult at rest produces approximately 200 mL of carbon dioxide per minute in the tissues (Leff and Schumacker, 1993). This gas must be transported back to the lung to be exhaled. Carbon dioxide enters the systemic capillaries because of the partial pressure gradient between the interstitial fluid and the plasma, which normally has a $PaCO_2$ of approximately 40 mm

Hg. As the gas diffuses into the capillaries, it raises the carbon dioxide tension (PCO_2) and the carbon dioxide content (CCO_2) of the blood. Normally the $P\bar{v}CO_2$ of blood leaving the systemic capillaries is raised to about 45 to 47 mm Hg by this transfer of gas. Following transport to the lung, CO_2 diffuses down its partial pressure gradient and enters the alveoli to be eliminated with expired gas. As the gas diffuses out of the pulmonary capillaries, both the carbon dioxide tension and carbon dioxide content of the pulmonary blood decrease.

Carbon dioxide is carried in the bloodstream in three different forms: *dissolved, carbamino compounds,* and *bicarbonate.* Dissolution of carbon dioxide accounts for approximately 10% of the total amount of gas transported, whereas carbamino forms of carbon dioxide are responsible for moving about 20% of the total. The bicarbonate form of transport moves approximately 70% of the total volume of carbon dioxide produced through cellular metabolism. Bicarbonate is generated in large amounts in the erythrocytes (see next section) but is primarily transported in the plasma. The **total carbon dioxide content** of the blood is the sum of the carbon dioxide dissolved in the plasma, the carbamino compounds formed when carbon dioxide combines with hemoglobin, the bicarbonate carried by the red blood cells, and the bicarbonate transported by the plasma (Fig. 13–8).

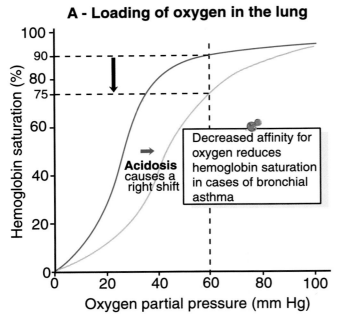

A - Loading of oxygen in the lung

Hemoglobin saturation (%)

Oxygen partial pressure (mm Hg)

Acidosis causes a right shift

Decreased affinity for oxygen reduces hemoglobin saturation in cases of bronchial asthma

B - Unloading of oxygen in the tissues

Blood O_2 content (mL/dL)

Oxygen partial pressure (mm Hg)

Acidosis causes a right shift

Decreased affinity for oxygen enhances the unloading of oxygen in the tissues in cases of bronchial asthma.

FIGURE 13–7. Right shifts of the oxyhemoglobin dissociation curve under abnormal conditions. In cases of bronchial asthma, alveolar and arterial oxygen tension is typically depressed (e.g., $Po_2 = 60$ mm Hg). A right shift of the oxyhemoglobin dissociation curve results in decreased loading of oxygen in the lung, and a decrease in hemoglobin saturation from approximately 90% to 75%. In the tissues, oxyhemoglobin gives up its oxygen readily because of reduced affinity under acidic conditions. (This is the Bohr effect.) In order to release 5 mL of oxygen per dL of blood, the partial pressure must normally change by about 25 mm Hg in the person with asthma (60–35 mm Hg). With a right-shifted curve, however, a greater partial pressure change of only 20 mm Hg is required to unload an equivalent amount of oxygen (60–40 mm Hg).

NOTE: Other minor transport modes, such as carbon dioxide dissolved in red blood cells and the carbamino compounds formed when carbon dioxide combines with plasma proteins, do not appear in the graph in Figure 13–8 but are shown schematically in Figure 13–9.

A series of steps occurs in the systemic capillaries following production of carbon dioxide by the cells of the body (Fig. 13–9). These stages are summarized in Table 13–3 and outlined below.

FORMATION OF BICARBONATE

Carbon dioxide generated through cellular metabolism builds up in the interstitial fluid and then enters the plasma. The presence of carbon dioxide in the venous blood causes an increase in the $P\bar{v}co_2$ to approximately 45 mm Hg. Once CO_2 accumulates in the plasma, it quickly enters the erythrocytes, where it is rapidly hydroxylated by the water inside red blood cells and converted to carbonic acid by the enzymatic action of *carbonic anhydrase*. The velocity of the reaction is accelerated about 12,000 to 13,000 times by the action of carbonic anhydrase (Beachey, 1998; Leff and Schumacker, 1993). Carbonic acid, in turn, ionizes to hydrogen ions (H^+) and bicarbonate ions (HCO_3^-). As the red blood cells become saturated with HCO_3^-, the bi-

carbonate ions diffuse into the plasma and combine with sodium ions (Na^+) which are carried to the lungs as sodium bicarbonate ($NaHCO_3$).

This mechanism is the **bicarbonate transport** mode responsible for about 70% of the total CO_2 car-

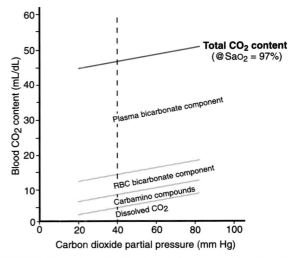

Blood CO_2 content (mL/dL)

Carbon dioxide partial pressure (mm Hg)

Total CO₂ content (@SaO_2 = 97%)

Plasma bicarbonate component

RBC bicarbonate component

Carbamino compounds

Dissolved CO₂

FIGURE 13–8. Carbon dioxide dissociation curve. The dissociation curve shows the relationship between arterial carbon dioxide partial pressure ($Paco_2$) and arterial carbon dioxide content ($Caco_2$) when the blood is fully oxygenated (arterial oxygen saturation, Sao_2 = 97%). The total carbon dioxide content is the sum of the dissolved carbon dioxide content, carbamino content, bicarbonate transported within RBCs, and bicarbonate transported by the plasma.

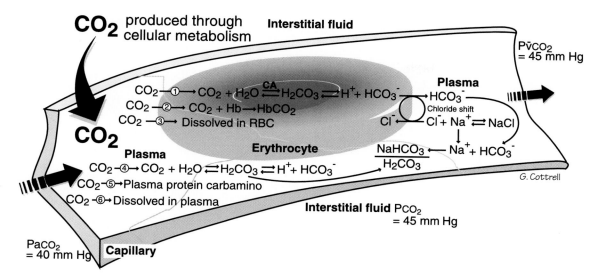

FIGURE 13–9. Carbon dioxide transport. Schematic showing the various transport modes for carbon dioxide. The capillary wall has been opened to reveal the interior of the blood vessel. Notice that both the RBC and the plasma function in carbon dioxide transport. Although most of the carbon dioxide is generated in the RBC through the formation of bicarbonate, transport occurs in the plasma as a result of the chloride shift that exchanges ions between the RBC and the plasma. (1) Bicarbonate transport within the RBC accounts for most of the carbon dioxide transport because of the enzymatic action of carbonic anhydrase (CA). Bicarbonate ions enter the plasma in large numbers to maintain the 20:1 ratio of the sodium bicarbonate/carbonic acid buffer system. (2) Carbaminohemoglobin is formed when carbon dioxide combines reversibly with binding sites on hemoglobin molecules. (3) A small volume of carbon dioxide is transported dissolved in the intracellular fluid of the RBC. (4) Formation of bicarbonate in the plasma occurs slowly when carbon dioxide combines with water without enzyme assistance. (5) Formation of carbamino compounds occurs when carbon dioxide combines with the amino group on plasma proteins. (6) Carbon dioxide dissolves in small amounts in the plasma and exerts carbon dioxide tension in the bloodstream.

ried by the bloodstream. A coupled ion transporter in the RBC membrane is responsible for exchanging anions between the plasma and the interior of the red blood cell. In this mechanism called the **chloride shift,** bicarbonate ions (HCO_3^-) leave the red blood cells and chloride ions (Cl^-) enter from the plasma. The ratio of bicarbonate to carbonic acid is normally 20:1 in order to maintain blood pH in the homeostatic range of 7.35 to 7.45. The *sodium bicarbonate/carbonic acid buffer* is one of several important physiologic buffer systems that function to maintain blood pH. Others include the *phosphate buffer system* and the *hemoglobin buffer system.* (The role of physiologic buffers in acid-base balance is discussed in Chapter 24.) The ratio of sodium bicarbonate to carbonic acid is approximately 20:1 because carbonic anhydrase greatly accelerates the production of bicarbonate ions in the red blood cells. Therefore, large quantities of HCO_3^- are continuously produced and are available for exchange with the virtually unlimited number of sodium ions in the plasma.

Bicarbonate is also formed in the plasma as carbon dioxide slowly combines with water (see Fig. 13–9). Carbonic anhydrase is lacking in the plasma; therefore, the reaction proceeds slowly and only accounts for approximately 5% of the total CO_2 transported by the bloodstream.

FORMATION OF CARBAMINO COMPOUNDS

Some of the carbon dioxide generated in the tissues enters the plasma, where it passes into the red blood cells and chemically combines with hemoglobin to form a carbamino compound called **carbaminohemoglobin** (see Fig. 13–9). Carbon dioxide combines reversibly with hemoglobin at a different site than where oxygen is bound. These binding sites allow hemoglobin to transport about 20% of the total CO_2 produced by the cells. A small amount of carbon dioxide (approximately 1%) also combines chemically with the amino groups of plasma proteins to form additional *carbamino compounds*. This transport mode plays a relatively minor role in overall **carbon dioxide transport.**

DISSOLVED CARBON DIOXIDE

Figure 13–9 also shows a quantity of carbon dioxide reaching the bloodstream and entering plasma dissolution. This mode of CO_2 transport is responsible for only about 5% of the carbon dioxide produced by the cells. Interestingly, it is this small volume of CO_2 in the venous blood that is assessed clinically to determine a patient's carbon dioxide partial pressure. Recall that it is

TABLE 13-3	Carbon Dioxide Loading in the Tissues

Carbon dioxide produced in the cells accumulates in the interstitial fluid and diffuses into the plasma, raising the partial pressure to approximately 45 to 47 mm Hg. From here, it is transported in a variety of modes, as follows:

Transport Mode	Summary of Steps
Bicarbonate Transport	CO_2 rapidly enters RBCs and is converted to H_2CO_3 by carbonic anhydrase.
	H_2CO_3 ionizes into H^+ and HCO_3^- in the RBC.
	HCO_3^- builds up in the RBCs and diffuses into the plasma.
	Chloride shift (anion exchange) mechanism moves HCO_3^- out of the RBCs in exchange for Cl^- in the plasma.
	HCO_3^- combines with Na^+ in the plasma to form $NaHCO_3$.
	Accumulation of HCO_3^- in the plasma (to form $NaHCO_3$) helps maintain the 20:1 ratio of the sodium bicarbonate/carbonic acid buffer system in the plasma.
	CO_2 also combines slowly with H_2O in the plasma to form H_2CO_3 (not assisted by carbonic anhydrase).
	H_2CO_3 ionizes into H^+ and HCO_3^- in the plasma.
Carbamino Transport	CO_2 rapidly enters the RBCs and combines with hemoglobin to form carbaminohemoglobin, which is transported to the lungs.
	CO_2 also combines with the amino group of plasma proteins to form carbamino compounds, which are transported to the lungs.
Transport as Dissolved Carbon Dioxide	No chemical reaction occurs between CO_2 and other compounds in the *dissolved* form of gas transport.
	CO_2 enters RBCs and is dissolved in the intracellular fluid.
	CO_2 also dissolves in plasma and is responsible for exerting the carbon dioxide partial pressure of blood (P_{CO_2}).

RBC = red blood cell (erythrocyte).

only those gases that do *not* combine chemically with other compounds that are capable of exerting a partial pressure in a fluid. A small volume (approximately 5%) of carbon dioxide also dissolves within red blood cells but does not contribute to carbon dioxide tension in the bloodstream.

CARBON DIOXIDE DISSOCIATION CURVE

The relationship between carbon dioxide tension (P_{CO_2}) and carbon dioxide content (C_{CO_2}) is basically linear and direct, rather than nonlinear (see Fig. 13–8). Therefore, the curve that results when the data are plotted is nearly a straight line, rather than a sigmoid curve characteristic of the oxyhemoglobin dissociation curve.

Unloading of oxygen from oxyhemoglobin along systemic capillaries causes the carbon dioxide dissociation curve to be shifted upward (Fig. 13–10). This shift indicates that the blood can take up more carbon dioxide at a given P_{CO_2} and is due to the ability of deoxygenated hemoglobin to form carbamino compounds (Leff and Schumacker, 1993). Because more deoxygenated hemoglobin is formed as blood gives up oxygen during its passage through systemic capillaries, the bloodstream is able to load even more carbon dioxide at any given carbon dioxide tension. The change occurs rapidly, causing the carbon dioxide dissociation curve

to shift dynamically upward as blood moves along the capillary.

This inverse relationship between oxygen saturation and the carbon dioxide content of blood is termed the **Haldane effect,** named after the physiologist J. S. Haldane. It deals with the effect oxyhemoglobin saturation has on the relationship of carbon dioxide content and carbon dioxide tension in the bloodstream. The Haldane effect is analogous to the Bohr effect, in which the oxyhemoglobin dissociation curve shifts dynamically to the right in response to the effects of changing P_{CO_2}. The Haldane effect contributes to the efficiency of both internal and external respiration as shown by the graph in Figure 13–10. At a depressed hemoglobin oxygen saturation (e.g., $S_{aO_2} = 75\%$), the carbon dioxide dissociation curve is shifted slightly upward, indicating an *increase* in the affinity of hemoglobin for carbon dioxide, and enhanced loading of CO_2 in the tissues through the Haldane effect. In the lung, however, elevated hemoglobin oxygen saturation (e.g., $S_{aO_2} = 97\%$) causes a *decrease* in the affinity of hemoglobin for carbon dioxide and a downward shift in the carbon dioxide dissociation curve (see Fig. 13–10). Thus, oxygenated blood enhances the unloading of CO_2 in the lung through the Haldane effect. In quantitative terms, the Haldane effect is more important in carbon dioxide transport than is the Bohr effect in oxygen transport (Guyton and Hall, 1996).

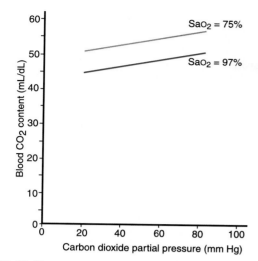

FIGURE 13–10. Haldane effect. The carbon dioxide dissociation curve is affected by the saturation of hemoglobin. As the arterial oxygen saturation (SaO_2) increases, the carbon dioxide content ($CaCO_2$) decreases at any given carbon dioxide partial pressure, thus enhancing the loading of carbon dioxide into the bloodstream in the tissues. This mechanism is known as the *Haldane effect*.

Summary

In this chapter we examined the mechanisms responsible for the carriage of oxygen and carbon dioxide by the bloodstream. We also studied the synergistic relationship between the two gases that facilitates their uptake and release in both the pulmonary and systemic capillaries. From the interactions studied in this chapter it is clear that changes in affinity of hemoglobin toward oxygen and the resulting increase or decrease in the volume of oxygen loaded in the lung and unloaded in the tissues have important consequences for the patient with hypoxia. These interactions, along with those associated with carbon dioxide transport, are studied as part of *arterial blood gas* (ABG) interpretation. This diagnostic technique is important in the assessment of pathophysiologic conditions, and will be reinforced and expanded upon in clinical courses. This chapter was designed to give the reader the basic physiologic background required to understand the clinical applications of gas transport principles.

BIBLIOGRAPHY

Beachey W: Respiratory Care Anatomy and Physiology: Foundations for Clinical Practice. Mosby-Year Book, St. Louis, 1998.

Des Jardins T: Cardiopulmonary Anatomy and Physiology: Essentials for Respiratory Care, ed 3. Delmar Publishers, Albany, NY, 1998.

Ganong WF: Review of Medical Physiology, ed 17. Appleton & Lange, Norwalk CT, 1995.

Guyton AC and Hall JE: Textbook of Medical Physiology, ed 9. WB Saunders, Philadelphia, 1996.

Leff AR and Schumacker PT: Respiratory Physiology: Basics and Applications. WB Saunders, Philadelphia, 1993.

Martini FH: Fundamentals of Anatomy and Physiology, ed 4. Prentice Hall, Upper Saddle River, NJ, 1998.

Mines AH: Respiratory Physiology, ed 3. Raven Press, New York, 1993.

Thomas CL (ed): Taber's Cyclopedic Medical Dictionary, ed 18. FA Davis, Philadelphia, 1997.

West JB: Respiratory Physiology: The Essentials, ed 6. Williams & Wilkins, Baltimore, 1998.

CHAPTER 14

Ventilation-Perfusion Relationships

chapter objectives

After studying this chapter the reader should be able to:

☐ Describe the ventilation-perfusion ratio as it applies to a single alveolus and
    to the entire lung.

☐ Explain how the alveolar oxygen tension is altered by changes in the
    following variables:
    Alveolar ventilation, cardiac output, inspired oxygen tension, mixed
        venous oxygen tension.

☐ Explain how the alveolar carbon dioxide tension is altered by changes in the
    following variables:
    Alveolar ventilation, cardiac output, inspired carbon dioxide tension, mixed
        venous carbon dioxide tension.

☐ Describe the concept of the ideal lung in terms of homogeneous ventilation-
    perfusion ratios.

☐ State the ideal alveolar oxygen equation and define the variables used in the
    calculation.

☐ Define the following terms:
    Respiratory exchange ratio (R), metabolic respiratory quotient (RQ).

☐ Explain the concept of balance of oxygen supply and demand in the alveolus
    by describing how alveolar oxygen tension is affected by alveolar ventilation,
    inspired oxygen tension, and oxygen uptake by the tissues.

☐ Explain how the alveolar-arterial oxygen tension gradient is useful as an
    index of efficiency of oxygen loading in the lung and state the disadvantages
    associated with use of the measurement.

☐ Calculate the alveolar-arterial oxygen tension gradient when the barometric pressure, body temperature, arterial blood gas values, and respiratory exchange ratio are known.

☐ Describe the concept of the nonideal lung in terms of nonhomogeneous ventilation-perfusion ratios.

☐ Discuss how the ventilation, blood flow, and ventilation-perfusion ratios change from the apical to the basal regions of the upright lung.

☐ Explain why the lung in a vertical (upright) position is less homogeneous than the lung in the horizontal position.

☐ Describe the concept of lung compartments and differentiate between a single-compartment lung model and a two-compartment lung model.

☐ Explain how the end-capillary oxygen tension is affected by a lung having two compartments with markedly different ventilation-perfusion ratios.

☐ Explain the concept of a flow-weighted average for the systemic arterial oxygen tension in a nonideal normal lung.

☐ Describe how a multicompartment lung model accurately simulates the gas-exchange function of the real lung.

☐ Define the following terms:
  Intrapulmonary shunt, shunt compartment.

☐ Explain the effect that intrapulmonary shunting has on the ventilation-perfusion relationships in a three-compartment lung model.

☐ Describe how the flowrate of oxygen is determined by the oxygen content and blood flowrate through a particular lung compartment.

☐ State the classic shunt equation and define the variables used in the calculation.

☐ Explain why the classic shunt equation provides the most accurate assessment of oxygen-loading efficiency in the lung.

☐ Calculate the shunt fraction for a patient given the necessary hematologic values for blood gas tensions, hemoglobin saturation, and hemoglobin amounts.

☐ State an estimated shunt equation and describe the advantages and disadvantages of the index as a measure of oxygen-loading efficiency.

☐ Define extrapulmonary shunting and explain how bronchial and thebesian vein venous drainage affect ventilation-perfusion ratios.

☐ Define the following terms:
  Hypoxemia, hypoxia, anoxia.

☐ Describe how the following conditions contribute to hypoxemic hypoxia:
  Low alveolar oxygen tension, diffusion impairment, intrapulmonary
    shunting, extrapulmonary shunting.

☐ Differentiate between physiologic shunts classified as relative shunts and those classified as absolute shunts.

☐ Explain why relative and absolute shunts differ in their response to supplemental oxygen therapy.

☐ Differentiate between absolute shunts classified as anatomic shunts and those classified as capillary shunts.

☐ Explain the difference between relative capillary shunts and absolute capillary shunts.

☐ Compare and contrast the following types of tissue hypoxia:
  Hypoxemic hypoxia, anemic hypoxia, stagnant hypoxia, histotoxic
    hypoxia.

key terms

absolute shunt; true shunt
  anatomic shunt
  capillary shunt
alveolar-arterial oxygen tension gradient; P(A–a)O$_2$
anoxia
classic shunt equation
estimated shunt equations
extrapulmonary shunting
hypoxemia
hypoxia
  anemic hypoxia
  histotoxic hypoxia

hypoxic hypoxia; hypoxemic hypoxia
  stagnant hypoxia; ischemic hypoxia
ideal alveolar oxygen equation
ideal lung; homogeneous lung
intrapulmonary shunting; pulmonary shunting
metabolic respiratory quotient (RQ)
nonideal lung; nonhomogeneous lung
physiologic shunt
relative shunt
respiratory exchange ratio (R)
shunt compartment
ventilation-perfusion ratio ($\dot{V}A/\dot{Q}$)

In previous chapters we discussed the details of both ventilation of the lung and blood flow through the lung, including the differences in gas distribution and regional blood flow caused by postural changes. These topics were treated as more or less separate issues. The focus of this chapter is on the introductory aspects of the *relationships* between ventilation and blood flow, especially on the complex interaction of ventilation and perfusion on gas exchange in the lung.

This chapter is not meant to provide the last word on arterial blood gas abnormalities, nor is it intended to be a comprehensive guide to clinical blood gas measurement and interpretation. Instead, it introduces basic physiologic principles associated with the complex interactions that occur between gas and blood in the normal lung. Through an understanding of the ventilation-perfusion relationships affecting gas exchange, the reader will be better able to understand the management of oxygenation in patients as well as the clinical implications of inequalities of ventilation and blood flow in the lung.

Ventilation-Perfusion Ratio

THE RATIO OF ALVEOLAR VENTILATION TO BLOOD FLOW

Recall that the diffusion of a gas is dependent on its partial pressure gradient—gases always diffuse from an area of high partial pressure to an area of lower partial pressure (see Chap. 11). In the alveolar-capillary system this partial pressure gradient is maintained by the dynamic nature of both *ventilation* and *perfusion*. As gas exchange occurs across the respiratory membrane, the partial pressure differential is maintained by constant alveolar ventilation and by continued pulmonary blood flow. Without blood flow, equilibration of gas remaining in the pulmonary capillaries with that in the alveoli would quickly occur and gas exchange would cease. Similarly, if ventilation of the alveoli stopped, the alveolar gas would quickly equilibrate with mixed venous blood and gas exchange would cease. In each case, gas exchange comes to an abrupt halt because partial pressure gradients disappear. Clearly, the partial pressure differential is a critical factor driving gas exchange.

The ratio of ventilation to blood flow is known as the **ventilation-perfusion ratio ($\dot{V}A/\dot{Q}$).** The relationship is used to describe the ratio of ventilation to blood flow for a single alveolus, a group of alveoli, or the entire lung. For a single alveolus, the ventilation-perfusion ratio is the ventilation of the alveolus divided by the capillary blood flow. For the whole lung, the ventilation-perfusion ratio is the total alveolar ventilation ($\dot{V}A$) divided by the entire pulmonary blood flow ($\dot{Q}$, cardiac output or C.O.). An adult standing upright and at rest has a ventilation-perfusion ratio of 0.8 when the alveolar ventilation is 4 L/min and the cardiac output is 5 L/min, as shown by the following calculation. Thus:

$$\dot{V}A/\dot{Q} = \frac{4 \text{ L/min}}{5 \text{ L/min}} = 0.8$$

Note that the ventilation-perfusion ratio is dimensionless because both ventilation and blood flowrates are expressed in the same units. Notice also that the *overall* gas exchange function of the lung is not necessarily revealed by the ventilation-perfusion ratio. For example, large numbers of alveoli can be adequately ventilated but receive no blood flow, while others can be perfused normally but not be ventilated. If these two groups of dysfunctional alveoli are approximately equal in number, the ventilation-perfusion ratio of the lung appears "normal" ($\dot{V}A/\dot{Q}$ ratio $\approx$ 0.8). The overall gas exchange function, however, is severely impaired under such conditions.

Arterial blood oxygen and carbon dioxide contents (Cao_2 and $Caco_2$) are determined by the respective tensions of the gases in the end-capillary blood of the lung. In other words, the Po_2 and Pco_2 of blood exiting from the end of the alveolar capillaries play an important role in determining the overall gas-transporting ability of the bloodstream. But what determines the Po_2 and Pco_2 of this blood in the alveolar capillaries?

Under normal conditions, the transit time of blood through the alveolar-capillary system allows the equilibration of oxygen and carbon dioxide to occur along the pulmonary capillary. In Chapter 11 it was pointed out that the equilibration rate for these gases is rapid enough in the short time available (0.75 second), to ensure that blood in the pulmonary capillary will have the same Po_2 and Pco_2 as its alveolar gas. The most important factor influencing alveolar Po_2 and Pco_2 is the ratio of ventilation to perfusion. Overall, this relationship between the ventilation-perfusion ratio and the gas-transporting ability of the bloodstream can be shown as follows:

$$\dot{V}A/\dot{Q} \text{ ratio} \rightarrow PAo_2 \text{ and } PAco_2 \rightarrow Pao_2$$
$$\text{and } Paco_2 \rightarrow Cao_2 \text{ and } Caco_2$$

ALVEOLAR GAS EXCHANGE

In Chapter 11 it was pointed out that the exchange of oxygen and carbon dioxide along the pulmonary capillary is perfusion-limited, as indicated by the equilibration between alveolar and arterial gas tensions. In other words, under normal circumstances, the transfer of these two gases into and out of pulmonary circulation is dependent upon the *rate* of blood flow through the alveolar-capillary system, not upon the diffusion characteristics of the gases across the exchange membrane. Changes in alveolar ventilation, blood flow through the lung, or a combination of both factors, dramatically affect such an interdependent system.

Oxygen

A given alveolar oxygen tension (PAo_2) is the result of the balance between two flowrates and two gas tensions affecting the alveolus. An illustrative analogy is the concept of each alveolus as a small "mixing tank" that receives a continuous flow of both hot and cold water through separate supply pipes, as shown schematically in Figure 14–1. The resulting temperature of the mixture of water in the tank is analogous to the partial pressure of oxygen in a single alveolus. Changes in alveolar ventilation ($\dot{V}A$) or cardiac output ($\dot{Q}$), as well as changes in inspired oxygen tension (PIo_2) or mixed venous oxygen tension ($P\bar{v}o_2$), continuously modify the partial pressure of oxygen in each alveolus. In such a dynamic system the end-capillary blood oxygen tension is equal to the alveolar oxygen tension.

When $\dot{V}A$ and $\dot{Q}$ are approximately equal, the alveolar and arterial Po_2 values are about 100 mm Hg. However, if the $\dot{V}A/\dot{Q}$ ratio is decreased by decreasing the alveolar ventilation or by increasing the blood flow, then the PAo_2 decreases toward the $P\bar{v}o_2$. If, on

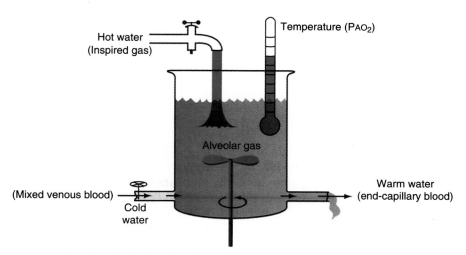

FIGURE 14–1. Alveolar gas composition in a single alveolus. Effect of the ventilation-perfusion ratio on the alveolar gas composition in a single alveolus in the lung. Each alveolus behaves like a mixing tank, where the alveolar Po_2 is analogous to the temperature of the water in the tank. Hot water pours in at the top (analogous to alveolar ventilation), and cold water is pumped in at the bottom (analogous to mixed venous blood flow). The temperature of the hot water supply is analogous to the inspired Po_2, and the temperature of the cold water supply is analogous to the mixed venous blood flow Po_2. The Po_2 in an alveolus is determined by the balance between ventilation (hot water flow) and perfusion (cold water flow). Note that for any given $\dot{V}A/\dot{Q}$ ratio, the alveolar Po_2 (water temperature in the tank) will also be influenced by the inspired and mixed venous Po_2 (temperatures of hot and cold water supplies). (From Leff AR and Schumacker PT: Respiratory Physiology: Basics and Applications. WB Saunders, Philadelphia, 1993, p 94, with permission.)

the other hand, the $\dot{V}A/\dot{Q}$ ratio is increased by increasing the alveolar ventilation or by decreasing the blood flow, the PAO_2 increases toward the PIO_2. An alveolus with an infinite $\dot{V}A/\dot{Q}$ ratio, that is, an alveolus having ventilation but no blood flow, has a PAO_2 equal to the inspired PO_2. Finally, if alveolar ventilation ceases completely, the $\dot{V}A/\dot{Q}$ ratio decreases towards zero and the PAO_2 decreases to match the $P\bar{v}O_2$. The PAO_2, however, does not decrease to zero. In general, the PAO_2 in any alveolus is a value between the PIO_2 and the mixed venous oxygen tension $P\bar{v}O_2$. The actual value depends on the $\dot{V}A/\dot{Q}$ ratio existing at the time.

Carbon Dioxide

Unlike the oxygen tension of inspired gas, the inspired carbon dioxide tension ($PICO_2$) is extremely low. (The low value is due to the very low tension of atmospheric carbon dioxide, typically about 0.2 to 0.3 mm Hg.) As a result of this factor, the carbon dioxide tension in a single alveolus ($PACO_2$) is determined by the mixed venous carbon dioxide tension ($P\bar{v}CO_2$) and the $\dot{V}A/\dot{Q}$ ratio of the alveolus. Recall that the $P\bar{v}CO_2$ is in the range 45 to 47 mm Hg. Normally the $PACO_2$ and the end-capillary blood are in equilibrium because the transfer of carbon dioxide is perfusion-limited. As a result of this perfusion-limited exchange, the carbon dioxide tension of end-capillary blood lies somewhere between the $P\bar{v}CO_2$ and zero.

As pointed out previously, the $PACO_2$ is profoundly affected by the prevailing $\dot{V}A/\dot{Q}$ ratio of the alveolus. If the $\dot{V}A/\dot{Q}$ ratio is close to zero, as occurs when alveolar ventilation is severely impaired, the $PACO_2$ rises, approaching the $P\bar{v}CO_2$. As the $\dot{V}A/\dot{Q}$ ratio increases, the $PACO_2$ decreases until it equals the $PICO_2$. The $PICO_2$ is virtually zero in an alveolus with infinite $\dot{V}A/\dot{Q}$ ratio, mainly as a result of the extremely low partial pressure of atmospheric carbon dioxide.

Gas Exchange in the Ideal Lung

HOMOGENEOUS VENTILATION-PERFUSION RATIOS

We have now considered the effect of the ventilation-perfusion ratio on gas exchange in a single alveolus. What would happen to gas exchange if _all_ of the alveoli in a lung had the same $\dot{V}A/\dot{Q}$ ratio? (This situation does not occur in the actual lung, by the way.) In such a fictitious scenario, the lung is considered **homogeneous** with respect to ventilation-perfusion ratios. In the **ideal lung** having an identical $\dot{V}A/\dot{Q}$ ratio for each alveolus, the alveolar oxygen tension is the same in each alveolus because the $P\bar{v}CO_2$ and the PIO_2 supplying each alve-

olus are the same. Similarly, the end-capillary blood oxygen tension and content are the same for blood exiting from each alveolus because equilibration with PAO_2 has occurred. Finally, systemic arterial oxygen tension (PaO_2) is equal to PAO_2 because the blood flowing out of the lung is a mixture of the end-capillary blood from each identically perfused and ventilated alveolus.

The gas exchange and transport of carbon dioxide in the ideal lung is affected by the same factors that influence the transfer and movement of oxygen, resulting in a systemic arterial carbon dioxide tension ($PaCO_2$) equal to the carbon dioxide tension within each alveolus ($PACO_2$) of the homogeneous lung.

IDEAL ALVEOLAR GAS EQUATION

A convenient way to discuss the homogeneous lung is to describe it as if it were composed of a single alveolus with blood flow equal to the entire cardiac output and alveolar ventilation equivalent to the total alveolar ventilation (Fig. 14–2). The arterial blood PO_2 and PCO_2 in such a _single-compartment lung model_ is identical to the alveolar gas PO_2 and PCO_2 for the reasons outlined in the preceding section. How can we determine the alveolar gas tension in the homogeneous lung represented as a large single alveolus?

The alveolar oxygen tension (PAO_2) in a homogeneous lung is calculated using the **ideal alveolar oxygen equation:**

$$PAO_2 = FIO_2 \times (PBAR - PH_2O) - \frac{PACO_2}{R}$$

where:

$PACO_2$ = alveolar carbon dioxide tension
FIO_2 = inspired oxygen fraction (percentage composition divided by 100)
$PBAR$ = barometric pressure (760 mm Hg at sea level)
PH_2O = water vapor partial pressure (47 mm Hg at 37°C)
R = respiratory exchange ratio

The relationship $FIO_2 \times (PBAR - PH_2O)$ represents the inspired oxygen tension (PIO_2) in this equation. Recall that water vapor partial pressure is due to humidity within the alveoli. The value for this vapor pressure is temperature-dependent and is normally around 47 mm Hg at a body temperature of 37°C. The inspired oxygen tension for a person breathing room air at sea level is approximately 150 mm Hg, as shown by the following calculation:

$$PIO_2 = FIO_2 \times (PBAR - PH_2O)$$
$$= 0.21 \times (760 \text{ mm Hg} - 47 \text{ mm Hg})$$
$$= 149.73 \text{ mm Hg}$$

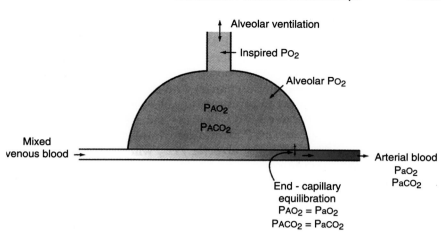

FIGURE 14–2. Single-compartment lung model (ideal lung). The *ideal lung* represented as a single alveolus. When all alveoli in a lung have the same ratio of ventilation to blood flow, the lung is homogeneous with respect to $\dot{V}_A/\dot{Q}$. In this ideal situation, the lung can be represented as if it were a single large alveolus receiving all the blood flow and all of the ventilation. This is an ideal lung because the arterial blood leaving it has the same P_{aO_2} and P_{aCO_2} as the ideal alveolar gas (P_{AO_2} and P_{ACO_2}). Thus the $P(A–a)O_2$ for this lung would be zero. (From Leff AR and Schumacker PT: Respiratory Physiology: Basics and Applications. WB Saunders, Philadelphia, 1993, p 96, with permission.)

Because we are dealing with the equilibration of gases that occurs in an ideal lung model, the value for alveolar carbon dioxide tension (P_{aCO_2}) used in the ideal alveolar oxygen equation is approximately equal to the arterial carbon dioxide tension (P_{aCO_2}). (It should be noted that some reference sources use the arterial P_{CO_2} factor, rather than the alveolar P_{CO_2} factor, in the ideal alveolar oxygen equation.)

The **respiratory exchange ratio (R)** is the ratio of carbon dioxide eliminated ($\dot{V}_{CO_2}$) from the tissues relative to the oxygen taken up ($\dot{V}_{O_2}$) by the lungs. Therefore:

$$R = \dot{V}_{CO_2}/\dot{V}_{O_2}$$

In the homeostatic state, the respiratory exchange ratio is normally *equal* to the **metabolic respiratory quotient (RQ)**. The RQ is defined as the number of carbon dioxide molecules produced by the tissues relative to the oxygen molecules consumed by the tissues. Although the metabolic respiratory quotient is affected by diet, a person in normal nutritional status will have an RQ (and R) value that ranges between 0.7 and 1.0 (Leff and Schumacker, 1993).

ALVEOLAR P_{O_2}—A BALANCE OF SUPPLY AND DEMAND

At any given time the alveolar oxygen tension reflects a balance between the rate of oxygen delivered to the alveoli and the rate at which oxygen is transferred into pulmonary capillary blood. Oxygen delivery depends on both alveolar ventilation and P_{IO_2}. The rate that oxygen is taken up by alveolar capillary blood depends on the oxygen demands of the tissues, and is represented by $\dot{V}_{O_2}$. For a given ventilation rate, therefore, the P_{AO_2} increases if the P_{IO_2} increases while the metabolic rate remains the same. On the other hand, during strenuous exercise the oxygen requirements of the tissues increase. Under such conditions of increased

metabolic stress, the P_{AO_2} decreases when the P_{IO_2} remains constant. Recall:

$$P_{IO_2} = F_{IO_2} \times (P_{BAR} - P_{H_2O})$$

and

$$P_{AO_2} = F_{IO_2} \times (P_{BAR} - P_{H_2O}) - \frac{P_{ACO_2}}{R}$$

Therefore, the ideal alveolar oxygen equation can be rearranged as:

$$P_{AO_2} = P_{IO_2} - \frac{P_{ACO_2}}{R}$$

The P_{IO_2} term in the equation represents the rate at which oxygen is delivered to the alveoli; the P_{ACO_2}/R term reflects the rate at which oxygen leaves the alveoli and enters the capillaries to satisfy the metabolic demands of the tissues. Again, alveolar oxygen tension reflects a *balance* between the amount of oxygen supplied to the alveoli and the amount of oxygen delivered to the alveolar capillaries and consumed by the tissues. How is this relationship revealed by the ideal alveolar oxygen equation?

ALVEOLAR-ARTERIAL OXYGEN TENSION GRADIENT

The alveolar oxygen tension calculated by the previous equation represents a theoretical *maximum* oxygen tension that can be attained in the systemic arteries. In other words, when the actual P_{aO_2} is equal to the P_{AO_2} calculated by the ideal alveolar oxygen equation, the lung is assumed to be operating at highest efficiency. Optimal gas exchange at the alveolar-capillary membrane results in the equilibration of the partial pressure of oxygen in both the alveoli and the bloodstream. In fact, the only way to increase the arterial P_{O_2} in such an ideal system is to increase the delivery of oxygen to the alveoli (P_{IO_2}) or to decrease the rate at which oxygen moves out of the alveoli into the blood ($P_{A}CO_2/R$). Increasing the amount of oxygen reaching the alveoli can be accomplished only via artificial means by raising the ambient barometric pressure through the use of a *hyperbaric chamber,* or by raising the inflowing concentration of oxygen (F_{IO_2}). Therefore, in an ideal lung operating under normal atmospheric conditions, the difference between alveolar and arterial partial pressures of oxygen is *zero.* This partial pressure differential is known as the **alveolar-arterial oxygen tension gradient,** or **$P(A–a)O_2$.** The value represents the difference between the theoretical and actual values for PO_2 and is obtained by subtracting the arterial value from the "ideal" alveolar value.

The *ideal* alveolar PO_2 is obtained from the ideal alveolar oxygen equation. This alveolar oxygen tension is the theoretical value the lung would have if no ventilation-perfusion inequality existed and the lung was exchanging gas at optimal efficiency, that is, at the same respiratory exchange ratio (R) as the real lung (West, 1998). The calculated value for $P(A–a)O_2$ gives a general indication of lung efficiency in terms of oxygen loading. The greater the value, the less efficient the lung as a gas exchanger. Consider the following example:

EXAMPLE

Arterial blood gas (ABG) analysis of a patient reveals $PaO_2 = 45$ mm Hg and $PaCO_2 = 80$ mm Hg when breathing room air. Assume that the patient's temperature is 37°C and the ambient barometric pressure is 760 mm Hg. Calculate the alveolar-arterial oxygen tension gradient when the respiratory exchange ratio (R) is 0.8.

First we need to calculate the theoretical alveolar PO_2 using the ideal alveolar oxygen equation under these conditions: (Assume that the alveolar and arterial carbon dioxide tensions are the same in this patient.)

$$P_{AO_2} = F_{IO_2} \times (P_{BAR} - P_{H_2O}) - \frac{P_{ACO_2}}{R}$$

$$= 0.21 \times (760 \text{ mm Hg} - 47 \text{ mm Hg}) - \frac{80 \text{ mm Hg}}{0.8}$$

$$= (0.21 \times 713 \text{ mm Hg}) - 100 \text{ mm Hg}$$

$$\therefore P_{AO_2} = 49.73 \text{ mm Hg}$$

To determine the $P(A–a)O_2$ for this patient, we simply subtract the ABG value for arterial oxygen tension from the calculated value for alveolar oxygen tension:

$$P(A–a)O_2 = 49.73 \text{ mm Hg} - 45 \text{ mm Hg}$$

$$= 4.73 \text{ mm Hg}$$

The maximum P_{AO_2} that can be achieved in this patient is 49.73 mm Hg, whereas the measured value for PaO_2 is only 4.73 mm Hg less than the theoretical maximum. Recall that the lower the $P(A–a)O_2$ value, the more efficient the lung as a gas exchanger. Therefore, on the basis of the relatively small alveolar-arterial oxygen tension gradient, it can be concluded that the patient's lung is operating near peak efficiency.

This level of efficiency, however, does not relieve the abnormal arterial blood gas values reported for the patient (e.g., $PaO_2 = 45$ mm Hg and $PaCO_2 = 80$ mm Hg). Because the ambient barometric conditions and inspired fraction of oxygen are constant, it can be assumed that the low alveolar PO_2 is caused by inadequate alveolar ventilation and is responsible for the patient's low arterial PO_2. Overall, the rate of oxygen movement into the alveoli relative to its transfer into the capillary blood has caused a decrease in alveolar ventilation, adversely affecting the patient's arterial blood gas status. Unfortunately, the $P(A–a)O_2$ index does not always give a clear indication of the progression of pulmonary disease at various values of F_{IO_2}. Not only does considerable variation exist among patients but also normal $P(A–a)O_2$ values do not remain constant at different F_{IO_2} levels (Malley, 1990).

Gas Exchange in the Nonideal Lung

$\dot{V}/\dot{Q}$ INEQUALITY IN A NORMAL LUNG

Although it is convenient to discuss ventilation-perfusion relationships that exist in an ideal lung model, it should be noted that the 300 million alveoli in a normal lung are neither ventilated nor perfused in a homogeneous manner. In fact, the normal lung is rather **nonhomogenous** in terms of both air flow and blood flow. The normal lung, therefore, is more accurately described as a **nonideal lung** with respect to ventilation and perfusion. Significant regional differences in both ventilation and perfusion exist in the apical and basal portions of the lung (see Chap. 11). Recall that groups of alveoli in the apex of the upright lung are not as well ventilated as those in the middle regions or those in the base. The disparity is due to the effects of gravity on the distribution of pleural and transpulmonary pressures going from superior to inferior regions of the upright lung (see Fig. 11–6). Similarly, the effects of gravity on the recruitment and distension of blood vessels near the base of the vertical lung cause the alveoli near the base to receive more blood flow than their counterparts near the apex of the lung (see Fig. 11–11). In general, there is an increase in ventilation and an increase in perfusion from the top to the bottom of the upright lung (see Fig. 11–6).

If the change in ventilation and perfusion of alveoli were constant throughout the vertical gradient, the ventilation-perfusion ($\dot{V}_A/\dot{Q}$) ratios for alveoli in the different zones would remain the same. However, the increase in blood flow because of gravity is more marked than the increase in ventilation along the hydrostatic gradient. Put another way, the alveoli in the apex of the lung receive less ventilation than those in the base, but they receive *far less* blood flow. As a result of this disparity, the $\dot{V}_A/\dot{Q}$ ratios of alveoli in different parts of the lung are not the same, thus contributing to the heterogeneity of the healthy lung. In general, the $\dot{V}_A/\dot{Q}$ ratios decrease going from top to bottom in the upright lung (Fig. 14–3). Alveoli in the apex receive far more ventilation than blood flow and thus have $\dot{V}_A/\dot{Q}$ ratios in the range of 1 to 10, whereas alveoli in the base of the lung receive more blood flow than ventilation, resulting in $\dot{V}_A/\dot{Q}$ ratios less than 1.0 (Leff and Schumacker, 1993). Because the lung is taller than it is wide, the distances are greater when the lung is in the vertical position. Consequently, the effects of gravity on ventilation and perfusion, as well as on $\dot{V}_A/\dot{Q}$ heterogeneity, are greater in the upright lung. When a subject lies down, there is still a vertical hydrostatic gradient affecting the distribution of gas and blood in the lung. However, the vertical distance is smaller and the lung becomes much more homogenous in regard to $\dot{V}_A/\dot{Q}$ ratios.

Clearly the presence of large numbers of alveoli with

vastly different $\dot{V}_A/\dot{Q}$ ratios contributes to the inefficiency of gas exchange in the nonhomogenous lung. Such lack of uniformity in $\dot{V}_A/\dot{Q}$ ratios is reflected in the alveolar-arterial oxygen tension gradient. Recall that a difference of *zero* represents optimal efficiency of gas exchange in the ideal lung. By contrast, the mean normal $P(A–a)O_2$ is approximately 10 mm Hg in adults younger than 60 years old breathing room air (Malley, 1990). This slightly elevated $P(A–a)O_2$ value tells us that alveoli in different regions of the nonideal lung have $\dot{V}_A/\dot{Q}$ ratios that decrease oxygen loading, thereby reducing the overall efficiency of the lung as a gas exchanger. In some types of lung disease, abnormalities of ventilation, perfusion, or both can result in $\dot{V}_A/\dot{Q}$ ratios among alveoli that differ by a factor of 1000 or more (Leff and Schumacker, 1993). Because the blood entering systemic arteries is always a mixture of blood from alveoli having nonuniform ventilation-perfusion ratios, the alveolar-arterial oxygen tension gradient may increase dramatically if the amount of blood coming from underventilated or overperfused alveoli is extensive. Such an increase in $P(A–a)O_2$ indicates a reduction in the efficiency of gas exchange in external respiration and may lead to *arterial hypoxemia* if not corrected.

$\dot{V}/\dot{Q}$ INEQUALITY IN A TWO-COMPARTMENT LUNG MODEL

Although an appreciation of regional differences in the distribution of gas and blood flow through the lung is of physiologic interest, it also provides the basis for understanding the outcome of mismatches between ventilation and perfusion. Of critical importance to the body as a whole, however, is whether inequalities in gas and blood flow seriously impair the overall ability of the lung to load oxygen into the bloodstream and remove carbon dioxide from the bloodstream. In this section we examine the effect of uneven ventilation and blood flow on the partial pressure and content of arterial blood gases.

Lung models made up of groups of alveoli comprising separate "compartments" in the nonhomogenous lung are used in classical physiologic studies of ventilation-perfusion inequalities (Leff and Schumacker, 1993; West, 1998). These models provide conceptual ways of studying one of the more difficult topics in pulmonary physiology and pathophysiology. It is assumed that all of the alveoli in a given compartment have the same $\dot{V}_A/\dot{Q}$ ratio, but that the $\dot{V}_A/\dot{Q}$ ratios in different compartments have different values.

In Figure 14–4 the nonideal lung is depicted as a *two-compartment lung model*, with a group of alveoli that are normally ventilated and perfused forming one compartment (Compartment A) and another group of alveoli underventilated and underperfused making up the second compartment (Compartment B). Alveolar

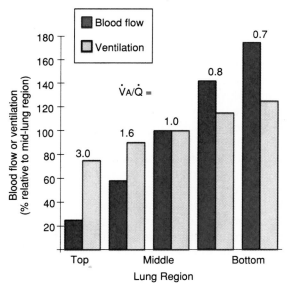

FIGURE 14–3. Ventilation-perfusion gradient in different regions of the upright lung. Relative ventilation, blood flow, and $\dot{V}_A/\dot{Q}$ ratio from the base to the apex of a vertical lung. Alveoli at the bottom of the lung receive more blood flow than ventilation and thus have $\dot{V}_A/\dot{Q}$ ratios of less than 1.0. Alveoli near the top of the lung normally receive somewhat less ventilation than at the base, but they receive much less blood flow. Hence alveoli near the top have $\dot{V}_A/\dot{Q}$ ratios in the range of 1 to 10. Under some circumstances (e.g., hemorrhage), alveoli at the apex may receive some ventilation but no blood flow at all, giving rise to alveoli with $\dot{V}_A/\dot{Q} = \infty$. (From Leff AR and Schumacker PT: Respiratory Physiology: Basics and Applications. WB Saunders, Philadelphia, 1993, p 109, with permission.)

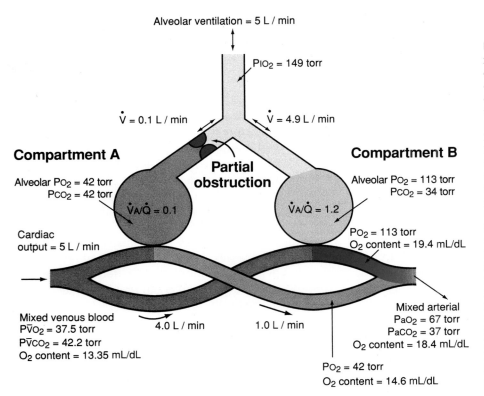

FIGURE 14–4. Two-compartment lung model (nonideal lung). A lung composed of two functional subpopulations of alveoli. The $\dot{V}_A/\dot{Q}$ ratio is the same for all alveoli within each group, but is different between groups. One group of alveoli ($\dot{V}_A/\dot{Q} = 1.2$) receives a blood flow of 4 L/min and an alveolar ventilation of 4.9 L/min. The second group ($\dot{V}_A/\dot{Q} = 0.1$) receives a blood flow of 1.0 L/min and an alveolar ventilation of 0.1 L/min. Because their $\dot{V}_A/\dot{Q}$ ratio is higher, the first group will have an alveolar P_{O_2} closer to the inspired P_{O_2}, while the second group has an alveolar P_{O_2} closer to the mixed venous P_{O_2}. End-capillary blood exiting from the two populations combines to form systemic arterial blood, with $Pa_{O_2} = 67$ torr and $Pa_{CO_2} = 37$ torr. Note that the systemic arterial blood oxygen *content* represents a blood flow–weighted average of the oxygen *contents* exiting from the two populations of alveoli. (From Leff AR and Schumacker PT: Respiratory Physiology: Basics and Applications. WB Saunders, Philadelphia, 1993, p 99, with permission.)

ventilation in this model is 5.0 L/min but the distribution of gas is uneven, with 4.9 L/min of the inspired gas reaching Compartment A and only 0.1 L/min reaching Compartment B because of a partial obstruction of the airway supplying the compartment. Similarly, blood flow through the two compartments is uneven as a result of partial occlusion of blood vessels supplying Compartment B. The cardiac output is 5.0 L/min with 80% (4.0 L/min) of the total flow reaching the normally ventilated lung compartment and 20% (1.0 L/min) of the blood flow reaching the underventilated compartment. Ventilation-perfusion ratios for the two populations of alveoli are calculated as follows (see Fig. 14–4):

Compartment A	Compartment B
$\dot{V}_A/\dot{Q} = \dfrac{4.9 \ \text{L/min}}{4.0 \ \text{L/min}}$	$\dot{V}_A/\dot{Q} = \dfrac{0.1 \ \text{L/min}}{1.0 \ \text{L/min}}$
$\dot{V}_A/\dot{Q} = 1.2$	$\dot{V}_A/\dot{Q} = 0.1$

Because of the higher $\dot{V}_A/\dot{Q}$ ratio in Compartment A, its alveolar P_{O_2} will be significantly higher than that in the other compartment. In fact, the alveolar P_{O_2} of Compartment A will be close to the inspired P_{O_2}, whereas the alveolar P_{O_2} in Compartment B will be closer to the mixed venous P_{O_2} entering the lung. The arterial oxygen tension (Pa_{O_2}) of the blood exiting from the alveoli of the two compartments will reflect

the respective alveolar oxygen tensions in the two compartments. As a result of this uneven gas exchange, the arterial oxygen *saturation* (Sa_{O_2}) of the blood draining the nonideal lung will be a mixture of the blood having an elevated Sa_{O_2} from the high $\dot{V}_A/\dot{Q}$ ratio compartment and blood having a depressed Sa_{O_2} from the low $\dot{V}_A/\dot{Q}$ ratio compartment. The important concept here is that the final systemic arterial oxygen tension reflects a *flow-weighted* contribution from the oxygen contents of the two compartments of the lung model. Compartment A receives most of the blood flow and ventilation and is responsible for most of the systemic arterial oxygen tension and hemoglobin saturation. By contrast, Compartment B receives a very small percentage of the ventilation and blood flow and, therefore, contributes relatively little to the arterial oxygen tension and content. The flow-weighted aspect of the interaction between dissimilar lung compartments produces a total oxygen saturation that is a *mixture* of arterial contents—*not* a numerical *average* of the end-capillary P_{O_2} values (Leff and Schumacker, 1993).

If the Pa_{CO_2} and the respiratory exchange ratio (R) are known, along with the barometric pressure and temperature, the ideal alveolar gas equation can be used to calculate the theoretical alveolar P_{O_2} for the ideal lung. (Recall that this value is found in a homogeneous lung, that is, a lung composed entirely of alveoli having identical $\dot{V}_A/\dot{Q}$ ratios.) The actual arterial P_{O_2} is subtracted from this calculated value to determine the alveolar-arterial oxygen tension gradient. Recall that large $P(A-a)O_2$ values indicate inefficient gas exchange in the lung. In this two-compartment lung model, the alveolar-arterial oxygen tension gradient occurs because of the ventilation-perfusion inequality between compartments. Do any compensatory mechanisms exist? For instance, can a normal arterial PO_2 be attained by overventilating some alveoli to compensate for the low oxygen content coming from poorly ventilated alveoli?

Nonideal lungs with multiple compartments of alveoli having different $\dot{V}A/\dot{Q}$ ratios are less efficient than ideal lungs, as we have seen. The nonlinear shape of the oxyhemoglobin dissociation curve and the resulting partial pressure-oxygen content relationship of blood is useful for illustrating the inefficiency that occurs when alveoli do not have homogeneous $\dot{V}A/\dot{Q}$ ratios (Leff and Schumacker, 1993; West, 1998). For example, compartments with low $\dot{V}A/\dot{Q}$ ratios have low alveolar oxygen tensions. The blood exiting from these alveoli has a relatively low oxygen content because the saturation of hemoglobin is incomplete. Recall that low PO_2 values fall on the lower portion of the oxyhemoglobin dissociation curve (see Fig. 13–4). As this blood mixes with that coming from compartments having higher $\dot{V}A/\dot{Q}$ ratios, the *overall* oxygen content is lowered.

In contrast, alveoli with normal $\dot{V}A/\dot{Q}$ ratios between approximately 0.3 and 10 have alveolar PO_2 values high enough that the hemoglobin in the end-capillary blood from these compartments is almost fully saturated. Recall that PO_2 values in the range of 10 to 60 mm Hg lie on the steep part of the oxyhemoglobin saturation curve. Changes in these PO_2 values generate large incremental changes in the content of arterial blood (see Fig. 13–4). On the other hand, alveoli with high $\dot{V}A/\dot{Q}$ ratios (greater than 10) have alveolar PO_2 values close to the inspired PO_2 but contribute little additional oxygen content to blood because most of the oxygen is added as a small volume of dissolved gas (Leff and Schumacker, 1993; West, 1998). These high PO_2 values intercept the oxyhemoglobin dissociation curve on the elevated plateau portion (see Fig. 13–4). From these relationships it can be seen that overventilating those alveoli with high $\dot{V}A/\dot{Q}$ ratios does not offset the low arterial oxygen content produced by poorly ventilated alveoli with low $\dot{V}A/\dot{Q}$ ratios. In other words, the decrease in arterial oxygen content caused by low $\dot{V}A/\dot{Q}$ ratios is greater than the improvement in arterial oxygen content brought about by high $\dot{V}A/\dot{Q}$ ratios.

$\dot{V}/\dot{Q}$ INEQUALITY IN A MULTICOMPARTMENT LUNG MODEL

If we take the idea of different alveolar compartments in the lung further, we can devise a *multicompartment lung model* composed of eight or more separate compartments, each with a unique $\dot{V}A/\dot{Q}$ ratio (Fig. 14–5A). All of the alveoli with a similar $\dot{V}A/\dot{Q}$ ratio are considered part of the compartment. It turns out that such a multicompartment lung model accurately simulates a real lung and provides a reliable conceptual means of analyzing ventilation-perfusion relationships (Leff and Schumacker, 1993).

In this multicompartment model, $\dot{V}A/\dot{Q}$ ratios are arranged on a logarithmic scale (Fig. 14–5B). The range of physiologic values extends from $\dot{V}A/\dot{Q} = 0$ (blood flow but no ventilation) to $\dot{V}A/\dot{Q} = \infty$ (ventilation but no blood flow). As can be seen in Figure 14–5B, most of the blood flow in a normal, healthy lung is directed to alveoli that are adequately ventilated, with $\dot{V}A/\dot{Q}$ ratios of approximately 1.0. Proportionately less blood perfuses alveoli with $\dot{V}A/\dot{Q}$ ratios substantially greater than or less than this value.

If the distribution of both blood flow and ventilation in a multicompartment model of the normal lung is compared, the two are very similar ($\dot{V}A/\dot{Q} = 1.0$). This finding tells us that adequate blood flow and ventilation is occurring in most of the alveoli of the normal lung. Such a lung is nearly homogenous with respect to $\dot{V}A/\dot{Q}$ ratios and behaves much like the single-compartment lung model discussed with the ideal alveolar oxygen equation (Leff and Schumacker, 1993). Because the gas exchange efficiency in an homogeneous lung is optimal, the alveolar-arterial oxygen tension gradient is quite small. By comparison, the ventilation and blood flow distribution patterns for a multicompartment lung model with nonhomogenous characteristics are *not* similar. Much of the blood flow in the nonhomogenous lung is directed to alveoli that are poorly ventilated. Similarly, the majority of the ventilation is directed to alveoli that are poorly perfused. As a result of these functional mismatches, the resulting $\dot{V}A/\dot{Q}$ ratios in the compartments of the lung are quite different. Consequently, the alveolar and arterial oxygen tensions, as well as the hemoglobin saturation and arterial oxygen content, vary widely in this nonhomogenous lung. The inefficiency of gas exchange, therefore, will be reflected by a large $P(A-a)O_2$ value.

Shunt

INTRAPULMONARY SHUNTING

Up to this point, we have talked about the detrimental effect of nonuniform ventilation and perfusion on arterial oxygen tension and content without actually *naming* the effect—**intrapulmonary shunting,** or simply, **pulmonary shunting.** When blood is delivered to an underventilated alveolus, or to a group of alveoli that are not properly ventilated, the end-capillary blood from that alveolus or compartment will have an oxy-

A.

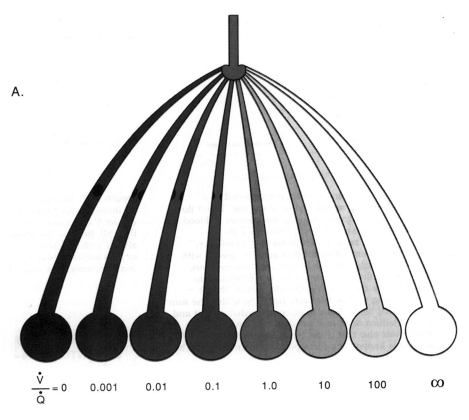

B.

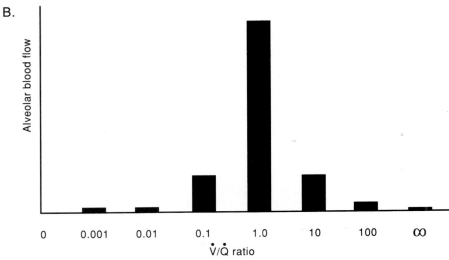

FIGURE 14–5. (A) Multicompartment lung model. A multicompartment lung model, allowing for the possible existence of alveoli with widely varying $\dot{V}A/\dot{Q}$. With the use of this model, a relatively normal lung is described by the histogram. Note that there are no alveoli in this normal lung with $\dot{V}A/\dot{Q}$ less than 0.1. Most of the blood flow is distributed to alveoli with nearly the same $\dot{V}A/\dot{Q}$, which happens to lie near 1.0. Only small amounts of blood flow are distributed to alveoli with $\dot{V}A/\dot{Q}$ near 0.1 or 10.0. Hence most of the "potential compartments" are unused in this example. (B) Histogram of ventilation-perfusion. A relatively homogeneous lung. This histogram describes how much blood flow travels to alveoli with $\dot{V}A/\dot{Q}$ ratios corresponding to the compartment values. Note that most of the blood flow is distributed to alveoli with nearly the same $\dot{V}A/\dot{Q}$ ratio. (From Leff AR and Schumacker PT: Respiratory Physiology: Basics and Applications. WB Saunders, Philadelphia, 1993, p 101, with permission.)

gen tension and an oxygen content very close to that of mixed venous blood entering the alveolar-capillary system. In other words, very little change in blood gases occurs when blood is distributed to a **shunt compartment.** The lack of ventilation of a group of alveoli could occur as a result of an airway obstruction, atelectasis (collapse) of the alveoli, or the accumulation of fluid within alveoli (alveolar edema). Blood exits from these low $\dot{V}A/\dot{Q}$ ratio alveolar compartments, and mixes with blood from normally ventilated alveoli. The resulting blend is called a *venous admixture,* also known as a *phys-*

iologic shunt or *wasted blood flow* (West, 1998). The P_{O_2} of this blood is greater than the P_{O_2} of mixed venous blood, but less than the P_{O_2} of arterial blood coming from normally ventilated compartments.

Figure 14–6 shows a multicompartment lung model composed of three separate groups of alveoli representing compartments with three different ventilation-perfusion relationships. This simplified multicompartment lung model is useful for discussing the effects of intrapulmonary shunting on the partial pressure and content of arterial blood gases. In this model a fraction of the to-

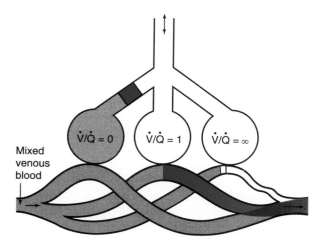

FIGURE 14–6. Three-compartment lung model (nonhomogeneous lung). Three-compartment model of the lung, which allows for the existence of alveoli with blood flow but no ventilation ($\dot{V}A/\dot{Q} = 0$), normal blood flow and ventilation ($\dot{V}A/\dot{Q} \approx 1$), and ventilation but no blood flow ($\dot{V}A/\dot{Q} = \infty$). Note that all gas exchange in this lung occurs in the middle compartment. (From Leff AR and Schumacker PT: Respiratory Physiology: Basics and Applications. WB Saunders, Philadelphia, 1993, p 103, with permission.)

tal cardiac output ($\dot{Q}T$) is distributed to the shunt compartment, that is, to the group of alveoli not ventilated ($\dot{V}A/\dot{Q} = 0$). Oxygen will not be loaded into the blood flowing through this compartment (see Fig. 14–8). A portion of the $\dot{Q}T$ is also distributed to the normally ventilated, or nonshunted, compartment. This group of alveoli behaves much like the ideal, or homogenous, lung discussed previously ($\dot{V}A/\dot{Q} = 0.3$ to 10.0). Finally, a fraction of the cardiac output fails to reach some alveoli in this three-compartment model ($\dot{V}A/\dot{Q} = \infty$). Obviously, no oxygen will be loaded in this compartment representing *alveolar dead space* (see Fig. 14–6). In summary, the only compartment in this model in which gas exchange takes place is the middle compartment where ventilation is closely matched to perfusion. As noted previously, the gas tension and content in the end-capillary blood exiting from the lung will be an admixture that represents the flow-weighted average of the effluent blood emerging from each compartment.

Determination of the fraction of cardiac output perfusing nonventilated lung compartments compared with normally ventilated compartments provides a useful index of gas exchange efficiency in the lung. For example, if a large percentage of the total blood flow is directed to lung regions that are not properly ventilated, rather than to alveoli with optimal $\dot{V}A/\dot{Q}$ ratios, overall gas exchange in the lung will be adversely affected and arterial hypoxemia may result.

The total amount of oxygen flowing into the systemic arteries (milliliters per minute) is the sum of the oxygen flows from each lung compartment. The oxygen flowrate for each compartment is the product of the

oxygen content of the blood exiting from the compartment and the *blood flowrate* for the compartment. Therefore, the total flow of oxygen in arterial blood ($\dot{Q}T \times CaO_2$) must equal the flow of oxygen from the shunt compartment ($\dot{Q}s \times C\bar{v}O_2$) plus the flow of oxygen from the nonshunt compartment [$(\dot{Q}T - \dot{Q}s) \times Cc'O_2$]. Recall that $Cc'O_2$ refers to the oxygen content of capillary blood exiting from normally ventilated alveoli, and that the saturation of this end-capillary blood is assumed to be 100%. The various oxygen flow relationships can be combined in the following equation:

$$\dot{Q}T \times CaO_2 = [\dot{Q}s \times C\bar{v}O_2] + [(\dot{Q}T - \dot{Q}s) \times Cc'O_2]$$

where:

$\dot{Q}T$	= total cardiac output
$\dot{Q}s$	= blood flow through shunt compartment
$\dot{Q}T - \dot{Q}s$	= blood flow through nonshunt compartment
CaO_2	= oxygen content of arterial blood
$C\bar{v}O_2$	= oxygen content of mixed venous blood
$Cc'O_2$	= end-capillary ideal oxygen content

This equation can be rearranged and solved for the fraction of cardiac output that perfuses the shunt compartment ($\dot{Q}s/\dot{Q}T$). The following **classic shunt equation** provides an index of gas exchange efficiency in the lung and is commonly used in respiratory physiology in arterial blood gas calculations (Leff and Schumacker, 1993; Malley, 1990; West, 1998).

$$\dot{Q}s/\dot{Q}T = \frac{Cc'O_2 - CaO_2}{Cc'O_2 - C\bar{v}O_2}$$

EXAMPLE

Calculate the *shunt fraction* for a patient breathing 100% oxygen using the following data:

$$P_{BAR} = 760 \text{ mm Hg}$$
$$\text{Body temp} = 37°C$$
$$PaO_2 = 80 \text{ mm Hg}$$
$$PaCO_2 = 40 \text{ mm Hg}$$
$$P\bar{v}O_2 = 40 \text{ mm Hg}$$
$$SaO_2 = 90\%$$
$$S\bar{v}O_2 = 65\%$$
$$Hb = 14 \text{ g\%}$$

To determine the shunt fraction in this patient, we need to use the ideal alveolar oxygen equation; therefore, we must first calculate the oxygen content of the blood. Recall from Chapter 13 that the oxygen content of blood is determined by the volume of oxygen bound to hemoglobin and the volume of oxygen dissolved in plasma. Furthermore, the values of the oxygen content of blood in different locations must be added together to arrive at the *total* oxygen content. With this patient, we have enough data to directly calculate both the arterial and the mixed venous oxygen contents:

- Arterial blood:

$$Ca_{O_2} = \frac{(1.34 \text{ mL O}_2 \times x \text{ g\% Hb} \times Sa_{O_2})}{1 \text{ g\% Hb}}$$

$$+ \frac{(0.003 \text{ mL O}_2/100 \text{ mL}}{1 \text{ mm Hg } Pa_{O_2}} \times x \text{ mm Hg } Pa_{O_2})$$

$$= \frac{(1.34 \text{ mL O}_2 \times (14 \text{ g\% Hb} \times 0.9)}{1 \text{ g\% Hb}}$$

$$+ \frac{(0.003 \text{ mL O}_2/100 \text{ mL} \times 80 \text{ mm Hg } Pa_{O_2})}{1 \text{ mm Hg } Pa_{O_2}}$$

$$= 16.884 \text{ mL} + 0.24 \text{ mL}/100 \text{ mL}$$

$$Ca_{O_2} = 17.12 \text{ mL}/100 \text{ mL}$$

- Mixed venous blood:

$$C\bar{v}_{O_2} = \frac{(1.34 \text{ mL O}_2 \times x \text{ g\% Hb} \times S\bar{v}_{O_2})}{1 \text{ g\% Hb}}$$

$$+ \frac{(0.003 \text{ mL O}_2/100 \text{ mL} \times x \text{ mm Hg } P\bar{v}_{O_2})}{1 \text{ mm Hg } P\bar{v}_{O_2}}$$

$$= \frac{(1.34 \text{ mL O}_2 \times 14 \text{ g\% Hb} \times 0.65)}{1 \text{ g\% Hb}}$$

$$+ \frac{(0.003 \text{ mL O}_2/100 \text{ mL} \times 40 \text{ mm Hg } P\bar{v}_{O_2})}{1 \text{ mm Hg } P\bar{v}_{O_2}}$$

$$= 12.194 \text{ mL} + 0.12 \text{ mL}/100 \text{ mL}$$

$$C\bar{v}_{O_2} = 12.31 \text{ mL}/100 \text{ mL}$$

In these calculations the volume of oxygen bound to hemoglobin is expressed in milliliters (mL), whereas the fraction dissolved in plasma is shown as milliliters of oxygen per 100 mL of blood (mL/100 mL, or vol% O_2). It is convenient to think of oxygen as the *solute*, whereas the 100 mL (1 dL) volume of blood is the *solution* in which the solute is found. Therefore, when additional solute (oxyhemoglobin) is added to the blood solution, the total concentration of oxygen in the bloodstream increases. Keep in mind, however, that the fraction of oxygen bound to hemoglobin is not, itself, freely dissolved in plasma—instead, it is the oxyhemoglobin molecules that are dissolved in, and transported by, the plasma component of blood.

The oxygen content of blood exiting from the ideal compartment (Cc'_{O_2}) can be determined using the ideal alveolar oxygen equation. When breathing pure oxygen ($FiO_2 = 1$), the alveoli contain only carbon dioxide, oxygen, and water vapor. Therefore, the ideal alveolar oxygen tension (PA_{O_2}) is calculated by subtracting the alveolar carbon dioxide tension (PA_{CO_2}) and the water

vapor pressure (PH_2O) from the barometric pressure ($PBAR$). Water vapor pressure is equal to 47 mm Hg at 37°C body temperature. Assume that equilibration of carbon dioxide occurs between the alveolus and the bloodstream, making the PA_{CO_2} equal to the Pa_{CO_2} value given for this patient. Further, assume that the respiratory exchange ratio (R) is equal to 1. Therefore, applying the ideal alveolar oxygen equation:

$$PA_{O_2} = FiO_2 \times (PBAR - PH_2O) - \frac{PA_{CO_2}}{R}$$

$$= 1 \times (760 \text{ mm Hg} - 47 \text{ mm Hg}) - \frac{40 \text{ mm Hg}}{1}$$

$$\therefore PA_{O_2} = 673 \text{ mm Hg}$$

Finally, assume that hemoglobin is 100% saturated when the P_{O_2} is above 150 mm Hg and calculate the oxygen content of end-capillary blood coming from the ideal compartment:

$$Cc'_{O_2} = \frac{(1.34 \text{ mL O}_2 \times x \text{ g\% Hb} \times 1)}{1 \text{ g\% Hb}}$$

$$+ \frac{(0.003 \text{ mL O}_2/100 \text{ mL} \times x \text{ mm Hg } PA_{O_2})}{1 \text{ mm Hg } Pa_{O_2}}$$

$$= \frac{(1.34 \text{ mL O}_2 \times 14 \text{ g\% Hb} \times 1)}{1 \text{ g\% Hb}}$$

$$+ \frac{(0.003 \text{ mL O}_2/100 \text{ mL} \times 673 \text{ mm Hg } PA_{O_2})}{1 \text{ mm Hg } PA_{O_2}}$$

$$= 18.76 \text{ mL} + 2.019 \text{ mL}/100 \text{ mL}$$

$$Cc'_{O_2} = 20.78 \text{ mL}/100 \text{ mL}$$

Now that we have calculated the oxygen content of arterial blood, mixed venous blood, and end-capillary blood from the ideal compartment, we can calculate the shunt fraction:

$$\frac{\dot{Q}s}{\dot{Q}T} = \frac{Cc'_{O_2} - Ca_{O_2}}{Cc'_{O_2} - C\bar{v}_{O_2}}$$

$$= \frac{20.78 \text{ mL}/100 \text{ mL} - 17.12 \text{ mL}/100 \text{ mL}}{20.78 \text{ mL}/100 \text{ mL} - 12.31 \text{ mL}/100 \text{ mL}}$$

$$= \frac{3.66 \text{ mL}/100 \text{ mL}}{8.47 \text{ mL}/100 \text{ mL}}$$

$$\therefore \dot{Q}s/\dot{Q}T = 0.43$$

This shunt fraction tells us that approximately 43% of the cardiac output went to the nonfunctional shunt compartment, while about 57% perfused the nonshunted ideal alveoli. The resulting decrease in gas exchange efficiency in this patient is reflected in the large alveolar-arterial oxygen tension gradient:

$$P(A–a)_{O_2} = 673 \text{ mm Hg} - 80 \text{ mm Hg}$$

$$= 593 \text{ mm Hg}$$

Although the classic shunt equation is somewhat cumbersome, it provides a sophisticated and accurate measure of gas exchange efficiency. A technical drawback of the classic shunt equation is the requirement for oxygenation data from mixed venous blood samples. These measurements must be obtained via an indwelling pulmonary artery catheter, a device not always readily available for all patients.

To address the practical limitation of obtaining mixed venous blood samples, modified versions of the classic shunt equation have been developed. **Estimated shunt equations** are used when sampling of mixed venous blood is unavailable or not practical. These derived equations assume a given arteriovenous oxygen content difference, or $C(a - \bar{v})O_2$, in their calculations. Some versions of the modified shunt equation use 5 vol%, while others use 3.5 vol% for the $C(a - \bar{v})O_2$ assumption. The classic shunt equation is rearranged as an estimated shunt equation to accommodate the arteriovenous oxygen content difference factor, as in the following example:

$$\dot{Q}s/\dot{Q}T = \frac{Cc'O_2 - CaO_2}{(Cc'O_2 - CaO_2) + 5.0}$$

NOTE: In addition to the alveolar-arterial oxygen tension gradient, classic shunt equation, and estimated shunt equations, other indices of gas exchange efficiency are employed in clinical studies of ventilation-perfusion relationships (e.g., PaO_2/PAO_2 ratio and PaO_2/FIO_2 ratio), and in clinical studies of oxygenation status of patients (e.g., PaO_2 and SaO_2). Each index has unique advantages and disadvantages that are discussed in textbooks specializing in the measurement and interpretation of clinical blood gases (see chapter bibliography for suitable references).

EXTRAPULMONARY SHUNTING

Up to this point we have discussed ventilation-perfusion inequalities produced when blood undergoes pulmonary shunting—that is, when blood in the pulmonary circuit bypasses normally ventilated areas of the lung and fails to load oxygen. *Shunt,* then, refers to blood that enters systemic arteries without going through ventilated regions of the lung. Can blood be diverted from ventilated areas of the lung *before* it even reaches the lung? In other words, can blood be shunted away from the lung itself?

Extrapulmonary shunting refers to mechanisms whereby a portion of desaturated blood enters the systemic arteries without first passing through the pulmonary arteries. As we have seen with intrapulmonary shunting, *extra*pulmonary shunting results in an overall decrease in hemoglobin saturation. The

shunt itself, however, is found outside the lung. In the healthy lung, this interesting mechanism is responsible for approximately 1% to 2% of the reduction in arterial oxygen saturation from its theoretical maximum of $SaO_2 = 100\%$ (Leff and Schumacker, 1993).

Several sources of extrapulmonary shunts are found in the normal lung. For example, bronchial circulation delivers systemic arterial blood to the bronchi and large airways. After gas exchange occurs in these organs, a portion of the desaturated blood is returned to pulmonary circulation "downstream" from the alveolar capillaries. The *bronchial veins* empty this mixed venous blood directly into the pulmonary veins, which contain end-capillary blood exiting from the alveoli. As a result of this extrapulmonary shunt, the oxygen tension of blood in the left atrium is reduced. In a similar way, a portion of the mixed venous blood coming from the myocardium is returned directly to the chamber of the left ventricle by several *thebesian veins.* Although the flowrate through thebesian veins is small, the blood itself has a very low mixed venous oxygen tension, thereby causing a reduction in the arterial oxygen content of blood in the left ventricle (Leff and Schumacker, 1993). Most of the desaturated blood emptying the heart muscle drains into the coronary sinus located on the posterior side of the right atrium. (The coronary sinus returns most of the desaturated blood to the right side of the heart where it is pumped through the pulmonary circuit to the alveoli of the lung.) In the healthy lung, venous drainage via the bronchial and thebesian veins is responsible for a small alveolar-arterial oxygen tension gradient of approximately 10 mm Hg.

In addition to normal circulatory structures located peripheral to the pulmonary circuit, abnormal cardiovascular structures may contribute to extrapulmonary shunting. For example, *congenital heart defects,* such as an opening in the interventricular septum, result in desaturated blood mixing with systemic arterial blood. The resulting venous admixture has a lower arterial oxygen content than would occur in the absence of the extrapulmonary shunt. Similarly, a *patent ductus arteriosus* in a newborn allows desaturated blood from the right heart to mix with systemic arterial blood pumped out of the left heart, thus lowering the oxygen content of the blood entering the systemic circuit (see Chap. 16).

Hypoxia

Hypoxemia is the condition that results when low PO_2 levels are found in arterial blood. Various conditions such as *hypoventilation, diffusion impairment, ventilation-perfusion inequalities (relative shunting),* and *absolute* or *true shunting* contribute to hypoxemia. In this section, we briefly discuss how these conditions produce different types of hypoxemia that may lead to oxygen deficit in the tissues. The section, however, is not designed to cover all of the pathophysiologic conditions that affect oxygenation of the tissues. Subsequent courses in respiratory pathophysiology and clinical blood gas analysis will fill that requirement.

Certain terms need to be clarified. **Hypoxia** refers to low or inadequate oxygen or a relative deficiency of oxygen for cellular metabolism. The renowned physiologist J. S. Haldane (1919) observed, "Hypoxia not only breaks the machine, it wrecks the machinery." The prevention, detection, and treatment of tissue hypoxia is one of the most important goals in the management of patients with cardiopulmonary disease (Malley, 1990). For this reason, the respiratory care practitioner needs to have a solid background in the relevant physiologic mechanisms affecting internal respiration and the oxygenation of tissues.

The degree of hypoxemia in an individual is an indicator of the likelihood of hypoxia developing in the tissues. Mild hypoxemia usually does not lead to hypoxia, whereas moderate hypoxemia *may* lead to tissue hypoxia if increased cardiac output does not compensate to deliver additional oxygen to the tissues. Severe hypoxemia generally leads to true tissue hypoxia (Malley, 1990). Clearly, there is a functional link between hypoxemia and hypoxia. Indeed, the whole *point* of breathing is to oxygenate the tissues. If vital organs such as the heart and brain are not oxygenated, the combined processes of ventilation of the lung, oxygen extraction from the air, and transport of oxygen to the tissues, are in vain. **Anoxia** refers to a complete lack of oxygen, a condition that can technically exist for only a very brief period.

Several classification schemes exist to describe various types of hypoxia, but the traditional four-type system is used in this section (Ganong, 1995). The four types of hypoxia are as follows:

- *Hypoxemic hypoxia* caused by reduced arterial Pa_{O_2}
- *Anemic hypoxia*, in which the Pa_{O_2} is normal but the amount of hemoglobin is reduced
- *Stagnant hypoxia*, a condition whereby the Pa_{O_2} and hemoglobin amounts are normal but the blood flow is so low that tissue oxygenation does not occur
- *Histotoxic hypoxia*, a condition in which a normal volume of oxygen is delivered to the tissues but the cells are unable to utilize the oxygen, usually because of failure of a critical enzyme system (Table 14–1)

HYPOXEMIC HYPOXIA

Clinically, **hypoxic hypoxia** is commonly referred to as **hypoxemic hypoxia,** a state of oxygen deficiency in the bloodstream. Hypoxic hypoxia is a condition of relative oxygen deficiency in the tissues caused by low arterial oxygen tension, which in turn, can result from a variety of causes including:

- *Low alveolar oxygen tension:* A low Pa_{O_2} may lead to a decrease in the Pa_{O_2} and Ca_{O_2}; low alveolar oxygen tension may be caused by (1) *hypoventilation* as a result of chronic obstructive pulmonary diseases (COPDs) such as emphysema that impair gas exchange in the lung, drug overdose via central nervous system depressants such as narcotics or barbiturates that depress central ventilatory (hypercapnic) drive, neuromuscular diseases such as myasthenia gravis that weaken muscles of breathing; (2) *high altitude* that reduces barometric pressure and inspired oxygen tension; and (3) *suffocation* caused by anesthetic gas mixtures containing low concentrations of oxygen.
- *Diffusion impairment:* Pathophysiologic conditions that alter the structure and function of the blood-gas interface include: (1) *interstitial fibrosis*, (2) *alveolar fibrosis*, (3) *interstitial edema*, and (4) *alveolar edema*. These pathophysiologic conditions slow gas transfer at the alveolar-capillary membrane and are considered diffusion-limited problems.
- *Intrapulmonary shunting:* Blood that exits from nonventilated alveoli mixes with that from normally ventilated alveoli to form a venous admixture with a reduced, flow-weighted average of Pa_{O_2} and Ca_{O_2}. The greater the $\dot{V}_A/\dot{Q}$ ratio mismatch, the less homogeneous the lung and the greater the hypoxemia produced. This type of shunt is called a **relative shunt.**
- *Extrapulmonary shunting:* Blood that reaches the left ventricle without coming into contact with the pulmonary circulation causes mixed venous blood to be blended with oxygenated blood entering the systemic arteries. This type of shunt is called an **absolute shunt** or a **true shunt.**

A **physiologic shunt** occurs when blood is not properly oxygenated. As pointed out previously, the result of the shunting is reduced arterial oxygen content in the systemic arteries. In general, two types of physiologic shunt are recognized: *relative shunt* and *absolute shunt.*

Relative Shunt

During intrapulmonary shunting, a portion of the pulmonary bloodstream enters the lung but is not saturated with oxygen from the alveoli. This type of physiologic shunt is a *shuntlike* effect called a *relative shunt.* The implication here is that the reduction in arterial oxygen tension and content occurs "as if" an actual structure was present that was responsible for causing a portion of the blood stream to bypass the lungs and thus not be oxygenated (Leff and Schumacker, 1993;

TABLE 14-1	Types of Hypoxia	
Hypoxia	**Description**	**Causes**

Hypoxemic hypoxia	Oxygen deficiency in the bloodstream (i.e., low Pa_{O_2}) that may lead to *hypoxic hypoxia,* or a deficiency of oxygen in the tissues	• Low Pa_{O_2} as a result of:
		Hypoventilation (COPD, CNS depressant overdose, head injury, neuromuscular disease)
		High altitude (low P_{BAR} results in decreased $P_{I_{O_2}}$ and Pa_{O_2})
		Suffocation (e.g., anesthetic gas mixtures with insufficient oxygen)
		
		• Diffusion impairment (reduced efficiency of gas exchange at the A-C membrane) caused by:
		Interstitial fibrosis
		Alveolar fibrosis
		Interstitial edema
		Alveolar edema
		
		• Intrapulmonary shunting (or a relative shunt) is a type of physiologic shunt described as a *shuntlike effect* caused by blood from nonventilated alveoli mixing with blood from ventilated alveoli to form a venous admixture with reduced Pa_{O_2} and Ca_{O_2}. Causes include:
		Bronchospasm
		Mucus plugging
		Pulmonary vasodilator drugs
		Diffusion defects (e.g., alveolar fibrosis, alveolar edema)
		
		• Extrapulmonary shunting (or absolute shunt or true shunt) is a type of physiologic shunt caused by blood reaching the left ventricle without being oxygenated by passage through the pulmonary circulation. The result is a venous admixture with reduced Pa_{O_2} and Ca_{O_2}:
		Anatomic shunts normally occur due to the introduction of desaturated blood from bronchial and thebesian veins into the systemic circulation. Abnormal anatomic shunts are caused by:
		  ○ Congenital heart defects (e.g., persistent foramen ovale, persistent ductus arteriosus)
		  ○ Vascular lung tumors
		Capillary shunts occur with severe functional or structural impairment of the A-C membrane:
		  ○ Alveolar consolidation
		  ○ Atelectasis
		  ○ Pulmonary edema

Anemic hypoxia	Oxygen deficiency in the tissues caused by reduced amount of hemoglobin in circulation (reduction in the number of RBCs, Hb, or both)	• Reduced number of RBCs caused by: Pernicious anemia (vitamin B_{12} deficiency) Acute hemorrhage Aplastic anemia (as a result of bone marrow damage) • Reduced Hb caused by: Iron-deficiency anemia Sickle cell anemia Carboxyhemoglobinemia Methemoglobinemia
Stagnant hypoxia or ischemic hypoxia	Severely reduced blood flow to the tissues results in a relative deficiency of oxygen in spite of normal Pa_{O_2} and Ca_{O_2} levels.	• Decreased cardiac output • Vascular insufficiency • Arteriovenous shunts • Imbalance between metabolic demand for oxygen and oxygen supplied by the blood (e.g., angina pectoris)
Histotoxic hypoxia	Poisoning of key enzymes needed in cellular respiration and utilization of oxygen in spite of normal Pa_{O_2} and Ca_{O_2} levels	• Cyanide poisoning • Strychnine poisoning

A-C = alveolar-capillary membrane; COPD = chronic obstructive pulmonary disease; CNS = central nervous system; Hb = hemoglobin; RBC = red blood cell.

West, 1998). Lungs with a high degree of ventilation-perfusion inequality, that is, lungs that are heterogeneous with respect to $\dot{V}A/\dot{Q}$ ratios, exhibit a high degree of relative shunting. Relative shunting is probably the most common clinical hypoxemic mechanism observed in patients, and is especially prevalent in patients with uncomplicated COPD (Malley, 1990).

Relative shunting may be caused by *bronchospasm, mucus plugging,* or both. In these conditions, ventilation is unevenly distributed, resulting in ventilation-perfusion mismatches. Relative shunting can also develop suddenly following administration of drugs that cause dilation of pulmonary blood vessels, including common bronchodilators such as albuterol (salbutamol) and vasodilators such as nitroglycerin. *Diffusion defects* in which the alveolar-capillary membrane is partially impaired also contribute to relative shunt. Conditions in which the membrane is thickened (e.g., alveolar fibrosis), or accumulated fluid is present (e.g., alveolar edema), slow the diffusion of oxygen and contribute to ventilation-perfusion inequality. In these conditions, the alveolus is adequately ventilated, but the normal capillary transit time (0.75 s) does not permit equilibration of gases to occur.

> **NOTE:** If the diffusion defect is extensive enough to totally block gas transfer at the air-blood interface, the shunt is referred to as a *true capillary shunt*—see next section.

Unlike absolute shunting, relative shunting is exquisitely sensitive to supplemental oxygen therapy. In other words, there is a good PaO_2 response when oxygen therapy is initiated. The alveoli of the shunt compartment—the lung region receiving perfusion in excess of ventilation—become more efficient in gas transfer because their inspired oxygen tension (PIO_2) is elevated by the higher FIO_2 values achieved via supplemental oxygen. Conversely, the PaO_2 falls dramatically in patients with relative shunt when oxygen therapy is discontinued. This marked response of arterial oxygen tension to therapeutic oxygen is caused by the fact that the high levels of hemoglobin saturation produced by supplemental oxygen occur on the elevated plateau region of the oxyhemoglobin dissociation curve (see Fig. 13–4). Therefore, a small change in hemoglobin saturation corresponds to a large incremental change in the arterial oxygen tension.

True Shunt

A physiologic shunt in which desaturated blood mixes with oxygenated blood without contacting the pulmonary bloodstream is called a *true shunt* or an *absolute shunt.* True shunts are refractory (resistant) to oxygen therapy. Because oxygen does not come in contact with the shunted blood, alveoli are unable to accommodate any improvement in ventilation brought about by therapeutic oxygen. Hypoxemic hypoxia, therefore, is not relieved by supplemental oxygen in patients with absolute shunt. True shunts are further subdivided into two groups—*anatomic shunts* and *capillary shunts* (Malley, 1990; West, 1998).

Anatomic Shunts

True Shunt

Recall that the healthy lung normally exhibits a small amount of anatomic shunting (1% to 2% of cardiac output) as a result of desaturated blood entering into systemic circulation through the bronchial and thebesian veins. An abnormal amount of anatomic shunting, however, occurs with the following conditions:

- *Congenital heart defects:* Congenital cardiovascular anomalies such as ventricular septal defects that allow blood to move from the right heart to the left heart are called **anatomic shunts.** Similarly, newborns with persistent fetal circulation have anatomic shunting that allows blood to bypass the pulmonary circuit in the lung. Abnormal fetal structures accompanied by anatomic shunting include a persistent foramen ovale, which allows blood to move from the right atrium to the left atrium, and a patent ductus arteriosus, which allows blood to move from the pulmonary circuit into the systemic circuit (see Chap. 16). According to Malley (1990), decreasing the pulmonary vascular resistance (PVR) in cases of persistent fetal circulation may greatly improve arterial PO_2 (Box 14–1). Pulmonary intervention is generally ineffective in cases of anatomic shunting. Such conditions often require surgical methods to produce satisfactory results (Malley, 1990). In general, structural defects of the cardiovascular system allow mixing of desaturated and reoxygenated blood, thus producing a venous admixture that contributes to hypoxemic hypoxia
- *Vascular lung tumors:* Highly vascularized tumors may permit desaturated blood to flow from the lung into pulmonary veins, creating a venous admixture that is returned to the left atrium to be pumped into systemic arteries by the left ventricle.

Capillary Shunt

If pathophysiologic conditions affecting the gas-blood interface are severe enough to totally block gas exchange in the alveolar-capillary system, they are classified as true **capillary shunts.** These conditions include *alveolar consolidation* (fluid accumulation) and *atelectasis.* In addition, pulmonary edema accompanying cardiogenic conditions such as left-sided heart fail-

P E R S P E C T I V E S

BOX 14-1

Improvement of V̇a/Q̇ Inequality through Selective Vasodilation

Dilation of blood vessels, either precapillary arterioles, postcapillary veins, or both, is an effective way to reduce vascular resistance and lower blood pressure. A variety of antihypertensive drugs (e.g., β_2- and α_1-adrenergic blockers, calcium channel blockers, angiotensin-converting enzyme inhibitors, aldosterone antagonists) either bring about dilation or prevent contraction of blood vessels. What if a decrease in PVR is desirable *without* a corresponding decrease in systemic vascular resistance (SVR)? None of the traditional antihypertensive drugs listed above is suitable because they change vascular resistance in *both* circulatory loops. Their lack of specificity is especially troublesome in the treatment of ARDS and persistent pulmonary hypertension of the newborn (PPHN).

In ARDS, acute lung injury results in physiologic derangements that include loss of surfactant function, pulmonary arterial hypertension caused by vasoconstriction, and intrapulmonary shunting that results in arterial hypoxemia. Acute pulmonary hypertension may lead to pulmonary edema and increased stress on the right ventricle. In some neonates with congenital heart defects such as persistent ductus arteriosus, PPHN may develop. In this syndrome, there is a state of fetal circulation complete with right-to-left shunting, elevated pulmonary vascular resistance, and reduced pulmonary blood flow. These conditions lead to *ventilation-perfusion inequalities,* hypoxemia, and a vicious cycle, as pulmonary vasculature constricts further and pulmonary hypertension increases.

In theory, vasodilator therapy should improve the hemodynamic dysfunctions associated with ARDS and PPHN. The traditional drugs, however, cause widespread dilation of pulmonary blood vessels throughout the entire pulmonary circuit, thus increasing the perfusion of underventilated regions. The increased flow to areas of intrapulmonary shunting worsens the ventilation-perfusion (V̇a/Q̇ ratio) mismatch and further reduces arterial oxygen tension (PaO_2).

Nitric oxide (NO), on the other hand, shows great promise as a pulmonary vasodilator drug in the treatment of pulmonary hypertension. NO is administered as an inhaled gas that rapidly diffuses out of the alveoli. Its vasodilating effects are highly localized and limited to *ventilated areas* of the lung. In addition, it binds to oxyhemoglobin and is rapidly inactivated. As a result of these actions, systemic vascular effects are minimized. By reducing PVR and selectively improving blood flow to damaged regions of the lung in cases of pulmonary hypertension associated with ARDS and PPHN, nitric oxide improves the matching of ventilation and perfusion, reduces intrapulmonary shunting, and increases PaO_2 without affecting systemic vascular resistance.

- Bone RC: A new therapy for the adult respiratory distress syndrome (editorial). N Engl J Med 328:431–432, 1993.
- Hudson LD: Pharmacologic approaches to respiratory failure. Respiratory Care 38:754–764, 1993.
- Malinowski C: Persistent pulmonary hypertension of the newborn. In Wilkins RL and Dexter JR (eds): Respiratory Disease: Principles of Patient Care, ed 2. FA Davis, Philadelphia, 1997.
- Maunder RJ and Hudson LD: Pharmacologic strategies for treating the adult respiratory distress syndrome. Respiratory Care 35:241–246, 1990.
- McCarty KD: Adult respiratory distress syndrome. In Wilkins RL and Dexter JR (eds): Respiratory Disease: Principles of Patient Care, ed 2. FA Davis, Philadelphia, 1997.
- Pison U et al: Inhaled nitric oxide reverses hypoxic pulmonary vasoconstriction without impairing gas exchange. J Appl Physiol 74:1287–1292, 1993.
- Roberts JD et al: Inhaled nitric oxide in congenital heart disease. Circulation 87:447–453, 1993.
- Rossaint R et al: Inhaled nitric oxide for the adult respiratory distress syndrome. N Engl J Med 328:399–405, 1993.

ure, as well as noncardiogenic conditions such as adult respiratory distress syndrome (ARDS), is associated with true capillary shunting. Pulmonary edema is responsible for much of the severe, absolute capillary shunting seen in critical care units (Malley, 1990).

Like other absolute shunts, true capillary shunts are unresponsive to oxygen therapy; therefore, hypoxemia persists in these cases. Keep in mind that these abnormal conditions may be moderately severe, in which case partial gas exchange occurs at the alveolar capillaries. Under such circumstances the physiologic shunt is classified as a relative shunt and will, therefore, be somewhat responsive to oxygen therapy. Differentiation of relative and true capillary shunting is based on the degree of change observed in the arterial oxygen tension following administration of supplemental oxygen. A marked increase in PaO_2 following an increase of FIO_2 suggests *relative* capillary shunting, whereas a small increase in PaO_2 in response to supplemental oxygen therapy is typical of *absolute* capillary shunting. The $P(A–a)O_2$ is normally less than 50 mm Hg at an FIO_2 of 1.0 (100% oxygen). Therefore, an alveolar-arterial oxygen tension gradient less than 50 mm Hg indicates a relative shunt effect, whereas, an increase in $P(A–a)O_2$ above 50 mm Hg indicates the presence of an absolute shunt effect (Malley, 1990). Breathing FIO_2 of 1.0 leads *in itself* to pulmonary problems such as an increase in true capillary shunting and atelectasis; therefore, the "100% oxygen test" is rarely done (Malley, 1990). The principle, however, is valid for differentiating relative from absolute capillary shunting.

Figure 14–7 summarizes the classification of the various physiologic shunts discussed in this section.

ANEMIC HYPOXIA

In a condition known as **anemic hypoxia** the amount of hemoglobin available for oxygen transport is reduced. In Chapter 13 we examined the form and function of hemoglobin in relation to gas transport. Because hemoglobin is found within red blood cells, the *hematocrit* (Hct), or volume of formed elements by volume, is a measure of potential oxygen-carrying ability

and is, therefore, a useful indicator of anemia. Recall that red blood cells (RBCs) make up most of the Hct, which is normally about 45% (see Fig. 13–1).

In general, the presence of anemia in a patient indicates either that there is a decrease in the production of RBCs or hemoglobin, or that RBCs or hemoglobin are being destroyed at an increased rate. Several types of anemia are recognized. The reader is encouraged to consult appropriate pathophysiology references for additional information. Reduction in the actual number of erythrocytes in circulation occurs with conditions such as *pernicious anemia,* caused by vitamin B_{12} deficiency; *acute blood loss* caused by severe hemorrhage; and *aplastic anemia* caused by bone marrow damage. Reduction in the synthesis of hemoglobin, or in the loss of function of hemoglobin is seen in conditions such as *iron-deficiency anemia* caused by low levels of iron, which is needed for the production of heme units in hemoglobin; *sickle cell anemia,* caused by formation of sickle cell hemoglobin (HbS) that causes deformation of RBCs; and production of abnormal species of hemoglobin such as *carboxyhemoglobin* (COHb) and *methemoglobin* (MetHb). Hemoglobin bound to carbon monoxide (CO) exhibits a marked reduction in the oxygen-binding capacity. Similarly, *methemoglobinemia* occurs when iron is oxidized to the ferric (Fe^{3+}) form, thus rendering hemoglobin molecules nonfunctional with respect to oxygen transport.

If any of the previous conditions are severe enough, anemic hypoxia occurs because of the overall reduction in the amount of functional hemoglobin available for oxygen transport to the tissues. Mild anemia (e.g., Hb = 10 g%) generally does *not* result in hypoxia (Malley, 1990). This surprising finding is due to the large reserve of oxygen normally present in the blood and to the compensatory mechanisms of the cardiovascular system. Only about 25% of the oxygen in arterial blood is normally extracted by the tissues, leaving a substantial reserve supply in the bloodstream (Malley, 1990). Compensatory mechanisms include increased cardiac output and increased production of 2,3-diphosphoglycerate (2,3-DPG) in red blood cells. An increase in the concentration of 2,3-DPG in RBCs causes a decrease in the affinity of hemoglobin for oxygen and a rightward

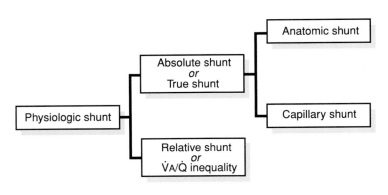

FIGURE 14–7. Types of physiologic shunt. Absolute shunts are also called *extrapulmonary shunts,* a classification that can be misleading in the case of capillary shunts because alveolar capillaries are clearly located *within* the lung. When the structure or function of the alveolar-capillary membrane is severely impaired, a true shunt develops that is unresponsive to supplemental oxygen therapy. In this way, capillary shunts are like other types of absolute or true shunts. Relative shunts are also called *intrapulmonary shunts* and are capable of producing shuntlike effects that are responsive to supplemental oxygen.

shift in the oxyhemoglobin dissociation curve (see Fig. 13–7). This change in affinity enhances the unloading of oxygen in the tissues and offsets the effects of mild hypoxia. At hemoglobin concentrations below 6 g%, however, the capabilities of the compensatory mechanisms are exceeded, and anemic hypoxia results.

STAGNANT HYPOXIA

When blood flow to the tissues is so low that oxygenation does not occur, in spite of adequate arterial oxygen tension and hemoglobin concentration, a condition of *ischemia* exists in the tissues. This type of relative oxygen deficiency in the tissues is known as **stagnant hypoxia** or **ischemic hypoxia.**

Causes of stagnant hypoxia include *decreased cardiac output* or *vascular insufficiency.* In such conditions, sluggish blood flow results in increased time for oxygen unloading at the tissues, but the oxygen supply in the systemic arteries progressively decreases as cellular metabolism continues. As a result of these changes, the P_{O_2} gradient between the blood and tissues decreases, thus contributing to tissue hypoxia. Other causes of stagnant hypoxia include *arteriovenous shunts* and *increased cellular metabolic needs.* A local arterial or venous obstruction can impede the flow of blood into or out of tissue capillaries, causing blood to bypass the cells and empty into the venous system without delivering its oxygen (Fig. 14–8). Increased oxygen demand in the tissues compared to the oxygen supply, can also produce a relative deficiency of oxygen, or tissue hypoxia. Such an imbalance of oxygen supply and demand occurs in *angina pectoris,* an ischemic condition that develops in heart muscle when the metabolic demand for oxygen is not met by the oxygen supplied by the coronary arteries. (A common cause of the imbalance is the partial narrowing of the blood vessels supplying the heart muscle.)

HISTOTOXIC HYPOXIA

A relatively rare type of hypoxia called **histotoxic hypoxia** is caused by the poisoning of cellular enzymes by toxic agents such as cyanide. In this disorder, cells are unable to utilize the oxygen delivered to them by the bloodstream because a mitochondrial enzyme called cytochrome oxidase is inactivated by the toxic agent. Cytochrome oxidase is a key enzyme in cellular respiration, the final pathway for oxygen utilization. When this enzyme is blocked, the cells are essentially "suffocated" at a cellular level. Blood gas analysis reveals that the arterial oxygen tension (PaO_2) and arterial oxygen content (CaO_2) are normal, but that the mixed venous oxygen tension ($P\bar{v}O_2$), mixed venous oxygen content ($C\bar{v}O_2$), and the mixed venous oxygen saturation ($S\bar{v}O_2$) are all elevated. These findings suggest that oxygen-laden blood passes through the tissue capillaries without giving up appreciable amounts of oxygen. The tissues simply are unable to utilize the oxygen in the bloodstream, therefore, widespread hypoxia rapidly develops. This situation is an interesting, but unusual, example of severe hypoxia occurring in the complete *absence* of hypoxemia. Clearly, a variety of interrelated factors are involved in the determination of both hypoxemia and hypoxia.

Summary

In preceding chapters we examined the movement of both air and blood to and from the alveolar-capillary membrane. In addition, we explored the gross and microscopic anatomy of the lung and associated structures, the mechanics of lung movement, the dynamics of air flow, and the diffusion characteristics of the blood-gas interface. If all of these cardiopulmonary structures and functions are normal, one would natu-

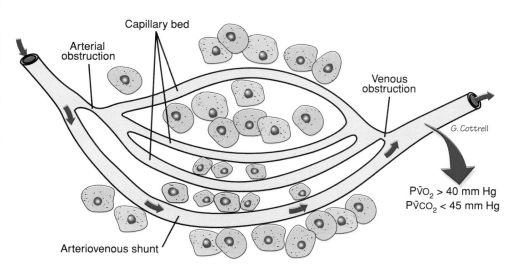

FIGURE 14–8. Arteriovenous shunt and stagnant hypoxia. Obstruction of the arterial supply (arterioles) or the venous drainage (venules) of capillary beds can lead to a state of stagnant hypoxia in the cells normally supplied by the capillary bed. An arteriovenous shunt is a type of vascular bypass around the obstruction. Such a vascular shunt results in the mixed venous blood having a P_{O_2} greater than normal and a P_{CO_2} less than normal. With normal gas exchange in the capillary beds, the mixed venous P_{O_2} should be reduced to approximately 40 mm Hg, and the mixed venous P_{CO_2} should be raised to approximately 45 to 47 mm Hg.

Capillary bed

Arterial obstruction

Venous obstruction

G. Cottrell

Arteriovenous shunt

$P\bar{v}O_2 > 40$ mm Hg
$P\bar{v}CO_2 < 45$ mm Hg

rally assume that optimal gas exchange will occur in the lung, but it turns out that this is not necessarily true. Instead, the *matching* of ventilation and perfusion within lung regions emerges as a critical factor governing gas transfer. In fact, the *mismatching* of ventilation and perfusion in the lung is the cause of much of the impairment in gas exchange associated with respiratory diseases.

This chapter considered the various factors that affect uneven matching of ventilation and blood flow in the lung, with particular emphasis on ventilation-perfusion ratios in both the ideal and the nonideal lung. The chapter concluded with an examination of several indices of gas exchange efficiency and with a brief discussion of various types of physiologic shunt and tissue hypoxia.

BIBLIOGRAPHY

Haldane JS: Symptoms, causes, and prevention of anoxemia. Br Med J 2:65, 1919.

Leff AR and Schumacker PT: Respiratory Physiology: Basics and Applications. WB Saunders, Philadelphia, 1993.

Levitzky MG: Pulmonary Physiology, ed 4. McGraw-Hill, New York, 1995.

Malley WJ: Clinical Blood Gases: Application and Noninvasive Alternatives. WB Saunders, Philadelphia, 1990.

Mines AH: Respiratory Physiology, ed 3. Raven Press, New York, 1993.

Shapiro BA, Peruzzi WT, and Kozelowski-Templin R: Clinical Application of Blood Gases, ed 5. Mosby–Year Book, St. Louis, 1994.

West JB: Pulmonary Pathophysiology: The Essentials, ed 5. Williams & Wilkins, Baltimore, 1997.

West JB: Respiratory Physiology: The Essentials, ed 6. Williams & Wilkins, Baltimore, 1998.

CHAPTER 15

Aging of the Respiratory System

chapter objectives

After studying this chapter the reader should be able to:

☐ Define senescence.

☐ Explain two current theories of aging by briefly describing the cellular changes observed with advancing age.

☐ Describe the general effects of aging on the bones of the skeleton by describing the processes of demineralization and reduced collagen synthesis.

☐ Explain how the thorax becomes more rigid with advancing age and explain how this change affects compliance.

☐ Describe how aging affects the microscopic structure of muscle.

☐ Explain what is meant by the *force-developing capacity* of muscle.

☐ Compare the effects of aging on limb muscles, the abdominal muscles, and the diaphragm.

☐ Explain why the elderly patient is at increased risk of airborne microbial infections by discussing the changes in lung defenses brought about through the aging process.

☐ Discuss the changes in the statics of breathing that occur in response to aging by describing changes in alveoli, elasticity, lung compliance, thorax compliance, and lung capacity.

☐ Discuss the changes in the dynamics of breathing and pulmonary mechanics that occur in response to aging by describing changes in airway closure and maximal expiratory air flow.

☐ Describe the change in the control of breathing associated with advancing age.

☐ Explain why low arterial oxygen tension occurs in response to age-related changes in the structure and function of the lung.

key term

senescence (sç-nes'-ens)

In this unit we explored various structures and functions that comprise the normal respiratory system. The overall contribution of the respiratory system to homeostatic balance in the body is overwhelming. For instance, the normal operation of the respiratory system ensures that blood is continually oxygenated and relieved of carbon dioxide, thus meeting the metabolic needs of all cells of the body. In addition, the respiratory system contributes to blood buffering through the elimination of carbon dioxide as bicarbonate, and contributes to overall protection of the body by housing immune cells in lymphoid organs such as the tonsils and phagocytic cells in the interior of alveoli. In summary, all organ systems of the body are totally dependent on the normal functioning of the respiratory system. Therefore, respiratory system health is a primary concern throughout the aging process. In this concluding chapter of the unit that began with the embryologic development of the respiratory system, we complete the life cycle by briefly examining the effects of aging on the respiratory system.

Theories of Aging

Although relatively little is currently understood regarding the precise mechanisms involved in aging, the sequence is generally considered a normal physiologic process. **Senescence** (L. *senescens,* the process of growing old, or a period of old age) is characterized by the progressive decline in form and function of the various organ systems of the body, including the *respiratory system.* This inevitable decline in the structure and activity of the body affects all its components, but not necessarily at the same rate. Aging affects all cells, tissues, organs, and systems of the body, probably through programmed genetic control of cell death (Ganong, 1995). Despite intensive research, the mechanism or mechanisms controlling aging are not properly understood. Numerous theories, however, have been advanced to help explain the phenomenon. The following paragraphs give a brief outline of a few of them (Ganong, 1995).

One theory of senescence is that the introduction of cumulative abnormalities in cells is responsible for the aging of cells, and that the abnormalities result from random mutation in the DNA of somatic cells. Another theory ascribes the cumulative abnormalities within cells to the gradual cross-linkage of collagen and other proteins over time. A third theory attributes the detrimental effects of aging to the cumulative result of tissue damage by free radicals formed within the tissues. Free radicals are cytotoxic (cell-destroying) molecules such as abnormal oxygen species (e.g., ozone). These damaging molecules are normally inactivated in the tissues by molecules functioning as free-radical scavengers (Box 15–1). It is postulated that the body's inability to neutralize free radicals may contribute to the aging process. Finally, there is speculation that a hormonal biologic clock, possibly located in the hypothalamus, is responsible for aging. Clearly, additional research needs to be done to fully understand senescence.

A series of cumulative degenerative changes affect both the microscopic and gross anatomy of the lung and associated structures. These structural changes are closely linked with the progressive decline in lung function observed in elderly patients. Although the changes in the respiratory system as a result of the effects of aging are conveniently organized into useful categories and presented in the following section, the reader should keep in mind that they are interdependent. For instance, a decrease in the mobility of the ribs alters the elastic recoil properties and compliance of the thorax. This change, in turn, limits the expansion of the lungs, thus decreasing the maximum voluntary inspiration attained by the subject. Prolonged hypoventilation can lead to ventilation-perfusion inequality and arterial hypoxemia. In addition, age-related changes in the cardiovascular system such as anemia or a decrease in cardiac reserve, can impact the overall functioning of the respiratory system. With such complex interrelationships in mind, we now consider the effects of aging on the respiratory system. Chapter 22 covers the effects of aging on the cardiovascular system.

Bony Thorax

The bones of the thorax—ribs, sternum, and thoracic vertebrae—are prone to the generalized changes caused by aging that affect other bones of the skeleton. The two major effects of senescence on bony tissue are (1) *demineralization* of bone matrix, and (2) *decreased rate of protein synthesis.* Demineralization, or the loss of calcium and phosphorous salts from the bony matrix, begins af-

PERSPECTIVES

BOX 15-1

Fast-Living Mice

A common animal model used in the study of aging is a special strain of mouse known as the *senescence-accelerated mouse* (SAM). SAM strains of mice provide good models for studying both physiologic and pathologic aging. SAMP2 is a senescence-prone strain bred to show the characteristics of premature aging; the SAMR1 strain is senescence-resistant and exhibits relatively normal aging. Through the use of these special strains of mice, researchers are able to design controlled experiments that test the effects of stresses such as cigarette smoking on the lungs and other organs of mice of different ages. Cigarette smoke is an oxidant stress that may affect the antioxidant capacity of both humans and animals. Antioxidants such as *glutathione* are found in limited supply in the liver. Such molecules reduce cellular damage caused by oxidants. The function of antioxidants, therefore, may play an important role in preventing age-related disorders. A limited number of animal studies using senescence-accelerated mice suggest that glutathione metabolism may be impaired by cigarette smoking and that the lungs of aged mice are more susceptible to cigarette smoke than those of young mice.

- Teramoto S et al: Effect of age on alteration of glutathione metabolism following chronic cigarette smoke inhalation in mice. Lung 174:119–126, 1996.
- Teramoto S et al: Effects of chronic cigarette smoke inhalation on the development of senile lung in the senescence-accelerated mouse. Res Exp Med Berl 197:1–11, 1997.

ter age 30 in women and accelerates around age 40 to 45 as levels of estrogen decline with the onset of menopause. The process of bone loss continues until as much as 30% of the stored calcium is lost by the age of 70 (Tortora and Grabowski, 1996). In men, the calcium loss from bones usually does not begin until after age 60. With demineralization, the density of bones is reduced, rendering them fragile. Aging also contributes to a decline in the rate at which the collagen protein framework of bony matrix is formed. The reduction in protein synthesis is probably linked to a decrease in human growth hormone (hGH) activity that accompanies aging. The collagen matrix gives bone its tensile strength; without it, bones become brittle and susceptible to fracture (Tortora and Grabowski, 1996). Because of the weight-bearing function of the thoracic vertebrae of the thorax, and the protective function of the ribs and sternum, this susceptibility to fracture as a result of demineralized and brittle bones becomes especially troublesome in the elderly patient.

In general, the chest wall becomes more rigid with advancing age (Marieb, 1998; Saladin, 1998). This loss of flexibility results from several anatomical changes, such as decreased movement of the costovertebral and sternocostal joints of the thorax, generalized deterioration of elastic tissue, and calcification of the costal cartilages (Levitzsky, 1995; Martini, 1998). In addition, the spaces between thoracic vertebrae become narrower and a greater degree of thoracic curvature, or

kyphosis, develops (Levitzsky, 1995). These changes in the thoracic spine contribute to a more rigid thorax with an increased anteroposterior dimension. In total, the age-related structural changes in the bony thorax lead to a decrease in compliance of the chest wall and an increase in static lung compliance. Because of decreased elasticity of the chest wall structures, the older individual must exert more effort to ventilate the lungs at a given respiratory minute volume.

Respiratory Muscles

Specific data on the effects of aging on respiratory muscles is scarce. Much of what is available is derived from studies of other skeletal muscle. In senescence, there is a general deterioration of skeletal muscles and strength (Brooks and Faulkner, 1995; Saladin, 1998; Tortora and Grabowski, 1996). The *force-developing capacity* of muscles is proportional to the total muscle fiber cross-sectional area (Brooks and Faulkner, 1995). Muscle *atrophy,* or a decrease in muscle mass, is due to a decrease in this fiber cross-sectional area, rather than to a decrease in the actual number of fibers. This decrease in muscle mass has not been reported for the diaphragm of elderly subjects. However, muscle fiber atrophy, and a general decrement in strength, is associated with aging and is seen in virtually all muscle groups in the body, including the abdominal group of accessory respiratory muscles. Data does not exist for other accessory muscles of breathing, but it appears that the respiratory muscles, other than the diaphragm, lose at least as much strength as the trunk and limb muscles (Brooks and Faulkner, 1995).

Elderly subjects generally exhibit a decrease in maximum voluntary inspiration and expiration mouth pressures. Such results provide an indirect way of assessing the maximum strength of respiratory muscles, but the results may lack accuracy. For example, the results can be affected by respiratory system factors unrelated to respiratory *muscle* function. These factors include airway narrowing, decreased lung compliance, or a combination of such factors. Age-related effects progressively cause a progressive decrease in the functional capacity of most of the muscles of breathing, but the deficit does not seriously interfere with normal respiration (Brooks and Faulkner, 1995). One of the reasons normal respiration is generally not compromised in the healthy older person is that the decrease in *limb muscle* function limits the person's ability to maintain a physically active lifestyle during old age. This decline is more or less matched by the decline in respiratory muscle capability.

In spite of the concurrent decline in muscle function in the limbs and in the accessory respiratory muscles, an older person is at increased risk for developing pulmonary insufficiency because of factors such as (1) changes in chest wall mechanics that increase the effort required to ventilate the lungs, and (2) decreased force-developing capacity of the muscles, making it more difficult to develop the strength needed to overcome the added resistance in the respiratory system. Therefore,

additional physiologic stress such as respiratory tract infections or long-term degeneration leading to chronic obstructive pulmonary diseases (COPDs), can seriously impair the ability of the elderly patient to ventilate the lungs (Brooks and Faulkner, 1995).

Lung Defenses

Recall that the respiratory system exposes an enormous surface area (70 to 80 m^2) to the external environment. This contact places the entire body at considerable risk for airborne microbial infections, inhalation of pollutants, and exposure to antigenic substances. For these reasons the lung and associated structures are well equipped with defensive structures such as nasal hairs, lymphoid tissue, mucus linings, and phagocytic cells, and with defensive mechanisms such as the mucociliary escalator and reflexes such as the bronchoconstriction reflex, cough reflex, and sneeze reflex. With advancing age, however, the effectiveness of these lung defenses decreases, thus placing the older person at increased risk for pulmonary disorders such as bronchitis, emphysema, and respiratory tract infections (Tortora and Grabowski, 1996). Pneumonia and influenza are especially prevalent in the older population (Marieb, 1998; Saladin, 1998).

Deterioration of the lung defenses with age includes changes such as (1) decreased efficiency of the mucociliary escalator, rendering the elderly person less capable of clearing the lungs of irritants and pathogens; and (2) decreased scavenging activity of alveolar macrophages (Marieb, 1998; Tortora and Grabowski, 1996).

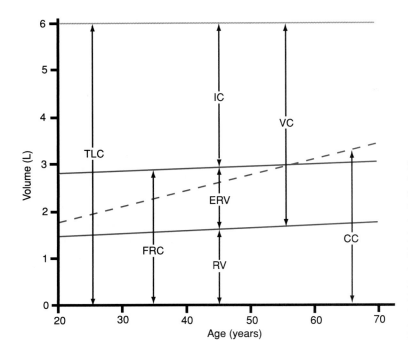

FIGURE 15–1. Age-related changes in standard lung volumes and capacities. Age-related changes in lung and thorax mechanics generally result in an increase in static lung compliance and a decrease in chest wall compliance. These changes typically cause an increase in functional residual capacity. Total lung capacity, adjusted for a decrease in height in an older person, normally remains unchanged. Vital capacity and inspiratory capacity decrease with advancing age. (TLC = total lung capacity; FRC = functional residual capacity; IC = inspiratory capacity; ERV = expiratory reserve volume; RV = residual volume; VC = vital capacity; CC = closing capacity). (Adapted from Levitzky MG: Pulmonary Physiology, ed 17. Appleton & Lange, Norwalk, 1995, p 79, with permission.)

Statics of Breathing

As the thoracic wall becomes more rigid with advancing age, the lungs gradually lose elasticity. In general, the airways and tissues of the respiratory system become less elastic, thus diminishing the older person's ability to ventilate the lungs (Marieb, 1998; Saladin, 1998; Tortora and Grabowski, 1996). The loss of elastic recoil in the lung is due to a combination of factors such as a decrease in elastic tissue in the lung interstitium, a reduction in the number of alveoli, and an overall loss of alveolar recoil. As a result of these changes in the mechanics of the lung and chest wall in elderly persons, the static lung compliance increases and the chest wall compliance decreases (Levitzsky, 1995). Thus, the older person's lungs are often overdistended, which leads to reduced efficiency of ventilation.

Measurements of static lung volumes and capacities performed during pulmonary function testing reflect a progressive decline in respiratory system efficiency caused by age-related changes in the compliance of the lung and thorax (Fig. 15–1). For example, the inspiratory capacity (IC) decreases with age, and the vital capacity (VC) may decrease by as much as 35% by age 70 (Marieb, 1998; Tortora and Grabowski, 1996). In addition, as discussed subsequently, the respiratory minute volume decreases, as well as the forced expiratory flow. Functional residual capacity (FRC), however, *increases* as the lungs distend as a result of loss of elastic recoil (see Fig.15–1). Interestingly, the total lung capacity (TLC), adjusted for the decrease in height seen in most older people, remains constant with age (Levitzsky, 1995).

TABLE 15–1	Age-Related Changes in the Respiratory System
Structure	**Changes**
Bony Thorax	• Demineralization of bone matrix and increased porosity • Decreased rate of collagen protein synthesis in bone • Calcification of costal cartilages • Decreased mobility of costovertebral and sternocostal joints in the thorax • Decreased space between thoracic vertebrae • Greater degree of thoracic curvature (kyphosis) and increased anteroposterior diameter of thorax • Increased rigidity/decreased elasticity of thorax • Increased outward elastic recoil of chest wall
Respiratory Muscles	• Loss of muscle mass and strength • Decreased cross-sectional diameter of muscle fibers • Decreased force-developing capacity of muscles
Lung Defenses	• Decreased efficiency of the mucociliary escalator • Decreased phagocytic activity of alveolar macrophages
Parenchyma and Interstitium	• Decreased alveolar elastic recoil/loss of radial traction • Decreased number of alveoli leading to decreased alveolar surface area • Decreased pulmonary capillary blood volume
Pulmonary Function (Functional changes associated with aging occur as a result of the combined effects of alveolar and bony thorax changes.)	• Increased static lung compliance • Decreased chest wall compliance • Increased functional residual capacity • Decreased inspiratory capacity • Decreased vital capacity • Decreased respiratory minute volume • Decreased forced expiratory flow • Increased residual volume • Increased closing volume • Decreased maximal expiratory airflow
Control of Breathing	• Decreased sensitivity of hypercapnic drive mechanism
Blood Gases	• Ventilation-perfusion inequalities (due to alveolar and circulatory changes) • Decreased volume of oxygen taken up by tissues during aerobic metabolism

Dynamics of Breathing and Pulmonary Mechanics

With the loss of alveolar elastic recoil that accompanies aging, there is decreased radial traction on small airways (Levitzsky, 1995). Mechanical tethering of small-diameter airways to the lung interstitium normally opposes dynamic compression during forced expirations. When this mechanism is impaired by advancing age, however, airway closure occurs at higher lung volumes (see Fig. 15–1). The higher closing volumes, combined with decreased respiratory muscle strength, leads to an increase in residual volume (RV) and a decrease in maximal expiratory air flow, as measured by forced expiratory flow between 25% and 75% of FVC ($FEF_{25\%-75\%}$), and by forced expiratory volume in one second (FEV_1) (Levitzsky, 1995). Airway closure may occur in dependent airways at lung volumes above the FRC.

Control of Breathing

An elderly person's hypercapnic drive, or sensitivity to arterial carbon dioxide tension ($Paco_2$), decreases with age (Marieb, 1998). This reduced response is especially evident when the person is in the reclining or supine position. Therefore, some older people may tend to become hypoxemic during sleep and exhibit *sleep apnea* symptoms, a condition of temporary cessation of breathing during deep sleep.

Blood Gases

In general, age-related changes in the respiratory system contribute to a decrease in arterial oxygen tension (Pao_2). With higher closing volumes, the elderly person may have substantially more ventilation of the upper regions than does a younger person. However, if dependent regions are overperfused, ventilation-perfusion inequalities may develop, leading to low Pao_2 values. The decrease in arterial oxygen tension is also related to a loss of alveolar surface area and a decrease in pulmonary blood flow, both of which result in decreased pulmonary diffusing capacity (Levitzsky, 1995). Other blood gas-related changes associated with aging include a steady decrease in the volume of oxygen ($\dot{V}o_2$) taken up by the tissues during aerobic metabolism. The value for $\dot{V}o_2$ decreases approximately 9% per decade in sedentary (inactive) people, beginning in their mid-20s. For active people, the $\dot{V}o_2$ value declines at a slower rate during aging, and is equivalent to that in a person 20 years younger (Marieb, 1998).

Table 15–1 summarizes the age-related changes of the respiratory system.

Summary

This chapter briefly explores the respiratory system's age-related changes in form and function. The complex interrelationships of the various structures and functions were stressed to reinforce the idea of an integrated system. Because changes in the respiratory system brought about by aging can affect mechanisms and structures other than those directly associated with the lung, the overall status, or *health,* of the respiratory system in the elderly takes on critical importance.

BIBLIOGRAPHY

Brooks SV and Faulkner JA: Effects of aging on the structure and function of skeletal muscle. In Roussos C (ed): The Thorax—Part A: Physiology, ed 2. Marcel Dekker, New York, 1995.

Ganong WF: Review of Medical Physiology, ed 17. Appleton & Lange, Norwalk, CT, 1995.

Levitzky MG: Pulmonary Physiology, ed 4. McGraw-Hill, New York, 1995.

Marieb E: Human Anatomy and Physiology, ed 4. Benjamin/Cummings, Menlo Park, CA, 1998.

Martini FH: Fundamentals of Anatomy and Physiology, ed 4. Prentice Hall, Upper Saddle River, NJ, 1998.

Saladin KS: Anatomy and Physiology: The Unity of Form and Function. WCB/McGraw-Hill, Boston, 1998.

Tortora GJ and Grabowski SR: Principles of Anatomy and Physiology, ed 8. HarperCollins, New York, 1996.

UNIT TWO

The Cardiovascular System

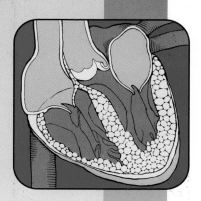

Although it seems fairly straightforward from an organizational standpoint to separate the study of respiratory system function from cardiovascular system function, in practice it is difficult or impossible. Clearly, the *structures* associated with the organ systems are different—one is designed to expose thin-walled blood vessels to a large surface area of the external environment; the other is designed to move blood throughout the body. Accordingly, the respiratory system possesses an extensive membrane system that forms an effective blood-gas interface, while the cardiovascular system consists of blood, a muscular pump, and an extensive vascular distribution system. Unlike their respective and separate structures, however, the *functions* of the two systems are inextricably linked through the common goal of maintaining normal oxygen and carbon dioxide levels in the tissues. This interdependency is exactly what makes it so difficult to separate the two systems in a specialized anatomy and physiology textbook. It is also the reason the function of the combined *cardiopulmonary system* has been stressed throughout this book. In the preceding chapters of Unit 1, numerous examples exist where a pertinent cardiovascular structure or function had to be discussed and integrated into the discussion of a respiratory system structure or function. For example, *gas exchange* in the lung (see Chap. 12) makes sense only if pulmonary circulation is discussed in conjunction with the topic; *gas transport* by hemoglobin in red blood cells (see Chap. 13) has obvious functional links with the blood of the cardiovascular system; and *extrapulmonary shunting* (see Chap. 14) has a clearer meaning if bronchial circulation and fetal circulation are examined along with the concept of physiologic shunt.

The foregoing are only a few examples of the integral nature of respiratory system and cardiovascular system function. In short, we have already discussed most of the relevant features of the cardiovascular system that affect respiratory system function. This unit provides an introduction to additional cardiovascular topics such as developmental aspects of the cardiovascular system, the cardiac cycle and cardiac output, electrophysiology of the heart, hemodynamics, blood pressure control, and the effects of aging on cardiovascular system structure and function.

CHAPTER 16

Development of the Cardiovascular System

chapter objectives

After studying this chapter the reader should be able to:

☐ Describe the embryologic development of blood vessels from embryonic blood islands.

☐ Describe the embryologic development of blood and list the various tissues that serve as hemopoietic sites.

☐ Describe the unique oxygen-transporting characteristics of fetal hemoglobin and fetal hematocrit that improve the efficiency of placental gas exchange.

☐ Review the partitioning of the thoracic cavity that occurs through the growth of the pleuroperitoneal folds, the transverse septum, and the pleuropericardial folds.

☐ Explain how the following pericardial structures develop in the embryo:
  Pericardial cavity, parietal pericardium, visceral pericardium.

☐ Define the following terms:
  Epicardium, myocardium, endocardium.

☐ Trace the sequence of heart development by describing the following structures:
  Mesodermal cells, endothelial (endocardial) tubes, primitive heart tube.

☐ Describe the function of the following subdivisions of the primitive heart tube:
  Sinus venosus, atrium, ventricle, bulbus cordis, truncus arteriosus.

☐ Describe the changes in the curvature and orientation of the primitive heart tube that reorient the pumping chambers so the atrium is superior to the ventricle.

☐ Explain septation of the heart by describing the development of the interatrial septum and interventricular septum.

☐ Describe the organization of the placenta into cotyledons.

☐ Explain how maternal and fetal circulatory routes are arranged within a cotyledon by describing the function of the following structures:
  Chorionic villi, intervillous spaces.

☐ Explain the concept of the transplacental barrier.

☐ Describe the function of the following fetal circulatory structures:
  Umbilical cord, umbilical vein, ductus venosus, umbilical arteries.

☐ Define the term *venous admixture* as it applies to fetal circulation.

☐ Trace the flow of blood through the fetal heart.

☐ Describe the function of the following fetal shunt structures:
  Foramen ovale, ductus arteriosus.

☐ Differentiate between functional closure and anatomic closure as the terms apply to fetal shunt structures.

☐ Outline the changes that occur to fetal circulatory structures in the perinatal period that help establish postnatal circulation following the infant's first breath.

☐ Name the fetal circulatory structures that give rise to the following postnatal structures:
  Ligamentum arteriosum, fossa ovalis, ligamentum teres, medial umbilical ligaments, ligamentum venosum.

key terms

blood islands; angiogenic clusters
bulbus cordis (bul′bus kor′dus)
chorionic villi (kō-rē-on′-ik vil′ē)
cotyledon (cot″-i-lē′don)
ductus arteriosus (duk′tus ar-tē″-rē-ō′-sus)
ductus venosus (duk′ tus ven ō′-sus)
endocardium
endothelial (endocardial) tubes
epicardium
fetal hemoglobin (HbF)
foramen ovale
fossa ovalis (fos′-a ō-val′-iss)
interatrial septum
interventricular septum
intervillous spaces
ligamentum arteriosum (lig″ a-men′-tum ar-tē″-rē-ō′-sum)

ligamentum teres; round ligament of the liver (lig″ a-men′-tum te′rēz)
ligamentum venosum (lig″ a-men′-tum ven ō′-sum)
medial umbilical ligaments
myocardium
parietal pericardium
pericardial cavity
placenta
primitive heart tube
sinus venosus (sī′nus ven ō′-sus)
transplacental barrier
truncus arteriosus
umbilical arteries
umbilical cord
umbilical vein
visceral pericardium (epicardium)

Because of the extensive distribution system that must be formed to meet the gaseous, nutritional, and waste requirements of widely scattered cells in a complex organism, the various elements of the cardiovascular system—heart, blood vessels, and blood—*must* begin developing within days of conception. This chapter introduces the basics of the embryologic development of the cardiovascular system and focuses on the fetal circulatory structures essential for oxygenation of the blood during the period when the lung is nonfunctional. The chapter also examines the cardiovascular changes that occur in the fetal-neonatal transition period and discusses the postnatal fate of fetal circulatory structures.

Development of Blood Vessels

Immediately following conception, a small volume of fluid in the uterus sustains the newly formed mass of undifferentiated cells that implants on the uterine wall. The *yolk sac, chorion, amnion,* and *placenta* are embryonic membranous structures that form shortly afterward to supply the nutrient needs of the young embryo. Unlike animals such as birds, however, the human yolk sac has relatively little yolk to provide nourishment for the rapidly dividing embryo. Instead, nourishment must be supplied by maternal circulation and transferred to the embryo via the placenta, a specialized exchange organ that develops from embryonic tissue. Blood vessels comprising the future circulatory system of the fetus distribute these maternally derived nutrients to the embryo, return waste products to the placenta, and transport gases between the placenta and embryo.

The development of blood vessels and blood begins around 15 to 16 days in the *mesoderm* of the yolk sac, chorion, and body stalk that attaches the embryo to the placenta (Tortora and Grabowski, 1996). Mesoderm is one of three basic embryonic germ layers from which specialized tissues such as smooth, skeletal, and cardiac muscle develop. Mesoderm consists of undifferentiated mesenchymal cells. Isolated masses and cords of these mesenchymal cells known as **blood islands** are responsible for the formation of blood vessels. Blood islands are also known as **angiogenic clusters** (Koff, 1993). The formation of blood vessels begins with the appearance of small spaces in the blood islands. The spaces enlarge, fuse together, and become organized into openings that form the tubelike interior, or *lumen*, of a future blood vessel (Marieb, 1998; Tortora and Grabowski, 1996).

As the openings are developing in the interior of the young blood vessels, the blood islands are sprouting branches that extend toward adjacent blood islands as well as toward the developing embryonic heart (as discussed subsequently). These branches form the primitive vascular system that connects the embryo to the placenta, as well as all parts of the embryo (Marieb, 1998). During this extensive period of development, the vascular system must expand, grow, reroute, and reform again as the embryo grows in size (Netter, 1969). Entire circulatory channels supplying different parts of the embryo are established, abandoned, and regrown again to keep pace with the embryo's breathtaking rate of development. Meanwhile, heart growth and development must continue to keep up with general development of the embryo, an amazing feat in itself. (For an in-depth account of the embryologic development of the cardiovascular system, the reader is directed to the classic treatment of the subject by Dr. Frank Netter. The detailed text description is accompanied by numerous full-color illustrations (Netter, 1969).

Mesenchymal cells immediately adjacent to the spaces within the blood islands form the *endothelium*, or lining of blood vessels. Mesenchymal cells peripheral to these endothelial cells form the muscular and fibrous *tunics* (layers) found in the medium- to large-diameter blood vessels (Marieb, 1998; Tortora and Grabowski, 1996). The organization of blood vessel layers is discussed in Chapter 21. As scattered blood islands with enlarging lumina fuse together throughout the rapidly-growing embryo, an extensive distribution network forms, eventually covering 100,000 km in the adult circulatory system (Marieb, 1998).

Specialized fetal vascular structures include the *fora-men ovale* and *ductus arteriosis* that allow blood to bypass the nonfunctional lungs, the *umbilical vein* and paired *umbilical arteries* that connect the placenta to the embryo, and the *ductus venosus* that permits blood to bypass the liver and enter directly into the inferior vena cava of the fetus. These structures and their functions are examined in the subsequent section on fetal circulation.

Development of Blood

Endothelial cells lining primitive blood vessels in the yolk sac and allantois are initially responsible for the production of *blood plasma* and *primitive blood cells*. In the second month of gestation, however, blood formation (*hemopoiesis*) begins in the liver and spleen of the embryo, followed many months later by production in bone marrow and lymph nodes (Tortora and Grabowski, 1996). Interestingly, if an unusual need for blood cell production arises in later life, the liver and spleen resume their hemopoietic function (Marieb, 1998).

As was discussed with gas transport (see Chap. 13), several different species of hemoglobin exist. During fetal life, **fetal hemoglobin (HbF)** is produced and incorporated into newly formed red blood cells. This unique type of hemoglobin has a higher affinity for oxygen than does adult hemoglobin (HbA). Fetal hemoglobin, therefore, causes a leftward shift in the oxyhemoglobin dissociation curve (see Fig. 13–5) (Aloan and Hill, 1997; Ganong, 1995; Koff, 1993). The P_{50} for fetal hemoglobin is normally around 20 mm Hg, compared with 27 mm Hg for adult hemoglobin (Aloan and Hill, 1997).

Recall that the P_{50} for hemoglobin represents the oxygen tension at which hemoglobin is 50% saturated. Fetal hemoglobin, therefore, exhibits a higher saturation than adult hemoglobin at a given oxygen tension. This decrease in the P_{50} value for fetal hemoglobin is typical of a left-shifted oxyhemoglobin dissociation curve, meaning that HbF readily binds oxygen but releases it less readily. The increased affinity of HbF for oxygen compensates for the less efficient gas-transferring ability of the placenta, compared with that of the postnatal lung. Structurally, HbF consists of two alpha (α) and two gamma (γ) polypeptide chains per globin molecule ($\alpha_2\gamma_2$), instead of the paired α and beta (β) chains of adult hemoglobin ($\alpha_2\beta_2$). The γ chains in fetal hemoglobin are responsible for the increased ability of the molecule to transport oxygen at a given oxygen tension. Fetal hemoglobin does not bind 2,3-diphosphoglycerate (2,3-DPG) as effectively as adult hemoglobin (Ganong, 1995; Aloan and Hill, 1997). The binding of 2,3-DPG to hemoglobin reduces the ability of hemoglobin to combine with oxygen. Recall that there is an inverse relationship between 2,3-DPG concentration in red blood cells and the affinity of hemoglobin for oxygen (see Chap. 13). Therefore, since the γ polypeptide chains of fetal hemoglobin are unable to bind 2,3-DPG effectively, the affinity of HbF for oxygen increases, causing a leftward shift in the oxyhemoglobin dissociation curve and enhanced oxygen loading at the placenta (Ganong, 1995). The concentration of 2,3-DPG increases throughout the gestation period, thus maintaining the affinity of fetal hemoglobin for oxygen, as well as the leftward shift of the oxyhemoglobin dissociation curve.

Although only about 20% of the hemoglobin present at birth is the HbA variant, by the age of 4 to 6 months, 90% of the circulating hemoglobin in the infant is HbA (Ganong, 1995). No additional HbF is produced after birth. Instead, fetal red blood cells containing HbF are rapidly destroyed immediately after birth as the newborn begins producing replacement red blood cells containing HbA. During the first year of life, the oxyhemoglobin dissociation curve of the infant gradually shifts toward the right as the concentration of HbA increases (Aloan and Hill, 1997).

In addition to the presence of fetal hemoglobin to compensate for relatively inefficient placental gas transfer, fetal red blood cells and hemoglobin are simply present in higher concentrations compared with those of the adult. For example, fetal and newborn hematocrit is typically 55% to 60%, compared with approximately 45% in the adult (Aloan and Hill, 1997). As a result of the elevated numbers of red blood cells, fetal hemoglobin concentration is in the range of 16 to 19 g%, compared with 12 to 15 g% for the older child and adult (see Table 13–1) (Aloan and Hill, 1997). Because most of the oxygen in the bloodstream is transported as oxyhemoglobin, the presence of *high-affinity* fetal hemoglobin at a *high concentration* of 16 to 19 g per 100 mL of blood contributes to improved oxygen loading at the placenta.

Development of the Heart and Pericardium

THE PACE OF CHANGE

To circulate the primitive blood cells through the newly formed and rapidly expanding system of blood vessels, and thus meet the metabolic needs of the growing embryo, a muscular pump is needed. This obvious requirement presents a formidable challenge in the young embryo because the placenta, which represents a proportionally large mass of extraembryonic tissue, must also be supplied with blood by the rudimentary heart. Typically, about 55% of the fetal cardiac output goes through the placenta (Ganong, 1995).

Within a matter of weeks, the embryonic heart must be transformed from a single, simple muscular tube into a complex, four-chambered organ with four valves. Although other body systems such as the nervous system

begin *structural* development sooner, the pace of change in the embryonic heart is characteristic of the cardiovascular system in general—a system that reaches an advanced *functional* state long before any of the other developing body systems (Netter, 1969). In the following section we first examine the development of the pericardial cavity and then trace the astounding changes that transform a muscular tube into a multichambered pump.

PERICARDIAL CAVITY

Recall that a sequence of partitioning occurs in the embryo to subdivide the primitive coelomic cavity into a future thoracic and peritoneal cavity, and to subdivide the thoracic cavity into separate compartments for the lungs and heart (see Chap. 1). The right and left *pleuroperitoneal folds,* along with the *transverse septum* fuse in the horizontal plane to form the diaphragmatic partition between the future thorax and peritoneal cavities (see Figs. 1–3 and 1–5). Meanwhile, the *pleuropericardial folds* project medially in the vertical plane to divide the common pleuropericardial cavity into separate pleural cavities for each lung and a separate *pericardial cavity* for the heart (see Figs. 1–4 and 1–7).

The mesoderm in the region of the developing *heart tubes* (see next section) splits into parietal and visceral layers that form the **pericardial cavity,** a double-walled membranous structure that protects, anchors, and lubricates the heart. The **parietal pericardium** lines the cavity, whereas the **visceral pericardium** covers the heart itself. Between the two layers is found the *pericardial space,* or *pericardial cavity,* which contains a lubricating *pericardial fluid.* This structural arrangement is reminiscent of the pleural membranes surrounding and protecting the lungs. In fact, the development of the pericardial structures is similar to what we have already seen with the pleural structures. Namely, the membranes are *not* "wrapped around" the organ after it develops in a particular place. Instead, the membranes are already present as a lining of the cavity to be occupied. The organ, in this case the heart, pushes into the cavity formed by the separation of visceral and parietal layers, and is enveloped by the lining material. Thus, the visceral pericardium makes initial contact with the heart and literally becomes the outer layer of the wall of the heart, or **epicardium.** The middle layer of the wall of the heart contains heart muscle and is called the **myocardium.** The lining of the chambers of the heart is known as the **endocardium,** and is continuous with the endothelium of developing blood vessels.

A useful analogy to visualize this "double wrapping" of the heart in a continuous membrane is to picture a fist pushed into a medium-sized balloon that has been tied with a very small amount of air in it. As the fist goes into the pliant material, the balloon folds on itself so that two layers of the material engulf the fist, leaving a narrow space between them. The space represents the fluid-filled "pericardial cavity," or space *around* the heart, while the two continuous layers represent the covering of the heart ("visceral pericardium") and the lining of the space ("parietal pericardium"). The point at the wrist where the balloon reflects back on itself is the region where the great vessels such as the aorta and venae cavae enter and exit at the base of the heart.

HEART

Development of the heart begins at about the same time as that of the blood vessels and blood (approximately week 2), with the appearance of a pair of **endothelial (endocardial) tubes** that develop from mesoderm (Tortora and Grabowski, 1996). Shortly afterward, the thin-walled muscular tubes unite to form the **primitive heart tube** beneath the floor of the future pharynx (Marieb, 1998; Martini, 1998; Saladin, 1998). By $3^1/_2$ weeks, the heart tube begins to differentiate into future pumping chambers, identified by slight bulges (Fig. 16–1). Marieb (1998) describes four regions with the **truncus arteriosus** as the cranial extension of the **bulbus cordis,** while Saladin (1998) and Tortora and Grabowski (1996) recognize five separate subdivisions of the primitive heart tube. For our purposes, the distinction is not important. From the caudal to the cranial end of the heart tube, in the order in which blood is pumped through the tube, the following regions are identified:

- *Sinus venosus:* At an early stage of development the **sinus venosus** receives all the deoxygenated blood from the embryo. The great veins (*superior vena cava* and *inferior vena cava*) eventually develop from this venous end of the heart tube. Much later, the sinus venosus becomes the smooth-walled part of the *right atrium* as well as the *coronary sinus*, a structure that will function to return most of the coronary blood flow to the right atrium. The sinus venosus also gives rise to the *sinoatrial node* (SA node), which begins to pace the heart early in its embryonic development and continues to control heart rate throughout life.
- *Atrium:* This bulged part of the heart tube eventually forms the remainder of the *right atrium* as well as the *left atrium.*
- *Ventricle:* The ventricle begins development as the strongest chamber of the young heart tube, functioning to pump primitive blood cells throughout the embryo as soon as the primitive heart tube forms. The embryonic ventricle continues in this role as the powerful *left ventricle* of the developed heart. The less powerful *right ventricle* also develops from the embryonic ventricle.

- *Bulbus cordis and truncus arteriosus:* These cranial portions of the heart tube differentiate to produce the *pulmonary trunk*, which arises from the right ventricle and eventually supplies blood to the lungs; the *proximal (ascending) aorta*, which originates in the left ventricle and sends blood into systemic arteries; and portions of the *right atrium*, which ultimately collects blood from the systemic veins. The **ductus arteriosus** is a temporary vascular structure that connects the pulmonary trunk and aorta. (The shunt function of the ductus arteriosus will be discussed under "Fetal Circulation.")

By $3^1/_2$ weeks the miniature heart is pumping blood through an embryo that is less than 6 mm long, a length about the same as the diameter of an average-sized pencil (Marieb, 1998).

During the embryonic period, the heart undergoes drastic changes in morphology and size, being converted from a simple muscular tube to a four-chambered double pump. Throughout this developmental period, as the very shape and design of the heart changes, the organ must continue to supply blood to the placenta and the growing embryo, *all without missing a beat*—a truly amazing feat.

During the next 3 weeks, various contortions of the heart tube occur (see Fig. 16–1). For example, during week 4 the ventricle and bulbus cordis grow rapidly, causing the developing heart tube to bend upon itself, first into a U shape, and later into an S shape as differential growth in the tube continues (Saladin, 1998; Tortora and Grabowski, 1996). Essentially, the heart enlarges more rapidly than its inferior and superior attachments. The resulting flexures reorient the portions of the tube so that the atrium and sinus venosus come to lie superior to the ventricle, bulbus cordis, and truncus arteriosus (Saladin, 1998; Tortora and Grabowski, 1996). In general, the looping of the heart causes the ventricle to move caudally while the atrium moves cranially. This reorientation of future pumping chambers is accompanied by *septation* (septum formation) and marked *growth* of the embryonic heart.

In week 5, folds of tissue called *septa* begin to divide the interior of the heart into its familiar four-chambered design (Fig. 16–2; see also Color Plate 11). The future **interatrial septum** begins as two folds of tissue that divide the single atrium into a right and a left atrium. The upper and lower parts of the interatrial septum do not fuse together. Instead, they overlap to form a valvelike flap over an oval opening called the *foramen ovale*. The role of this important fetal circulatory structure is covered in the following section. Also during week 5, the future **interventricular septum** begins to divide the single large ventricle of the primitive heart into a thin-walled right ventricle and a thicker-walled left ventricle (see Fig. 16–2). The thick-

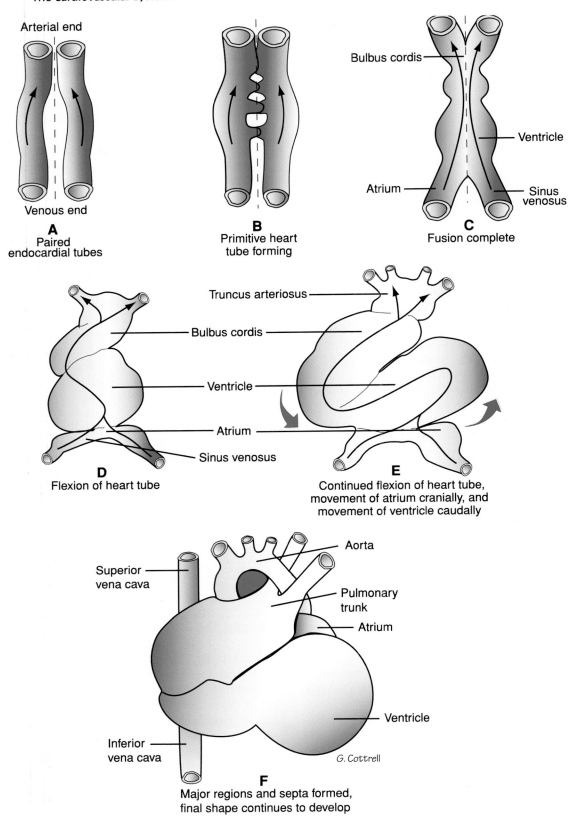

FIGURE 16–1. Development of heart from endocardial tubes. Dotted lines represent the midline of the original paired endocardial tubes; arrows indicate the flow of blood through the embryonic structures.

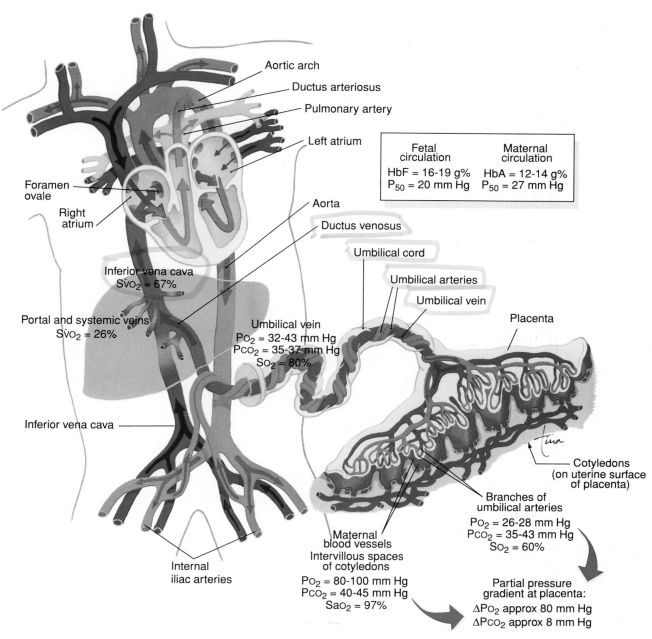

FIGURE 16–2. Fetal circulation. Note that the separate oxygenated and deoxygenated circulatory routes are not seen in the fetus. Instead, several different *venous admixtures* are found. The umbilical vein admixture contains the highest amount of oxygen following gaseous exchange at the placenta ($So_2 = 80\%$). Maternal blood values in the intervillous spaces of the placenta are typical of those found in systemic arteries. (Adapted from Scanlon VC and Sanders T: Essentials of Anatomy and Physiology, ed. 3. FA Davis, Philadelphia, 1999, p 290, with permission.) (See also Color Plate 11.)

ness of the myocardium in the developing chambers is proportional to the force developed by the chamber of the heart, a feature that is constant throughout life. Interestingly, the difference in wall thickness between the thin-walled atrium and the thicker-walled ventricle is visible even at the early two-chamber stage of heart development (Martini, 1998). Unlike the intera-

trial septum that remains *unfused* in the fetal state, the two parts of the interventricular septum *fuse* together, thus completing the partitioning of the single ventricle into two separate pumping chambers.

Table 16–1 summarizes the highlights of the chronological development of blood vessels, blood, pericardium, and the heart during the embryonic period.

TABLE 16-1	Time Line of Development of Cardiovascular Structures
Week	**Developmental Event**
0–3	• Masses of mesenchymal cells called blood islands (angiogenic clusters) derived from mesoderm of yolk sac, chorion, and body stalk develop small spaces that enlarge, fuse together, and form lumina of future blood vessels. • Sprouting from groups of blood islands establishes the branching network of blood vessels. • Cells lining the lumina form the endothelium of blood vessels; mesenchymal cells in deeper layers form the muscular and fibrous tunics of blood vessels. • Foramen ovale, ductus arteriosus, umbilical vein, umbilical arteries, and ductus venosus begin to form. • Primitive blood cells derived from lining of yolk sac and allantois begin to be circulated. • Paired endocardial tubes unite to form the primitive heart tube. • Partitioning of thorax begins with appearance of the pleuroperitoneal folds and pleuropericardial folds to form the future pericardial cavity.

3–4	• Primitive heart tube differentiates into future pumping chambers and regions:
	  ○ *Sinus venosus* eventually gives rise to the SVC, IVC, RA, coronary sinus, and sinoatrial node.
	  ○ *Atrium* develops into the RA and LA.
	  ○ *Ventricle* gives rise to the RV and LV.
	  ○ *Bulbis cordis* and *truncus anteriosus* produce the pulmonary trunk, ascending aorta, RA, and ductus arteriosus.

4	• Heart tube flexes upon itself because of rapid growth in the ventricle and bulbus cordis. The looping of the tube reorients the heart so that the ventricle moves caudally and the atrium moves cranially.

5–7	• Septation divides the heart into the future four pumping chambers:
	  ○ Interatrial septum produces the RA and LA but is incomplete, thus forming the foramen ovale.
	  ○ Interventricular septum divides the single ventricle into the future RV and LV.
	• Hemopoiesis begins in the liver and spleen.

Note: All time periods shown above are approximate.
IVC = inferior vena cava; SVC = superior vena cava; RA = right atrium; LA = left atrium; RV = right ventricle; LV = left ventricle.

Fetal Circulation

PLACENTA

The **placenta** is a fetal-derived exchange organ found at the interface between maternal and fetal bloodstreams. The structure of the placenta allows blood gases, wastes, and nutrients to transfer between the microcirculation of the two blood streams. In this way, the functions of the placenta mimic those of the lung, digestive system, and urinary system. Typically, the 0.5-kg placenta is organized into 15 to 20 functional units called **cotyledons.** These convex, bean-shaped structures project from the uterine (maternal) surface of the placenta, where they mesh with shallow concave depressions in the lining of the uterus. Within a single cotyledon fetal blood enters through microscopic branches of the *umbilical arteries.* These arterial branches are distributed into structures known as **chorionic villi,** small fingerlike projections that help increase the surface area of the blood-blood interface. Maternal blood enters the cotyledon via small branches of the *uterine arteries* and percolates in the **intervillous spaces** found around the chorionic villi. Maternal blood is returned via systemic veins to general circulation in the mother.

An analogy that may prove useful to visualize such a blood-to-blood interface is that of a glove placed inside a mitten. If one fluid is found inside the "chorionic villi," or fingers of the glove, and a different fluid is contained within the "intervillous spaces" represented by the interior of the mitten, the two fluids do not actually *contact* each other—they are separated by the material of the glove. Depending on the nature of the material (e.g., pore size) and the makeup of the substances contained in the two fluids (e.g., size of molecules), movement of substances will occur because of exchange mechanisms such as osmosis and diffusion.

This interface between the bloodstream of the mother and that of the fetus forms the **transplacental barrier.** The series of membranes comprising the barrier restrict the entry of red blood cells and most large molecules, but plasma-borne substances, including some drugs and antibodies, cross the barrier with relative ease. It is here at the transplacental barrier that exchanges normally take place between maternal and fetal circulation. The arrangement of squamous endothelial cells of the fetal capillaries found in close proximity to squamous epithelial cells of the chorionic villi is similar to that found in the alveolar-capillary membranes of the lung. The structures in the placenta, however, are much thicker than their counterparts in the alveolar-capillary system. Furthermore, the total surface area of the blood-blood exchange structures in the placental is significantly smaller than that of the postnatal lung. Consequently, the gas exchange *efficiency* of the placenta, or diffusing capacity, is less than that of the alveolar-capillary system in the functional lung. Compensatory mechanisms that minimize the impact on oxygenation caused by reduced placental gas-exchange efficiency include (1) fetal hemoglobin (HbF) with a high affinity for oxygen ($P_{50} \approx$ 20 mm Hg); (2) a high concentration of fetal hemoglobin (16 to 19 g%); and (3) a maternal-fetal oxygen tension gradient that is substantial ($\Delta Po_2 \approx 80$ mm Hg).

CONNECTIONS BETWEEN PLACENTA AND FETUS

The reference point for naming blood vessels associated with fetal circulation is the *fetal* heart. Recall that veins transport blood toward the heart; therefore, the unpaired **umbilical vein** functions to carry blood from the placenta toward the fetal heart. The umbilical vein, along with the paired umbilical arteries (discussed below), is found in the **umbilical cord,** the external connection between the fetus and placenta (see Fig. 16–2). Oxygenated blood enters the umbilical vein after being collected from the capillaries of the chorionic villi. Although blood gas values continually change with the age and metabolic needs of the fetus throughout the gestation period, the Po_2 of the umbilical vein normally ranges between 32 and 43 mm Hg, and the Pco_2 ranges between 35 and 37 mm Hg after gas exchange with maternal circulation has occurred (Koff, 1993). The oxygen saturation in the umbilical vein is normally around 80%, compared with approximately 97% in the adult (Ganong, 1995). Blood gas values in the maternal circulation of the intervillous spaces of the cotyledons is characteristic of systemic arterial values; that is, $Pao_2 = 80$ to 100 mm Hg and $Paco_2 = 40$ to 45 mm Hg. As the umbilical vein enters the fetus, it splits into two branches carrying roughly equal amounts of blood. One branch joins the *hepatic portal vein* draining the fetal gastrointestinal (GI) tract, thus transporting blood to the fetal liver for processing. This blood contains maternal-derived nutrients; therefore, it mimics the nutrient-rich venous blood that will drain the GI tract when foodstuffs begin to be taken by mouth by the infant.

The other branch of the umbilical vein is known as the **ductus venosus.** This important fetal circulatory structure joins the inferior vena cava (IVC) and thus diverts about one-half of the oxygenated blood from the placenta directly into the systemic circulatory system of the fetus (see Fig. 16–2). The blood transported by the ductus venosus blends with that of the IVC, producing a *venous admixture* with an oxygen saturation of approximately 67% (Ganong, 1995). This blood is returned to the right atrium. By com-

parison, the $S\bar{v}o_2$ in portal and systemic veins is only about 26% (Ganong, 1995). Note that fetal circulation does not have separate "oxygenated" and "deoxygenated" circulatory routes; there is no clear distinction between "arterial" and "venous" blood.

The placental-derived blood is delivered to the fetal heart and pumped out again into systemic circulation through the *aorta,* which bifurcates into a *right* and *left common iliac artery* in the inguinal region. Each of these arteries branches into an *external iliac artery* that supplies blood to superficial structures such as the skin and an *internal iliac artery* that sends blood to deeper muscles. The internal iliac arteries, in turn, give off small branches known as the **umbilical arteries** (see Fig. 16–2). The paired umbilical arteries return blood to the placenta for gas exchange. The blood returning to the placenta has a Po_2 of approximately 26 to 28 mm Hg and a Pco_2 of about 35 to 43 mm Hg (Koff, 1993). The oxygen saturation (So_2) of this returning blood is approximately 60% (Ganong, 1995). Upon entering the chorionic villi, blood gases exchange with maternal circulation once again, and the entire process repeats. Note that a considerable oxygen tension gradient of approximately 80 mm Hg is present between maternal and fetal circulatory systems, thus increasing the efficiency of oxygen loading at the placenta.

FETAL SHUNT STRUCTURES

The fluid-filled, atelectic lungs in the fetal state offer extremely high resistance to flow through the normal pulmonary circulatory route. Therefore, relatively little blood enters the right ventricle from the right atrium to be pumped against this high pulmonary vascular resistance (PVR). Instead, most of the blood entering the right atrium bypasses the nonfunctional fetal lungs by passing through the **foramen ovale** and entering the left atrium (see Fig. 16–2). Recall that the foramen ovale is formed because the two portions of the interatrial septum do not normally fuse in the fetal heart. The overlapping, flaplike arrangement of the septal segments forms a crude valve that prevents blood movement from the left atrium to the right atrium. The pressure within the left atrium tends to be low because relatively little blood returns to the heart from the high-resistance pulmonary vascular beds. The low pressure in the left atrium enhances the right-to-left movement of blood through the foramen ovale, thus providing an effective anatomical shunt around the nonfunctional lungs.

The ductus arteriosus is a vascular structure that links the pulmonary trunk to the aorta and provides an additional shunt that allows blood to bypass the lungs (see Fig. 16–2). The pressure in the pulmonary trunk is normally several mm Hg higher than it is in the aorta; therefore, most of the blood flow in the pulmonary trunk passes through the ductus arteriosus into the aorta (Ganong, 1995). As described above, the PVR is elevated when the fetal lungs are collapsed and fluid-filled. The collapse of alveoli causes pulmonary blood vessels to be compressed, thus restricting blood flow through the pulmonary circuit. As a result of these limitations, most of the blood flow coming out of the right ventricle is directed into the ductus arteriosus to join the blood pumped into the aorta by the left ventricle. Normally, only about 10% of the fetal cardiac output reaches the lung because of the effective right-to-left shunts that are operating (Koff, 1993). The volume of blood perfusing the lung primarily functions to sustain the developing structures in the fetal lung.

In addition to serving as a fetal shunt structure to allow blood to bypass the lungs, the ductus arteriosus functions as a *compensatory exercising channel* for the right ventricle (Gardiner, Gray, and O'Rahilly, 1967). The ductus arteriosus allows the right ventricle to develop its muscular pumping power throughout the gestation period. By contracting in unison with the left ventricle, and trying to pump blood into the high-resistance pulmonary vascular beds, the right ventricle becomes stronger. Most of the right ventricular output, however, is directed into the aorta. These contractions prepare the right ventricle so that it is capable of assuming its postnatal role as the right-sided pump responsible for sending blood to the lungs for gaseous exchange.

POSTNATAL FATE OF FETAL CIRCULATORY STRUCTURES

The negative inspiratory pressure developed during the infant's first breath (e.g., -30 to -50 mm Hg), plus constriction of the umbilical vein, draws about 100 mL of oxygenated blood out of the placenta. This mechanism, known as "placental transfusion," helps raise the Po_2 of the newborn's blood stream (Ganong, 1995). Once the placenta is delivered and the umbilical cord is clamped, less blood is returned to the right side of the heart, causing the pressure to decrease. At the same time, loss of the low-pressure placental circuit causes the systemic vascular resistance to increase, along with the pressure in the left side of the heart (Aloan and Hill, 1997). The newborn's heart must now increase its output in order to perfuse both the newly opened pulmonary circuit and the higher-resistance systemic circuit.

The infant's first breath initially inflates alveoli throughout the lung. Assuming the lung has reached maturity, adequate amounts of pulmonary surfactant will be present to reduce alveolar surface tension and ensure that the alveoli remain inflated (see Fig. 1–13). With inflation of the alveoli, compression of pulmonary blood vessels is reduced, thus decreasing pulmonary vascular resistance to less than 20% of its in utero value

(Ganong, 1995). The reduced PVR allows pulmonary blood flow to increase substantially, initiating a sequence of events that ultimately causes the foramen ovale and ductus arteriosus to disappear. As more blood is pumped by the right ventricle to the lower-resistance vascular beds of the postnatal lungs, two important changes in the blood flow pattern emerge: less blood passes through the ductus arteriosus, and more blood returns to the heart from the lungs. The flow of blood to ventilated lungs results in a rise in arterial oxygen tension. Although the mechanism of the vascular response is not completely understood, elevated Pao_2 levels cause *dilation* of pulmonary vascular beds, but *constriction* of the ductus arteriosus. *Functional closure* of the ductus arteriosus does not occur immediately at birth. Instead, the ductus gradually closes over a period of several hours.

Obliteration of the ductus arteriosus (and the umbilical vessels) is aided by *bradykinin,* a powerful tissue hormone released during birth (Aloan and Hill, 1997). Bradykinin also causes dilation of the pulmonary vascular beds. As the ductus arteriosus is progressively deprived of more and more blood, *avascular necrosis* causes the vessel to undergo *anatomic closure* and finally be converted into a nonfunctional cordlike structure known as the **ligamentum arteriosum.** Such a structure is complete by age 3 weeks and is no longer capable of transporting blood (Aloan and Hill, 1997). The birth process (*parturition*) also triggers the production of tissue hormones such as *prostaglandin $F_{2\alpha}$* ($PGF_{2\alpha}$), a powerful vasoconstrictor that aids in the closure and conversion of the ductus arteriosus to a nonfunctional fibrous cord connecting the pulmonary trunk and aorta (Box 16–1).

With increased blood flow to the lungs, more blood returns to the heart. Therefore, as the blood pressure of the left atrium increases, the flaplike portion of the unfused interatrial septum closes over the foramen ovale, reducing the entry of blood from the right atrium. Functional closure of the foramen ovale occurs almost immediately after birth, whereas anatomic closure takes place over several weeks or months (Aloan and Hill, 1997). Anatomic closure culminates in the formation of the **fossa ovalis,** a shallow, oval-shaped depression in the interatrial septum. Closure of the foramen ovale restricts the shunting of blood from the right atrium to the left atrium, and helps establish the postnatal flow of blood into the right ventricle and pulmonary circuit.

As blood flow is reduced or halted in other fetal circulatory structures, vascular spasm results, which further narrows the lumen size of the vessels and further reduces blood flow. Through such positive feedback mechanisms, the fetal vascular structures are converted into nonfunctional tissues. (These vascular changes are also aided by the vasoconstricting action of bradykinin.) The umbilical vein external to the liver is converted into

P E R S P E C T I V E S

BOX 16–1

Opening and Closing the Ductus Arteriosus without Opening and Closing the Infant

A group of tissue hormones known as the *prostaglandins* (PGs) have been the subject of intense study since the 1930s. They were originally recovered from seminal fluid and were believed to be produced solely by the *prostate gland,* hence their name. Different prostaglandins have since been identified in a variety of body fluids and tissues, where they mediate functions such as the relaxation and contraction of smooth muscle. Prostaglandins with smooth muscle–contracting properties include $PGF_{2\alpha}$ and PGD_2, while those with smooth muscle–relaxing effects include PGE_1, PGE_2, and PGI_2.

Prostaglandins are involved in the regulation of the patency of the ductus arteriosus. A balance of these tissue hormones helps to keep the ductus arteriosus open in the fetal circulation, and aids in the closure of the ductus immediately after birth. Prostaglandin I_2 (PGI_2) is also known as *prostacyclin* or *epoprostenol.* This mediator maintains patency of the ductus arteriosus prior to birth to provide the needed right-to-left shunt that restricts blood flow through the fetal lung. Following birth, the ductus arteriosus normally closes functionally as a result of an increase in arterial oxygen tension and a decrease in the levels of PGI_2.

Occasionally, however, a congenital defect causes the ductus arteriosus to remain open after birth. This condition, called a patent ductus arteriosus (PDA), is seen either as an isolated defect, or in combination with other cardiac anomalies. Because of the anatomic shunt, a PDA causes mixing of oxygenated and deoxygenated blood, which results in arterial hypoxemia in the newborn. The infant with a large PDA will also develop pulmonary hypertension as a result of (1) the large volume of blood moved into pulmonary circulation, and (2) the direct transfer of systemic pressure into pulmonary circulation through the defect. Sustained pulmonary hypertension may lead to *cor pulmonale,* a condition characterized by enlargement of the right ventricle caused by increased functional stress on the chamber. This condition, in turn, may progress to right ventricular failure, systemic venous hypertension, tricuspid valve insufficiency, decreased cardiac output, and generalized edema. Surgical closure of a PDA had been the only means to correct the defect until the advent of drugs that alter prostaglandin levels in the newborn. For example, rectal administration of *indomethacin,* an inhibitor of prostaglandin, may reduce the levels of PGI_2 and allow the ductus arteriosus to close in many premature infants who would otherwise require surgery. Pharmacologic closure of a PDA is less effective in the full-term infant (Aloan and Hill, 1997).

Closure of the ductus arteriosus before birth causes pulmonary hypertension and severe $\dot{V}A/\dot{Q}$ inequalities. There is evidence (Ganong, 1995) that a high incidence of pulmonary hypertension occurs in children born to women given prostaglandin inhibitors to delay the onset of labor. Prostaglandins such as $PGF_{2\alpha}$ are naturally released during early stages of labor to initiate contraction of uterine smooth muscle. Prostaglandin inhibitor drugs are useful in slowing these contractions under certain circumstances. Unfortunately, PGI_2 is also inhibited by these drugs, thereby initiating premature closure of the ductus arteriosus.

The clinical use of *PGE_1* to maintain patency or to pharmacologically reopen the ductus arteriosus in certain types of congenital cardiac defects is also possible. For instance, in severe cardiac abnormalities such as the *tetralogy of Fallot* (TOF) and *transposition of the great vessels* (TGV), a vascular connection between the pulmonary and systemic circuits—a patent ductus arteriosus—provides the critical bypass that allows the infant's heart to send a venous admixture of blood into the systemic arteries.

continued

P E R S P E C T I V E S

BOX 16-1   ## Opening and Closing the Ductus Arteriosus without Opening and Closing the Infant (Continued)

Treatment with PGE_1 improves pulmonary blood flow until the cardiac abnormality can be surgically corrected. The defects included in the TOF syndrome include a large ventricular septal defect, pulmonary valve stenosis (narrowing), right ventricular hypertrophy, and coarctation of the aorta. (In coarctation, the aorta is found in an overriding position at the interventricular septum, or it arises from the right side of the heart.) An artificially maintained PDA is beneficial in these cases because it allows additional mixing of blood to occur.

In the TGV defect, the aorta arises from the right ventricle and the pulmonary trunk originates in the left ventricle, producing two parallel circulations instead of the normal series arrangement. In other words, *oxygenated* blood from the pulmonary veins continuously circulates through the left atrium, left ventricle, and pulmonary circulation, while *deoxygenated* blood from systemic veins continuously circulates through the right atrium, right ventricle, and systemic circulation. Without some type of communication between pulmonary and systemic circulatory routes in the form of a septal defect, persistent foramen ovale, or a patent ductus arteriosus, oxygenated blood never reaches the cells of the body—the outcome of which is ultimately fatal. The use of PGE_1 to maintain or reopen the ductus arteriosus reduces arterial hypoxemia and cyanosis until surgical correction of the cardiac defect can be carried out.

Clearly, a delicate balance exists between different prostaglandins that mediate opposing physiologic actions. These complex interactions confound and intrigue researchers in physiology and pharmacology. Greater understanding of the role played by the prostaglandins in the control of body processes such as the opening and closing of the ductus arteriosus will undoubtedly lead to more effective clinical treatment of conditions such as congenital heart defects.

- Aloan CA and Hill TV: Respiratory Care of the Newborn and Child, ed 2. Lippincott-Raven, Philadelphia, 1997.
- Cottrell GP and Surkin HB: Pharmacology for Respiratory Care Practitioners. FA Davis, Philadelphia, 1995.
- Ganong WF: Review of Medical Physiology, ed 17. Appleton & Lange, Norwalk, CT, 1995.
- Salyer JW, Keenan JP, and Masi-Lynch J: Congenital cardiac defects. In Barnhart SL and Czervinske MP (eds): Perinatal and Pediatric Respiratory Care. WB Saunders, Philadelphia, 1995.

TABLE 16-2	Postnatal Fate of Fetal Circulatory Structures
Fetal Structure	**Postnatal Structure**
Shunt (Bypass) Structures	
Ductus venosus	Ligamentum venosum
Ductus arteriosus	Ligamentum arteriosum
Foramen ovale	Fossa ovalis
Placental Connections	
Umbilical vein (1)	Ligamentum teres (round ligament of the liver)
Umbilical arteries (2)	Medial umbilical ligaments
Placenta and Umbilical Cord	None (delivered as "afterbirth")

the **ligamentum teres** or **round ligament of the liver,** a fibrous cord that binds the liver to the umbilicus. The umbilical arteries are changed into fibrous cords called the **medial umbilical ligaments,** and the ductus venosus becomes the **ligamentum venosum,** another fibrous cord in the liver. The placenta and umbilical cord are delivered as *afterbirth,* and have no postnatal role in the newborn.

Table 16–2 summarizes the postnatal fate of fetal circulatory structures.

Summary

This chapter traced the remarkable transformation of the heart from a simple, undifferentiated muscular tube to a complex, multichambered pump. It also briefly outlined the development of the vascular system from a small, branched network of primitive blood vessels supplying a tiny embryo to a vast network of constantly adapting blood vessels that carry blood to and from the metabolically active tissues of a rapidly growing fetus. This chapter also outlined the physiologic events involved in the transitional period following the infant's first breath. These critical changes prepare the cardiovascular system for an independent extrauterine existence. Coupled with the physiologic changes occurring simultaneously in the newborn's respiratory system, the perinatal period in the young infant is marked by extraordinary changes unfolding at a breathtaking pace.

BIBLIOGRAPHY

Aloan CA and Hill TV: Respiratory Care of the Newborn and Child, ed 2. Lippincott-Raven, Philadelphia, 1997.

Ganong WF: Review of Medical Physiology, ed 17. Appleton & Lange, Norwalk, CT, 1995.

Gardner E, Gray DJ, and O'Rahilly R: Anatomy: A Regional Study of Human Structure, ed 2. WB Saunders, Philadelphia, 1967.

Koff PB: Development of the cardiopulmonary system. In Koff PB, Eitzman D, and Neu J (eds): Neonatal and Pediatric Respiratory Care, ed 2. Mosby–Year Book, St. Louis, 1993.

Marieb E: Human Anatomy and Physiology, ed 4. Benjamin/Cummings, Menlo Park, CA, 1998.

Martini FH: Fundamentals of Anatomy and Physiology, ed 4. Prentice Hall, Upper Saddle River, NJ, 1998.

Netter FH: Heart, Vol 5. In Yonkman FF (ed): The CIBA Collection of Medical Illustrations. CIBA Pharmaceutical Co., Summit, NJ, 1969.

Saladin KS: Anatomy and Physiology: The Unity of Form and Function. WCB/McGraw-Hill, Boston, 1998.

Tortora GJ and Grabowski SR: Principles of Anatomy and Physiology, ed 8. HarperCollins, New York, 1996.

CHAPTER 17

Gross Anatomy of the Heart

chapter objectives

After studying this chapter the reader should be able to:

☐ Describe the function of the great vessels of the heart.
☐ Define the following terms:
   Pulmonary circulation, systemic circulation, base, apex.
☐ Review the organization of the following pericardial structures:
   Visceral pericardium, parietal pericardium, pericardial space, pericardial fluid.
☐ Review the layers of the wall of the heart.
☐ Explain why the myocardium of the physiologic left heart is thicker than that of the physiologic right heart.
☐ Describe the structure of the fibrous skeleton of the heart.
☐ Name two functions of the fibrous skeleton of the heart.
☐ Describe the location and function of the following structures:
   Atria, ventricles, interatrial septum, interventricular septum.
☐ Describe the location of the following surface features of the heart:
   Atrioventricular (coronary) sulcus, anterior interventricular sulcus, posterior interventricular sulcus.
☐ Compare and contrast the structure and function of the semilunar and atrioventricular valves, including the function of the chordae tendineae and papillary muscles.
☐ Describe the pressure changes responsible for opening and closing heart valves.
☐ Explain the concept of oxygen supply and demand in the myocardium.
☐ Describe the unique functional characteristics of the myocardium in regard to resistance to fatigue, reliance on aerobic metabolism, and blood flow during the cardiac cycle.

□ Describe the arterial supply to the myocardium by naming the regions supplied and the branches of the left and right coronary arteries.

□ Describe the venous drainage of the myocardium by describing the role of the great cardiac vein, middle cardiac vein, coronary sinus, and thebesian veins.

key terms

anastomosis (a-nas″ tō-mō′ sis)
anterior interventricular sulcus (sul′ kus)
apex
atrioventricular sulcus; coronary sulcus
atrioventricular (AV) valves
   left atrioventricular valve; bicuspid valve; mitral valve
   right atrioventricular valve; tricuspid valve
base
chordae tendineae (kor′dē ten-din′ ē ē)
coronary circulation
coronary sinus
cusps
fibrous skeleton
great cardiac vein
great vessels
   aorta
   inferior vena cava (IVC)
   pulmonary trunk; pulmonary arteries
   pulmonary veins
   superior vena cava (SVC)
interatrial septum

interventricular septum
left atrium (LA)
left coronary artery
   anterior interventricular branch
   circumflex branch
left ventricle (LV)
middle cardiac vein
papillary muscles (pap′ i-lar-ē)
posterior interventricular sulcus
pulmonary circulation
right atrium (RA)
right coronary artery
   marginal branch
   posterior interventricular branch
right ventricle (RV)
semilunar (SL) valves
   aortic semilunar valve
   pulmonary semilunar valve
systemic circulation
thebesian veins (thē-bē′ zē-an)
trabeculae carneae (tra-bek′-ū-lē car′ nē-ē)

The cardiovascular system consists of the *heart, blood vessels,* and *blood.* The embryologic development of these components was outlined in the previous chapter. In terms of numbers of organs, the cardiovascular system is relatively uncomplicated, consisting of a muscular pump that propels blood through an extensive vascular network. The structure and function of the system, however, is extremely complex and, as we have seen in previous chapters, is intricately linked to the structure and function of the respiratory system. A brief overview of the gross anatomy of the heart follows, including a discussion of blood flow through the chambers of the heart, and blood flow through heart muscle.

The Great Vessels

The blood vessels of the cardiovascular system are organized into two separate circuits—the **pulmonary circulation** supplying deoxygenated blood to the lungs, and the **systemic circulation** responsible for distributing oxygenated blood to the tissues of the body *other than* the functional units of the lung. The arteries and veins attached to the heart on its superior aspect, or **base,** are called the **great vessels** because of their large diameters. The **apex** of the heart is the inferior portion adjacent to the diaphragm (Fig. 17–1; see also Color Plate 12). Mixed venous blood having low oxygen tension and high carbon dioxide tension is returned to the right side of the heart by systemic veins. The **superior vena cava (SVC)** returns blood from regions superior to the heart, whereas the **inferior vena cava (IVC)** brings blood back to the heart from those regions inferior to the heart. The *physiologic right heart* pumps this deoxygenated blood to the lungs through the **pulmonary trunk** that bifurcates into the right and left **pulmonary arteries** supplying the right and left lungs, respectively (see Fig. 17–1). After gas transfer has occurred in the pulmonary capillaries of the lung, oxygenated blood is returned to the left side of the heart by a pair of **pulmonary veins** from each lung. The *physiologic left heart*

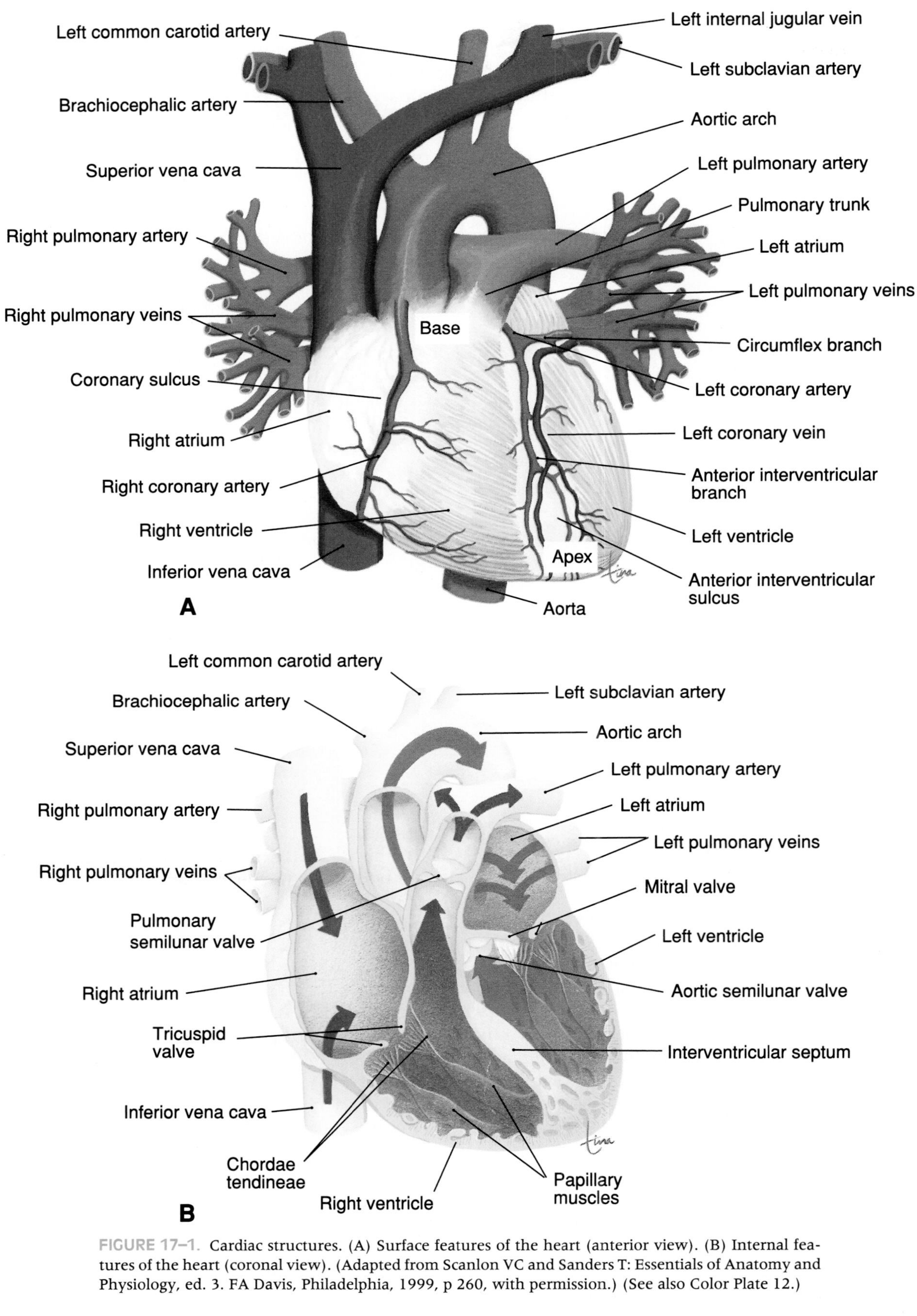

The Cardiovascular System

A

Left common carotid artery

Brachiocephalic artery

Superior vena cava

Right pulmonary artery

Right pulmonary veins

Coronary sulcus

Right atrium

Right coronary artery

Right ventricle

Inferior vena cava

Left internal jugular vein

Left subclavian artery

Aortic arch

Left pulmonary artery

Pulmonary trunk

Left atrium

Left pulmonary veins

Circumflex branch

Left coronary artery

Left coronary vein

Anterior interventricular branch

Left ventricle

Anterior interventricular sulcus

Base

Apex

Aorta

B

Left common carotid artery

Brachiocephalic artery

Superior vena cava

Right pulmonary artery

Right pulmonary veins

Pulmonary semilunar valve

Right atrium

Tricuspid valve

Inferior vena cava

Chordae tendineae

Right ventricle

Left subclavian artery

Aortic arch

Left pulmonary artery

Left atrium

Left pulmonary veins

Mitral valve

Left ventricle

Aortic semilunar valve

Interventricular septum

Papillary muscles

FIGURE 17–1. Cardiac structures. (A) Surface features of the heart (anterior view). (B) Internal features of the heart (coronal view). (Adapted from Scanlon VC and Sanders T: Essentials of Anatomy and Physiology, ed. 3. FA Davis, Philadelphia, 1999, p 260, with permission.) (See also Color Plate 12.)

pumps the oxygenated blood into the systemic arteries through the **aorta.**

Pericardium and Heart Wall

PERICARDIAL STRUCTURES

The heart is located in the *mediastinum,* a flexible mid-line partition found between the two lungs (see Chap. 1). As discussed with the developmental aspects of the heart (see Chap. 16), the mesodermal tissue in the vicinity of the future *pericardial cavity* separates into two layers, forming a space between them. The embryonic heart then pushes into this developing peri-cardial cavity, becoming enveloped by one of the membranes in the process. The layer that contacts and adheres to the heart becomes the *visceral pericardium;* whereas the layer that lines the cavity becomes the *parietal pericardium* (Fig. 17–2). The space between them is filled with a serous fluid known as *pericardial fluid.* Friction between pericardial layers is practically eliminated through the lubricating action of pericardial fluid. In addition to lubricating and anchoring the heart in the chest cavity, the double-walled arrange-ment of the pericardial sac isolates the heart from other

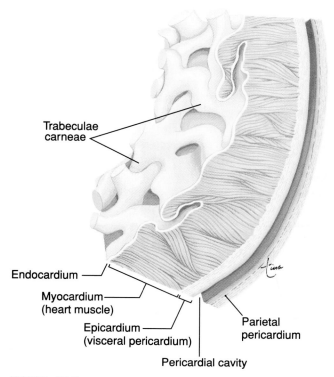

Trabeculae
carneae

Endocardium

Myocardium
(heart muscle)

Epicardium
(visceral pericardium)

Parietal
pericardium

Pericardial cavity

FIGURE 17–2. Heart wall and pericardial structures. The peri-cardium is a double-walled saclike structure that anchors, protects, and lubricates the heart. Pericardial fluid occupies the pericardial cavity and functions to reduce friction between the visceral and pari-etal layers of the pericardium during heart contractions. (Adapted from Scanlon VC and Sanders T: Essentials of Anatomy and Physiol-ogy, ed. 3. FA Davis, Philadelphia, 1999, p 258, with permission.)

thoracic organs, while allowing it to expand as it fills with blood.

ORGANIZATION OF THE HEART WALL

The visceral pericardium forms the outermost layer of the wall of the heart and is known as the *epicardium.* The middle layer is composed of heart muscle and is called the *myocardium.* (Details of the structure and function of myocardium are considered in Chapter 18.) The innermost layer, or *endocardium,* lines the chambers of the heart and valves (see Fig. 17–2). This layer of sim-ple squamous cells is continuous with the endothelial lining of blood vessels. Unlike the outermost and in-nermost layers of the wall of the heart, the thickness of the myocardium is not uniform. Cardiac muscle mass is proportional to the force that must be generated by dif-ferent regions of the heart. This force is required to overcome vascular resistance, which is different in dif-ferent parts of the circulatory system. Accordingly, the physiologic left heart is about three times as thick as the physiologic right heart, owing to the greater pressures that must be developed by the left heart. The muscle fibers of the myocardium are arranged in a spiral fash-ion; thus when the myocardium contracts, a twisting or "wringing" action results. The spiral myocardial fibers are interwoven with collagenous and elastic connective tissue fibers (Saladin, 1998). This unique structural arrangement forms the **fibrous skeleton** of the heart (Fig. 17–3).

The fibrous skeleton provides structural support for the heart, and is especially strong in the vicinity of the heart valves and great vessels. In addition to providing structural rigidity, the fibrous skeleton provides some-thing against which the myocardial fibers can pull. Fi-nally, this structure functions to electrically isolate the upper portions of the heart from the lower portions. By serving as a nonconductor of electrical impulses, the fi-brous skeleton limits the routes that electrical activity can take from the upper to the lower parts of the heart. This limitation, in turn, helps synchronize electrical ac-tivity in different parts of the heart. As discussed in Chapter 18, electrically isolating different parts of the heart requires a sophisticated electrical timing and con-duction system to link them together again. Such a con-trol system must operate flawlessly to coordinate the pumping activity of the different chambers of the heart.

Chambers of the Heart

INTERNAL FEATURES

The heart is organized as two pairs of pumping cham-bers. The pair of superior chambers consists of the *right atrium* and the *left atrium,* which simultaneously receive

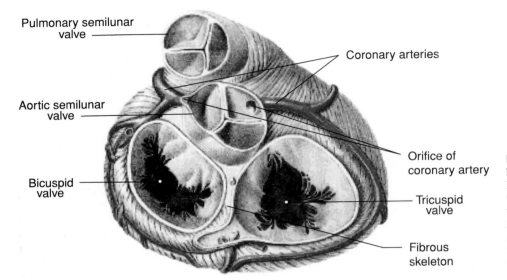

Pulmonary semilunar valve

Coronary arteries

Aortic semilunar valve

Bicuspid valve

Orifice of coronary artery

Tricuspid valve

Fibrous skeleton

FIGURE 17–3. Heart valves and fibrous skeleton of the heart. The atria have been removed in this superior view in order to show all four heart valves. Note the origin of the coronary arteries in the aorta. The fibrous skeleton of the heart provides added strength in the vicinity of the atrioventricular valves.

blood returning to the heart through the veins (see Fig. 17–1B). The **right atrium (RA)** receives deoxygenated blood from systemic circulation through the IVC, SVC, and the *coronary sinus,* a venous structure on the posterior wall of the RA that serves to collect deoxygenated blood from large veins draining the heart muscle. The **left atrium (LA)** receives oxygenated blood from the lungs through the four pulmonary veins. Each atrium has a small flaplike extension called an *auricle.* This small pocket of tissue resembles an ear and functions to slightly increase the overall volume of the atria. The paired atria contract in tandem to raise the pressure of blood in the chambers and pump this volume of blood a short distance into the inferior chambers. Because the blood does not have to overcome a great resistance in the ventricles, the force developed by the atria is relatively small—consequently, the myocardial layer is thin. The action of the combined RA and LA forming the *atrial pump* forces an extra volume of blood into the ventricles prior to ventricular contraction, thus serving to prime the ventricles and increase their volume just prior to ventricular contraction. (Changes in ventricular volume during the cardiac cycle are discussed in Chapter 19.)

The two lower chambers are the **right ventricle (RV)** and the **left ventricle (LV),** which function together as the *ventricular pump* to eject blood into the arteries (see Fig. 17–1B). As pointed out previously, ventricular walls are much thicker than those of the atria. Furthermore, the pressure developed by the left ventricle is approximately six times greater than the pressure generated by the right ventricle, a difference required to overcome the greater resistance of the systemic circuit compared with that of the pulmonary circuit.

Internally, the right and left sides of the heart are separated by a longitudinal septum. The development of various septa was described with the embryologic aspects of the heart (see Chap. 16). The **interatrial sep-**

tum divides the right and left atria. The shallow *fossa ovalis,* the postnatal remnant of the *foramen ovale,* is visible on the surface of the interatrial septum. The right and left ventricles are separated by the thick-walled **interventricular septum** (see Fig. 17–1B) The lining of both the right and left ventricle is marked by conspicuous internal ridges called **trabeculae carneae** (see Fig. 17–2).

SURFACE LANDMARKS

On the exterior of the heart are found shallow fat-filled grooves, or *sulci,* that contain the coronary blood vessels (see Fig. 17–1A). The external landmarks that serve as rough approximations of the location of internal divisions between the chambers of the heart are (1) the **atrioventricular (coronary) sulcus,** which encircles the heart and separates the atria from the ventricles; (2) the **anterior interventricular sulcus,** which extends vertically from the atrioventricular sulcus and separates the right and left ventricles on the anterior surface of the heart; and (3) the **posterior interventricular sulcus,** which is a vertical depression that marks the division between ventricles on the posterior surface of the heart.

Valves and Blood Flow Through the Heart

Heart valves are located where blood *exits* from each chamber; therefore, four separate heart valves control blood flow through the chambers to ensure an orderly, unidirectional flow pattern. The paired *atrioventricular valves* control the exit of blood from the atria to the ventricles, whereas the paired *semilunar valves* regulate the flow of blood out of the ventricles into the arteries (see Figs. 17–1B and 17–3).

ATRIOVENTRICULAR VALVES

Atrioventricular (AV) valves close when ventricular pressure exceeds atrial pressure. In general terms, this gradient is created when the downstream (distal) pressure is higher than the upstream (proximal) pressure. The artrioventricular pressure difference develops immediately following contraction of the paired ventricles. Because the right and left ventricles beat together as a unit and simultaneously raise pressures in the right and left ventricles, the two atrioventricular valves close at approximately the same time. Conversely, the two atrioventricular valves open together as the paired ventricles relax and ventricular pressure decreases in both ventricles. The **right atrioventricular valve,** also known as the **tricuspid valve,** consists of three irregular-shaped **cusps,** or flaps, that open and close to control the flow of blood from the right atrium to the right ventricle (see Fig. 17–3). Blood flow from the left atrium to the left ventricle is controlled by the operation of the **left atrioventricular valve,** also known as the **bicuspid valve,** or the **mitral valve.** The left AV valve has two irregular-shaped cusps (see Fig. 17–3). The closure of the AV valve cusps in both the tricuspid and mitral valves is limited by tough, threadlike fibers called **chordae tendineae** that insert on the lower (ventricular) aspect of the valve flaps.

These strong fibers are, in turn, anchored to muscular bundles called **papillary muscles** that project from the floor of the ventricles (see Fig. 17–1B).

When the ventricles are relaxed and dilated, the outward expansion of the ventricular wall applies tension to the papillary muscles and chordae tendineae. The increased tension assists in the opening of the atrioventricular valves, allowing blood to flow freely from the atria into the ventricles during the period of ventricular relaxation, or *diastole* (Fig. 17–4A). (Various phases of the cardiac cycle are discussed in Chapter 19.) Contraction of the ventricles (*systole*) causes the walls of the heart to squeeze inward, creating a smaller chamber volume and raising the pressure of the blood in the chamber. Because this inward movement of the heart wall relieves tension on the chordae tendineae, the flaps of the AV valves swing upward toward the opening into the atria (Fig. 17–4B). The mechanical arrangement provided by the chordae tendineae and papillary muscles effectively couples the AV valve flaps to the wall of the ventricle so that they move as a unit in response to contraction and relaxation of ventricular muscle. Prolapse (overclosure) of the AV valves is prevented by this structural arrangement. Without such a limiting mechanism, reflux (backflow) of blood into the atria occurs, severely reducing the pumping efficiency of the ventricles.

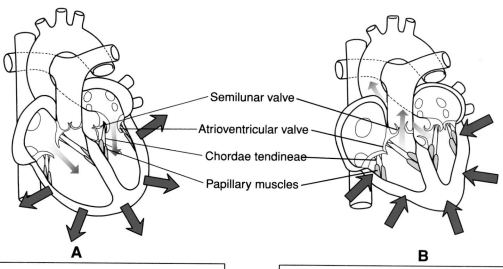

Semilunar valve

Atrioventricular valve

Chordae tendineae

Papillary muscles

A

Relaxation of ventricular wall
Tension on chordae tendineae increased
Opening of atrioventricular valves

B

Contraction of ventricular wall
Tension on chordae tendineae decreased
Closure of atrioventricular valves

FIGURE 17–4. Action of heart wall and atrioventricular valves. (A) During relaxation (*diastole*), the outward expansion of the heart wall increases the tension on the chordae tendineae because the structures are anchored to the ventricular wall by the papillary muscles. This action aids in the opening of the atrioventricular valves. (B) During contraction (*systole*), inward movement of the heart wall relieves the tension on the papillary muscles and the chordae tendineae, allowing the cusps of the atrioventricular valves to close. The rise in ventricular pressure aids in the opening of the semilunar valves to allow ejection of blood from both ventricles.

SEMILUNAR VALVES

The closure of **semilunar (SL) valves** is due to a combination of two events related to the cardiac cycle. An abrupt drop in ventricular pressure occurs immediately following relaxation of the paired ventricles. This decrease in pressure on the upstream (proximal) side of the SL valves closes the valve cusps. The closure is assisted by a temporary increase in pressure on the downstream (distal) side of the valves, caused by the elastic recoil of arterial walls. For example, the outward expansion of the wall of the aorta and the pulmonary trunk in response to contraction of the ventricles causes potential energy to be stored in the elastic fibers of the vessel wall. The rebound, or recoil, effect of the elastic fibers creates a pulse wave that propels blood forward, an action that is particularly noticeable in the aorta. The effect also raises arterial pressure, which helps to close the SL valves. The *aortic pump mechanism* thus functions in a passive way to improve the efficiency of the left heart, by operating during the brief period of time when the left ventricle is relaxed. Elastic recoil is also seen in the pulmonary arteries, but the pressures are only about one-sixth as great as those generated in the aorta. Contraction of the ventricles raises ventricular pressure above that in the arteries distal to the SL valves, thus causing the valves to open at approximately the same time that the AV valves close. Liquids are virtually incompressible; therefore, as the ventricles begin to squeeze inward, there is nearly a simultaneous closure of the AV valves and opening of the SL valves.

Semilunar valves are formed by three moon-shaped, symmetrical cusps that have shallow concave depressions on their vascular (distal) sides (see Fig. 17–3). As the ventricles relax, blood surges back toward the heart, pushing against these shallow depressions to help close the SL valve. The **pulmonary valve** is found at the origin of the pulmonary trunk, where it controls the exit of blood out of the right ventricle into the pulmonary circuit. The **aortic valve** is located at the origin of the aorta (see Fig. 17–1B). This valve governs the flow of blood out of the left ventricle into the systemic circuit (Box 17–1). Because the opening and closing of both semilunar valves is linked to the contraction and relaxation of the paired ventricles, the pulmonary and aortic valves operate together to control blood flow out of the heart.

Blood Flow Through the Myocardium

OXYGEN SUPPLY AND DEMAND

Some organs receive a flowrate of blood that is disproportionate to their size. These organs, such as the brain, kidneys, and heart, are said to be highly perfused. For example, the heart makes up only about 0.5% of the mass of the body, but it receives approximately 5% of the *cardiac output* (about 250 mL/min) to meet its considerable metabolic needs (Saladin, 1998). When this metabolic demand is not met, an imbalance of oxygen supply and oxygen demand rapidly develops, a condition known as *myocardial ischemia.* Such a condition can occur as a result of reduced blood flow in the vessels supplying the myocardium, or increased workload in the heart muscle.

Temporary ischemia produces *angina pectoris,* a cardiac condition described as a choking or crushing sensation in the chest. (*Angina* comes from the Latin word *angere,* which means "to choke.") Hypoxia in the myocardium results in anaerobic conditions and the production of lactic acid, a metabolic byproduct that accumulates in muscle tissue during periods of anaerobic metabolism. Although heart muscle is versatile enough to utilize a variety of fuels to power its contractions, it is very intolerant of metabolic waste products such as lactic acid—which causes the acute pain of angina pectoris.

If myocardial ischemia is untreated, the region of heart muscle deprived of blood undergoes *necrosis,* or tissue death. This area of tissue death is called a *myocardial infarction* (MI), and is responsible for producing a feeling of heavy pressure, or a squeezing pain in the chest. Infarctions are nonfunctional areas of tissue that weaken the heart wall and may disrupt electrical activity in the heart. Such destructive changes may lead to *cardiac arrest.*

FUNCTIONAL CHARACTERISTICS OF THE MYOCARDIUM

Cardiac muscle is unique in the following functional respects:

- Myocardial cells do not rely on anaerobic fermentation to any great degree, nor do they depend on the oxygen debt mechanism to eliminate metabolic waste products at a later time. As a result of these functional characteristics, myocardium is not prone to fatigue, as is skeletal muscle—an obvious benefit in a tissue that must perform continuously throughout our lifetimes.

- Dependence on aerobic metabolism requires that myocardial cells be continually supplied with oxygenated blood. This is the only way that the high oxygen demand resulting from the metabolic stress of repetitive contractions can be satisfied.

- Most of the blood flow to the heart muscle occurs during the relaxation period (*diastole*) when the blood vessels are dilated. Contraction of the heart muscle (systole) compresses the blood vessels supplying the heart and restricts blood flow. This situation is the opposite of that occurring in the systemic arteries, where more blood is delivered to

PERSPECTIVES

BOX 17–1   **Heart Valves and Breathlessness**

It is difficult or impossible to separate many of the functions of the respiratory and cardiovascular systems. Often, a structural defect in one will produce disordered function in the other. For example, *stenosis* (narrowing) of the aortic valve due to damaged valve cusps affects left ventricular function during both the contraction and relaxation phases of the cycle. The stenosed valve increases the resistance to outflow of blood from the left ventricle, causing the left ventricle to become larger (*cardiomegaly*) as it strains to push blood past the restricted opening. Stenosis also permits reflux of blood to occur as blood regurgitates into the left ventricle from the aorta during ventricular relaxation. The resulting increase in stress of the heart wall increases the oxygen demand of the myocardium. Clearly, the immediate effect of this valvular defect is reduced pumping efficiency of the heart. The *pathogenesis,* or progression, of the disorder, however, extends far beyond the heart.

Because a lower volume of blood is ejected by the left ventricle, the volume remaining in the chamber is greater than normal. This volume produces a damming effect that reduces the amount of blood that can enter the left atrium and pulmonary veins. As blood backs up into the pulmonary circuit, blood flow through the pulmonary capillaries becomes more and more sluggish. This pulmonary congestion causes edema, which reduces the efficiency of gas exchange. The reduced blood flow extends to the physiologic right heart and systemic veins, overloading the right heart and causing it to enlarge as it struggles to push blood through congested pulmonary blood vessels. A destructive positive feedback loop develops as the heart becomes larger and larger, and its walls become thinner relative to the size of its chambers. As a result, the heart cannot develop adequate force and its output progressively declines. Since less blood enters the right heart, blood backs into the systemic veins, causing generalized edema in the tissues of the body.

Taken together, these hemodynamic changes are responsible for clinical and laboratory findings such as *hypoxemia, hypercapnia, cardiomegaly, dyspnea, cyanosis,* and *edema* of the extremities (e.g., swollen ankles). These findings are indicative of heart failure, or the inability of the heart to adequately meet the gaseous needs of the tissues. A patient with this condition experiences marked breathlessness upon slight physical exertion, an indicator of respiratory distress. In actual fact, the structure and function of the respiratory system is *normal,* but is masked by the congestion and edema caused by the *abnormal* structure and function of the cardiovascular system. It is the heart valve defect that is responsible for the pathophysiologic changes in the combined cardiopulmonary system. The patient's breathing difficulties can be traced to the stenosis of the aortic valve. The respiratory problems generally disappear when the faulty heart valve is repaired or replaced—a perfect example of the interdependency of the two systems and the difficulties encountered when attention is confined to one or the other. Instead, awareness of the *integral* function of the combined cardiovascular and respiratory systems is needed in the study of cardiopulmonary physiology and pathophysiology.

the tissues during the systolic period. Notice in Figure 17–5 that the time period to complete systole is relatively uniform whether the heart is at rest beating 60 times per minute, or contracting at three times that rate. Therefore, the diastolic period must become progressively shorter to com-

plete more cardiac cycles per minute. Because blood flow to the myocardium is linked to diastole, oxygen delivery to heart muscle is reduced as the heart rate increases. In a healthy heart, this periodic reduction in blood flow is unnoticed, but in individuals with restricted blood flow in the *coro-*

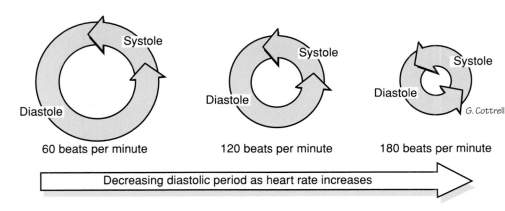

FIGURE 17–5. Coronary blood flow and heart rate. The systolic period remains relatively fixed as the heart rate fluctuates. Therefore, increases in heart rate are brought about by a decrease in the interval required to complete the diastolic period. Most coronary blood flow occurs during diastole.

nary arteries, higher heart rates brought about by exertion may cause myocardial ischemia and trigger an angina attack.

On the basis of these characteristics—intolerance to metabolic wastes, high oxygen demand, and vulnerability to reduced blood flow at faster heart rates—it can be seen that certain conditions may render the heart muscle susceptible to myocardial ischemia. Conditions such as obstructed blood vessels supplying the myocardium, coupled with exercise-related increases in oxygen demand, can place an enormous physiologic stress on myocardial tissue. For all of the foregoing reasons, the arteries and veins comprising **coronary circulation** must perform flawlessly to distribute blood throughout the myocardium and thus maintain the metabolic status of the pump itself.

ARTERIAL SUPPLY

Recall that blood returning to the left heart from the lungs has an oxygen tension (P_{O_2}) of approximately 100 mm Hg and a carbon dioxide tension (P_{CO_2}) of about 40 mm Hg. These blood gas values are at optimal levels at the instant the left ventricle pumps this blood into the aorta. Immediately adjacent to the cusps of the aortic valve, on the distal side of the valve, are found the openings into the *right* and *left coronary arteries*—the main arterial supply to the myocardium. Thus, the hardworking myocardium is the first tissue of the body to receive freshly-oxygenated blood from the lung.

The **left coronary artery** travels under the left auricle and divides into the *anterior interventricular branch* and the *circumflex branch* (Fig. 17–6A):

- The **anterior interventricular branch** of the left coronary artery travels in the anterior interventricular sulcus toward the apex of the heart and gives off small branches that supply the interventricular septum and the anterior wall of both ventricles.
- The **circumflex branch** of the left coronary artery circles the heart in the coronary sulcus and issues

smaller branches that supply the left atrium and the posterior wall of the left ventricle.

The **right coronary artery** supplies the right atrium and then travels along the coronary sulcus before branching into the *marginal branch* and the *posterior interventricular branch* (Fig. 17–6B):

- The lateral walls of the right atrium and right ventricle are supplied by branches of the **marginal branch** of the right coronary artery.
- The **posterior interventricular branch** of the right coronary artery travels along the posterior interventricular sulcus and issues smaller branches that supply the posterior walls of both ventricles.

Several important junctions of arteries exist in coronary circulation. At these junctions, blood flow from multiple routes joins together to form a common circulatory route called an **anastomosis.** This specialized circulatory structure provides *collateral circulation;* that is, an alternate pathway blood can take if one of the circulatory routes comprising the vascular network is blocked. This structural design minimizes the chance that tissue distal to the anastomosis will be completely deprived of blood. Collateral circulatory routes formed by arterial anastomoses are common in the heart and brain where interruption of blood flow can have immediate and dire consequences. Important coronary anastomoses are formed by the union of the (1) circumflex branch of the left coronary artery and the right coronary artery to supply blood to the posterior interventricular branch, and (2) anterior interventricular branch of the left coronary artery and the posterior interventricular branch of the right coronary artery at the apex of the heart (Saladin, 1998).

VENOUS DRAINAGE

Small veins drain most of the deoxygenated blood from the myocardium and return it to two larger-diameter veins known as the *great cardiac vein* and the *middle cardiac vein* (see Fig. 17–6B). The **thebesian veins** drain a small amount of deoxygenated blood di-

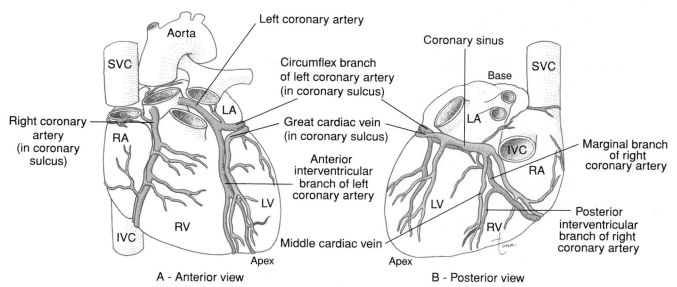

FIGURE 17–6. Coronary circulation. (A) Anterior view. (B) Posterior view. The larger coronary blood vessels are located within fat-filled grooves known as *sulci*. The *coronary sulcus* marks the separation between atria and ventricles and accommodates the right coronary artery, the circumflex branch of the left coronary artery, and the great cardiac vein; the *anterior* and *posterior interventricular sulci* separate right and left ventricles and accommodate the anterior interventricular branch of the left coronary artery and the posterior interventricular branch of the right coronary artery, respectively. Extensive anastamoses among various blood vessels provide an elaborate collateral circulatory system that can reroute blood around minor obstructions so that the myocardium is not deprived of blood. Several thebesian veins empty deoxygenated blood directly into the left ventricle (not shown). (IVC = inferior vena cava; SVC = superior vena cava; LA = left atrium; LV = left ventricle; RA = right atrium; RV = right ventricle.) (Adapted from Scanlon VC and Sanders T: Essentials of Anatomy and Physiology, ed. 3. FA Davis, Philadelphia, 1999, p 262, with permission.)

rectly from the myocardium and return it to the left heart:

- The **great cardiac vein** collects blood from the anterior side of the heart and travels within the anterior interventricular sulcus toward the *coronary sinus.*
- Venous drainage from the posterior aspect of the myocardium is collected by the **middle cardiac vein,** which is found in the posterior interventricular sulcus.

The great and middle cardiac veins, as well as several smaller-diameter veins, empty into the thin-walled venous sinus called the **coronary sinus,** located on the posterior wall of the right atrium (see Fig. 17–6B). The *thebesian valve* is a small flap of endocardial tissue at the entrance of the coronary sinus to the right atrium. Because the coronary sinus opens directly into the right atrium, *most* of the venous drainage from the myocardium is returned to the physiologic right heart to be pumped to the lung for gas exchange. However, the *thebesian veins* empty blood directly into the left ventricle. Several thebesian veins collect deoxygenated blood from the myocardium and return it to the left heart where it forms a venous admixture with the oxygenated blood already in the chamber. (Thebesian

veins are small venules named after the German physician, Adam Christian Thebesius [1686–1732].) As discussed in Chapter 14, this type of anatomic shunt contributes to a reduction in arterial oxygen saturation. Although the volume of venous blood entering the left ventricle through the thebesian veins is relatively small, its P_{O_2} is very low and its P_{CO_2} is very high because of the marked metabolic activity of heart muscle cells.

Summary

This chapter provides a brief overview of cardiac anatomy with the emphasis on gross anatomical structures such as the great vessels, pericardial sac, chambers, and valves. Organization of the pumping chambers and operation of the heart valves and their role in controlling blood flow through the heart was also considered. The chapter concludes with a discussion of coronary circulation, anastomoses, and the unique metabolic needs of myocardium. This chapter serves both as a review of general cardiac anatomy and as an introduction to a detailed study of heart muscle and its electrical characteristics, topics to be considered in the following chapter.

BIBLIOGRAPHY

Martini FH: Fundamentals of Anatomy and Physiology, ed 4. Prentice Hall, Upper Saddle River, NJ, 1998.

Saladin KS: Anatomy and Physiology: The Unity of Form and Function. WCB/McGraw-Hill, Boston, 1998.

Shier D, Butler J, and Lewis R: Hole's Human Anatomy and Physiology, ed 7. Wm C Brown, Dubuque, IA, 1996.

Thibodeau GA and Patton KT: Anatomy and Physiology, ed 3. Mosby–Year Book, St Louis, 1996.

Thomas CL (ed): Taber's Cyclopedic Medical Dictionary, ed 18. FA Davis, Philadelphia, 1997.

Tortora GJ and Grabowski SR: Principles of Anatomy and Physiology, ed 8. HarperCollins, New York, 1996.

Woodburne AM and Burkel WE: Essentials of Human Anatomy, ed 9. Oxford University Press, New York, 1994.

CHAPTER 18

Cardiac Muscle and the Cardiac Conduction System

chapter objectives

After studying this chapter the reader should be able to:

☐ Compare and contrast cardiac and skeletal muscle fibers on the basis of sarcoplasmic reticulum, calcium stores, and mitochondria.

☐ Describe the appearance of cardiac myocytes.

☐ Explain the function of the following cardiac myocyte structures:
Intercalated discs, desmosomes, gap junctions, ion channels.

☐ Discuss the concept of a functional syncytium as it applies to cardiac myocytes.

☐ Define the following terms:
Myogenic origin of heartbeat, autorhythmic, ectopic focus.

☐ Discuss the role of the cardiac conduction system by explaining the function of the following components:
Sinoatrial node, interatrial band, internodal pathways, atrioventricular node, atrioventricular bundle, bundle branches, conduction myofibers.

☐ Differentiate between sinus rhythm and nodal rhythm.

☐ Explain the concept of a "primary pacemaker" in the control of cardiac electrical activity.

☐ Define arrhythmia and differentiate between supraventricular arrhythmias and ventricular arrhythmias.

☐ Define the following terms related to cell membrane electrical events:
Voltage-gated ion channels, influx, efflux, polarization, depolarization, repolarization, resting membrane potential, action potential.

☐ Discuss the generation of a cardiac action potential in the sinoatrial node by describing the electrophysiologic characteristics and phases of the action potential.

☐ Discuss the generation of a cardiac action potential in conducting tissue such as conduction myofibers by describing the electrophysiologic characteristics and phases of the action potential.

☐ Discuss the generation of a cardiac action potential in ventricular muscle cells by describing the electrophysiologic characteristics and phases of the action potential.

☐ Define electrocardiogram (ECG).

☐ Explain what the following components of the electrocardiogram waveform represent in the cardiac cycle:

P wave, P-Q interval, QRS complex, S-T segment, T wave.

key terms

arrhythmias; dysrhythmias
atrioventricular bundle (A-V bundle); bundle of His
atrioventricular node; A-V node
autorhythmic
bundle branches (right and left)
cardiac action potential
    Phase 0—depolarization
    Phase 1—transient repolarization
    Phase 2—plateau phase
    Phase 3—repolarization
    Phase 4—polarization (resting membrane potential; RMP)
cardiac conduction system; intrinsic conducting system
cardiac electrophysiology
cardiac muscle cells; cardiac myocytes
conduction myofibers; Purkinje fibers
desmosomes
ectopic focus
electrocardiogram (ECG, EKG)
    P wave
    P-Q interval; P-R interval

QRS complex
S-T segment
T wave
functional syncytium
    atrial syncytium
    ventricular syncytium
gap junctions
interatrial band
intercalated discs
internodal pathways
myogenic origin
nodal rhythm
pacemaker potential
Purkinje system; His-Purkinje system (his′ pur-kin′-jē)
sinoatrial node; SA node; primary pacemaker
sinus rhythm
voltage-gated ion channels
    voltage-gated fast Na^+ channels
    voltage-gated slow Ca^{2+} channels
    voltage-gated slow K^+ channels
    voltage-gated slow Na^+ channels

In the previous chapter we discussed a few of the unique functional properties of the myocardium, such as its nearly total reliance on aerobic metabolism and its remarkable fatigue resistance in the face of repetitive contractions. Here we examine unique structural and electrophysiologic characteristics of myocardial cells and specialized conduction tissue. The chapter explores how electrical impulses are initiated and distributed rapidly and efficiently throughout the myocardium.

Structure and Organization of Heart Muscle Cells

Muscle cells, or *myocytes,* make up *muscle tissue,* one of the body's four basic tissue classifications. (Recall that connective, nervous, and epithelial tissues are the other three types of tissues.) Myocytes exhibit the characteristics of *irritability,* or the ability to respond to a stimulus, and *contractility,* the ability to shorten in length. The three subtypes of muscle tissue—*striated muscle, smooth muscle,* and *cardiac muscle*—exhibit these basic characteristics of muscle cells but differ in other ways such as motor control, response time to a stimulus, and fatigue resistance.

The morphology of **cardiac muscle cells,** or **cardiac myocytes,** differs from that of striated (skeletal) muscle cells, although both appear somewhat thready, or "fibrous" when viewed under the microscope. Such cells are often called muscle *fibers.* Cardiac muscle fibers contain one nucleus per cell, and are branched and generally shorter and thicker than the multinucleated skeletal muscle fibers (Table 18–1). Within the *sarcoplasm* of the heart muscle cell, the *sarcoplasmic reticulum* (SR) is less well developed than that in skeletal muscle fibers. (Recall that *sarcoplasm* refers to the cytoplasm of muscle cells, and that the *sarcoplasmic reticulum* is the intracellular communication network of microtubules found within muscle cells. For a review of basic structure and function of muscle tissue, consult any of the general anatomy and physiology texts listed in the chapter bibliography.) The SR of heart muscle cells releases far fewer calcium ions (Ca^{2+}) to the myocytes, compared with the SR of skeletal muscle fibers; therefore, the myocardium is almost totally dependent on *extracellular* stores of Ca^{2+} to power its contractions. The SR of heart muscle cells is designed to rapidly admit Ca^{2+} from the extracellular fluid during excitation of the cell.

In contrast, the SR of skeletal muscle cells provides abundant stores of *intra*cellular Ca^{2+}; therefore, the contraction of skeletal muscle is not affected to the same degree by fluctuations in the extracellular concentration of Ca^{2+}. Because of the demanding aerobic activity of heart muscle, cardiac myocytes are equipped with a large number of very large mitochondria. Mitochondria occupy approximately 25% of the volume of a heart muscle cell, compared with about 2% of the volume of a typical skeletal muscle cell (Saladin, 1998). These complex cytoplasmic organelles provide exten-

sive internal membranes and metabolic enzymes for *cellular respiration,* and serve as the sites of adenosine triphosphate (ATP) production for the cell (Box 18–1).

Heart muscle cells are joined together by thick connections called **intercalated discs.** These unique structures are characterized by interdigitating margins of adjacent myocytes that increase the surface area for contact between cells. Intercalated discs contain cell connection structures known as *desmosomes* and *gap junctions.* **Desmosomes** provide strong connections between myocytes to keep them from pulling apart during contraction (Fig. 18–1). These structures function as "spot welds" to stabilize adjacent cells by anchoring them to each other by means of interlocking filaments, much as the nylon hooks and fabric loops of Velcro fasten objects together securely. **Gap junctions** function as *electrical synapses* that permit muscle action potentials to spread rapidly and allow the vast network of muscle fibers to contract in unison as a single group of cells. Within gap junctions are found ion channels that provide a direct pathway for communication from one cell to the next; therefore, cardiac myocytes can electrically stimulate *each other* instead of having to be stimulated individually by neurochemicals (see Fig. 18–1).

In contrast, in skeletal muscle *each* individual muscle fiber must be stimulated by a nerve impulse. Because of the rapid operation of gap junctions, electrical impulses travel very quickly throughout the myocardium, thus allowing cardiac muscle cells to act in concert as a single unit. Cardiac muscle cells, therefore, are connected to each other mechanically, chemically, and electrically so that they operate together as a single, large, interconnected "muscle cell." Such an arrangement is called a **functional syncytium.** A true *syncytium,* such as skeletal muscle, is composed of a multinucleate mass formed by the fusion of several cells. On the other hand, cardiac muscle is made up of cells having one nucleus each (see Table 18–1). The unified and

TABLE 18-1	**Comparison of Cardiac and Skeletal Muscle Fibers**	
Feature	Cardiac Muscle Fibers	Skeletal Muscle Fibers
Appearance of fibers	• Short, thick, branched	• Very long, thin, branched
Nucleus	• One nucleus per cell	• Multiple nuclei per cell
Sarcoplasmic reticulum (SR)	• Higher degree of structural organization	• Lower degree of structural organization
	• Small amount of Ca^{2+} stored intracellularly	• Large amount of Ca^{2+} stored intracellularly
	• Extracellular Ca^{2+} enters rapidly for excitation of cell	• Less dependence on extracellular Ca^{2+} for excitation of cell
Mitochondria	• More numerous (e.g., 25% of cell volume)	• Less numerous (e.g., 2% of cell volume)
Electrochemical characteristics	• Gap junctions function as *electrical synapses* for direct cell-to-cell ionic stimulation	• Each cell stimulated individually by a *neurochemical synapse*
	• Functional syncytium formed by rapid intracellular communication	• True syncytium formed by multinucleated mass of cells

Source: Data from Saladin (1998).

PERSPECTIVES

BOX 18–1

Hitchhikers in Our Cells

It is a good thing for the entire enterprise that mitochondria and chloroplasts have remained small, conservative, and stable, since these two organelles are, in a fundamental sense, the most important living things on earth. Between them they produce the oxygen and arrange for its use. In effect, they run the place.

LEWIS THOMAS, "ORGANELLES AS ORGANISMS" IN *A LONG LINE OF CELLS* (1990)

When cells first appeared on the earth around 3.5 to 4 billion years ago, no atmospheric oxygen was present. Oxygen is a *product* of life. Therefore, all early cells were adapted for anaerobic (oxygen-free) metabolism. Certain bacteria today are classified as obligatory (strict) anaerobes. Such life forms are extremely sensitive to the cell-damaging effects of highly reactive chemicals formed when oxygen enters a cell. Presumably, ancient anaerobic cells would also have been harmed by toxic oxygen species such as the superoxide ion (O_2^-), the hydroxyl radical (OH^-), or hydrogen peroxide (H_2O_2). Where did the oxygen come from?

Around 2 billion years ago ancient photosynthetic microorganisms, the cyanobacteria, began to utilize the radiant energy of the sun to extract the hydrogen they required for self-replication and other cellular functions. This reaction resulted in the creation of molecular oxygen (O_2) and caused a rise in atmospheric oxygen. Early eukaryotic cells, our direct ancestors, were adapted for an anaerobic environment, and were threatened by this rising level of atmospheric oxygen. An explanation of their (and our) survival is presented by Christian de Duve and other biologists. Dr. de Duve discovered lysosomes in 1952, and in 1974 shared the Nobel Prize for Physiology or Medicine with Albert Claude and George E. Palade for discoveries related to the structural and functional organization of the cell. Christian de Duve suggested in 1982 that the survival of our ancestral cells was directly linked to the development of primitive oxygen detoxification systems. Modern *mitochondria* perform this job for us, converting potentially toxic oxygen into harmless water and generating energy-rich ATP molecules in the process. Precursors of mitochondria are now thought to have stemmed from primitive bacteria. These prokaryotic cells were incorporated into much larger eukaryotic cells where they essentially functioned as metabolic prisoners, detoxifying reactive oxygen compounds. Such "cellular hitchhikers" are called *endosymbionts* (Gk *endon-*, within; *syn*, together; *bioun*, to live).

For the most part, endosymbionts such as mitochondria and chloroplasts (derived from cyanobacteria) have retained DNA and RNA separate from that of the nucleus and carry out some replication independently. The idea that mitochondria might be endosymbionts was presented as long ago as 1885 but was not seriously considered until comparatively recently. Proof of the theory has been growing steadily since the mid-1960s.

Some evidence suggests that endosymbionts were not *engulfed* by the phagocytic action of an evolving eukaryotic cell but instead *invaded* the eukaryotic cell and have maintained a more or less separate existence ever since. Lewis Thomas—doctor, scientist, and brilliant essayist—describes endosymbionts from such a perspective in his essay, "Organelles as Organisms":

continued

BOX 18-1   **Hitchhikers in Our Cells (Continued)**

. . . the organelles might be viewed as having learned early how to have the best of both possible worlds, with least effort and risk to themselves and their progeny. Instead of evolving as we have done, manufacturing longer and elaborately longer strands of DNA, and running ever-increasing risks of mutating into evolutionary cul-de-sacs, they elected to stay small and stick to one line of work. To accomplish this, and to assure themselves the longest possible run, they got themselves inside all the rest of us.

LEWIS THOMAS, "ORGANELLES AS ORGANISMS" IN *A LONG LINE OF CELLS* (1990)

- de Duve C: The birth of complex cells. Sci Am, 274:50–57, Apr 1996.
- Thomas L: A Long Line of Cells: Collected Essays. BOMC, Camp Hill, PA, 1990 (by arrangement with Viking Penguin). "Organelles as Organisms" originally appeared in *The New England Journal of Medicine*, Massachusetts Medical Society, 1971–1973.

coordinated action of a functional syncytium allows a pair of pumping chambers to work in unison to effectively move blood through the heart; therefore, an **atrial syncytium** ("atrial pump") and a **ventricular syncytium** ("ventricular pump") are found in the heart. The two syncytia are separated by the fibrous skeleton of the heart, which electrically isolates the two pumps.

Overview of the Cardiac Conduction System

MYOGENIC ORIGIN OF HEARTBEAT AND AUTORHYTHMICITY

In humans, each heartbeat arises within the myocardium itself, rather than in a pacemaker area located in the nervous system. This unique property is called the **myogenic origin** of heartbeat (*myo*, muscle; *genesis*, a beginning). External (extrinsic) factors such as autonomic nerve impulses or hormones such as *epinephrine* (*adrenaline*) can modify the basic rhythm generated by heart muscle cells but are not necessary to initiate the activity. The heart continues to beat even after all nerve connections are severed, and all chemical stimuli have been blocked. In fact, *pieces* of myocardium removed from certain parts of the heart continue to exhibit contractions when they are isolated in a nutrient bath of oxygenated physiologic saline. Clearly, the ability of some cardiac myocytes to contract is inherent within the cells themselves.

Certain cardiac myocytes are said to be **autorhythmic;** that is, they are capable of spontaneously depolarizing at a regular rate. These portions of the heart

no longer take part in the actual contractions of the myocardium. Instead, they become specialized cardiac tissue responsible for initiating, conducting, and distributing electrical activity throughout the heart in the form of cardiac *action potentials* (APs). Autorhythmicity is an intriguing electrophysiologic property that helps explain why different locations, or *foci*, in the myocardium have the potential to generate unique electrical rhythms. An area of spontaneously generated electrical activity, other than that originating in the *sinoatrial node*, is called an **ectopic focus.** These regions can develop abnormal self-excitability, and may become dominant to the heart's natural pacemaker (described subsequently). Common drugs such as *nicotine* and *caffeine* can trigger such ectopic electrical activity in the heart.

CARDIAC CONDUCTION SYSTEM

Specialized cardiac tissue exhibiting autorhythmicity comprises the **cardiac conduction system,** also known as the **intrinsic conducting system.** Briefly, the components of the system include the following:

Sinoatrial Node

Initiation of normal electrical activity occurs in a specialized mass of myocytes called the **sinoatrial (SA) node** (Fig. 18–2). This **primary pacemaker** is the site of the **sinus rhythm** that drives the rest of the heart. The sinoatrial node is located on the posterior wall of the right atrium, near the entrance of the superior vena cava. Automaticity in the SA node ranges from 60 to 100 impulses per minute. Because of the myogenic origin of heartbeat, other regions of the heart are capable

The Cardiovascular System

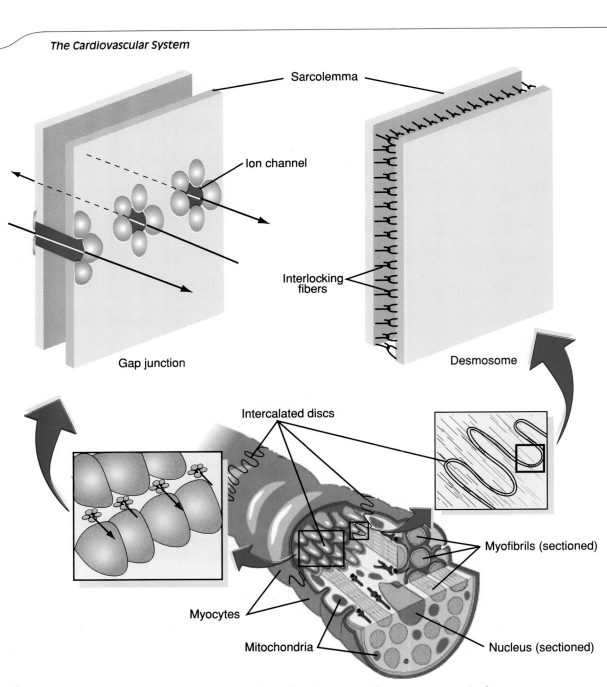

FIGURE 18–1. Cardiac myocytes. Intercalated discs between cardiac myocytes contain desmosomes and gap junctions. *Desmosomes* stabilize adjacent cells by anchoring them to each other through interlocking fibers. *Gap junctions* fuse the cell membranes together and provide for the direct transfer of ions between cells to allow for the rapid spread of action potentials. Arrows depict movement of ions through protein channels in the gap junction.

of generating APs, but at a slower rate. Although the interlaced muscle fibers of the atrial syncytium form a very effective distribution network for APs generated in the SA node, high-speed bundles of atrial muscle fibers also exist. For instance, the **interatrial band** passes through the walls of the atria to rapidly distribute impulses to the left atrium (see Fig. 18–2). Similarly, several **internodal pathways** provide a high-speed conduction link from the sinoatrial node to the atrioventricular node (see Fig. 18–2). These specialized conduction pathways in the atria conduct at velocities of 1 m/s, approximately three times faster than the conduction velocities observed in other atrial muscle fibers (Guyton and Hall, 1996). The specialized routes consist of bundles of atrial muscle fibers mixed with conduction fibers similar to those found in the very high-speed Purkinje fibers of the ventricles (discussed subsequently). In general, action potentials from the SA node stimulate other parts of the conducting system before those regions can generate APs of their own.

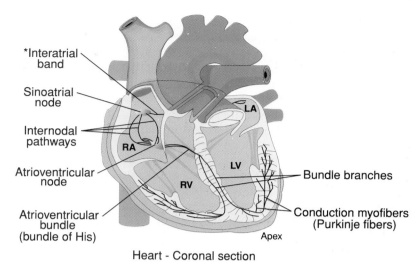

FIGURE 18–2. Intrinsic conducting system. (RA = right atrium; RV = right ventricle; LA = left atrium; LV = left ventricle.)

*The conducting fibers making up the interatrial band pass along the anterior wall of both atria to reach the left atrium. Therefore, the distribution of the fibers does not show in this coronal (frontal) section.

Heart - Coronal section

Atrioventricular Node

The APs initiated by the SA node spread via internodal pathways to the **atrioventricular (A-V) node,** a second mass of specialized cardiac myocytes located at the lower end of the interatrial septum near the tricuspid valve (see Fig. 18–2). The A-V node functions as a *secondary pacemaker,* having an intrinsic firing rate, or **nodal rhythm,** of approximately 40 to 50 beats per minute. Under normal conditions, the A-V does not pace the heart as long as a normal sinus rhythm is being generated by the SA node. Recall that the SA node paces the heart because it generates APs faster than other parts of the heart. Therefore, the rate of firing of the A-V node, like that of other components of the conducting system, is matched to the SA nodal rate under normal conditions. The A-V node acts as an electrical "gateway" into the ventricles, which are electrically isolated from the atria by the fibrous skeleton of the heart. The A-V node also delays electrical impulses before relaying them to the **atrioventricular (A-V) bundle,** the next component in the intrinsic conducting system. This delay of approximately 100 ms allows sufficient time for mechanical events such as atrial emptying and ventricular filling to be completed. Delay in the A-V node occurs because the impulse velocity of the myocytes comprising the A-V node is only around 0.05 m/s, a speed approximately 80 times slower than that of high-speed conduction fibers making up the A-V bundle (Saladin, 1998).

His-Purkinje System (A-V Bundle)

Synchronization between the electrically isolated atrial syncytium and the ventricular syncytium is essential to maintain pump efficiency. A high-speed conduction pathway penetrates the fibrous skeleton of the heart, thus electrically linking the two syncytia so that proper

timing of atrial and ventricular events occurs. Remember that no nervous tissue is found within the heart; these high-speed conduction fibers are composed of specialized *cardiac muscle* tissue. The conduction fibers connecting atria and ventricles collectively form the **Purkinje system** or **His-Purkinje system,** named after the physiologists Wilhelm His Jr. (1863–1934) and Johannes E. Purkinje (1787–1869). This conducting system is composed of the following structures (see Fig. 18–2):

- The A-V bundle, also known as the **bundle of His,** is a bundle of conduction fibers that leaves the A-V node and travels a short distance in the posterior part of the interatrial septum. The A-V bundle splits into the **right** and **left bundle branches** that enter the interventricular septum and travel towards the apex of the heart. These nervelike conducting fibers transmit electrical signals at very high velocities.

- As each bundle branch reaches the apex, it splits into a terminal network of very fine branches known as **conduction myofibers** or **Purkinje fibers** that function to distribute impulses throughout the myocardium. The functional syncytium arrangement of ventricular fibers also contributes to the rapid and efficient spread of cardiac APs in the ventricles.

The conduction velocity of the fibers of the Purkinje system is approximately 4 m/s, compared with around 0.3 to 0.5 m/s in the ventricular muscle fibers (Saladin, 1998). This rapid conduction of impulses out of the A-V node ensures that all parts of the ventricles receive the impulse at virtually the same instant. If conduction through the thick-walled ventricles were dependent upon the slower velocity of typical ventricular myocytes, some parts of the ventricles would begin to contract before others received the signal to do so. When an impulse arrives in the ventricles via the conduction myofibers, however, *coordinated* ventricular contraction begins. Meanwhile, atrial contraction has already occurred, due to the firing of the SA node. Recall that contraction of the atria forces an extra 30 to 40 mL of blood into the two lower chambers. This atrial contraction primes the ventricles just before they are stimulated to contract by the arrival of an electrical impulse in the conduction myofibers. Through these coordinated actions the intrinsic conducting system controls the rate, rhythm, and distribution routes of electrical impulses within the heart. Failure of any part of the intrinsic conducting system to transmit impulses is called *heart block* (Saladin, 1998). The classification of heart blocks is beyond the scope and needs of this textbook; however, the pathophysiologic outcome of many types of heart block is predictable from a basic knowledge of physiology. For instance, a *bundle branch block* resulting from disease or degeneration of conduction tissue, results in faulty transmission of electrical impulses from the atria to the ventricles. Consequently, the pumping activity of the two pairs of chambers becomes disorganized and uncoordinated, adversely affecting cardiac efficiency.

Types of Arrhythmias

Abnormal patterns or rates of firing in the conduction tissue or myocardial tissue of the heart are known as **arrhythmias** or **dysrhythmias.** The term "arrhythmia" literally means "without rhythm," a misleading concept because some dysfunctions such as *atrial tachyarrythmias* are characterized by *rhythmic* but very *fast* rates in excess of 200 beats per minute. The more precise term is "dysrhythmia," which means an "abnormal rhythm." Both terms, however, are used in an equivalent way.

In very simple terms, electrical abnormalities originating in the sinoatrial node, atrioventricular node, atrial musculature, or at a combination of these sites, are classified as *supraventricular arrhythmias*. *Atrial flutter* is an example of a supraventricular arrhythmia characterized by extremely rapid atrial rates of 200 to 400 beats per minute (Saladin, 1998). This pattern is caused by rapidly firing ectopic foci in the atria that initiate extra contractions. As a general rule, if supraventricular arrhythmias are not treated, they can lead to more serious *ventricular arrhythmias*. Electrical dysfunctions originating in regions inferior to the A-V node are known as ventricular arrhythmias. These arrhythmias include electrical abnormalities originating in the A-V bundle, bundle branches, conduction myofibers, ventricular musculature, or at a combination of these sites. *Ventricular fibrillation* is an example of a serious, life-threatening ventricular arrhythmia characterized by bizarre electrical activity, and a quivering, dilated heart incapable of co-ordinated contractions. As a result of the heart's inability to contract, the coronary arteries are not perfused and the myocardium rapidly becomes ischemic.

Cardiac Electrophysiology

OVERVIEW

To understand the mechanisms of **cardiac electrophysiology,** or the electrical events associated with contraction and relaxation of the heart, a basic understanding of cell membrane electrical properties is needed. The reader is encouraged to review appropriate sections of general anatomy and physiology textbooks so that terms such as *voltage-gated ion channel, influx, efflux, polarization, depolarization, repolarization, resting membrane potential,* and *action potential* are familiar.

Recall that a cell membrane AP is produced by an orderly but rapid sequence of electrophysiologic events triggered by a *threshold stimulus.* The electrical gradient across a membrane is known as the *resting membrane potential* (RMP). Cell membranes are said to be *polarized* when this condition exists. The polarization, or difference, in the two sides of the membrane is created by the concentration gradient of ions found in the extracellular fluid (ECF) and the intracellular fluid (ICF). Differences in the transmembrane rate of movement of sodium (Na^+) and potassium (K^+) cations through their respective *voltage-gated ion channels* in the cell membrane create the RMP, which is unique for different cells (Table 18–2). The loss of membrane polarity as a result of the rapid movement of ions down a concentration gradient from an area of high concentration to an area of low concentration is called *depolarization;* restoration of the polarized state of the membrane is known as *repolarization.*

Although the details of transmembrane movement (flux) of ions are different for different cells, the general sequence is similar. The opening and closing of selective voltage-gated ion channels controls the inward movement (*influx*) of ions such as Na^+ or Ca^{2+} ions, and the outward movement (*efflux*) of ions such as K^+ ions. The reader should note that most descriptions of these steps refer to the electrophysiologic events associated with the generation of *nerve cell* APs. For example, in neurons, depolarization occurs rapidly as **voltage-gated fast Na^+ channels** open, allowing rapid influx of Na^+ from the extracellular fluid. Opening of **voltage-gated slow K^+ channels** permits K^+ efflux to occur. Finally, repolarization occurs as the different voltage-gated ion channels close and active transport pumps move cations back to their respective sides of the cell membrane, thus restoring the RMP. We will see that the electrical events associated with a **cardiac action potential** are similar to those associated with a nerve cell AP, but that important differ-

TABLE 18-2	Electrophysiologic Properties of Different Cells	
Cell	**Resting Membrane Potential (mV)**	**Duration of Action Potential (ms)**
Nerve cell	Typical: −70	0.5–2.0
	Range: −40 to −90	
Skeletal muscle cell	−90	1.0–5.0
Smooth muscle cell*	−50 to −70	500–5000+
Heart muscle cell		
Nodal cell (e.g., sinoatrial node)	−65 to −70	200
Conductile cell (e.g., conduction myofiber)	−90 to −95	400
Contractile cell (e.g., ventricular fiber)	−80 to −90	300

*Highly variable; depends on type of cell.
Source: Data from Tortora and Grabowski (1996); Brody, et al (1989).

ences exist. In fact, the generation of cardiac APs is different in different parts of the heart itself.

ELECTROPHYSIOLOGY OF THE SINOATRIAL NODE

As pointed out previously, some parts of the heart, such as the SA node and A-V node, exhibit automaticity, the ability to spontaneously generate APs. For example, the **resting membrane potential** of an SA node cell is approximately −65 mV to −70 mV. This RMP value is less negative than that of other cardiac cells, as shown in Figure 18–3. Notice, however, that the RMP (**Phase 4** in the graph) does not remain stable as it does in a ventricular cell. Instead it spontaneously drifts upward. This gradual depolarization to-

ward threshold is called the **pacemaker potential** and is typical for the SA node. As soon as the resting membrane potential is established in an SA nodal cell, the RMP gradually decays until self-excitation occurs. At this point, an AP is generated and the process repeats. The mechanism responsible for the drifting RMP baseline and the pacemaker potential is not fully understood. According to Saladin (1998), one theory is that voltage-gated K^+ channels close in the cell membranes of the SA nodal cells; therefore, the slow influx of Na^+ without a corresponding efflux of K^+ causes a gradual depolarization of the SA node. At a critical point, a threshold of approximately −40 mV is reached, and the SA nodal cells depolarize.

Depolarization of the SA node is brought about through the opening of **voltage-gated slow Na^+**

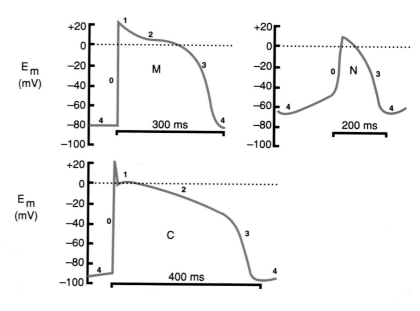

FIGURE 18–3. Cardiac action potentials. Cardiac action potentials have characteristic shapes resulting from differences in ion conductance across cell membranes in different parts of the heart. The phases of the cardiac action potential are labeled on the conductile cell cardiac action potential. Notice that spontaneous, pacemaker depolarization is absent in muscle cells (M); that the cells of the conduction system (C), specialized for high-velocity conduction, have very rapid upstroke and long duration; and that the nodal pacemaker cells (N) exhibit spontaneous depolarization but have a very slow upstroke, and therefore low conduction velocity. E_m = membrane potential (mV). (Adapted from Brody MJ, Feldman RD, and Hermsmeyer RK: Cardiovascular drugs. In Conn PM and Gebhart GF (eds): Essentials of Pharmacology. FA Davis, Philadelphia, 1989, p 238, with permission.)

M = muscle cell (eg. left ventrical cell)
N = nodal cell (eg. sinotrial node cell)
C = conductile cell (eg. conduction myofiber cell)

channels and **voltage-gated slow Ca²⁺ channels,** which allow Na⁺ and Ca²⁺, respectively, to flow into the SA nodal cells. This influx occurs because of the concentration gradient established during the polarization of the membrane (Phase 4). The slow entry of Na⁺ and Ca²⁺ brings about relatively slow **depolarization of the SA node (Phase 0).** The slow upstroke of the SA node depolarization curve is characteristic of this tissue. The interlaced atrial fibers rapidly spread the impulse throughout the atria to initiate atrial contraction. Meanwhile, the AP stimulates the A-V node, which relays the impulse into the rest of the conducting tissue.

As the voltage-gated slow ion channels close, the inward current of Na⁺ and Ca²⁺ ceases. This event is immediately followed by **repolarization (Phase 3).** Repolarization of the SA nodal cells occurs because of the opening of voltage-gated slow K⁺ channels, which allows K⁺ efflux to occur (see Fig. 18–3). The increase in membrane conductance to K⁺ delays depolarization of the SA node for a brief period, as shown by the downstroke of the SA action potential curve. However, as K⁺ conductance gradually tapers off, Na⁺ and Ca²⁺ influx once again erodes the RMP, thus exciting the cell. Because these electrophysiologic events can be completed faster by SA nodal cells than they can by other cells in the heart, the SA node *paces* the heart.

ELECTROPHYSIOLOGY OF CONDUCTING TISSUE

Many of the electrophysiologic characteristics of cell membranes of conducting tissue in the heart are similar to those of cell membranes of contractile tissue in the heart. Consequently, the overall *shape* of the cardiac action potential curve for conduction myofibers and ventricular muscle cells is nearly identical (see Fig. 18–3). However, subtle differences, however, are described in the following section.

The RMP of a conduction myofiber is approximately −100 mV to −95 mV, a value very close to that of a ventricular muscle fiber, but considerably more negative than the RMP of an SA node cell (see Table 18–2). Rapid transport of Na⁺ out of the cell and K⁺ into the cell by the active transport mechanism known as the *Na⁺-K⁺-ATPase pump* helps maintain the large ionic differential across the cell membrane. Notice that the RMP of the membrane in the polarized state (Phase 4) exhibits the upwardly drifting baseline indicative of tissue that is self-excitatory or autorhythmic (see Fig. 18–3). The slope of this line is more gradual than that of SA nodal cells; nevertheless, it unmistakably "creeps" upward to a critical threshold level of around −90 mV before depolarization occurs. Recall that this myogenic property is inherent in the conducting tissue itself, and does not require an external stimulus. Under normal circumstances, however, the conducting tissue cells *are*

stimulated by the arrival of electrical impulses generated intrinsically in the SA node and relayed to them by the A-V node.

The arrival of an impulse causes voltage-gated fast Na⁺ channels to open in the cell membranes of conducting tissue cells. This increase in membrane permeability to Na⁺ causes rapid Na⁺ influx and depolarization of the fiber (Phase 0). Note the nearly vertical upstroke characteristic of depolarization of conduction myofibers caused by the operation of *fast* Na⁺ channels, compared with the gradual upstroke and slow depolarization of SA nodal cells via *slow* Na⁺ channels (see Fig. 18–3).

As Na⁺ influx gradually decreases, the cell membranes repolarize briefly **(Phase 1),** but the process is delayed by an abrupt change in membrane permeability to Ca²⁺ (see Fig. 18–3). This initial phase of repolarization is known as **transient repolarization,** a phase abruptly halted by the inward movement of calcium ions due to the opening of voltage-gated slow Ca²⁺ channels. These cation channels allow Ca²⁺ to flow inward down a concentration gradient. Calcium ions also enter the sarcoplasm from limited storage sites in the sarcoplasmic reticulum. The accumulation of intracellular Na⁺ and Ca²⁺ maintains the cell membrane in an extended depolarized state called the **plateau phase (Phase 2),** thus contributing to most of the 400-ms duration typical of the AP of conducting cells. By comparison, the AP in neurons and in skeletal muscle cells only lasts about 1 millisecond (see Table 18–2).

The plateau phase is followed by repolarization (Phase 3) as shown in Figure 18–3. This phase is similar to repolarization of nerve cells or skeletal muscle cells, whereby voltage-gated slow K⁺ channels open, allowing K⁺ to diffuse out of the cell down a concentration gradient. At approximately the same time, Na⁺ and Ca²⁺ channels close, thus restricting the inflow of these cations. As more K⁺ exit from the cell and fewer Na⁺ and Ca²⁺ enter, the RMP of approximately −95 mV is restored (Phase 4).

ELECTROPHYSIOLOGY OF VENTRICULAR FIBERS

The resting membrane potential of a contractile fiber from the ventricles is typically around −80 mV to −90 mV. Like the electrophysiologic characteristics described previously for conduction myofibers, this value is more negative than that of a cell from the SA node but is similar to the RMP values of several other cells (see Table 18–2). The large negative potential is maintained through the operation of the Na⁺-K⁺-ATPase pump that selectively transports Na⁺ out of the cell and K⁺ into the cell.

The network of conduction myofibers (Purkinje fibers) in the ventricles causes an electrical impulse to be efficiently distributed throughout the tissue. These impulses cause voltage-gated fast Na^+ channels to open in the cell membranes of ventricular muscle cells, initiating rapid depolarization of the fibers (Phase 0). As seen with the depolarization of conduction myofibers, the vertical upstroke of Phase 0 in ventricular cells is characteristic of depolarization via fast Na^+ channels.

Ventricular muscle cell membranes begin to repolarize (Phase 1), as shown by the small downward deflection in the graph, but the opening of voltage-gated slow Ca^{2+} channels allow Ca^{2+} to enter and delay the process (see Fig. 18–3). As described previously with conduction myofibers, calcium ions also enter the sarcoplasm from limited storage sites in the sarcoplasmic reticulum. As the intracellular fluid temporarily becomes more positive with accumulated Na^+ and Ca^{2+}, depolarization is delayed, creating the characteristic plateau of Phase 2. Overall, the duration of the AP of a ventricular muscle fiber is around 300 milliseconds. As can be seen in Figure 18–3, much of this delay is caused by the plateau phase. As Ca^{2+} continue to enter the myocytes, the contraction continues. Thus, the development of ventricular contractile force begins immediately following depolarization and builds during the plateau phase. This unique characteristic allows the myocardium to develop the sustained contraction necessary to squeeze blood out of the chambers. By contrast, the normal contraction of a skeletal muscle fiber is a brief *twitch,* lasting approximately 1.0 to 5.0 milliseconds (see Table 18–2). The prolonged contraction of the ventricles is discussed with the *cardiac cycle* in the following chapter.

As described previously with the electrophysiology of conducting tissue, the plateau phase of the AP of ventricular muscle is followed by repolarization (Phase 3), caused by the opening of voltage-gated slow K^+ channels (see Fig. 18–3). As K^+ diffuse out of the myo-

cardial cell, the Na^+ and Ca^{2+} channels close, thus slowing the influx of these cations. This action restores the RMP of approximately -90 mV (Phase 4) and allows the muscle fiber to relax.

Table 18–3 summarizes the phases of the cardiac action potential.

CONTRACTION OF THE MYOCARDIUM

The duration of the plateau phase (Phase 2) allows ventricular muscle fibers to develop maximal tension over a 300-millisecond interval, thus contributing to efficient cardiac pumping. The physiologic events associated with the contraction itself are very similar to those occurring when skeletal muscle fibers contract. (Consult general anatomy and physiology texts listed in the chapter bibliography for a review of the excitation-coupling mechanism involved with muscle contraction.) In this mechanism, free Ca^{2+} in the cardiac muscle cell sarcoplasm bind to specific muscle proteins. These proteins activate others and initiate the *sliding filament* mechanism that shortens the length of the muscle fibers. Myocardial contraction can be affected by altering the amount of Ca^{2+} available, a mechanism of action exhibited by some cardiac drugs. For instance, *norepinephrine* enhances Ca^{2+} inflow through the voltage-gated slow Ca^{2+} channels and thus increases myocardial contraction; whereas, *verapamil* (Isoptin) is a calcium channel–blocker that decreases myocardial contraction by decreasing Ca^{2+} inflow.

Electrocardiogram

THE ECG WAVEFORM

During a single cardiac cycle several unique action potentials are produced. A blend of these APs results in the generation of an **electrocardiogram (ECG,**

TABLE 18-3	Phases of the Cardiac Action Potential	
Phase	**Name**	**Description**
0	Depolarization	• Sinoatrial node: Opening of voltage-gated *slow* Na^+ channels and opening of voltage-gated *slow* Ca^{2+} channels • Conducting tissue: Opening of voltage-gated *fast* Na^+ channels
1	Transient repolarization	• Initial decrease in the rate of Na^+ influx causes brief period of repolarization in ventricular muscle cells and in conducting cells.
2	Plateau phase	• Influx of Ca^{2+} through the open voltage-gated *slow* Ca^{2+} channels and accumulation of Ca^{2+} from intracellular stores halts the repolarization begun in Phase 1; accumulation of intracellular Ca^{2+} and Na^+ delays repolarization for most of the duration of the action potential in ventricular muscle cells and in conducting cells (300–400 ms).
3	Repolarization	• Opening of voltage-gated *slow* K^+ channels; closing of Na^+ channels begins
4	Polarization	• Restoration of the resting membrane potential (RMP) caused by complete closure of membrane ion channels and operation of the sodium-potassium active transport pump (Na^+-K^+-ATPase)

EKG), which is a pen-and-ink or oscilloscope recording of the electrical activity of the heart.

> **NOTE:** *EKG* is based on the German spelling for *Elektrokardiogramm.* "EKG" has a distinctive sound when spoken, and is not easily confused with the initials "EEG," which refer to an *electroencephalogram,* a recording of electrical activity in the brain.

A variety of electrocardiographic techniques employing pairs of recording electrodes, or *leads,* are used to produce diagnostic ECGs. By changing the placement of electrodes on the skin, the electrical pattern of the heart can be displayed from a different perspective. This versatility is caused by each recording electrode's different position relative to the heart, which makes it possible to measure the voltage between two points. For our purposes we will limit our discussion to a common lead configuration called a *Lead II ECG.* The configuration refers to the limb attachments of the electrodes that monitor the heart's electrical signals from the patient's right arm to left leg. In some diagnostic studies, complex ECG techniques using multiple chest electrodes are employed, but these will not be considered in this text.

LEAD II ELECTROCARDIOGRAM

In an electrocardiogram, a series of positive and negative waves are recorded that represent the electrical characteristics associated with different events of the cardiac cycle. A description of the lead II ECG waveform includes the following components.

P Wave

The **P wave** represents atrial depolarization (Fig. 18–4). As discussed with the microscopic anatomy of heart muscle, electrical activity from the SA node radiates rapidly throughout the thin-walled atrial syncytium by means of extensively branched muscle fibers and the electrical synapses of gap junctions. The atria begin to contract (atrial systole) shortly after the P wave begins. The **P-Q interval** extends from the start of the P wave to the start of the *QRS complex.* The R wave (discussed subsequently) is not always apparent in the ECG waveform; therefore, "P-Q interval" is a more accurate description of this period, than is **P-R interval.** The P-Q interval represents the conduction time required from the beginning of atrial stimulation to the start of ventricular stimulation.

QRS Complex

The **QRS complex** is formed by a sequence of both positive and negative waves that are blended together—a

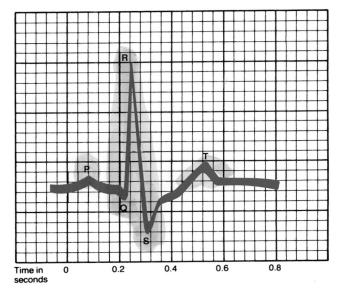

FIGURE 18–4. Lead II electrocardiogram. A heart beat is a series of electrical events that can be detected by placing electrodes on the surface of the body. The recording is called an *electrocardiogram (ECG, EKG).* Atypical lead II ECG is a waveform that consists of three distinct waves or deflections produced by specific electrical events in the heart: P wave = depolarization of the atria; QRS complex = depolarization of the ventricles; T wave = repolarization of the ventricles. (See text for full explanation.) (Adapted from Scanlon VC and Sanders T: Essentials of Anatomy and Physiology, ed. 3. FA Davis, Philadelphia, 1999, p 266, with permission.)

small downward deflection (Q); a tall, sharp positive peak (R); followed by another downward deflection (S). The QRS complex is the electrical "signature" representing ventricular depolarization, or the spread of an impulse through the ventricles (see Fig. 18–4). The complex shape of the waveform is a result of the fact that the two ventricles are different sizes and require different times in which to depolarize (Saladin, 1998). Shortly after the QRS complex begins, the ventricles begin to contract and eject blood. Atrial repolarization and diastole occur during ventricular depolarization, but the electrical signal corresponding to atrial repolarization is hidden within the QRS complex. The signal is weak and is, therefore, obscured by the powerful electrical events of the more muscular ventricles. The **S-T segment** is the period of time from the end of the S wave to the beginning of the T wave. It is during this period that the ventricular fibers are fully depolarized and ventricular systole begins. The S-T segment corresponds to the plateau phase (Phase 2) of the ventricular cell action potential (see Fig. 18–3).

T Wave

Repolarization of the ventricles is represented by the **T wave.** The ventricles require more time to repolarize than to depolarize, as can be seen by wider shape of the

T wave, compared to that of the QRS complex (see Fig. 18–4). The ventricles start to relax immediately after the T wave begins.

Because abnormalities in the initiation or conduction of impulses in the heart produce changes in the shape or pattern of the electrocardiogram, the recordings play an invaluable role in modern medicine. Cardiologists depend on ECGs in the diagnosis of dysfunctions such as conduction abnormalities or myocardial infarction. For example, multiple P waves displayed on an ECG may be caused by a rapidly firing SA node that triggers successive atrial contractions, a prolonged P-Q interval may indicate reduced conduction velocity between atria and ventricles, and a widened QRS complex in the ECG may indicate slow conduction velocity through the ventricles.

Summary

The first part of this chapter discussed the unique structure of cardiac myocytes that links them together and allows them to operate in unison as a functional syncytium. The second part of the chapter focused on the specialized tissue within the heart that functions to initiate, coordinate, and distribute electrical impulses.

The chapter concluded with an overview of a lead II electrocardiogram and a brief discussion of the components of the ECG waveform. Classification of different types of arrhythmias, lead configurations, and ECG interpretation is beyond the scope and needs of this textbook. Applied topics such as these are usually covered in clinical and diagnostics courses and texts.

BIBLIOGRAPHY

Brody MJ, Feldman RD, and Hermsmeyer RK: Cardiovascular Drugs. In Conn PM and Gebhart GF (eds): Essentials of Pharmacology. FA Davis, Philadelphia, 1989.

Cottrell GP and Surkin HB: Pharmacology for Respiratory Care Practitioners. FA Davis, Philadelphia, 1995.

Guyton AC and Hall JE: Textbook of Medical Physiology, ed 9. WB Saunders, Philadelphia, 1996.

Martini FH: Fundamentals of Anatomy and Physiology, ed 4. Prentice Hall, Upper Saddle River, NJ, 1998.

Saladin KS: Anatomy and Physiology: The Unity of Form and Function. WCB/McGraw-Hill, Boston, 1998.

Shier D, Butler J, and Lewis R: Hole's Human Anatomy and Physiology, ed 7. Wm C Brown, Dubuque, IA, 1996.

Thibodeau GA and Patton KT: Anatomy and Physiology, ed 3. Mosby–Year Book, St Louis, 1996.

Tortora GJ and Grabowski SR: Principles of Anatomy and Physiology, ed 8. HarperCollins, New York, 1996.

CHAPTER 19

The Cardiac Cycle and Cardiac Output

chapter objectives

After studying this chapter the reader should be able to:

☐ Define auscultation and state the mechanical event responsible for producing the two main heart sounds:
First heart sound (S1), second heart sound (S2).

☐ Describe the mechanical events associated with the third heart sound (S3) and the fourth heart sound (S4).

☐ Differentiate among the following phases of the cardiac cycle by describing valve action and heart sounds, as well as blood flow, electrocardiographic, and pressure changes associated with each phase:
Quiescent period, atrial systole, isovolumetric contraction, ventricular ejection, isovolumetric relaxation, ventricular filling.

☐ Define the following terms:
End-diastolic volume (EDV), end-systolic volume (ESV), stroke volume (SV), ejection fraction.

☐ Define cardiac output and explain the concept of cardiac reserve.

☐ Differentiate among the following terms:
Chronotropic, inotropic, dromotropic.

☐ Define the following terms:
Tachycardia, bradycardia.

☐ Describe the operation of the cardiac center in controlling heart rate by explaining the function of the cardioacceleratory center and the cardioinhibitory center.

☐ Describe how the following peripheral receptors are involved in the modification of heart rate:
Chemoreceptors, baroreceptors, proprioceptors.

☐ Describe how the following chemical effects alter heart rate:
Hormonal effects, drug effects, electrolytes.

☐ Describe how venous return effects change heart rate by explaining the function of the Bainbridge reflex.

☐ Discuss how myocardial contractility and stroke volume are changed by autonomic nervous system effects and by chemical effects such as hormones, drugs, and electrolytes.

☐ Explain the concept of ventricular preload and its effect on end-diastolic pressure (EDP) and stroke volume.

☐ Describe the length-tension relationship known as the Frank-Starling law and explain how this mechanism affects stroke volume.

☐ Define pulmonary capillary wedge pressure (PCWP) and explain how it provides an estimate of ventricular preload.

☐ Explain the concept of ventricular afterload and its effect on stroke volume.

key terms

auscultation (aws' kul-tā' shun)
Bainbridge reflex
baroreceptors
bradycardia (brad″ ē-kar' dē-a)
cardiac accelerator nerve
cardiac center
   cardioacceleratory center
   cardioinhibitory center
cardiac output (C.O., Q̇)
cardiac reserve
chemoreceptors
chronotropic; chronotropism (kron″ ō-trop' ik)
dromotropic; dromotropism (drō″ mō-trop' ik)
ejection fraction
end-diastolic pressure (EDP)
end-diastolic volume (EDV)
end-systolic volume (ESV)
Frank-Starling law; Starling's law of the heart
heart sounds
   first heart sound, S1

   second heart sound, S2
   third heart sound, S3
   fourth heart sound, S4
inotropic; inotropism (in″ ō-trop' ik)
phases of the cardiac cycle
   quiescent period
   atrial systole
   isovolumetric contraction
   ventricular ejection
   isovolumetric relaxation
   ventricular filling
proprioceptors
pulmonary capillary wedge pressure (PCWP)
stroke volume (SV)
tachycardia (tak″ ē-kar' dē-a)
vagus nerve
ventricular afterload
ventricular preload

Heart Sounds

In this chapter we examine the sounds of the heart and the pattern of blood flow through the chambers during the phases of a typical cardiac cycle. The chapter also explores physiologic factors that affect heart rate and stroke volume—the two variables that determine the amount of blood pumped by the heart per unit time. The blood flow concepts introduced in this chapter are explored further in the following chapter where we consider how blood flow, blood pressure, cardiac work, and vascular resistance are measured.

Vague sounds associated with the heart have been known since antiquity. However, with the invention of the stethoscope in 1816 by the French physician René Laënnec, clinicians have learned to accurately identify normal and abnormal sounds (*murmurs*), and have gained a deeper understanding of the relevance of these sounds to the contraction and relaxation phases of the cardiac cycle (Box 19–1). Listening to the sounds of the body is known as **auscultation,** and with the expert and practiced use of a stethoscope, clinicians are able to identify distinctive **heart sounds** that are audible during the course of a single cardiac cycle (Fig. 19–1). The diagnostic implications of this deceptively simple technique are enormous, ranging from the accurate assessment of heart rate to the early detection of valvular defects such as stenosis or prolapse.

Interestingly, the actual closure of heart valves does not create a sound (Saladin, 1998). However, the two principal heart sounds, called the **first** and **second**

PERSPECTIVES

BOX 19–1   ## Listening to the Body

It is the early 1800s in the smoke-filled, overcrowded slums of Paris. Picture a well-dressed doctor carrying a foot-long wooden cylinder with him whenever he works among the poor of the city. It must have been a curious sight, watching him bend down and carefully place the end of the crude wooden instrument—the forerunner of the modern *stethoscope*—on the heaving chests of victims wracked by the coughs of tuberculosis and other common ailments of the day. After listening intently to the sounds of the body (*auscultation*), he would then speak with the person, writing copious notes pertaining to the chest sounds he had just heard. Months or years later, after the patients had inevitably succumbed to disease, the doctor carefully correlated autopsy findings with his previous notes and observations of their illnesses.

Through this painstaking process, René-Théophile-Hyacinthe Laënnec came to be known as the "father of chest medicine." With his invention of the stethoscope in 1816 (Gr. *stethos*, chest + *skopein*, to examine), and with his extensive clinical experience, Dr. Laënnec accurately described a variety of lung and heart sounds, including *vesicular, bronchial,* and *adventitious lung sounds, first* and *second heart sounds*, cardiac irregularities caused by *ectopic beats*, and *murmurs* resulting from valvular disease.

Direct auscultation of the chest, that is, placing the ear directly on the chest, was an unsatisfactory and little-used diagnostic technique at the time. Laënnec himself observed, "Direct auscultation was as uncomfortable for the doctor as it was for the patient." Laënnec's invention changed all that. Although minor modifications such as an earpiece and trumpet-shaped chest piece were added in 1828, the basic stethoscope design remained unchanged until the beginning of the 20th century when a New York City physician named P .G. Cammann added *two* earpieces to produce the modern binaural stethoscope. This modification further improved the transmission of sound to the ears, making auscultation even more accurate. Many of the terms used in modern auscultation (e.g., *bruit, rale*) were developed and introduced by Laënnec in his two-volume masterpiece, *De l'auscultation médiate*. The classic work was published in 1819 and sold for 13 francs. For 19th century physicians eager to learn the new technique of auscultation, Laënnec's wooden stethoscope could be purchased *with* the reference book for an additional 2.50 francs—a clever piece of marketing for any century.

- Ornadel D: How to use a stethoscope [Historic account of invention and clinical use of stethoscope posted on the World Wide Web]. n.d./1998. Retrieved July 3, 1998 from the World Wide Web: URL http://www.bmjpg.com/studbmj/data/st09ed2.ht
- The New Encyclopædia Brittannica, ed 15: Micropædia, Vol 7. Robert McHenry (ed), Chicago, 1993.
- The New Illustrated Science and Invention Encyclopedia (Vol 19). Donald Clarke (ed), H.S. Stuttman Publishers, Westport, CT, 1987.
- Thomas CL (ed): Taber's Cyclopedic Medical Dictionary, ed 18. FA Davis, Philadelphia, 1997.

heart sounds, are associated with the turbulence created in the bloodstream by the closure of heart valves (see Fig. 19–1). The **first heart sound,** also known as **S1,** is associated with *ventricular systole* and is usually described as being louder and a little longer than the **second heart sound,** or **S2,** a softer and sharper sound associated with *ventricular diastole*. The description of such sounds is highly subjective, but the two main heart sounds are typically described as the familiar "lubb-dupp" rhythm of a beating heart. The **third heart sound (S3),** is sometimes audible in children and adolescents (Ganong, 1995; Saladin, 1998). This soft, low-pitched sound is associated with *rapid ventricular filling* during diastole, and is heard about one-third of the way through diastole (see Fig. 19–1). The origin of S3 is discussed subsequently with **phases of the cardiac cycle.** A **fourth heart sound (S4)** is sometimes faintly audible just before the first heart sound of the next cycle (see Fig. 19–1). This sound is rarely heard in normal hearts but may occur when atrial pressure is high or the ven-

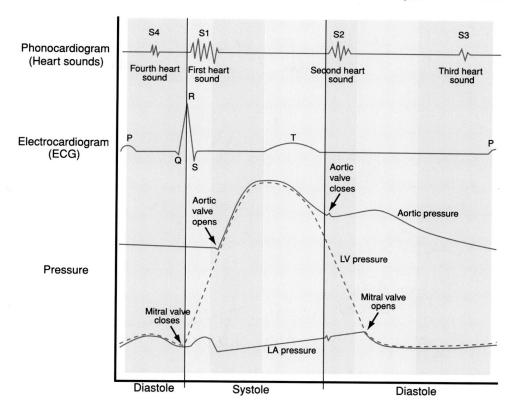

FIGURE 19–1. Composite graph of the cardiac cycle. Waveforms pertaining to heart sounds, electrical events, and pressure changes in the left heart and aorta during one cardiac cycle are shown on the same graph. (LA = left atrium; LV = left ventricle.)

tricle is stiff in conditions such as ventricular hypertrophy. The **fourth heart sound** is believed to be caused by atrial systole (Ganong, 1995).

Phases of the Cardiac Cycle

In the following section we examine the various **phases of the cardiac cycle**—*quiescent period, atrial systole, isovolumetric contraction, ventricular ejection, isovolumetric relaxation,* and *ventricular filling*—an orderly sequence of events completed in less than 1 second under resting conditions. The terms "systole" and "systolic" refer generally to contraction of heart muscle. However, the terms are assumed to pertain to *ventricular* events, unless stated otherwise. Similarly, the terms "diastole" and "diastolic" refer to relaxation of heart muscle but are usually employed to describe ventricular relaxation, unless stated otherwise.

QUIESCENT PERIOD

During the interval between beats, there is a brief period of time called the **quiescent period,** during which the heart prepares for the beginning of the next beat (see Fig. 19–1). Figure 19–2 shows this period (*Phase 1*), which is characterized by lack of contraction of the chambers of the heart. Note that both atrial and ventricular pressures are zero and that no sounds

(other than background noise) are produced by the heart. During this period of atrial diastole, blood returns to the atria through the veins, flows through the atria, and enters the ventricles through open atrioventricular (A-V) valves.

ATRIAL SYSTOLE

The period known as **atrial systole** is marked by the firing of the sinoatrial (SA) node, which triggers atrial depolarization and generation of the P wave of the ECG (see Fig. 19–1). Notice that atrial blood pressure rapidly peaks during this period and that the ventricular volume abruptly rises by about 40 mL (see Fig. 19–2). Recall that atrial systole is responsible for priming the ventricles just before they contract. At the end of *Phase 2* each ventricle contains an **end-diastolic volume (EDV)** of approximately 120 to 130 mL of blood—most of it added passively during the quiescent period, with the balance forced in during the period of atrial systole.

ISOVOLUMETRIC CONTRACTION

Following atrial systole, the atrial fibers relax and remain in diastole for the remainder of the cardiac cycle. Rapid transmission of an electrical impulse through the intrinsic conducting system of the heart causes the ventricles to depolarize, thus generating the QRS com-

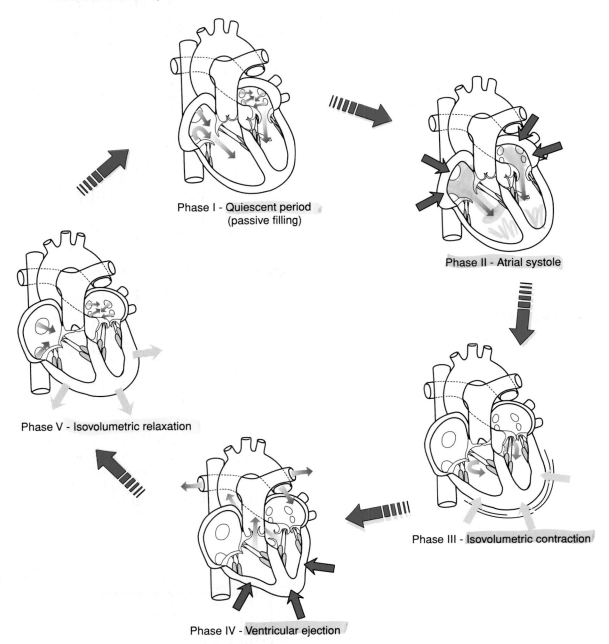

Phase I - Quiescent period
(passive filling)

Phase II - Atrial systole

Phase III - Isovolumetric contraction

Phase IV - Ventricular ejection

Phase V - Isovolumetric relaxation

FIGURE 19–2. Phases of the cardiac cycle. Ventricular filling (diastole) overlaps Phase I and Phase II of the cycle, and consists of three subphases: *rapid ventricular filling, diastasis* (slower filling of the ventricles), and *ventricular priming* brought about by the volume of blood pumped into the ventricles by the atria.

plex of the ECG (see Fig. 19–1). Note that the P-Q interval represents the time required for impulse transmission from the atria to the ventricles. The ventricles begin to contract shortly after the QRS complex, thus raising the ventricular pressure above atrial pressure. This extremely brief (0.05 s) contractile activity in the ventricles during *Phase 3* is termed **isovolumetric contraction** because the ventricular muscle fibers begin to generate tension but do not shorten appreciably (see Fig. 19–2). In other words, the intraventricular

pressure rises sharply as the myocardium begins to press inward on the blood in the ventricle (Ganong, 1995). The heart wall, however, is not moved inward enough to decrease the chamber volume and eject blood. As a result, the volume of the chamber essentially remains the same—it is *isovolumetric.* (This type of muscular action is an example of an *isometric contraction* because muscle force is being applied to an object, but no actual movement occurs. By contrast, an *isotonic contraction* results in the application of force and the movement of an object as muscle fibers shorten.) During the isovolumetric contraction phase, the blood pressure in the pulmonary trunk and aorta is higher than that in the right and left ventricles; therefore, the semilunar (SL) valves remain closed and no blood is ejected by the ventricles.

As ventricular pressure builds, the atrioventricular A-V valves close, thus creating turbulence and producing the S1 heart sound (see Fig. 19–1). Notice also in the pressure graph that there is an abrupt, but small, rise in atrial pressure during *Phase 3* of the cycle. This change is produced when the rising ventricular pressure causes the A-V valve cusps to bulge a short distance into the atria, thus briefly pressurizing the atria by a small amount. Recall that the chordae tendineae prevent complete prolapse of the A-V valves into the atria during ventricular contraction.

VENTRICULAR EJECTION

As the contraction builds in the ventricular fibers and intraventricular pressure increases, it reaches a critical point where it exceeds the blood pressure in the pulmonary trunk and aorta. At that instant, the pulmonary and aortic SL valves open and blood is forced out under pressure into the pulmonary and systemic circulatory routes (see Fig. 19–1). This period represents *Phase 4* of the cardiac cycle, and is known as **ventricular ejection** (see Fig. 19–2). During this phase ventricular pressure reaches a peak of approximately 25 mm Hg in the right ventricle, and about 120 mm Hg in the left (Ganong, 1995; Saladin. 1998). The duration of ventricular ejection is about the same as that of the plateau phase of the cardiac action potential in ventricular muscle fibers, around 300 milliseconds (see Fig. 18–3). Recall that the accumulation of calcium and sodium ions within ventricular myocytes is responsible for this prolongation of depolarization. The delay helps coordinate electrical and mechanical events, thus giving the ventricles sufficient time to develop the force necessary to expel blood during systole.

After the ventricles have expelled blood into the blood vessels, approximately 60 mL of blood remains in each chamber. This volume is called the **end-systolic volume (ESV)**. Even after the most powerful contraction, a volume of blood remains in the ventricles. The difference between the EDV and the ESV is the **stroke volume (SV),** or the volume of blood ejected into the arteries by the contraction of the ventricle. The **ejection fraction** is the SV expressed as a percentage of the EDV, as shown by the following calculation:

$$\text{Ejection fraction} = \frac{\text{stroke volume}}{\text{end-diastolic volume}}$$

$$= \frac{70 \; \text{mL}}{130 \; \text{mL}} \times 100$$

$$= 54\%$$

The ejection fraction is affected by conditions such as distensibility of the ventricles, diastolic filling, and systemic vascular resistance, and is an important indicator of cardiac health (Saladin, 1998). For example, in cases of heart failure, the output of blood does not match the metabolic needs of the tissues. The heart becomes enlarged and the EDV is increased. The SV, however, remains small because of weak contractions, obstructed outflow, or a combination of factors. The ejection fraction, therefore, is reduced in a patient with heart failure.

ISOVOLUMETRIC RELAXATION

Phase 5 represents the first part of ventricular diastole. During this period called **isovolumetric relaxation** the T wave is generated on the ECG as the ventricles repolarize (see Fig. 19–1). Notice that the ventricular pressure decreases during this period as the force of the contraction fades, but the volume of the ventricles does not begin to rise until very late in the period. During the period of isovolumetric relaxation, the A-V and SL valves are closed; therefore, no blood enters the ventricles (see Fig. 19–2).

Blood in the pulmonary trunk and the aorta surges back toward the closed pulmonary and aortic valves during this period of early ventricular diastole. Recall that elastic recoil of the large arteries not only helps propel blood through the blood vessels during the brief time the heart is relaxed but also assists in the closure of the SL valves as the ventricular pressure decreases (see Chap. 17). Blood in the aorta "rebounds" off the closed cusps of the aortic valve, creating the distinctive *dicrotic notch* of the aortic pressure curve (see Fig. 19–1). The abrupt closure of the SL valves creates the turbulence that is detected as the S2 heart sound.

VENTRICULAR FILLING

As the period of diastole continues, the pressure within the ventricles falls below that of the atria and the A-V valves open, allowing blood to fill the ventricles (see Fig. 19–2). **Ventricular filling** has three subphases that overlap with both the quiescent period (*Phase 1*) and the period of atrial systole (*Phase 2*) (Saladin, 1998):

- *Rapid ventricular filling*—In the early part of ventricular filling, vibration in the wall of the ventricles may produce the S3 heart sound (see Fig. 19–1). The vibrations are caused by blood from the atria streaming through open A-V valves and rapidly filling the chambers.

- *Diastasis*—This subphase is characterized by slower filling of the ventricles. The P wave is generated at the end of diastasis (see Fig. 19–1).
- *Ventricular priming*—During the last one-third of ventricular filling, atrial systole forces an additional 30 to 40 mL of blood into the ventricles to expand and prime the ventricular pump just before the electrical impulse arrives to trigger ventricular contraction.

Cardiac Output

FACTORS AFFECTING CARDIAC OUTPUT

The volume of blood ejected by each ventricle per minute is called the **cardiac output (C.O. or $\dot{Q}$).** This hemodynamic concept was considered in several chapters covering the respiratory system, most notably, Chapter 14. Cardiac output is the product of heart rate and stroke volume:

$$\text{C.O.} = HR \times SV$$

where:

C.O. = cardiac output
HR = heart rate
SV = stroke volume

Under resting conditions, the body's total volume of blood (4 to 6 L) passes through the heart each minute as shown by the following calculation:

$$\text{C.O.} = HR \times SV$$

$$= \frac{70 \text{ beats}}{1 \text{ min}} \times \frac{70 \text{ mL}}{1 \text{ beat}} \times \frac{1\text{L}}{1000 \text{ mL}}$$

$$= 4.9 \text{ L/min}$$

Cardiac output is not fixed. Instead it is automatically adjusted to match the metabolic requirements of the tissues. Most people have a physiologic reserve that allows the cardiovascular system to respond to increased demand. This functional reserve is called the **cardiac reserve,** and is normally expressed as a multiple of the resting cardiac output value. For example, the cardiac reserve is approximately three to four times the resting C.O. in a normal healthy person (approximately 15 to 20 L/min), and may rise to around seven or eight times the resting C.O. in an endurance-trained athlete such as a world-class marathoner or cyclist (35 to 40 L/min). Taken in perspective, this level of cardiac performance in an elite athlete represents a phenomenal amount of work—the equivalent of the entire blood volume of the body circulating through the heart

every 7 or 8 seconds! As we saw with patients having respiratory disease and reduced *respiratory reserve,* patients with severe heart disease and reduced cardiac reserve have little or no tolerance of physical exertion.

As a general rule, heart rate and stroke volume are interrelated (Fig. 19–3). We explore these relationships with a discussion of the control of blood pressure in Chapter 21. Although both heart rate and stroke volume can increase or decrease together under some conditions, it is common for the two conditions to move in different directions. For example, it is sufficient to state at this point that cardiac output can be maintained at a given level by increasing one variable while the other decreases. Terms related to *heart rate, force of contraction,* and *velocity of conduction* are useful in the following discussion of the effects of different variables on cardiac output:

- **Chronotropic** and **chronotropism** refer to conditions or agents that alter the *heart rate*. Positive chronotropic agents raise heart rate; negative chronotropic agents lower heart rate.
- **Inotropic** and **inotropism** are used to describe conditions or agents that affect the force of ventricular contraction, or *stroke volume*. Positive and negative inotropic agents increase and decrease the stroke volume, respectively.
- **Dromotropic** and **dromotropism** refer to conditions or agents that change the *velocity of impulse conduction* in the heart, thus affecting heart rate. Positive dromotropic agents increase the speed of impulse transmission, whereas negative dromotropic agents slow impulse velocity.

HEART RATE

General Remarks

Heart rate is influenced by a number of chronotropic effects controlled by the autonomic nervous system and by chemical effects mediated through neurotransmitters, hormones, and drugs. For instance, sympathetic and parasympathetic *neuronal impulses* can modify the basic sinus rhythm of the heart, *hormonal influences* such as the secretion of adrenaline can increase cardiac activity, and autonomic drugs known as *sympathomimetics* and *parasympathomimetics* simulate autonomic effects by either increasing or decreasing cardiac activity. In addition, heart rate can be affected by the returning volume of blood to the heart.

Positive chronotropic effects raise the heart rate above a normal value of approximately 70 beats per minute (bpm). A persistent, resting rate in excess of 100 bpm in the adult heart is termed **tachycardia.** Such an increase in heart rate occurs in response to strenuous exercise, elevated body temperature (hyperthermia), stress, anxiety, heart disease, and sympa-

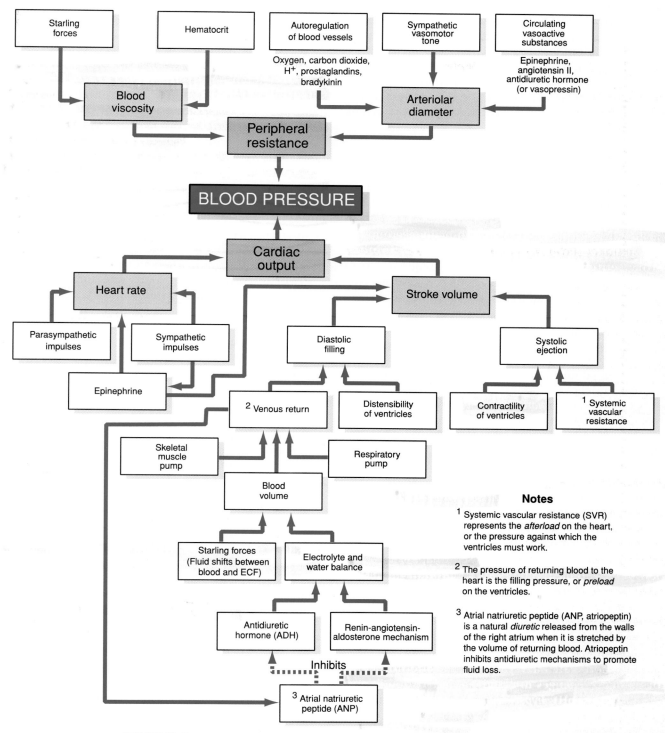

FIGURE 19–3. Factors affecting blood pressure, cardiac output, and peripheral resistance.

thomimetic drugs. At a given stroke volume, tachycardia increases the cardiac output. Tachycardia also occurs as a compensatory mechanism in instances where the stroke volume has been seriously reduced—in severe hemorrhage, for example. Through this mechanism, cardiac output to the tissues can be temporarily maintained, even though the returning volume of

blood to the heart is decreased. However, if the hemorrhaging is not controlled, tachycardia will simply accelerate the blood loss until a condition of irreversible *hypovolemic shock* develops and death occurs.

A resting heart rate that is persistently below 60 bpm in the adult is termed **bradycardia.** This condition is observed with depressed body temperature (hypothermia), parasympathomimetic drugs, and in response to endurance training. Athletes who attain high levels of aerobic conditioning through endurance training generally have hearts that develop very large stroke volumes; therefore, adequate tissue perfusion can be maintained even at a low heart rate. As a general rule, bradycardia decreases the cardiac output at a given stroke volume.

Autonomic Effects

Although extrinsic nervous stimuli are not required to initiate myocardial contractions, they can *modify* the basic sinus rhythm of the heart. Neuronal pools located in the medulla are organized into two functional groups—the **cardioacceleratory center** and the **cardioinhibitory center.** Collectively, these groupings comprise the **cardiac center** of the brain stem. The cardiac center receives sensory inputs from a variety of receptors located in the aortic arch, carotid arteries, muscles, and joints.

Motor outflow from the cardioacceleratory center is transmitted to the SA node and A-V node of the heart by sympathetic adrenergic fibers making up the **cardiac accelerator nerve.** The postganglionic fibers of these motor pathways secrete *norepinephrine* (NE), which stimulates β_1-adrenergic receptors, depolarizing them and producing a positive chronotropic effect.

Parasympathetic motor outflow from the cardioinhibitory center is transmitted to the SA and A-V nodes by cholinergic fibers in the **vagus nerve.** These fibers release the neurotransmitter *acetylcholine* (ACh), which binds to M_3-muscarinic receptors and causes chemically-gated potassium (K^+) channels to open. The resulting K^+ efflux hyperpolarizes the cells and produces a negative chronotropic effect. (See Chap. 4 for a review of autonomic receptors and neurotransmitters.)

Sensory receptors are found in a variety of peripheral locations where they send afferent information to the cardiac center. The function of some of these receptors has been previously discussed in regard to control of respiratory system activity (see Chap. 10). For example, aortic arch and carotid sinus **chemoreceptors** monitor changes in blood chemistry. Conditions of *acidosis* (low pH), *hypercapnia* (elevated arterial carbon dioxide tension, $PaCO_2$), or *hypoxemia* (decreased arterial oxygen tension, PaO_2) are indicative of increased metabolic activity in the tissues. Such conditions stimulate the chemosensitive cells of the aortic arch and carotid sinus, causing them to discharge and send impulses to the cardiac center. The cardioacceleratory center responds by initiating motor impulses that increase heart rate, cardiac output, and perfusion of hard-working tissues, thus restoring homeostasis of blood pH, $PaCO_2$, and PaO_2. Opposite blood conditions

result in a decrease in heart rate, cardiac output, and perfusion of tissue.

Aortic arch and carotid sinus **baroreceptors** are mechanoreceptors that monitor the degree of stretch in major arterial walls, thus providing an indirect measurement of blood pressure. Stated briefly, a fall in blood pressure causes the baroreceptors to send relatively few impulses to the cardiac center. The cardioacceleratory center responds by sending motor impulses through the accelerator nerves to the heart to increase heart rate and restore blood pressure to a normal range. Conversely, a rise in blood pressure stimulates the baroreceptors, which transmit sensory impulses to the cardiac center. The cardioinhibitory center responds by sending inhibitory (vagal) impulses to the heart to slow heart rate and lower blood pressure towards the homeostatic range.

Proprioceptors in the joints and muscles detect changes in position and tension in muscle fibers. These sensations are often associated with physical exertion. The sensory impulses from the various proprioceptors are relayed to the cardiac center, which increases heart rate and cardiac output to compensate for the increased metabolic demand that accompanies exercise.

Chemical Effects

A variety of chemical influences such as hormones, drugs, and electrolytes can change the heart rate and, therefore, alter the cardiac output.

Hormone Effects

Catecholamine hormones such as *norepinephrine* and *epinephrine* are synthesized by the adrenal medulla. Stimuli such as exercise and anxiety cause the adrenal medulla to secrete these hormones. Epinephrine (adrenaline) is released in large quantities in response to stress during the alarm reaction. The catecholamines exhibit very powerful positive chronotropic effects.

Drug Effects

Many catecholamines employed as therapeutic agents mimic sympathetic stimulation of the heart and thus exhibit a positive chronotropic effect. For example, adrenergic agonist bronchodilators such as *albuterol* (also known as salbutamol) and *salmeterol* are commonly used as inhaled drugs in the treatment of bronchial asthma. These drugs primarily cause relaxation of bronchiolar smooth muscle, but they also produce the unwanted side effect of cardiac stimulation. Cholinergic drugs such as *Urecholine* mimic parasympathetic stimulation and are routinely used to initiate smooth muscle activity in the gastrointestinal tract or the bladder. Unfortunately, this nonselective mechanism of action also causes vagal effects in the heart, including negative chronotropism. Most of the autonomic drugs used to treat cardiac conditions work by enhancing or inhibiting either sympathetic or parasympathetic impulses.

Electrolyte Effects

Abnormal levels of certain electrolytes can also affect heart rate. For example, elevated blood levels of sodium ions, a condition called *hypernatremia,* block the inflow of calcium ions (Ca^{2+}) into the SA node, thus stabilizing the node and reducing its firing rate. *Hyperkalemia* is an abnormally high concentration of K^+ ions in the blood stream. Such an electrolyte disturbance hyperpolarizes the SA node and prevents it from firing. Finally, an excess of calcium ions in the blood stream, a condition known as *hypercalcemia,* causes tachycardia because the increased concentration gradient enhances the inflow of Ca^{2+} into cardiac myocytes, thus causing myocardial contractions to occur at a faster rate.

Venous Return Effects

The returning volume of blood (*venous return*) causes the heart wall to expand, or bulge outward. In Chapter 21, various factors that affect venous return are discussed in detail. Stretching of the sinoatrial node in the wall of the right atrium has a direct affect on the rate and rhythm of the SA node itself, increasing the heart rate by approximately 10% to 15% (Guyton and Hall, 1996). Passive stretching of the right atrium also triggers a nervous response called the **Bainbridge reflex.** The sensory component of this reflex passes to the vasomotor center of the medulla, and then back to the heart via the sympathetic accelerator nerves and the parasympathetic vagal nerves. The motor response of the Bainbridge reflex results in an increase in heart rate and cardiac output, which helps expel the extra blood that initially caused the stretching of the SA node and right atrial wall.

Table 19–1 summarizes the heart rate responses caused by autonomic, chemical, and venous return effects. Keep in mind that positive and negative chronotropic effects produce positive and negative effects on cardiac output, *at a given stroke volume.* We now consider the changes in cardiac output caused by changes in stroke volume.

STROKE VOLUME

General Remarks

In the adult resting heart, approximately 70 mL of blood is ejected from the ventricle with each beat. This volume is known as the *stroke volume* and is affected by

myocardial contractility, ventricular preload, and *ventricular afterload* (see Fig. 19–3).

Myocardial Contractility

The strength of myocardial contraction, or inotropism, can be affected by a variety of neural and chemical factors. There is also a length-tension relationship operating in the heart that affects the force of contraction and stroke volume. This effect on contractility is discussed separately.

Autonomic Effects

Autonomic effects influence stroke volume in much the same way they affect heart rate. Sympathetic impulses transmitted from the medullary cardioacceleratory center through cardiac accelerator nerves to the heart produce a positive inotropic effect, whereas parasympathetic impulses from the cardioinhibitory center travel through the vagus nerve to the heart and produce a negative inotropic effect. *Sympathetic dominance* during the fight-or-flight response causes a marked increase in the force of contraction that results in a corresponding increase in cardiac output and tissue perfusion.

Chemical Effects
Hormone Effects

Catecholamine hormones such as norepinephrine, epinephrine, and *glucagon* exhibit a positive inotropic effect on the heart by promoting the entry of Ca^{2+} into cardiac myocytes. Passive stretching of the wall of the right atrium in response to an elevated venous return causes the heart wall to release the hormone *atrial natriuretic peptide* (ANP) or *atriopeptin* (see Fig. 19–3). This hormone has a diuretic effect to aid in the elimination of excess plasma volume, thus reducing the volume of returning blood to the heart. Atriopeptin increases glomerular filtration rate, and inhibits antidiuretic factors such as renin, aldosterone, and antidiuretic hormone.

Drug Effects

Similarly, catecholamines employed as therapeutic agents produce positive inotropism, as do drugs such as *digitalis.* Digitalis is classified as a cardiotonic drug, a drug that increases the "tone," or force of contraction of heart muscle. Digitalis improves myocardial contraction by blocking the Na^+-K^+-ATPase pumps in heart muscle, which raises the intracellular concentration of Na^+. Sodium ions are then exchanged for Ca^{2+}, which raises the intracellular concentration of Ca^{2+} in the sarcoplasm, initiating a contraction.

TABLE 19–1 Factors Causing Chronotropic Effects in the Heart

Factor	Increased Heart Rate	Decreased Heart Rate
Autonomic Effects (affected by sensory inputs from chemoreceptors, baroreceptors, and proprioceptors)		
• Cardiocelleratory center—cardiac accelerator nerves (sympathetic)	√	
Chemoreceptors:		
○ ↓ pH, ↑ $Paco_2$, Pao_2	√	
Baroreceptors		
○ ↓ BP	√	
Proprioceptors		
○ ↑ proprioceptor activity	√	
• Cardioinhibitory center—vagus nerve (parasympathetic)		√
Chemoreceptors:		
○ ↑ pH, ↓ $Paco_2$, ↑ Pao_2		√
Baroreceptors		
○ ↑ BP		√
Proprioceptors		
○ ↓ proprioceptor activity		√
Chemical Effects		
• Hormone effects (e.g. catecholamines—epinephrine, norepinephrine)	√	
• Drug effects		
○ Adrenergic stimulants (with β_1-adrenergic activity)	√	
○ β_1-Adrenergic blockers (e.g., Propranolol)		√
○ Cholinergic stimulants (with M_3-muscarinic activity)		√
• Electrolyte effects		
○ Hypernatremia ↓		√
○ Hyponatremia ↑	√	
○ Hyperkalemia ↓		√
○ Hypokalemia ↑	√	
○ Hypercalcemia ↑	√	
○ Hypocalcemia ↓		√
Venous Return Effects		
• Passive stretch of SA node and wall of RA—direct effect on heart rate	√	
• Bainbridge reflex (passive stretch of wall of RA)—indirect effect on heart rate via cardiocelleratory center	√	

BP = blood pressure; SA = sinoatrial node; RA = right atrium.

Electrolyte Effects

As explained previously with the effects of electrolyte disturbances on heart rate, abnormal concentrations of sodium, potassium, or calcium can change the force of contraction and stroke volume. Hyponatremia, hypokalemia, and hypercalcemia produce positive inotropic effects, whereas hypernatremia, hyperkalemia, and hypocalcemia produce negative inotropic effects.

Table 19–2 summarizes the cardiac effects of autonomic and chemical influences on stroke volume. Positive and negative inotropic effects produce positive and negative effects on cardiac output, *at a given heart rate.* We now consider how stroke volume is affected by changes in ventricular preload and afterload.

Ventricular Preload

Recall that the volume of blood returning to the heart contributes to the end-diastolic volume (EDV) of the heart. This volume is affected by *distensibility* of the ventricles and *venous return* factors such as the arterial-venous pressure gradient. (This gradient is discussed with hemodynamic principles of pressure and flow in Chapter 21.) The pressure of the returning blood in the atria creates a filling pressure on the ventricles called the **ventricular preload.** Ventricular preload is determined by the degree of stretch of myocardial fibers prior to contraction, and is increased when venous return increases. A moderate amount of stretch in cardiac myocytes causes them to generate more tension

TABLE 19–2 Factors Causing Inotropic Effects in the Heart

Factor	Increased Stroke Volume	Decreased Stroke Volume
Autonomic Effects (affected by sensory inputs from chemo-receptors, baroreceptors, and proprioceptors)		
• Cardioaccelleratory center—cardiac accelerator nerves (sympathetic)	√	
Chemoreceptors:		
○ ↓ pH, ↑ $Paco_2$, ↓ Pao_2	√	
Baroreceptors		
○ ↓ BP	√	
Proprioceptors		
○ ↑ proprioceptor activity	√	
• Cardioinhibitory center—vagus nerve (parasympathetic)		√
Chemoreceptors:		
○ ↑ pH, ↓ $Paco_2$, ↑ Pao_2		√
Baroreceptors		
○ ↑ BP		√
Proprioceptors		
○ ↓ proprioceptor activity		√
Chemical Effects		
• Hormone effects		
○ Catecholamines—epinephrine, norepinephrine	√	
○ Glucagon	√	
• Drug effects		
○ Adrenergic stimulants (with β_1-adrenergic activity)	√	
○ β_1-Adrenergic blockers (e.g., Propranolol)		√
○ Cholinergic stimulants (with M_3-muscarinic activity)		√
○ Cardiac glycosides (e.g., digitalis)	√	
• Electrolyte effects		
○ Hypernatremia ↓		√
○ Hyponatremia ↑	√	
○ Hyperkalemia ↓		√
○ Hypokalemia ↑	√	
○ Hypercalcemia ↑	√	
○ Hypocalcemia ↓		√

BP = blood pressure; SA = sinoatrial node; RA = right atrium.

when they begin to contract—in other words, the increased force of contraction expels more blood, thus automatically adjusting stroke volume to increased venous return.

Because ventricular preload is a function of the pressure of returning blood to the ventricle during diastole, ventricular preload is reflected in the ventricular **end-diastolic pressure (EDP),** which is in turn directly influenced by the ventricular EDV. As the EDV changes, so does the EDP and the cardiac output. The relationship between the degree of myocardial stretch (represented by EDP) and the cardiac output (represented by SV), is the length-tension relationship known as **Starling's law of the heart** or the **Frank-Starling law,**

named after physiologists Otto Frank (1865–1944) and Ernest Starling (1866–1927). This relationship states that within homeostatic limits, the heart tends to pump all the blood returning to it without allowing excessive damming of blood in the veins.

Direct measurement of the pressure within the left ventricle, or even the left atrium, provides an accurate assessment of left ventricular preload. Such direct pressure measurements, however, are not practical in a clinical setting. Instead, the left ventricular pressure is assessed with a special balloon-tipped catheter used to measure the **pulmonary capillary wedge pressure (PCWP).** In this procedure, a catheter is threaded into a systemic vein, where it is carried downstream by the flow of blood (Leff and Schumacker, 1993). The catheter is advanced into the pulmonary artery but does not enter the small-diameter pulmonary capillaries (see Fig. 20–1). When the balloon is inflated, a static "column" of blood extends distally from the tip of the catheter occluding the pulmonary artery, through the pulmonary capillaries and pulmonary veins, and all the way into the left atrium. Because the left atrium communicates with the left ventricle, the value recorded for the pulmonary artery occlusion pressure also provides an indirect measurement of the left ventricle pressure.

Ventricular Afterload

Stroke volume is influenced by factors such as myocardial *contractility* and *vascular resistance*. Vascular resistance is the pressure against which the ventricles must work. This resistance represents the **ventricular afterload** on the heart, which opposes the opening of the semilunar valves. An increase in ventricular afterload reduces stroke volume and cardiac output (see Fig. 19–3). For example, an increase in pulmonary vascular resistance (PVR) increases right ventricular afterload and puts increased stress on the right ventricle, usually causing hypertrophy and weakening of the heart wall. Failure of the right ventricle caused by obstructed pulmonary circulation results in the condition known as *cor pulmonale*, a common finding in chronic obstructive pulmonary diseases (COPDs) such as emphysema and chronic bronchitis (Saladin, 1998).

Summary

This chapter correlated information from several other chapters to show the interrelationships among pressures generated by contraction of the heart, volumes of blood ejected, blood flow through the chambers, the sounds produced by turbulence of the blood, and the electrophysiologic changes coinciding with these mechanical events. The chapter began with a consideration of the four sounds produced by the heart during one cycle and continued with a discussion of the distinct phases of the cardiac cycle—quiescent period, atrial systole, isovolumetric contraction, systolic ejection, isovolumetric relaxation, and ventricular filling. The chapter concluded with an examination of heart rate and stoke volume factors that affect cardiac output.

BIBLIOGRAPHY

Ganong WF: Review of Medical Physiology, ed 17. Appleton & Lange, Norwalk, CT, 1995.

Guyton AC and Hall JE: Textbook of Medical Physiology, ed 9. WB Saunders, Philadelphia, 1996.

Leff AR and Schumacker PT: Respiratory Physiology: Basics and Applications. WB Saunders, Philadelphia, 1993.

Martini FH: Fundamentals of Anatomy and Physiology, ed 4. Prentice Hall, Upper Saddle River, NJ, 1998.

Saladin KS: Anatomy and Physiology: The Unity of Form and Function. WCB/McGraw-Hill, Boston, 1998.

Shier D, Butler J, and Lewis R: Hole's Human Anatomy and Physiology, ed 7. Wm C Brown, Dubuque, IA, 1996.

Tortora GJ and Grabowski SR: Principles of Anatomy and Physiology, ed 8. HarperCollins, New York, 1996.

CHAPTER 20

Hemodynamic Measurements

chapter objectives

After studying this chapter the reader should be able to:

☐ Define the term *hemodynamics.*

☐ Describe how the pulmonary artery catheter is used in right heart catheterization studies.

☐ List the pressures that can be recorded with the pulmonary artery catheter.

☐ Explain how the concept of pulmonary capillary wedge pressure (PCWP) provides an indirect measurement of left atrial pressure.

☐ Explain how thermodilution studies are used with the pulmonary artery catheter to obtain values for cardiac output.

☐ Describe how the body surface area (BSA) affects hemodynamic measurements.

☐ State the formulas used to calculate the following hemodynamic measurements based on cardiac output:
   Stroke volume (SV), stroke volume index (SVI), cardiac index (CI).

☐ Explain the concept of stroke work.

☐ State the formulas used to calculate the following hemodynamic measurements of ventricular stroke work:
   Left ventricular stroke work index (LVSWI), right ventricular stroke work index (RVSWI).

☐ State the formulas used to calculate the following hemodynamic measurements of vascular resistance:
   Systemic vascular resistance (SVR), systemic vascular resistance index (SVRI), pulmonary vascular resistance (PVR), pulmonary vascular resistance index (PVRI).

key terms

body surface area (BSA)
cardiac index (CI)
cardiac output (C.O., $\dot{Q}$)
central venous pressure (CVP)
hemodynamics
left ventricular stroke work index (LVSWI)
mean pulmonary artery pressure (MPAP)
pulmonary artery catheter
pulmonary capillary wedge pressure (PCWP)
pulmonary vascular resistance (PVR)

pulmonary vascular resistance index (PVRI)
right atrial pressure (RAP)
right heart catheterization
right ventricular stroke work index (RVSWI)
stroke volume (SV)
stroke volume index (SVI); stroke index (SI)
systemic vascular resistance (SVR)
systemic vascular resistance index (SVRI)
thermodilution studies

Physiologic factors affecting cardiac output were discussed in the previous chapter. In this chapter we examine measurements of cardiac output as well as direct hemodynamic measurements based on cardiac output. The chapter also considers calculated, or derived, hemodynamic measurements of ventricular work and vascular resistance. This chapter is not designed to provide an in-depth account of hemodynamic measurement techniques encountered by the respiratory care practitioner. Instead, it is meant to introduce a few key hemodynamic concepts to give the reader a glimpse of how physiologic principles can be *applied* to monitor the cardiopulmonary status of the critically ill patient.

Hemodynamics—Overview

Hemodynamics is concerned with the study of those functions that influence the circulation of blood through the heart and vessels. Fluid dynamics principles dealing with resistance, flow, and pressure apply to the behavior of both gases and liquids and have already been discussed in relation to air flow in the respiratory system. In the following section we consider hemodynamic factors primarily affecting the heart; however, hemodynamics associated with the blood vessels are introduced here and discussed in greater detail in the following chapter. Both *direct* and *indirect* (*calculated*) measurements are used in hemodynamic studies, as described in the following sections.

Direct Hemodynamic Measurements

RIGHT HEART CATHETERIZATION

Right heart catheterization forms the basis for obtaining direct hemodynamic measurements of cardiac

blood flow. In this procedure a 2- to 3-mm-diameter, balloon-tipped **pulmonary artery catheter** (e.g., Swan-Ganz catheter) with multiple recording capabilities and separate injection ports is inserted into a systemic vein. When the balloon at the catheter tip is inflated, the catheter is carried downstream by the flow of blood, advancing through the superior vena cava (SVC), right atrium (RA), right ventricle (RV), and then into the pulmonary trunk and pulmonary artery (Fig. 20–1). A pressure transducer records the pressure in the RA, RV, and pulmonary artery as the catheter passes through the different areas. Some pulmonary artery catheters are also equipped with an injectate port and a fast-response thermistor to record rapid temperature changes in the bloodstream (discussed subsequently). The pulmonary artery catheter has revolutionized the physiologic monitoring of the critically ill patient, providing a wealth of physiologic information and continuous monitoring of hemodynamic factors such as cardiac output.

As introduced in the previous chapter with the measurement of left ventricular (LV) pressure and assessment of ventricular preload, the **pulmonary capillary wedge pressure (PCWP)** represents the pressure of blood distal to the pulmonary artery (see Fig. 20–1). Inflation of the balloon at the tip of the catheter "wedges" the catheter into the pulmonary artery and creates a continuous column of blood from the distal tip of the catheter occluding the pulmonary artery, all the way into the left atrium and left ventricle. Therefore, the PCWP recorded when the balloon is inflated indirectly represents the pressure in the left atrium.

The pulmonary artery catheter provides direct hemodynamic measurements of **right atrial pressure (RAP)** and **mean pulmonary artery pressure (MPAP)** as it is advanced through the right heart. As a general rule it is difficult to measure pressures in the pulmonary circuit because all the vessels are located in the chest (Leff and Schumacker, 1993). The pulmonary artery catheter, al-

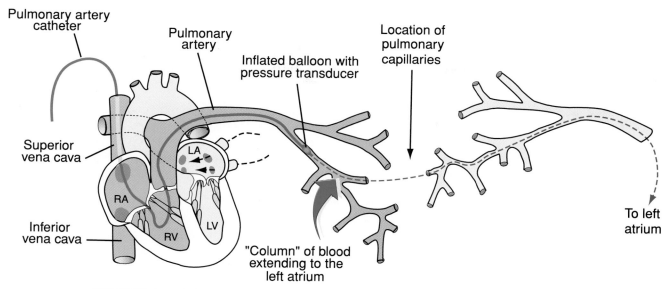

FIGURE 20–1. Right heart catheterization. A pulmonary artery catheter equipped with a balloon and a pressure transducer at its tip is advanced through a systemic vein into the superior vena cava, right atrium, right ventricle and pulmonary artery. As the tip of the catheter passes through the different regions, the pressures are recorded. When the catheter "wedges" into a branch of the pulmonary artery, the blood flow distal to the catheter ceases, forming a continuous column of blood, (dotted line) that reaches to the left atrium. The pulmonary capillary wedge pressure (PCWP) detected at the catheter tip approximates the left atrial pressure. (RA = right atrium; RV = right ventricle; LA = left atrium; LV = left ventricle.)

though somewhat invasive, has made this task much easier. **Central venous pressure (CVP)** is recorded as the initial pressure when the pulmonary artery catheter is inserted into a systemic vein. CVP can also be measured directly by the insertion of a pressure catheter into the thoracic great veins. According to Ganong (1995), *peripheral venous pressure* correlates well with CVP. For instance, one of the clinical findings associated with congestive heart failure is an increase in peripheral venous pressure and CVP because of the inability of the right heart to effectively pump blood. This increase in CVP is often manifested as a bulging in the neck veins just above the clavicles, a condition called *jugular vein distention* (JVD).

THERMODILUTION

Some multilumen pulmonary artery catheters used in right heart catheterization studies are equipped with a sensitive thermistor, or temperature probe. The rapid-response thermistor records the temperature of blood flowing past the distal tip of the catheter. This device is used in **thermodilution studies** to estimate the **cardiac output (C.O., or $\dot{Q}$)** of the heart. In the procedure a small quantity of chilled saline or dextrose and water solution is injected into the blood stream through a port in the catheter that opens through a lumen into the right atrium. The cold injectate mixes with blood in the right ventricle before being pumped into the pulmonary

trunk. The resulting drop in blood temperature is recorded as the blood flows past the tip of the catheter lodged in the pulmonary artery. In this technique it is assumed that heat is neither gained nor lost by the blood through the walls of the heart or blood vessels (Leff and Schumacker, 1993).

Because the temperature and volume of the bolus of chilled injectate is known, the change in blood temperature per unit time can be calculated. The temperature change is inversely proportional to the amount of blood flowing through the pulmonary artery. The resulting temperature-time data yield an area under the curve that represents the cardiac output (Fig. 20–2). A large decrease in temperature implies that blood is moving very slowly through the heart and the chilled injectate has sufficient time to decrease the temperature of the blood. Conversely, a small drop in temperature is indicative of rapid blood flow, or increased cardiac output. In other words, the temperature of fast-flowing blood is not appreciably lowered in the right ventricle before it streams past the catheter tip. Because the computation of cardiac output by the thermodilution method involves complex mathematical integration and numerous calculations, a *cardiac computer* is generally used to analyze the data obtained by the pulmonary artery catheter (Leff and Schumacker, 1993).

Table 20–1 summarizes the direct hemodynamic values obtained by right heart catheterization.

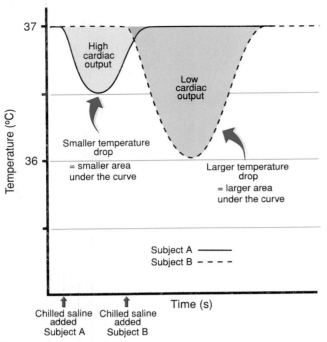

FIGURE 20–2. Determination of cardiac output by thermodilution. A pulmonary artery catheter is advanced into the right heart, with the catheter tip wedged into a branch of the pulmonary artery and the lumen of an injectate port residing in the right atrium. When a chilled solution of dextrose and water or saline is added to the catheter of subject A, a relatively small drop in temperature is detected by the thermistor at the tip of the catheter. The temperature drop and the area under the curve is much greater for subject B, indicating a lower cardiac output. (Modified from Leff AR and Schumacker PT: Respiratory Physiology: Basics and Applications. WB Saunders, Philadelphia, 1993, p 61, with permission.)

Derived Hemodynamic Measurements

BODY SURFACE AREA

Hand-held, programmable calculators are often used with computed hemodynamic measurements. Note that several of the derived, or calculated, measurements are affected by the size of the person and are therefore indexed to the **body surface area (BSA),** which is around 1.5 to 2 m² for the normal adult. Through indexing, comparisons can be made of the hemodynamic measurements obtained for people of differing sizes. For instance, a large person has a much larger cardiac output than a person of smaller size. However, when the cardiac outputs of these two people are indexed to their respective body surface areas, the resulting *cardiac index* for each person is very similar. Body surface area estimates are determined by height-weight nomograms such as the DuBois Body Surface Chart (see Appendix B). Note that a normal person with a mass of 70 kg has a BSA of approximately 1.7 m² (Guyton and Hall, 1996).

CALCULATIONS BASED ON CARDIAC OUTPUT

Several derived hemodynamic measurements such as *stroke volume, stroke volume index,* and *cardiac index* are based on cardiac output values obtained by direct hemodynamic methods such as thermodilution.

Stroke Volume

The **stroke volume (SV)** is the amount of blood pumped out of each ventricle. As discussed previously, it is affected by myocardial contractility, ventricular preload, and ventricular afterload (see Fig. 19–3). Since cardiac output is determined by the product of stroke volume and heart rate, stroke volume can be calculated by dividing the cardiac output by the heart rate:

$$SV = \frac{C.O.}{HR}$$

where:

SV = stroke volume
C.O. = cardiac output
HR = heart rate

EXAMPLE 1

Thermodilution studies indicate the cardiac output of a patient is 4800 mL/min. Calculate the stroke volume for this individual when the pulse rate is 60 beats per minute (bpm).

$$SV = \frac{C.O.}{HR}$$

$$= \frac{4800 \text{ mL}}{1 \text{ min}} \times \frac{1 \text{ min}}{60 \text{ beats}}$$

$$= 80 \text{ mL/beat}$$

Stroke Volume Index (SVI)

Stroke volume can be affected by body size; therefore, it is often indexed to the body surface area as the **stroke volume index (SVI)** or the **stroke index (SI):**

$$SVI = \frac{SV}{BSA}$$

where:
SVI = stroke volume index

TABLE 20-1	Direct Hemodynamic Measurements

(Obtained by right heart catheterization method using a pulmonary artery catheter)

Measurement	Comments
Central venous pressure (CVP)	• CVP is recorded when the pulmonary artery catheter is first inserted into a systemic vein. • Peripheral venous pressure correlates well with CVP.
Right atrial pressure (RAP)	• RAP is measured as the catheter is advanced through the right atrium.
Mean pulmonary artery pressure (MPAP)	• MPAP is measured as the catheter is advanced through the pulmonary trunk into the pulmonary artery.
Pulmonary capillary wedge pressure (PCWP)	• PCWP is recorded when the catheter tip wedges into a distal branch of the pulmonary artery, obstructing the flow of blood through the branch. • A static column of blood reaching from the catheter tip to the left atrium is formed when the balloon is inflated. • Experimental studies reveal that the PCWP detected by the pulmonary artery catheter correlates well with the left atrial pressure.
Cardiac output (C.O., $\dot{Q}$)	• Thermodilution studies obtained via the introduction of chilled saline injectate through the pulmonary artery catheter provide indirect measurement of cardiac output. • The degree to which chilled saline is warmed by blood as it passes from the right atrium to the tip of the catheter in the pulmonary artery indicates the flow rate of blood through the heart, a measure of cardiac output.

SV = stroke volume
BSA = body surface area (in m²)

EXAMPLE 2

Assume that the subject in Example 1 has a body surface area of 1.6 m². Calculate the stroke index for the patient.

$$SVI = \frac{SV}{BSA}$$

$$= \frac{80 \text{ mL/beat}}{1.6 \text{ m}^2}$$

$$= 50 \text{ mL/beat per m}^2$$

Cardiac Index

Cardiac output is another hemodynamic measurement affected by body size. The **cardiac index (CI)** shows the correlation between C.O. and the BSA. For example, the cardiac output per square meter of body surface is around 3.0 to 3.2 L/min in an average-sized individual (Ganong, 1995; Guyton and Hall, 1996).

$$CI = \frac{C.O.}{BSA}$$

where:
CI = cardiac index
C.O. = cardiac output
BSA = body surface area (in m²)

EXAMPLE 3

Thermodilution studies reveal that the cardiac output of a patient is 5 L/min. Calculate the cardiac index for this patient having a body surface area of 1.6 m².

$$CI = \frac{C.O.}{BSA}$$

$$= \frac{5 \text{ L}}{1 \text{ min}} \times \frac{1}{1.6 \text{ m}^2}$$

$$= 3.12 \text{ L/min per m}^2$$

In general, a low cardiac index and stroke index indicate a state of low blood flow and poor peripheral circulation which, in turn, imply that a condition of poor myocardial contractility or reduced blood volume exists.

CALCULATIONS OF VENTRICULAR WORK

A *stroke work index* is a measurement of the amount of work a ventricle must perform to move blood through blood vessels. An increase in vascular resistance increases ventricular afterload as well as the ventricular stroke work index. For the ventricles to perform *work*, a "force" (represented by the pressure generated by ventricular contraction) must move a mass a given "distance" (represented by the stroke volume) (Beachey, 1998). Therefore, since *work = force × distance*, we can calculate ventricular work by multiplying the pressure generated through ventricular contraction by the stroke volume index, and then adjust the units as necessary. The pressures used in the determination of ventricular work are derived from direct hemodynamic measurements obtained by the pulmonary artery catheter.

Left Ventricular Stroke Work Index

The pressure generated by the left ventricle is the difference between the mean arterial pressure (MAP) and the left ventricular end-diastolic pressure (represented by PCWP):

$$LVSWI = SVI \times (MAP - PCWP) \times \text{conversion factor}$$

> *where:*
> LVSWI = **left ventricular stroke work index**
> *SVI* = stroke volume index, or stroke index (SI)
> *MAP* = mean arterial pressure
> *PCWP* = pulmonary capillary wedge pressure

NOTE: To express the LVSWI in the proper cardiac work units, we must first multiply the answer by a factor that will convert the pressure units ("millimeters of mercury," mm Hg) into the desired "g-m/m² per beat" units used with the ventricular stroke work index. Some sources simply show this factor as the dimensionless quantity, "0.0136," referring to it as the "density of mercury factor." The reader must then remember that the stroke work index units are always expressed as "g-m/m² per beat". Using the dimensionless factor "0.0136," however, will *not* actually generate the final units. If this is mathematically true, where *do* the stroke work index units come from? The following example shows the derivation of the stroke work index units and may prove helpful in understanding the concept of cardiac work.

EXAMPLE 4

Calculate the LVSWI for a patient having a stroke volume of 70 mL/beat, BSA of 2.0 m², MAP equal to 105 mm Hg, and a pulmonary capillary wedge pressure of 5 mm Hg.

First, calculate the SVI for this patient. Recall that this value represents the "distance" that a mass of blood is moved in the *work = force × distance* equation:

$$SVI = \frac{SV}{BSA}$$

$$= \frac{70 \text{ mL/beat}}{2.0 \text{ m}^2}$$

$$\therefore SVI = 35 \text{ mL/beat per m}^2$$

Next, we calculate the LVSWI. Recall that the pressure gradient generated by the contraction of the left ventricle (MAP − PCWP = 100 mm Hg) is the "force" in the *work = force × distance* equation. We also introduce a conversion factor to change the *mm Hg* pressure units to the standard units used to express cardiac work.

NOTE: The density of mercury is given as $d = 13.6$ g/mL.

$$LVSWI = SVI \times (MAP - PCWP) \times \text{conversion factor}$$

$$= \frac{35 \text{ \sout{mL}}}{\text{beat/m}^2} \times 100 \text{ \sout{mm Hg}} \times \frac{13.6 \text{ g}}{1 \text{ \sout{mL}}}$$

$$\times \frac{1 \text{ m}}{1000 \text{ \sout{mm}}}$$

$$\therefore LVSWI = 47.6 \text{ g-m/m}^2 \text{ per beat}$$

NOTE: It is common to see the formula for left ventricular stroke work index stated as:

$$LVSWI = SVI \times (MAP - PCWP) \times 0.0136$$

Remember that the conversion factor 0.0136 eliminates the pressure units based on the density of mercury but will not actually yield the final stroke work index units of *g-m/m² per beat*. The stroke work index units must be committed to memory when using this dimensionless conversion factor.

Right Ventricular Stroke Work Index

The **right ventricular stroke work index (RVSWI)** reflects the contractility of the right ventricle. The pressure generated by the right ventricle is the difference between the MPAP and the right ventricular end-diastolic pressure (represented by CVP):

$$RVSWI = SVI \times (MPAP - CVP) \times 0.0136$$

> *where:*
> RVSWI = right ventricular stroke work index
> *SVI* = stroke volume index, or stroke index (SI)
> *MPAP* = mean pulmonary artery pressure
> *CVP* = central venous pressure

NOTE: The conversion factor, 0.0136, eliminates the pressure units based on the density of mercury but will not generate the desired cardiac work units (g-m/m² per beat). As explained previously with the calculation of LVSWI, the stroke work index units for RVSWI must be memorized when using the dimensionless factor 0.0136.

CALCULATIONS OF VASCULAR RESISTANCE

As with previous derived hemodynamic measurements, determination of *vascular resistance* is based on pressures obtained via right heart catheterization studies.

Systemic Vascular Resistance

The **systemic vascular resistance (SVR)** and *systemic vascular resistance index* (discussed in the next section) indicate the magnitude of LV afterload. In other words, SVR represents the peripheral resistance that must be overcome by the left ventricle for the chamber to eject its stroke volume into systemic circulation. As we see in the following chapter, SVR is affected primarily by the vasomotor tone of small-diameter muscular arteries called *arterioles*. An increase in SVR increases LV afterload, which in turn lowers stroke volume and reduces cardiac output (see Fig. 19–3).

SVR is calculated by first determining the *driving pressure* that produces blood flow through the systemic circuit. The MAP in the systemic arteries represents the proximal pressure at the start of the systemic circuit, whereas the mean right atrial pressure (RAP) represents the pressure at the distal end of the systemic circuit where blood enters the right heart.

> NOTE: The distal pressure in the systemic circuit is sometimes stated as the central venous pressure, or CVP (Des Jardins, 1998).

The pressure gradient (MAP − RAP) is then divided by the blood flow, or cardiac output, to arrive at a resistance measurement. Resistance is measured in terms of *pressure per unit of flow* (e.g., mm Hg/L per minute). In the calculation of SVR, the resistance calculation is multiplied by a factor of 80 to convert the units of "mm Hg/L per minute" to "dynes · sec · cm^{-5}," which are standard units used in the clinical setting (Beachey, 1998; Des Jardins, 1998). Therefore, systemic vascular resistance is given as:

$$SVR = \frac{(MAP - RAP)}{C.O.} \times 80$$

where:
SVR = systemic vascular resistance
MAP = mean arterial pressure
RAP = right arterial pressure
C.O. = cardiac output

As explained previously, the SVR and the **systemic vascular resistance index (SVRI)** indicate the afterload of the left ventricle. Indexing allows accurate comparison of SVR values among individuals of different sizes. The units of SVRI are dynes · sec · cm^{-5}/m²:

$$SVRI = \frac{SVR}{BSA}$$

where:
SVRI = systemic vascular resistance index
SVR = systemic vascular resistance
BSA = body surface area (in m²)

Pulmonary Vascular Resistance

The **pulmonary vascular resistance (PVR)** and the **pulmonary vascular resistance index (PVRI)** (discussed in the next section) indicate the afterload in the pulmonary circuit against which the right ventricle (RV) must pump. This vascular resistance must be overcome for the RV to eject its stroke volume into the pulmonary circuit. Although the resistance in the systemic circuit is about 10 times greater than that of the pulmonary circuit, it must be remembered that the force-developing capability of the myocardium of the LV is much greater than that of the myocardium of the RV.

As described previously with SVR, the driving pressure, or pressure difference responsible for moving blood through the pulmonary circuit, is divided by the blood flow, and then adjusted for the proper units. The proximal pressure in the pulmonary circuit is the pressure where the system begins—the MPAP. The system ends distally where blood vessels enter the left heart. As described previously, the blood pressure in the left heart is represented indirectly by the PCWP. Subtracting these two pressures, dividing by the cardiac output, and multiplying by the conversion factor of 80 gives the pulmonary vascular resistance in the required clinical units of dynes · sec · cm^{-5}:

$$PVR = \frac{(MPAP - PCWP)}{C.O.} \times 80$$

where:
PVR = pulmonary vascular resistance
MPAP = mean pulmonary artery pressure
PCWP = pulmonary capillary wedge pressure
C.O. = cardiac output

Pulmonary Vascular Resistance Index

The pulmonary vascular resistance index (PVRI) expresses PVR as a function of body surface area. As with the systemic vascular resistance index, calculation of

TABLE 20-2	Derived Hemodynamic Measurements

Measurement and Formula	Comments

Calculations Based on Cardiac Output
 	
 Stroke volume (SV)
    SV = C.O./HR
 Stroke volume index (SVI)
    SVI = SV/BSA
 Cardiac index (CI)
    CI = C.O./BSA
	• Stroke volume is affected by myocardial contractility, ventricular preload, ventricular afterload, and other factors.
	 • SV expressed as a function of body surface allows comparison of values in individuals of differing sizes.
	 • C.O. expressed as a function of body surface allows comparison of values in individuals of differing sizes.
	 • CI is around 3 L/min per m^2 in an average-sized individual.

Calculations of Ventricular Work
 	
 Left ventricular stroke work index (LVSWI)
    LVSWI = SVI × (MAP − PCWP) × conversion factor*
 Right ventricular stroke work index (RVSWI)
    RVSWI = SVI × (MPAP − CVP) × conversion factor*
	• PCWP represents both the left atrial pressure and the left ventricular end-diastolic pressure.
	 • CVP represents the right ventricular end-diastolic pressure.

Calculations of Vascular Resistance
 	
 Systemic vascular resistance (SVR)
    SVR = (MAP − RAP/C.O.) × 80†
 Systemic vascular resistance index (SVRI)
    SVRI = SVR/BSA
 Pulmonary vascular resistance (PVR)
    PVR = (MPAP − PCWP/C.O.) × 80†
 Pulmonary vascular resistance index (PVRI)
    PVRI = PVR/BSA
	• The driving pressure in the systemic circuit is the difference between the proximal pressure (MAP) and the distal pressure (RAP).
	 • The distal pressure can be stated as CVP.
	 • SVR expressed as a function of body surface allows comparison of values in individuals of differing size.
	 • The driving pressure in the pulmonary circuit is the difference between the proximal pressure (MPAP) and the distal pressure (PCWP), representing left atrial pressure.
	 • PVR expressed as a function of body surface allows comparison of values in individuals of differing sizes.

*Conversion factor = 13.6 g/mL × 1 m/1000 mm = 0.0136 g-m.
†80 is needed to convert resistance units of mm Hg/L per minute to standard units of dynes · sec · cm^{-5}.
C.O. = cardiac output; SV = stroke volume; HR = heart rate; BSA = body surface area (in m^2); MAP = mean arterial pressure; PCWP = pulmonary capillary wedge pressure; MPAP = mean pulmonary arterial pressure; CVP = central venous pressure; RAP = right atrial pressure.

PVRI allows comparison of the pulmonary vascular resistance in individuals of differing size. The units of PVRI are dynes · sec · cm^{-5}/m^2:

$$PVRI = \frac{PVR}{BSA}$$

where:
PVRI = pulmonary vascular resistance index
PVR = pulmonary vascular resistance
BSA = body surface area (in m^2)

Table 20–2 summarizes the hemodynamic values

TABLE 20-3	Hemodynamic Parameters

Parameter	Normal Range	Indication
C.O.	4–8 L/min	Total blood flow
CI	2.5–4.0 L/min per m^2	Blood flow for size of patient
CVP	0–6 mm Hg	Right ventricular preload
PCWP	6–12 mm Hg	Left ventricular preload
SVR	900–1400 dynes · sec · cm^{-5}	Left ventricular afterload
PVR	200–450 dynes · sec · cm^{-5}	Right ventricular afterload
MAP	80–100 mm Hg	Perfusion pressure
PAP	20–30/6–15 mm Hg	Pulmonary artery pressure

C.O. = cardiac output; CI = cardiac index; CVP = central venous pressure; PCWP = pulmonary capillary wedge pressure; SVR = systemic vascular resistance; pulmonary vascular resistance; MAP = mean arterial pressure; PAP = pulmonary arterial pressure.

Source: Modified from Wilkins RL and Dexter JR: Hemodynamic Monitoring and Shock. In Wilkins RL and Dexter JR (eds): Respiratory Disease: A Case Study Approach to Patient Care, ed 2. FA Davis, Philadelphia, 1998.

obtained via computed values. The normal range of hemodynamic parameters, and the physiologic principle indicated by the parameter, is given in Table 20–3.

Summary

This chapter focused on two types of measurement of blood flow through the heart and vessels—direct hemodynamic measurements and derived hemodynamic measurements. It also briefly examined the effect that body surface area has on hemodynamic measurements. Direct hemodynamic measurements are based on the calculation of cardiac output; therefore, the thermodilution method of determining cardiac output was briefly discussed prior to a consideration of the measurements themselves. Derived hemodynamic measurements of ventricular stroke work and vascular resistance were also considered. The basic information presented in the chapter was designed to introduce the *concepts* of hemo-

dynamic measurement and monitoring of the critically ill patient.

BIBLIOGRAPHY

Beachey W: Respiratory Care Anatomy and Physiology: Foundations for Clinical Practice. Mosby–Year Book, St. Louis, 1998.

Des Jardins T: Cardiopulmonary Anatomy and Physiology: Essentials for Respiratory Care, ed 3. Delmar Publishers, Albany, NY, 1998.

Ganong WF: Review of Medical Physiology, ed 17. Appleton & Lange, Norwalk, CT, 1995.

Guyton AC and Hall JE: Textbook of Medical Physiology, ed 9. WB Saunders, Philadelphia, 1996.

Leff AR and Schumacker PT: Respiratory Physiology: Basics and Applications. WB Saunders, Philadelphia, 1993.

Malley WJ: Clinical Blood Gases: Application and Noninvasive Alternatives. WB Saunders, Philadelphia, 1990.

Shapiro BA, Peruzzi WT, and Kozelowski-Templin R: Clinical Application of Blood Gases, ed 5. Mosby–Year Book, St. Louis, 1994.

Wilkins RL and Dexter JR: Hemodynamic Monitoring and Shock. In Wilkins RL and Dexter JR (eds): Respiratory Disease: A Case Study Approach to Patient Care, ed 2. FA Davis, Philadelphia, 1998.

CHAPTER 21

Flow, Pressure, and Resistance in Blood Vessels

chapter objectives

After studying this chapter the reader should be able to:

☐ Discuss the distribution of blood in the body by stating typical percentages of blood found in the systemic circulation, pulmonary circulation, and heart.

☐ Describe the structure of blood vessel walls by explaining the organization of the following layers:
    Tunica externa, tunica media, tunica interna.

☐ Contrast the structure and function of the following arteries:
    Elastic arteries, muscular arteries, resistance arteries.

☐ Describe the structure and function of arterioles and metarterioles.

☐ Explain the concept of a *resistance vessel.*

☐ Describe the structure and function of capillaries and capillary beds.

☐ Explain how thoroughfare channels and precapillary sphincters operate to control the flow of blood in a capillary bed.

☐ Describe the structure and function of veins, venules, venous valves, and venous sinuses.

☐ Explain the concept of a *capacitance vessel.*

☐ State the relationship between pressure and resistance in the determination of blood flow.

☐ Differentiate between blood flow and perfusion.

☐ Compare and contrast the following pressures:
   Systolic pressure, diastolic pressure, pulse pressure, mean arterial blood pressure (MABP).

☐ Define peripheral vascular resistance.

☐ Explain how the following factors influence blood flow in a vessel:
   Viscosity, vessel length, vessel radius.

☐ Describe laminar flow by explaining the concept of a *parabolic velocity profile* of the moving blood.

☐ Describe turbulent flow and explain how the following variables affect Reynolds' number:
   Vessel diameter, blood velocity, blood density, blood viscosity.

☐ State the relationship between vascular resistance, conductance, and the diameter of blood vessels.

☐ Review Poiseuille's law and explain how the following variables affect the calculation of flowrate:
   Pressure gradient, vessel radius, blood viscosity, vessel length.

☐ Explain why the velocity of blood slows as blood travels away from the heart.

☐ Describe how arterioles regulate peripheral vascular resistance.

☐ Explain how local factors such as tissue hypoxia and autacoids contribute to the short-term control of vascular resistance and blood pressure.

☐ Explain how neural factors provide short-term control of vascular resistance and blood pressure by describing the operation of the following neural mechanisms:
   Baroreceptor reflex, chemoreceptor reflex, medullary ischemic reflex.

☐ Explain how hormonal factors provide long-term control of vascular resistance and blood pressure by describing the function of the following hormones:
   Angiotensin II, aldosterone, antidiuretic hormone (ADH), erythropoietin (EPO), atrial natriuretic peptide (ANP).

☐ Describe the operation of the renin-angiotensin-aldosterone mechanism (renal mechanism) in the control of vascular resistance, plasma volume, and blood pressure.

☐ Review capillary membrane fluid dynamics by describing filtration, reabsorption, and osmosis at the capillary membrane and explaining the significance and interrelationships of the four Starling forces (blood hydrostatic pressure, tissue fluid hydrostatic pressure, blood colloid osmotic pressure, tissue fluid colloid osmotic pressure).

☐ Describe how venous return is maintained by explaining the function of the following mechanisms:
   Arteriovenous pressure gradient, respiratory pump, skeletal muscle pump, hydrostatic (gravitational) effect.

key terms

aldosterone
angiotensin II
antidiuretic hormone (ADH); vasopressin
arteries
   conducting arteries; elastic arteries
   distributing arteries; muscular arteries

resistance arteries
arterioles
arteriovenous pressure gradient
atrial natriuretic peptide (ANP); (nã″ trē-ur-et′ ik); atriopeptin
autoregulation

blood flow
blood vessel length
blood vessel radius
blood viscosity
capacitance vessels
capillaries
capillary bed
conductance
diastolic pressure
erythropoietin (EPO) (e-rith" ró poy' e-tin)
hydrostatic effect
mean arterial blood pressure (MABP)
medullary ischemic reflex
metarterioles
perfusion
peripheral vascular resistance
precapillary sphincter

pulse pressure
renin-angiotensin-aldosterone mechanism; renal mechanism
resistance vessels
respiratory pump; abdominothoracic pump mechanism
skeletal muscle pump
systolic pressure
thoroughfare channel
tunica externa; tunica adventitia
tunica interna; tunica intima
tunica media
vasomotor center
veins
venous sinus
venous valves
venules

This chapter provides an introductory, but comprehensive, look at some of the factors affecting blood flow and blood pressure. Armed with this fundamental information, the reader can better understand the relationships between these factors and the determination of resistance in the circulatory system. Many of the concepts revisited here should be familiar by this time—namely, Reynolds' number and turbulent flow, Poiseuille's law and flowrate, and total cross-sectional area and convective acceleration. The reader is encouraged to review these basic fluid dynamics principles as necessary because they apply to the behavior of both gases and liquids.

The chapter begins with an introduction to the structure of blood vessels to help explain the role of vessels in controlling resistance, pressure, and flow. Different types of pressure are considered as well as the regulation of peripheral resistance and plasma volume in the short-term and long-term control of blood pressure. The chapter concludes with a brief look at mechanisms of capillary exchange and venous return.

Distribution of Blood

As discussed previously, the total blood volume in a normal adult is around 5 L, a volume that varies with age, body size, and sex. In the resting adult, this volume is distributed in different circulatory compartments: 70% to 75% is found in systemic circulation, 10% to 18% in pulmonary circulation, and approximately 12% to 18% in the heart (Des Jardins, 1998; Saladin, 1998). Overall, about 60% of the body's blood volume is distributed in

the systemic veins, with approximately 10% distributed in the systemic arteries. The balance is found in the heart, systemic capillaries, and pulmonary capillaries. Pulmonary capillaries, at rest, hold about 75 mL of blood but can accommodate approximately 200 mL during periods of increased activity (Des Jardins, 1998). Blood vessels not only have the ability to handle additional *blood capacity* (volume) but also can accommodate additional *blood flow* (volume/time). In fact, the blood flow through most tissues of the body exhibits remarkable changes during heavy work. Blood flow to skeletal muscle, for example, increases 10-fold during strenuous exercise as cardiac output increases and blood is redistributed to those tissues that require it most. The mechanisms that control this redistribution are discussed later in the chapter. We now examine how the structure of blood vessels helps determine the volume, flow, and pressure of blood. From measurements of blood flow and blood pressure, we can determine the resistance of blood vessels.

Structure of Blood Vessels

BLOOD VESSEL WALLS

Arteries and veins have similar structural features. The differences, however, result in differing capacities, flowrates, resistances, and pressures. Three distinct *tunics*, or layers, are found in the walls of both arteries and veins, but the composition of each tunic is slightly different (Fig. 21–1; see also Color Plate 13).

- The outermost layer is called the **tunica externa (tunica adventitia),** a layer composed of loose connective tissue. This tunic anchors the blood vessel to surrounding tissues and allows passage of structures such as nerves, lymphatics, and smaller blood vessels. The outer wall of larger blood vessels is supplied by blood delivered by very small vessels that penetrate the tunica externa. These small blood vessels are called *vasa vasorum.*

- The middle layer is the **tunica media,** a layer composed of smooth muscle, elastic tissue, and collagen. The wall thickness of blood vessels is determined primarily by the thickness of the tunica media. The middle layer of certain blood vessels plays a major role in the regulation of vascular resistance *(vasomotor tone)* and blood pressure because of changes in the tension of smooth muscle fibers brought about by chemical, hormonal, and neural influences.

- The innermost layer of blood vessels is the luminal surface. This layer is known as the **tunica interna (tunica intima),** and is composed of squamous epithelium called *endothelium.* The endothelium layer is supported by a thin *basement membrane,* and the *lamina propria,* a thin layer of smooth muscle and connective tissue. The endothelium is continuous with the endocardium that lines the chambers of the heart. The cells of the tunica intima not only provide a smooth layer for the passage of blood and a semipermeable barrier to substances transported by the blood but also secrete several vasoactive substances that will be discussed later.

ARTERIES

Arteries carry blood away from the heart and are designed to withstand the high-pressure surges characteristic of ventricular systole. This pulsatile flow is absorbed by the thick muscular layers and elastic connective tissue of the tunica media of the large- and medium-diameter arteries (see Fig. 21–1). The following classes of arteries are recognized:

- The larger arteries proximal to the heart, such as the aorta and pulmonary arteries, are designated **conducting arteries,** or **elastic arteries.** As the name implies, these arteries are characterized by substantial amounts of elastic tissue. Elastin protein fibers alternate with layers of smooth muscle to produce a thick, tough, resilient blood vessel capable of absorbing the fluctuations of powerful ventricular contractions. The elastic component of the vessels is responsible for the elastic recoil effect that helps damp the fluctuations of blood pressure on smaller-diameter arteries located distally. Recall that the *aortic pump mechanism* also helps propel blood through the systemic circuit during the brief period of ventricular diastole.

- Smaller branches of the conducting arteries are

known as **distributing** or **muscular arteries.** The muscular arteries are generally given names such as the bronchial arteries, femoral artery, and radial artery. About three-quarters of the wall of a distributing artery is composed of vascular smooth muscle. By comparison, only about one-third of the wall of a conducting artery is made up of smooth muscle (Saladin, 1998).

- Small-diameter arteries with a thick tunica media in proportion to the lumen of the vessels are designated **resistance arteries.** These blood vessels have up to 25 layers of smooth muscle and are capable of changing their diameters in response to various stimuli. The smallest of these **resistance vessels** have internal diameters ranging from 8 μm to as much as 30 μm and are known as **arterioles** (Guyton and Hall, 1996). These thin-walled vessels are composed of only one or two layers of vascular smooth muscle; therefore, slight changes in smooth muscle tone result in dramatic changes in blood vessel diameter because the muscular walls make up a large *proportion* of the vessel diameter (Guyton and Hall, 1996; Saladin, 1998). The importance of this class of artery in the control of vascular resistance and blood pressure is discussed later in the chapter. Finally, arterioles give off numerous, small-diameter vessels called **metarterioles,** which have circularly arranged, individual smooth muscle cells, rather than a continuous muscular layer within the tunica media (see Fig. 21–1). These short vessels connect arterioles directly to *capillary beds* composed of 10 to 100 *capillaries* and help control the flow of blood through the capillary beds, as discussed in the next section (Saladin, 1998).

CAPILLARIES

Capillary Beds

The structure of a typical **capillary** differs significantly from that of arteries and veins. The obvious difference is the extremely small diameter of most capillaries. The average diameter of capillaries is about 5 μm, whereas erythrocytes average approximately 7 μm in diameter. Consequently, red blood cells usually travel through capillaries in single file, often folding upon themselves, or becoming somewhat distorted, to be pushed through the smallest capillaries. This relatively slow progress of red blood cells through capillaries allows sufficient time for nutrient, gas, and waste exchange to occur. The exchange of these substances is aided by the extremely thin walls of capillaries. The wall structure consists of a single layer of squamous epithelial cells (endothelium) overlying a thin basement membrane (see Figs. 3–4 and 11–9). Because of the extensively branched network of blood vessels, the total *surface area* of the capillaries of

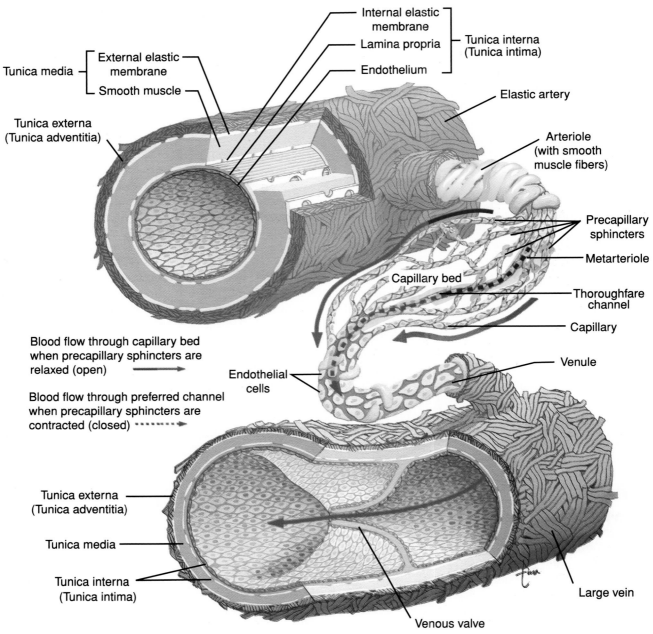

FIGURE 21–1. Blood vessel structure. Elastic artery and large vein connected by an arteriole, capillary bed, and venule. Note that the same three tunics are present in both arteries and veins, but that the thickness of the smooth muscle of the tunica media is much greater in arteries. Note also that arterioles have a high proportion of smooth muscle in their walls. The metarteriole and the thoroughfare channel form a *preferred channel* that provides a direct route for blood flow through the capillary bed when the precapillary sphincters are closed. (Adapted from Scanlon VC and Sanders T: Essentials of Anatomy and Physiology, ed. 3. FA Davis, Philadelphia, 1999, p 277, with permission.) (See also Color Plate 13.)

the body is estimated at approximately 6300 m² (Saladin, 1998). This surface area is substantially larger than a football field, thus providing an extensive exchange "membrane" between the bloodstream and the body's 60 trillion cells, most of which are within a few micrometers of a capillary. Certain tissues such as the epidermis of the skin and the retina and lens of the eye

lack capillaries. Such tissues are nourished by vascularized structures located nearby.

As explained previously, a single metarteriole supplies a group of 10 to 100 capillaries comprising a **capillary bed.** These clusters of capillaries supply groups of cells within tissues and are organized so that the flow of blood through the capillary bed can be regulated. The metarteriole continues through the capillary bed as the **thoroughfare channel,** a small blood vessel that connects distally to a *venule* (see Fig. 21–1). Individual capillaries arise from the proximal end of the metarteriole, branch extensively within the tissue being supplied by the capillary bed, and connect distally to the thoroughfare channel or to the venule. At the origin of each capillary is found a circular smooth muscle forming the **precapillary sphincter** (see Figs. 21–1 and 11–9). Through the constriction of individual capillaries, these sphincters regulate the perfusion of vascular beds in the body and are thus responsible for routing blood from one region to another. When the precapillary sphincters are closed (contracted), blood in the metarteriole is shunted directly into the thoroughfare channel and then into the venule, thus bypassing the capillaries. Such a circulatory route is activated in the fingers and toes in response to cold temperatures—the rapid closure of precapillary sphincters reduces the heat loss that would occur if blood entered the large surface area of a capillary bed exposed to low temperatures. When the precapillary sphincters are open (relaxed), blood leaves the metarteriole and perfuses the capillary bed. This transit of blood through the capillaries allows gas, nutrient, waste, and heat exchange to occur.

VEINS

Veins carry blood toward the heart. After leaving the distal end of the thoroughfare channel in the capillary beds, blood is collected by small-diameter venous structures called **venules.** These vessels are collected into small-diameter veins that join to form large-diameter veins. Veins are subjected to relatively low blood pressure and conditions of nearly pulseless flow compared to arteries. For example, average venous pressure is about 10 mm Hg, whereas average arterial pressure ranges from 90 mm Hg to approximately 100 mm Hg (Saladin. 1998). The wall of a typical vein has very little smooth muscle or elastic tissue; therefore, the inside diameter of a vein is much larger than that of an artery of equivalent outside diameter (see Fig. 21–1). Because of the large lumen and thin walls of a typical vein, the vessels can easily expand to accommodate more blood volume than an artery of the same diameter. Consequently, about 60% of the body's total blood volume can be stored in the systemic veins, which are often referred to as **capacitance vessels.**

The medium-diameter veins of the arms and legs are equipped with numerous **venous valves** that provide unidirectional flow of blood toward the heart. The mechanism known as the *skeletal muscle pump* passively compresses the thin-walled veins during skeletal muscle contraction. This action drives blood toward the heart. When the muscle relaxes, blood falls in the veins, closing the venous valves, thus preventing backflow. This mechanism, as well as several others that influence venous return to the heart, are examined at the end of the chapter. A **venous sinus** such as the coronary sinus (see Fig. 17–6) is a thin-walled structure with a large lumen and no smooth muscle. Such venous structures collect blood from specific circulatory routes such as coronary circulation.

Blood Flow

RELATIONSHIPS AMONG FLOW, PRESSURE, AND RESISTANCE

As discussed in previous chapters, hemodynamics is concerned with the principles that affect blood flow—namely, *pressure* and *resistance*. **Blood flow** refers to the volume of blood flowing through a blood vessel in a given time. In the resting state, total flow is equal to the cardiac output, typically about 5 L of blood per minute for an average-sized individual. As discussed later, blood can be rapidly shunted, or diverted, from one vascular bed to another as needs change; thus regional blood flow may be quite variable, even though total flow is relatively constant. Moreover, different flow patterns such as *laminar flow* and *turbulent flow* develop within blood vessels as the radii change.

Blood flow is directly proportional to the blood pressure difference between two points $(P_1 - P_2)$ in a conducting tube—in other words, flow varies directly with the driving pressure, or pressure gradient (ΔP) in a blood vessel. Blood flow is also indirectly proportional to the resistance in a blood vessel. The greater the resistance, the less will be the flow of blood through the vessel. These fluid dynamics relationships have already been explored in conjunction with gas flow through the conducting passages of the respiratory system. The principles apply equally well to the behavior of both gases and liquids:

$$F \propto \Delta P / R$$

where:
F = flow
ΔP = pressure gradient or driving pressure
 $(P1 - P_2)$
R = resistance

Because the total blood flow in the resting person is equal to the cardiac output, we can substitute $\dot{Q}$ for F in the preceding equation. Therefore:

$$\dot{Q} \propto \Delta P / R$$

PERFUSION OF TISSUES

Perfusion refers to the rate of blood flow per given mass of tissue, as in *mL/min per gram*. The perfusion of tissues is not uniform. Some tissues are said to be highly perfused, meaning that they receive a disproportionate flow of blood compared to their size or mass. The kidneys, for example, receive approximately 20% to 25% of the cardiac output but only represent a very small fraction of total body mass. In Chapter 10 we discussed control of respiration. In the section covering chemical control, it was pointed out that the tiny (2-mg) carotid and aortic bodies are among the most extensively perfused tissues in the body, receiving about 2000 mL of blood per minute per 100 g of tissue (Ganong, 1995). By comparison, the kidneys receive a blood flow of 1000 to 1200 mL/min, but are *perfused* at a rate of only 420 mL/min per 100 g of tissue.

Blood Pressure

As pointed out in Chapter 20, the pressure in a blood vessel or in a heart chamber can be determined with a pulmonary artery catheter that is inserted into a vessel or chamber. However, for routine monitoring purposes, blood pressure (BP) is measured clinically with a blood pressure cuff (*sphygmomanometer*) at an artery near the heart (e.g., brachial artery). The *systolic pressure* and *diastolic pressure* recorded by the device reflect the arterial pressures found elsewhere in the systemic circuit.

SYSTOLIC AND DIASTOLIC PRESSURES

The peak arterial pressure recorded during ventricular systole is the **systolic pressure,** typically about 120 mm Hg for an individual in his or her mid-20s. The **diastolic pressure** is the pressure recorded during ventricular diastole. This arterial value is approximately 75 to 80 mm Hg (Fig. 21–2D; see also Color Plate 14). Left ventricular pressure falls essentially to zero during relaxation of the heart; however, closure of the aortic valve normally prevents arterial pressure from dropping below 75 to 80 mm Hg (see Fig. 19–1). Arterial blood pressure is expressed as a ratio of systolic over diastolic pressure, as in *120/80*. Occasionally, these pressures are more accurately written as a *range* of values such as *118-123/75-80*.

Elastic recoil of arteries such as the aorta results in a damping effect that reduces the *pulsatile* flow pattern common in systemic arterial flow (see Fig. 21–2D). Such pressure fluctuations can stress the more delicate small-diameter blood vessels. As a result of the damping effect, the smaller distal arteries and capillaries are not subjected to damaging high-pressure surges of blood. The nearly pulseless flow pattern in capillaries is ideal for the exchange of gases, nutrients, and waste products. The elastic recoil effect also helps propel blood in the arterial circuit and close the semilunar valves of the heart during the brief relaxation phase of the cardiac cycle. With advancing age, however, arteries become stiffer, thus reducing the elastic recoil effect. Therefore, the modulating effect of the rhythmic distention and recoil of the arterial wall during systole is lessened and the blood pressure rises.

PULSE AND MEAN PRESSURES

The difference between systolic and diastolic pressure is known as the **pulse pressure** (see Fig. 21–2D). For an individual with a BP of 120/80, the pulse pressure is 40 mm Hg. Notice in the graph that as blood travels out from the heart and back again, not only do the systolic and diastolic pressures decrease, but the *difference* between them also decreases to a point where the pulse pressure is virtually imperceptible. In other words, the 40 mm Hg pulse pressure typically found in an artery makes it relatively easy to determine an individual's pulse in beats per minute. This occurs because the pressure differential between the systolic and diastolic pressures is so great that one can easily detect the bounding sensation beneath the fingertips. The sensation marks the passage of a mechanical pulse wave caused by the "bulge" of blood and the elastic recoil of the arterial wall. At a greater distance from the heart, however, the difference between systolic and diastolic pressures becomes less distinct, and detection of the pulse pressure becomes more difficult. This is the reason, of course, that a pulse cannot be detected in a vein, even in a large-diameter superficial vein (see Fig. 21–2D). The differential between the high-pressure and the low-pressure phase of the cardiac cycle is so slight—because of the damping effect of elastic recoil and the distance from the heart—that the blood flow through a vein feels essentially pulseless to our fingertips.

Blood pressure taken at regular intervals throughout the cardiac cycle yields the **mean arterial blood pressure (MABP).** As discussed in Chapter 17, diastole lasts substantially longer than systole; therefore, MABP is not simply the average of the two pressures. Instead, it has been determined that a reliable estimate of the MABP is given by the sum of the diastolic pressure and one-third of the pulse pressure. Therefore, in an individual with a blood pressure of 120/80, the MABP will be:

$$MABP = 80 + 40/3 \approx 93 \text{ mm Hg}$$

Mean arterial blood pressure values of approximately 90 mm Hg are common in arteries at the level of the heart in the standing adult; however, MABP varies directly with the effect of gravity. For instance, MABP is

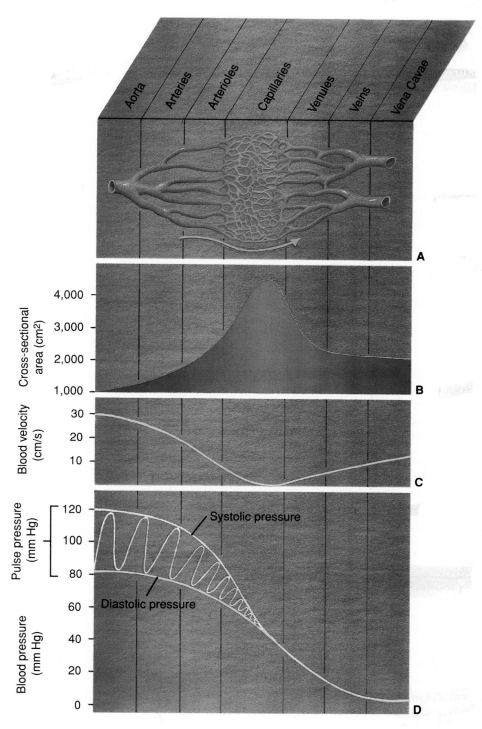

FIGURE 21–2. Characteristics of the vascular system. (A) Schematic of the branching vessels. (B) Cross-sectional area. (C) Blood velocity. (D) Systemic blood pressure changes. (Adapted from Scanlon VC and Sanders T: Essentials of Anatomy and Physiology, ed. 3. FA Davis, Philadelphia, 1999, p 291, with permission.) (See also Color Plate 14.)

about 62 mm Hg in the major arteries of the head, but increases to approximately 180 mm Hg in the arteries of the ankle in the upright adult (Saladin, 1998).

Blood pressure is affected by *cardiac output, peripheral resistance,* and *blood volume.* Factors affecting cardiac output were considered in Chapter 19 (see Fig. 19–3). In the following section we examine factors that affect peripheral resistance and blood volume.

Resistance

PERIPHERAL VASCULAR RESISTANCE

To understand how blood pressure is affected by resistance, we need to first examine some of the factors that influence resistance to flow. Recall that blood flow varies inversely with resistance. To begin, it should be understood that pressure is directly proportional to resistance ($P \propto R$). In fact, fluids have no pressure unless they encounter resistance, as explained subsequently. **Peripheral vascular resistance** is the resistance that blood encounters within blood vessels. This impediment to blood flow in a vessel cannot be measured directly. Instead, resistance is derived from measurements of blood flow and blood pressure.

Vascular resistance is subdivided into *pulmonary vascular resistance* (PVR) and *systemic vascular resistance* (SVR), and in each case, blood pressure varies directly with resistance (see Chap. 20). Peripheral resistance results from the cumulative friction of blood against the walls of blood vessels and is affected by *blood viscosity, vessel length,* and *vessel radius*. Changes in variables such as blood viscosity or vessel length occur very slowly. Changes in vessel radius, on the other hand, can change rapidly, thus providing an immediate way of altering resistance, pressure, and flow in blood vessels.

BLOOD VISCOSITY

Viscosity is a measure of the resistance of a fluid to flow. **Blood viscosity** directly affects peripheral resistance; however, the viscosity of blood is fairly constant and does not change rapidly. Under normal conditions the viscosity of blood is about three times greater than that of water (Guyton and Hall, 1996). Certain conditions can change blood viscosity, but usually do so over an extended period of time. For example, *polycythemia* increases the number of formed elements in the blood, whereas *dehydration* reduces the amount of plasma suspending the formed elements. Either way, blood viscosity increases as the blood becomes thick, sluggish, and more difficult to move. As a result of the increased viscosity, peripheral resistance increases, thus raising blood pressure. If all other factors are held constant, the greater the viscosity of blood, the less the flow through a blood vessel. Conversely, *anemia,* which reduces the number of red blood cells, and *hypoproteinemia* caused by a reduction in the blood protein albumin, reduce blood viscosity and decrease peripheral resistance and blood pressure. Blood flow increases as the viscosity decreases because the "thinned" blood exhibits less friction and moves more easily through blood vessels.

VESSEL LENGTH

Changes in the **blood vessel length** generally occur very slowly as blood vessels advance into newly repaired or growing tissues. Such development of blood vessels is known as *angiogenesis.* As length is added to a vascular system, increased friction is encountered by blood traveling through the expanded system.

VESSEL RADIUS

Of the variables capable of changing peripheral resistance, only alterations in **blood vessel radius** can produce the *rapid* changes required for immediate and precise control of pressure and flow of blood to the tissues. The fluid dynamics principles at work here have been studied in depth in previous chapters dealing with the flow of gases through the conducting passages of the respiratory system. However, we briefly revisit the basics that govern the behavior of fluids flowing in tubes.

Laminar Flow and Parabolic Velocity Profile

Recall that *laminar flow* refers to the smooth, steady, longitudinal movement of fluid in a tube. Blood flowing in a vessel of given radius flows in *streamlines,* with each layer of blood maintaining the same distance from the wall of the vessel (see Fig. 8–1A). By contrast, in *turbulent flow,* the streamlines are not present, and the blood flows in all directions, continually mixing within the tube (see Fig. 8–1B). In laminar flow in a large-diameter vessel, blood has the fastest velocity near the center of the tube. Here, frictional forces with the walls of the tube are nonexistent, and the only frictional forces are those encountered as the different components of blood slide past one another at slightly different velocities. In fact, if the velocity profiles of the different layers of blood are analyzed, a *parabolic velocity profile* results. The appearance resembles a three-dimensional cone, or series of telescoping cylinders with the central core moving at a faster velocity, and thus projecting further along the vessel (see Fig. 8–3). The layer of blood making contact with the endothelial lining of the blood vessel encounters the greatest friction and thus moves very slowly. The second layer slightly away from the wall slides over the first layer and moves a little faster, the third slides over the second, and so on. In this way, the fluid in the middle of the vessel moves very rapidly because of the many layers of slipping molecules between it and the endothelial lining of the vessel.

Turbulent Flow and Reynolds' Number

Turbulence occurs in the blood stream when blood velocity increases significantly, or when an obstruction, sharp turn, or rough surface is encountered. Under these circumstances, at a constant vessel diameter, the smooth streamline flow becomes interrupted and the apparent viscosity of the blood increases. In *turbulent flow,* blood begins to flow in nonuniform ways, often moving perpendicular to the long axis of the vessel and forming *eddy currents* (see Fig. 8–1B). These swirling eddy currents impart great resistance to flow because of the added friction among blood layers and between layers and the walls of the vessel. In general, turbulent flow requires more driving pressure to maintain the same flowrate of blood because the potential energy of the flow is being dissipated in the swirls and eddies (see Fig. 8–3).

The development of random turbulence varies directly with the *diameter* (D) of the blood vessel, the *average velocity* of the blood (μ), and the *density* (ρ) of the blood. It is inversely proportional to the *viscosity* (η) of the blood. These variables are combined into the equation we used to calculate Reynolds' number (Re) in the determination of turbulent flow in the airways (see Chap. 8). As Reynolds' number rises above 200 to 400, turbulent flow will occur at some branches of blood vessels, but will smooth out again and become laminar through the straighter portions (Guyton and Hall, 1996). A Reynolds' number in excess of 2000, however, generally indicates that the laminar flow pattern will be disrupted and break into a *randomly oriented* turbulent flow. Interestingly, streamline flow may also break into *organized* swirls of turbulence (see Fig. 8–1C). This type of turbulence is responsible for the sounds produced by blood moving within the blood vessels (Box 21–1).

Notice in the following equation that Reynolds' number itself is dimensionless:

$$Re = \frac{D \times \mu \times \rho}{\eta}$$

where:
Re = Reynolds' number (dimensionless)
D = diameter of the vessel (cm)
μ = average velocity (*mu*) of the blood (cm/s)
ρ = density (*rho*) of the blood (g/mL)
η = viscosity (*eta*) of the blood (g/s · cm)

At a constant blood viscosity and density, notice that blood flowing through larger-diameter, higher-velocity blood vessels such as the aorta will have a larger Reynolds' number indicative of turbulent flow.

CONDUCTANCE, RESISTANCE, AND CHANGES IN BLOOD VESSEL DIAMETER

The measure of flow through a blood vessel for a given pressure difference (ΔP) is known as **conductance.** In other words, if the resistance in a blood vessel is great, the conductance of blood through the vessel will be slight. This measurement is normally expressed in units of *liters/second per mm Hg.* Conductance is the reciprocal of resistance, as shown by the following relationship:

$$Conductance = \frac{1}{resistance}$$

When the blood flow within blood vessels of different diameters is compared, remarkable differences are noted. For example, at the same driving pressure, vessels with relative diameters of 1 and 2 exhibit relative flowrates of 1 and 16, respectively. Figure 8–2 shows this dramatic relationship between conductance and blood vessel diameter. The conductance of the vessel varies directly with the *fourth power* of the diameter; thus:

$$Conductance \propto diameter^4$$

What relationship is responsible for this dramatic increase in conductance with an increase in blood vessel diameter? Actually, we have already studied this fluid dynamics relationship in the lung as part of the *Hagen-Poiseuille law* (see Chap. 3). The following section briefly reviews the highlights of Poiseuille's law as it applies to the flow of blood in the circulatory system.

Poiseuille's Law

BLOOD FLOW IN A SINGLE VESSEL

Recall that in laminar flow, concentric rings of moving blood travel in a straight line at a fixed distance from the vessel wall. The flowrate of each layer, or ring, of blood is different from that of the other rings, increasing towards the central core. In a large-diameter vessel, this sequence results in a large proportion of the blood flowing at a relatively fast velocity. But what of a smaller-diameter blood vessel? The same laminar flow principles apply, but most of the blood is flowing very near the wall of the vessel. Consequently, a high-velocity central core of blood does not exist. Frictional forces affect a greater percentage of the total volume of blood in a small vessel, essentially because fewer concentric rings are present to slide over one another.

Poiseuille's law is derived by integrating the velocities of all the concentric rings of blood flowing in the vessel and multiplying these by the areas of the rings (Guyton and Hall, 1996). The resulting equation shows that the blood flow is directly proportional to the driving pressure and blood vessel radius, and indirectly proportional to the viscosity of blood and the length of the blood vessel:

$$\dot{Q} = \frac{\Delta P \pi r^4}{8 \eta l}$$

where:
$\dot{Q}$ = flowrate of blood
ΔP = driving pressure (pressure gradient, $P_1 - P_2$)
π = *pi* (mathematical constant)
r = radius of blood vessel
η = *eta* (viscosity of blood)
l = length of blood vessel

PERSPECTIVES

BOX 21-1

Æolian Harps, Fluttering Flags, and Meandering Streams

In contrast to classic Reynolds' turbulence caused by laminar flow breaking into a *randomly oriented flow pattern*, laminar flow may also break into an *organized flow pattern of swirls and vortices*. Such a pattern results in Æolian turbulence, also known as fluttering turbulence. The production of Æolian (ee-oh'-lee-uhn) *tones* occurs at flow velocities lower than those causing random turbulence. The term is taken from Æolus, the mythic Greek god of the winds, who was believed to live in the Æolian Islands of Greece. The term is also used to describe a remarkable stringed instrument called the Æolian harp, which was recreated in the 17th century. When this zither-like instrument is placed in the wind, the action of moving air currents over the strings produces haunting, eerie sounds with constantly changing chords, overtones, and harmonics. The 12 to 16 strings are all of the same length but are strung with different gauge wire. All are tuned in unison to the same note. Changes in sound are related to the intensity of the wind "playing" the strings. When a breeze sets the strings in motion, the wind velocity and different diameters of the strings cause *eddies* and *vortices* of air downwind to vary considerably. These changes are responsible for the variations in tone and the ghostly harmonies produced by the harp. So what do strange sounds coming from an ancient harp played by the wind have to do with blood flow in the circulatory system?

When an obstacle is placed in the path of a flow stream—either a gas or liquid—a slight disturbance in the streamline causes the flow wake to be diverted toward one side of the obstacle. Inertial forces cause the stream to continue into the lower pressure, higher velocity region. This movement then forces the flow back in the opposite direction, creating another low-pressure area where the flow wake overshoots and is forced back in the opposite direction. With this repeating, fluctuating type of positive feedback mechanism, vortices are created, shed, and carried downstream, and created again as the flow wake swings back and forth. Oscillations in the flow wake within a blood vessel cause lateral pressure fluctuations on the wall of the vessel. If these lateral fluctuations are of sufficient magnitude and intensity, audible sounds are produced. In fact, relatively more sound is produced by this organized turbulent flow (at a given driving pressure) than is produced by the disorganized, randomly oriented turbulent flow observed with Reynolds' turbulence.

The murmurs heard in a blood vessel wall, the fluttering of a flag in a stiff breeze, the alternating path of a meandering stream, and the harmonics of an ancient harp, are all examples of Æolian tones and fluttering turbulence.

- Rothe CF: Fluid dynamics. In Selkurt EE (ed): Physiology, ed 2. Little, Brown and Co., Boston, 1966.
- The New Encyclopædia Brittannica, ed 15: Micropædia, Vols 1 and 4. Robert McHenry (ed), Chicago, 1993.

An important feature to note in this equation is that the rate of blood flow is directly proportional to the fourth power of the radius of the blood vessel. Although blood viscosity and vessel length can affect blood flow, changes in the radius of blood vessels are clearly the most important means of altering the flowrate—doubling the radius of the blood vessel results in a 16-fold increase in the flowrate. In the following section we examine the special role of arterioles in the regulation of blood vessel radius, vascular resistance, pressure, and flow.

BLOOD FLOW IN THE CIRCULATORY SYSTEM

The extremely large lumen diameter of the aorta (about 2.5 cm) allows a flow velocity of approximately 300 to 1200 mm/s (see Fig. 21-2C; see also Color Plate 14). By contrast, the extremely small lumen diameter of a typical capillary (about 5μm to 7μm) severely restricts blood flow velocity to approximately 0.4 mm/s (Saladin, 1998). As we noted with air flow within branching conducting passages of the lung, blood flow is dramatically affected by the extensively branched vascular system (see Fig. 21–2A; see also Color Plate 14). In other words, even though the radii of blood vessels become smaller and smaller as blood travels away from the heart, the blood flows into a *conducting system* with an ever-enlarging total cross-sectional area. For instance, the aorta is a very large blood vessel with a cross-sectional area of 3 to 5 cm²—but it is only *one* vessel. By comparison, the innumerable capillaries of the body possess a total cross-sectional area of 4500 to 6000 cm² (see Fig. 21–2B; see also Color Plate 14) (Saladin, 1998). This tubular system is analogous to that formed by the trachea and the distal bronchioles (see Chap. 8). Just as the velocity of gas is reduced as it moves into the large total cross-sectional area formed by the bronchiolar system, the velocity of blood decreases as it flows into the expanded system formed by branched arterioles and capillaries.

In summary, the velocity of blood progressively slows from the aorta to the capillaries because (1) the *length* of the blood vessels has imparted friction to the blood as it moves further away from the heart, (2) the *smaller radii* of arterioles and capillaries offer greater resistance to flow, and (3) the *convective acceleration (Bernoulli) effect* slows the forward velocity of the blood as it moves into the greater total cross-sectional area formed by the arteriolar-capillary network. As blood continues back toward the heart in the venous system, it is collected into progressively fewer, but larger diameter, blood vessels. This transit through the veins causes the velocity of blood to increase. However, its velocity is not restored to that of the large arteries because of the considerable distance from the head of pressure in the left ventricle.

Regulation of Peripheral Resistance and Plasma Volume

THE ROLE OF ARTERIOLES

Unlike the larger resistance arteries that have thick muscular walls, the tunica media of arterioles is composed of only one or two layers of smooth muscle. This thin-walled section, combined with a small internal diameter (8 to 30 μm), results in the arterial equivalent of a "muscle-bound capillary." Slight changes in vascular tone rapidly change the lumen diameter of such vessels by as much as *four-fold* (Guyton and Hall, 1996). The fourth power law associated with blood flow and blood vessel diameter dictates that an increase in lumen

diameter of this magnitude will theoretically result in a 256-fold increase in flowrate through the arteriole. Of course, a decrease in arteriolar diameter will cause a correspondingly dramatic decrease in blood flow. According to Guyton and Hall (1996), approximately two-thirds of the resistance in the systemic circulation is in the small arterioles. Therefore, the overall importance of this class of blood vessel in the regulation of blood flow to the capillary beds cannot be overemphasized:

- Arterioles are *numerous* and represent a large cross-sectional area.
- They have *strong* muscular walls that respond rapidly to neural and local tissue signals.
- The *fourth power* relationship between diameter and flow results in dramatic changes in tissue perfusion and the redistribution of blood to different capillary beds with only slight changes in arteriolar diameter.

We now examine the factors that affect blood vessel diameter and vascular resistance—*local control, neural control,* and *hormonal control.* These controls of vascular resistance contribute to the control of blood pressure. Recall that pressure varies directly with resistance.

LOCAL CONTROL

Metabolic activity in tissues that are poorly perfused results in hypoxia and the accumulation of carbon dioxide (CO_2), hydrogen ions (H^+), and lactic acid. The presence of these waste products in the tissues causes vasodilation of local blood vessels, which improves the perfusion and removes the metabolites. As the concentration of metabolites decreases, vasoconstriction occurs to reduce the blood flow to the tissue. This self-adjusting negative feedback mechanism for the control of blood vessel diameter and local perfusion is known as **autoregulation.**

Various autacoids, or tissue hormones, exert local control over blood vessel tone to change the volume of blood flowing into tissues under conditions such as exercise, trauma, or inflammation. For example, *histamine, prostaglandins,* and *bradykinin* are powerful autacoids released or synthesized during the inflammatory response. Histamine, prostaglandin E_2 (PGE_2), and bradykinin are potent vasodilators, whereas prostaglandin $F_{2\alpha}$ ($PGF_{2\alpha}$) and prostaglandin D_2 (PGD_2) are vasoconstrictors (see Chap. 5).

Endothelial cells and thrombocytes (platelets) also produce vasoactive substances that produce localized effects in the tissues. For example, endothelial cells produce the vasodilator known as *nitric oxide* (NO), a substance originally named *endothelium-derived relaxing factor* (EDRF). Another vasodilator synthesized by endothelial cells is *prostacyclin,* also known as *prostaglandin I_2 (PGI_2).* Platelets release vasoconstrictors in response to tissue in-

The Cardiovascular System

jury. These vasoactive substances include *thromboxane A_2* (TXA_2) and *serotonin,* also known as *5-hydroxytryptamine* (*5-HT*).

Table 21–1 summarizes the chemical control of vasomotor effects.

NEURAL CONTROL

The autonomic nervous system (ANS) controls blood vessel diameters via sympathetic motor impulses transmitted by the **vasomotor center** of the medulla. The arterioles of the vascular system are especially well supplied with sympathetic fibers. (Blood vessels are singly innervated, and thus do not receive impulses from *both* divisions of the ANS.) Different subtypes of adrenergic receptors are located on vascular smooth muscle of arterioles found in different tissues. Such receptors respond differently when stimulated. For example, sympathetic impulses directed to these adrenergic receptors produce either vasodilation or vasoconstriction to increase or decrease the perfusion of a given capillary bed. Since blood takes the path of least resistance, the change in arteriolar diameter and the fourth-power relationship with blood flow cause blood to be redistributed among the different vascular beds of the body. For example, during the fight-or-flight response, sympathetic dominance occurs. The motor outflow of sympathetic impulses from the vasomotor center stimulates α_1-adrenergic receptors in cutaneous and gastrointestinal blood vessels, which results in vasoconstriction. Simultaneously, sympathetic impulses stimulate β_2-adrenergic receptors in skeletal muscle blood vessels, which results in vasodilation. As a result of these sympathetic impulses during times of stress, blood is diverted from nonessential regions such as the skin and digestive organs, and redirected to essential areas such as the skeletal muscles. The vasomotor center integrates the following neural reflexes that control vascular resistance and pressure: *baroreceptor reflex, chemoreceptor reflex,* and *medullary ischemic reflex.*

The short-term, or acute, control of vessel diameter and blood pressure is provided by the baroreceptor reflex, also known as the pressoreceptor reflex. This neural control of vessel resistance is a negative feedback mechanism based on the detection of mechanical stretching in the walls of major arterial vessels. Specialized nerve cells called *baroreceptors* function as mechanoreceptors to monitor the amount of mechanical stretch during cardiac pumping. The *aortic arch* and *carotid sinus baroreceptors* are located in strategic locations to detect changes in the distention of the aorta and the carotid sinus, a thin-walled saclike structure located at the bifurcation of the common carotid artery (see Fig. 10–6). A rise in arterial blood pressure expands the walls of the arteries and stimulates the baroreceptors located within them. As these receptors depolarize, they fire sensory impulses into the medulla. The incoming impulses cause (1) decreased cardioacelleratory center activity, which reduces sympathetic outflow to the heart and reduces rate and force; (2) increased cardioinhibitory center activity, which increases parasympathetic (vagal) outflow to the heart to slow the rate and force; and (3) decreased vasomotor center activity, which reduces sympathetic tone to the arterioles. As a result of the reduction in sympathetic motor tone to the blood vessels, reflex dilation occuŨs, causing a fall in vascular resistance and blood pressure. When blood pressure falls below normal, the baroreceptors are not stimulated as intensely, and the opposite responses occur to raise blood pressure back to the homeostatic range. Elevated systemic blood pressure not only causes the baroreceptors to decrease the cardiovascular response but also reduces the rate of ventilation. Con-

TABLE 21–1	Chemical Control of Vasomotor Effects		
Stimulus	**Response**		
	Vasodilation		**Vasoconstriction**
Metabolic Products			
CO_2, H^+, lactic acid	√		
Autacoids			
Histamine	√		
Prostaglandin E_2	√		
Bradykinin	√		
Nitric oxide (NO)	√		
Prostaglandin I_2 (prostacyclin)	√		
Prostaglandin $F_{2\alpha}$			√
Prostaglandin D_2			√
Thromboxane A_2			√
Serotonin (5-hydroxytryptamine, 5-HT)			√

versely, a fall in blood pressure increases the cardiovascular response and increases the rate of ventilation (see Chap. 10).

The chemoreceptor reflex was first discussed in Chapter 10 with examination of the role of peripheral *chemoreceptors.* These specialized cells are the sensory components of the hypoxic drive mechanism. They reside in the *aortic bodies* and *carotid bodies,* where their primary role is to monitor the blood chemistry of systemic arterial blood (see Fig. 10–6). In addition to the primary respiratory activity detailed in Chapter 10, the peripheral chemoreceptors are involved in cardiovascular activity. For example, when arterial hypoxemia, hypercapnia, or acidosis occur, the aortic and carotid bodies send sensory impulses to the vasomotor center which results in generalized vasoconstriction. The increase in vasomotor tone raises blood pressure and improves perfusion of the lungs. In this way, the increase in ventilation triggered by the aortic and carotid bodies is matched by an increase in perfusion to restore blood pH as well as the oxygen and carbon dioxide tension of the blood.

Hypoxia and hypercapnia resulting from inadequate perfusion of the brainstem stimulate the medullary vasomotor center, which responds by initiating vasoconstriction of blood vessels in the lowermost parts of the body. This mechanism, the **medullary ischemic reflex,** causes more blood to be distributed to the upper part of the body, thus improving cerebral blood flow and reducing the ischemic conditions of the brainstem.

Finally, the vasomotor center receives a variety of impulses from higher brain centers. For example, the *thermoregulatory center* of the hypothalamus responds to exercise and changes in body temperature by signaling the vasomotor center to alter the perfusion of tissues as required to maintain body temperature. Emotions such as fear or anger and activities such as exercise or sexual arousal stimulate the vasomotor center to result in vasoconstriction and an increase in blood pressure.

Table 21–2 summarizes the neural control of vasomotor effects.

HORMONAL CONTROL

In this final section covering the control of peripheral resistance, we look at long-term, or chronic, control of resistance and pressure by examining the role of hormones: the *renin-angiotensin-aldosterone mechanism, antidiuretic hormone,* and *atrial natriuretic peptide.*

Long-term control of blood pressure is accomplished through adjustments of plasma volume. For instance, as plasma volume increases, the returning volume of blood becomes greater, thus increasing the stroke volume via the Frank-Starling mechanism (see Chap. 19). The increase in stroke volume increases cardiac output, which restores blood pressure (see Fig. 19–3). We know that a fall in systemic blood pressure proportionately reduces the blood flow through renal arteries supplying the kidneys. The kidneys respond by conserving fluid— for example, by curtailing urine production and reabsorbing more salt and water. This reabsorption, in turn, restores plasma volume and blood pressure.

The **renin-angiotensin-aldosterone mechanism,**

TABLE 21–2	**Neural Control of Vasomotor Effects**		
Neural Control		**Response**	
		Vasodilation	**Vasoconstriction**
Medullary Vasomotor Center			
Sympathetic—α_1 (e.g., skin blood vessels)			√
Sympathetic—β_2 (e.g., skeletal muscle blood vessels)		√	
Increased temperature, emotions, exercise			√
Baroreceptor Reflex (aortic arch and carotid sinus baroreceptors)			
Increased stretch of arterial walls (i.e., high blood pressure)		√	
Decreased stretch of arterial walls (i.e., low blood pressure)			√
Chemoreceptor Reflex (aortic and carotid bodies)			
Decreased Pa_{O_2}, increased Pa_{CO_2}, decreased pH			
Impulses sent to medullary vasomotor center			√
Increased Pa_{O_2}, decreased Pa_{CO_2}, increased pH			
Impulses sent to medullary vasomotor center		√	
Medullary Ischemic Reflex			
Decreased P_{O_2}, increased P_{CO_2} in brainstem			
Impulses sent to medullary vasomotor center			√*

*Vasoconstriction of blood vessels in the lower part of the body improves *cerebral* blood flow.

also known simply as the **renal mechanism,** plays a primary role in the overall regulation of plasma volume (see Fig. 11–11). The kidneys respond to low blood pressure by secreting the hormone *renin,* which acts on a plasma precursor called *angiotensinogen.* This prohormone is converted to *angiotensin I* by the action of renin. As angiotensin I travels through the pulmonary circuit the endothelial cells of the pulmonary capillaries secrete *angiotensin-converting enzyme* (ACE), which transforms angiotensin I to a powerful vasoactive substance known as **angiotensin II** (see Chap. 11). This plasma-derived substance has a dual effect on blood pressure. First, angiotensin II exhibits a direct vasoconstrictor effect on resistance vessels to increase systemic vascular resistance (SVR). Second, angiotensin II has an indirect effect on plasma volume through stimulation of **aldosterone** release from the adrenal cortex. The potent salt-conserving action of aldosterone causes increased sodium and water reabsorption in the kidney, which decreases urine production and expands plasma volume (see Fig. 11–11). Restored plasma volume increases venous return and stroke volume, thereby increasing cardiac output and blood pressure (see Fig. 19–3).

Plasma volume and blood pressure are also regulated by **antidiuretic hormone (ADH)** (see Fig. 19–3). This hypothalamic hormone was originally known as **vasopressin,** a reference to its vasoconstricting effects on blood vessels when present in very high concentrations. Its primary target is the kidney, where it stimulates tubule cells to reabsorb water from glomerular filtrate. This action slows *diuresis* (urine production) and expands plasma volume, thus helping in the long-term maintenance of blood pressure.

Blood volume can also be altered in the long term by changes in the hematocrit. In response to hypoxia, the kidney secretes **erythropoietin (EPO).** This hormone targets stem cells in the bone marrow, stimulating them to increase the production and maturation of erythrocytes, a process called erythropoiesis. As the number of red blood cells in circulation increases, the blood volume increases and the condition of hypoxia is reduced as a result0of the improved oxygen-transporting capacity of the blood.

The long-term control of vascular resistance, plasma volume, and blood pressure is also accomplished by the secretion of a hormone from the right atrium of the heart. **Atrial natriuretic peptide (ANP),** also known as **atriopeptin,** is a naturally occurring *diuretic* hormone released when the atrial wall is stretched by the volume of returning blood (see Fig. 19–3). ANP causes the reduction of plasma volume and blood pressure by inhibiting the body's *antidiuretic* mechanisms and hormones such as renin, aldosterone, and ADH. In other words, ANP actually brings about an increase in urine production, thus unloading excess fluid from circulation. The decreased plasma volume reduces the returning volume of blood as well as the stretch of the atrial wall, thus completing the negative feedback loop.

Table 21–3 summarizes the hormonal control of vasomotor and blood volume effects on blood pressure.

TABLE 21-3	Hormonal Control of Vasomotor and Blood Volume Effects			
Hormones and Comments	**Vascular Effects**		**Blood Volume Effects**	
	Vasodilation	Vasoconstriction	Increased Volume	Decreased Volume
Renin-Angiotensin-Aldosterone Mechanism				
Reduced plasma volume and blood pressure stimulates the release of renin from the kidney, which results in the formation and release of:				
Angiotensin II		√		
Aldosterone			√	
Antidiuretic hormone (ADH)	√ (mild)		√	
Reduced osmotic pressure of blood stimulates production of ADH from the hypothalamus and its release from the posterior pituitary.				
Erythropoietin (EPO)			√*	
Hypoxia stimulates the release of EPO from kidney cells.				
Atrial Natriuretic Peptide (ANP)				√†
Passive stretch of heart wall stimulates release of ANP from the right atrium.				

*EPO brings about an increase in *red blood cell* volume, whereas aldosterone and antidiuretic hormone cause an increase in *plasma* volume.
†ANP is a *diuretic* hormone that inhibits antidiuretic mechanisms such as the release and synthesis of renin, aldosterone, and antidiuretic hormone.

Capillary Exchange Mechanisms

A variety of exchange mechanisms transport substances through capillary walls. The mechanisms of *diffusion, filtration,* and *osmosis* were discussed in Chapter 11 with the topic of the *Starling forces* and lung fluid balance. These exchange mechanisms are part of capillary membrane fluid dynamics, clearly a cardiovascular system topic. However, because of the integral nature of the cardiovascular and respiratory systems, the topic of fluid transfer into and out of capillaries was discussed in the context of *pulmonary* capillaries and fluid overload in the alveoli. The reader is encouraged to review appropriate sections of Chapter 11 to clearly understand capillary exchange mechanisms, lung fluid balance, and the role of pulmonary lymphatics.

Venous Return Mechanisms

Following exchange of gases, nutrients, and wastes in the systemic capillaries, blood returns to the heart by way of the veins. As discussed earlier, veins function as capacitance vessels because they can store a large percentage of the body's total blood volume. They also carry blood back to the heart at very low pressures and flowrates. Finally, much of the blood to be returned is found in regions *below* the heart. What mechanisms exist to enhance venous return under these conditions? In the following section we examine several mechanisms of venous return—*arteriovenous pressure gradient,* the *respiratory pump, skeletal muscle pump,* and the *hydrostatic effect.*

ARTERIOVENOUS PRESSURE GRADIENT

Recall that blood flow, as calculated by the Poiseuille equation, is directly proportional to the pressure gradient, or driving pressure, in a conducting tube. The proximal pressure in the systemic circuit is the pressure in the aorta; the distal pressure is the pressure found in the vena cavae. In a comparison of systolic pressures in the systemic circuit, the driving pressure exceeds 100 mm Hg under normal conditions. The **arteriovenous pressure gradient** is simply the difference in pressure between a blood vessel at the proximal end of the circuit and a blood vessel at the distal end of the circuit. At any given pair of points along the route, the downstream pressure in the blood vessel must be less than the upstream pressure. If a blockage of the blood vessel occurs, this pressure gradient is not present, and blood flow ceases. The concept of pressure differentials is very straightforward but still worth mentioning. Flu-

ids such as liquids and gases can only be made to flow between two points if there is a pressure gradient between the two points. All other things being equal, the greater the driving pressure acting on a fluid, the greater its velocity of flow.

Remember that the pressures in the circulatory system do not decrease linearly from arteries to veins; that is, the pressure drop from the aorta to the inferior vena cava does not occur in a straight line. Instead, systolic, diastolic, and pulse pressures are maintained at levels relatively close to those in the aorta throughout the medium- and small-diameter arteries, decreasing dramatically through the arterioles (see Fig. 21–2D). Recall that the enormous cross-sectional area of the arteriolar system offers relatively little resistance to blood flow; therefore, blood pressure plummets just as blood enters the capillary beds composed of extremely fragile, thin-walled capillaries. Low pressure, low flow, nearly pulseless conditions in capillary blood are ideal for the exchange of substances. The arteriovenous pressure gradient from the capillaries to the inferior vena cava follows more of a straight line function with a very gradual slope (see Fig. 21–2D). For instance, venule pressure is about 12 to 18 mm Hg, whereas central venous pressure (CVP) ranges between 2 mm Hg and approximately 6 mm Hg at the point where the inferior vena cava enters the heart (Saladin, 1998). (This fluctuation in CVP is explained in the next section.) The venous pressure gradient in the systemic circuit is approximately 7 to 13 mm Hg.

RESPIRATORY PUMP

As explained in Chapter 6, the downward movement of the diaphragm increases the height of the thorax, thus increasing the volume of the thorax and decreasing its pressure. This same diaphragmatic movement decreases the volume of the abdomen and increases its pressure. The simultaneous increase in abdominal pressure as the pressure in the thorax decreases assists in the venous return of blood to the heart during inspiration (see Fig. 19–3). The mechanism is called the **respiratory pump,** or the **abdominothoracic pump mechanism.** Because the inferior vena cava (IVC) passes through both cavities and the central tendon of the diaphragm, the pressure differential created during inspiration squeezes blood upward toward the heart (Fig. 21–3). During expiration, when the pressures reverse in the thorax and abdomen, blood is not forced downward into the legs because the valves of the veins in the legs close to prevent backflow. Because of this rhythmic pumping action, blood flow is faster during inspiration. The respiratory pump also causes the CVP to fluctuate between 2 mm Hg during inspiration to approximately 6 mm Hg during expiration (Saladin, 1998).

The Cardiovascular System

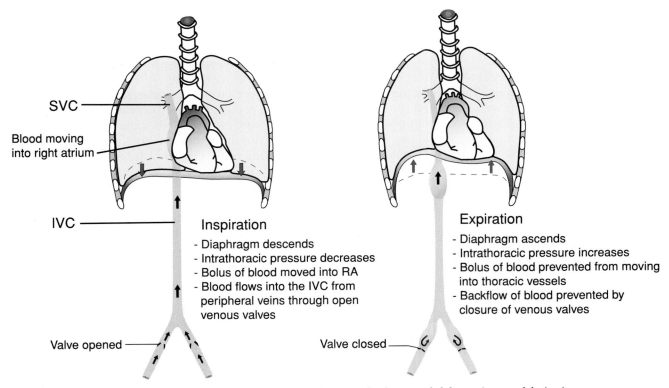

SVC

Blood moving
into right atrium

IVC

Inspiration
- Diaphragm descends
- Intrathoracic pressure decreases
- Bolus of blood moved into RA
- Blood flows into the IVC from
  peripheral veins through open
  venous valves

Valve opened

Expiration
- Diaphragm ascends
- Intrathoracic pressure increases
- Bolus of blood prevented from moving
  into thoracic vessels
- Backflow of blood prevented by
  closure of venous valves

Valve closed

FIGURE 21–3. Respiratory pump. The pressure between the thorax and abdomen is created during inspiration. The respiratory pump, or abdominothoracic pump mechanism, assists the return of blood to the heart through the inferior vena cava. Venous valves in the medium- to large-diameter veins ensure unidirectional flow of blood toward the heart. (SVC = superior vena cava; IVC = inferior vena cava; LA = left atrium; RA = right atrium.)

SKELETAL MUSCLE PUMP

Medium-sized veins in the arms and legs pass between adjacent muscles, usually in a *triad* that includes an artery and nerve. Thin-walled veins are thus surrounded by skeletal muscles and are rhythmically squeezed by them whenever skeletal muscles contract, a mechanism referred to as the **skeletal muscle pump** (see Fig. 19–3). Physical activity, therefore, massages blood out of the compressed part of a vein, assisting its movement toward the heart (Fig. 21–4). Closure of venous valves prevents backflow of blood.

HYDROSTATIC EFFECT AND VENOUS POOLING

When sitting or standing, regions such as the head and neck are superior to the heart. Venous return of blood from these regions is assisted by gravity, the **hydrostatic effect.** As a result of this gravitational effect, the venous pressure in the large veins of the neck is usually close to zero (Saladin, 1998).

Venous pooling in the veins of the legs can severely reduce venous return to the heart because of the distention of large-diameter veins. The action of venous valves and the combined effect of the other venous re-

turn factors normally offsets the risk for venous pooling in the large capacitance vessels. In a condition known as *varicose veins,* however, venous valves do not function properly, allowing blood to backflow into the large veins of the legs. This action results in venous pooling and reduced venous return. As can be seen by this example, the impairment of a single venous return mechanism can adversely affect the volume of blood returning to the heart. Recall that the returning volume is one of the most important determinants of cardiac output and adequate tissue perfusion. None of the venous return mechanisms on their own are particularly impressive. However, working together, they move venous blood back to the heart and ensure that the endless circulatory loop is not interrupted.

Summary

This chapter presented the structural features of blood vessels that allow them to transport blood and regulate its flow. The chapter focused on three areas—blood flow, blood pressure, and resistance in the vascular system. Considerable emphasis was placed on the factors that alter resistance and plasma volume in the circulatory system because it is through changes in peripheral

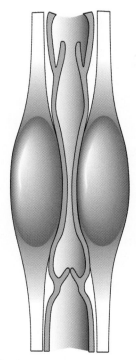

FIGURE 21–4. Skeletal muscle pump. Venous compression during contraction of skeletal muscles helps propel blood through the medium- and large-diameter veins. Venous valves provide unidirectional flow of blood toward the heart.

vascular resistance and in the volume of blood in circulation that blood pressure is controlled. Both acute (short-term) controls and chronic (long-term) controls of blood pressure were examined in depth. The chapter concluded with an examination of the factors that affect venous return. These factors were emphasized because venous return plays such an important role in the determination of stroke volume, cardiac output, and tissue perfusion.

BIBLIOGRAPHY

Carola R, Harley JP, and Noback CR: Human Anatomy and Physiology, ed 2. McGraw-Hill, New York, 1992.

Des Jardins T: Cardiopulmonary Anatomy and Physiology: Essentials for Respiratory Care, ed 3. Delmar Publishers, Albany, NY, 1998.

Ganong WF: Review of Medical Physiology, ed 17. Appleton & Lange, Norwalk, CT, 1995.

Guyton AC and Hall JE: Textbook of Medical Physiology, ed 9. WB Saunders, Philadelphia, 1996.

Martini FH: Fundamentals of Anatomy and Physiology, ed 4. Prentice Hall, Upper Saddle River, NJ, 1998.

Saladin KS: Anatomy and Physiology: The Unity of Form and Function. WCB/McGraw-Hill, Boston, 1998.

Shier D, Butler J, and Lewis R: Hole's Human Anatomy and Physiology, ed 7. Wm C Brown, Dubuque, IA, 1996.

Tortora GJ and Grabowski SR: Principles of Anatomy and Physiology, ed 8. HarperCollins, New York, 1996.

CHAPTER 22

Aging of the Cardiovascular System

chapter objectives

After studying this chapter the reader should be able to:

☐ Explain how arteriosclerosis affects the distensibility of blood vessels.
☐ Describe three outcomes in the vascular system resulting from arteriosclerosis of blood vessels.
☐ Contrast *arteriosclerosis* and *atherosclerosis*.
☐ Explain how atherosclerosis affects peripheral vascular resistance and blood flow.
☐ Describe the changes observed in systolic, diastolic, pulse, and mean arterial pressures with advancing age.
☐ Review the operation of the renin-angiotensin-aldosterone mechanism in the long-term control of blood pressure.
☐ Explain how the effectiveness of the renin-angiotensin-aldosterone mechanism declines with advancing age and how benign nephrosclerosis affects the long-term control of blood pressure.
☐ List the erythropoietic centers that are active during the following stages: Embryo, fetus, infant, adult.
☐ State three factors that may cause anemia in an older person.
☐ Describe how anemia affects blood viscosity, blood flow, venous return, ventricular preload, and cardiac output.
☐ Describe how age-related fibrotic changes in heart muscle affect compliance and contractility of the myocardium.
☐ Describe how age-related fibrotic changes in heart valves affect blood flow and cardiac output.
☐ Review the concept of cardiac index.
☐ Explain how venous return controls cardiac output.

☐ Describe the causal relationships among age, basal metabolic rate, venous return, and cardiac output.

☐ Discuss the reasons that cardiac reserve declines with advancing age.

☐ Review the following terms:

Collateral circulation, coronary circulation, arterial anastamoses.

☐ Describe the stages in the revascularization of myocardium that has been deprived of blood because of blockage of a small blood vessel.

☐ Name two age-related changes that may affect the cardiac conduction system.

key terms

arteriosclerosis (ar-tē″ rē-ō-skle-rō′ sis)

atherosclerosis (ath″ er-ō′-skle-rō′ sis)

In this chapter on aging we conclude our unit of the study of the cardiovascular system. All of the basic ideas, terms, mechanisms, and relationships are in place. Here we examine the outcome that degenerative changes in the blood vessels, blood, and heart, have on mechanisms such as vascular resistance, blood flow, blood pressure, compliance, contractility, cardiac output, cardiac reserve, and cardiac conduction.

In many ways this chapter is ideally situated to reinforce the intimate relationships and inseparable functions associated with an integrated study of the respiratory and cardiovascular systems. For instance, although all tissues of the body depend on the respiratory system to extract oxygen from the external environment and make it available for cellular use, it should be remembered that cells do *not* pick up oxygen from the *lungs,* but rather from the *blood,* which is pumped by the heart through the blood vessels to supply the metabolic needs of the body. Therefore, the respiratory system is concerned primarily with gas *exchange,* whereas the cardiovascular system plays a critical role in the *delivery* of oxygen. Both systems are vital to the body as a whole, but useless without each other. Thus, failure of the combined *cardiopulmonary system,* resulting from accident, disease, or the cumulative effects of aging, threatens homeostasis of the internal environment and the very existence of the individual.

Blood Vessels, Vascular Resistance, and Blood Pressure

CHANGES IN BLOOD VESSELS AND VASCULAR RESISTANCE

Arteriosclerosis is a disease of blood vessels characterized by thickening, hardening, and loss of elasticity of the arterial wall. These changes are associated with advancing age but are not limited to older persons. The degenerative changes may occur in the tunica intima, tunica media, or both. A variety of outcomes may occur in response to arteriosclerosis. For example, blood vessels affected in this way are less able to withstand sudden pressure changes; consequently, they are more prone to the development of *aneurysms,* weakened areas in the vessel wall that may rupture under stress (Martini, 1998). This rupture may result in a cerebral vascular accident (CVA, or stroke), myocardial infarction (MI), or massive blood loss, depending on the blood vessel affected. Second, when arterial walls become hard, they lose elasticity, causing blood pressure to rise. Diastolic pressure in particular is affected by this increase in rigidity of the vessel wall. Loss of compliance of major arteries such as the aorta reduces the effectiveness of the elastic recoil mechanism ("aortic pump") that damps the high-pressure surges of systole, and helps propel blood through the circulatory system during the low-pressure phase of diastole. Consequently, the heart must work harder to pump the same amount of blood. As a result of the stress of increased loadings, the heart may enlarge. Finally, arteriosclerosis of cerebral arteries results in reduced blood flow to the brain, which may impair memory of recent events or cause difficulty in speaking (Carola, Harley, and Noback, 1992; Tortora and Grabowski, 1996).

Blood flow through the circulatory system in older persons is also impaired by decreased effectiveness of venous valves leading to increased venous pooling in veins of the legs, and decreased venous return (Martini, 1998). Recall that the Starling mechanism, which regulates the strength of myocardial contraction, is controlled by venous return. Therefore, faulty venous valves have the overall effect of decreasing stroke volume and cardiac output.

Atherosclerosis is a type of arteriosclerosis involving the deposition of fatty, plaquelike material on the luminal wall of blood vessels.

NOTE: The terms *arteriosclerosis* and *atherosclerosis* are not interchangeable; they are distinct terms that refer to two different varieties of vascular disease.

As a result of the accumulation of plaque, the lumen diameter of blood vessels decreases, dramatically increasing peripheral vascular resistance to blood flow (Shier, Butler, and Lewis, 1996). According to Marieb (1998), atherosclerosis begins in childhood but is accelerated by factors such as a sedentary lifestyle, smoking, and stress. Consequences of atherosclerotic changes in the blood vessels include increased risk for heart attack and stroke. Part of the risk can be explained by the increased incidence of thrombus (clot) formation at sites of atherosclerotic plaque. A thrombus can detach from the vessel wall and be carried downstream to lodge in smaller blood vessels such as pulmonary capillaries, possibly occluding them and obstructing blood flow to distal tissues (Martini, 1998).

ELEVATED BLOOD PRESSURE AND AGING

Because of a variety of vascular factors such as arteriosclerosis in general, and atherosclerosis in particular, blood pressure increases progressively with advancing age. Part of the increase is due to the increased rigidity and decreased lumen diameter of blood vessels, and part is due to the progressive decline in effectiveness of control mechanisms that normally respond to elevated blood pressure, lowering it to restore homeostasis. Note

in Figure 22–1 that systolic, diastolic, and pulse pressures all increase over time. Also notice that changes in systolic pressure increase faster than changes in diastolic pressure. Recall from Chapter 21 that the *mean arterial blood pressure* (MABP) is not simply an average of systolic and diastolic pressures but is, instead, a "blend" of the two given by the following equation:

$$MABP = \text{diastolic pressure} + \frac{\text{pulse pressure}}{3}$$

Therefore, MABP is determined about 60% by the prevailing diastolic pressure and 40% by the systolic pressure. Throughout the age spectrum, MABP rises, but at all ages it is closer to the diastolic than to the systolic pressure. This effect is especially evident in advanced age (see Fig. 22–1).

CHANGES IN THE LONG-TERM CONTROL OF BLOOD PRESSURE

The increases in blood pressure shown in Figure 22–1 are due primarily to the effects of aging on long-term blood pressure control mechanisms. Recall that the long-term control of blood pressure is accomplished through the action of the *renin-angiotensin-aldosterone mechanism*, also commonly known as the *renal mechanism* (see Fig. 11–11). Recall that in this mechanism, kidney cells release the enzyme *renin* in response to low blood pressure. Renin converts a circulating prohormone called *angiotensinogen* into *angiotensin I*, a mild vasoconstrictor. After passing through the pulmonary circulation and being acted upon by *angiotensin-converting enzyme* (ACE), angiotensin I is changed into *angiotensin II*, a powerful vasoactive substance. These vasoconstrictors are activated within 30 minutes of the

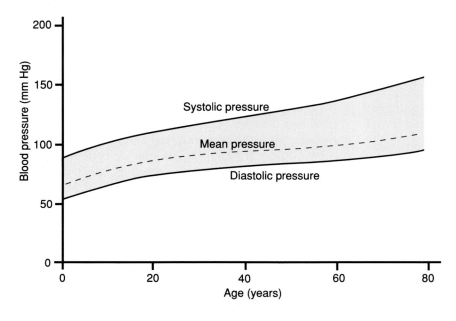

FIGURE 22–1. Changes in systolic, diastolic, and mean pressures at different ages. Mean arterial blood pressure (MABP) is shown by the dotted line. Pulse pressure is represented by the shaded area between the systolic and diastolic pressures. Note that all pressures tend to increase steadily with age. (Adapted from Guyton AC and Hall JE: Textbook of Medical Physiology, ed. 9. WB Saunders, Philadelphia, 1996, p 176, with permission.)

release of renin and circulate throughout the body, where they promote contraction of vascular smooth muscle, thus increasing vascular resistance and blood pressure. Such vasoconstrictor effects provide *intermediate* pressure control that sustains blood pressure for several hours to several days. By this time, the *rapidly acting* neurologic control mechanisms such as the *baroreceptor, chemoreceptor,* and *medullary ischemic reflexes,* have fatigued and are no longer providing blood pressure control.

Release of the corticosteroid *aldosterone* from the adrenal cortex in response to circulating angiotensin II results in *long-term* control of blood pressure through adjustment of salt and water reabsorption by the kidneys. An increase in water reabsorption increases plasma volume, venous return, stroke volume, cardiac output, and, finally, blood pressure. A decrease in water reabsorption causes more fluid to be eliminated by the kidneys, thus decreasing plasma volume and blood pressure through the same sequence of changes described previously. The operation of the renin-angiotensin-aldosterone system is especially important in the daily, long-term control of blood pressure. For example, salt intake can vary dramatically from day to day, ranging from 1/10 normal to as much as 10 to 15 times normal. Regulation of arterial pressure via a properly functioning renal mechanism, however, maintains the mean arterial blood pressure within only a few millimeters of mercury. Without the renin-angiotensin-aldosterone system, excessive salt intake produces an effect on MABP that is *10 times as great* (Guyton and Hall, 1996). This is one of the reasons that dietary salt intake and fluid levels are especially important in the control of arterial pressure in older persons. How does the effectiveness of the renin-angiotensin-aldosterone system, and the long-term control of blood pressure, change with age? Because age-related degenerative changes in renal function are common, especially after the age of 50, we must answer this question by briefly considering pathophysiologic conditions affecting the kidneys.

As occurs with most body systems, kidney function progressively declines with age. In most persons in old age, degenerative changes in the kidney gradually reduce the number of *nephrons*—the functional units of the kidney (see Chap. 23). There are several million of these units, so the decline in their number and function is usually gradual; however, the following process occurs, at least to some extent, in most persons.

Various types of vascular lesions can reduce blood flow and lead to renal ischemia and necrosis of renal tissue. Such tissue death can result from (1) *atherosclerosis* of larger renal arteries with progressive sclerotic constriction of the blood vessels; or (2) *benign nephrosclerosis,* a condition characterized by sclerotic lesions of the small arteries and arterioles of the kidney (Guyton and

Hall, 1996). *Sclerosis* of blood vessels involves the deposition of a plaquelike material on the luminal surface of a blood vessel, thus increasing the stiffness of the vessel, narrowing its diameter, and reducing the flow of blood through it (Gr. *sklerosis,* hardness).

Progressive destruction of blood vessels in the kidney via sclerosis gradually destroys large numbers of nephrons. In effect, kidney tissue becomes replaced by multiple areas of nonfunctional fibrotic tissue, reducing the overall size and effectiveness of the kidney. As the functional reserve of the kidney declines, its ability to clear (eliminate) substances from the bloodstream diminishes, along with its ability to secrete renin, the critical starting point in the long-term control of blood pressure. When the renin-angiotensin-aldosterone mechanism is impaired, MABP cannot be effectively stabilized through adjustments in plasma volume and urine output. Therefore, blood pressure becomes closely linked to salt intake, fluctuating erratically each time the plasma volume increases or decreases in response to changing salt concentrations.

Erythropoiesis and Anemia

ERYTHROPOIESIS AND AGING

Sites of red blood cell formation, or *erythropoietic centers,* change several times during the course of a lifetime. As discussed with the embryologic development of the cardiovascular system, initial formation of primitive red blood cells occurs in the yolk sac of the embryo. During the middle trimester of pregnancy, erythropoiesis occurs primarily in the liver, spleen, and lymph nodes of the developing fetus, finally switching to the marrow cavities of most bones during the latter part of gestation. Postnatally, up to the age of about 5 years, red blood cells continue to be produced in the marrow cavities of most bones. After age 20, however, the membranous bones of the skeleton—vertebrae, sternum, and ribs—become the primary sites for erythropoiesis (Guyton and Hall, 1996). The marrow cavities of other bones, such as the femur and humerus, become filled with fatty tissue, thus converting productive *red marrow* to nonproductive *yellow marrow.* According to Guyton (1991), even the marrow cavities of the primary erythropoietic bones become less productive with increasing age; thus red blood cell counts steadily decline and contribute to *anemia,* a common finding in older persons.

Anemia may result from nutritional deficiencies, inadequate exercise, inability of the hemopoietic system to respond to stressors, degenerative changes in other organ systems, or to a combination of such factors (Saladin, 1998). For example age-related degenerative changes in the kidneys reduce the overall number of functioning nephrons, as we have seen. As the number of nephrons decline, the ability of the kidney to synthesize and secrete the hormone *erythropoietin* (EPO) diminishes. Recall that this hormone directly stimulates erythropoiesis in bone marrow and is normally released in response to arterial hypoxia. Another possible cause of anemia is that there may be a limit as to how many times hemopoietic stem cells can divide to produce new blood cells (Saladin, 1998).

ANEMIA, VISCOSITY, AND CARDIAC WORKLOAD

To understand the effect anemia has on cardiovascular performance in the older person, consider the following sequence. Typically, the older person has a decreased *hematocrit*, an indicator of the relative volumes of formed elements and plasma in a sample of whole blood (see Fig. 13–1) (Martini, 1998). As anemia progresses, the viscosity of the blood is reduced from approximately three times that of water to about one-and-a-half times (Guyton and Hall, 1996). Viscosity is one of the variables used in the Poiseuille equation to calculate flowrates of liquids (see Chap. 21). Recall that blood flow is inversely proportional to the viscosity of blood. Therefore, anemia causes blood flow through the tissues to increase, thus increasing both venous return and ventricular preload. Increased blood returning to the heart stretches the heart wall, causing blood to be pumped out again with increased vigor, in accordance with the Frank-Starling law of the heart.

Anemia also elevates ventricular preload and increases the workload on the aging heart through a second mechanism. Fewer red blood cells means that the total amount of hemoglobin available for oxygen transport is less than normal. Because the majority of oxygen in the bloodstream is bound to hemoglobin as oxyhemoglobin, the arterial oxygen tension (Pao_2) decreases, resulting in hypoxemic hypoxia and contributing to potential tissue hypoxia (see Chap. 14). The development of local tissue hypoxia, in turn, leads to the accumulation of metabolic wastes such as carbon dioxide (CO_2), hydrogen ions (H^+), and lactic acid, triggering reflex vasodilation through the local blood flow control mechanism of autoregulation (see Chap. 21). As metarterioles relax and additional capillary beds open, peripheral vascular resistance decreases markedly, thus increasing flowrates and venous return. Factors such as these that increase ventricular loadings can stress the heart to the point of heart failure (Guyton and Hall, 1996). In addition, the reduction in oxygen-transporting ability caused by anemia contributes to general atrophy of tissues throughout the body (Saladin, 1998).

Heart Muscle and Heart Valves

Age-related changes in the heart and heart valves collectively reduce the ability of the heart to maintain adequate cardiac output and tissue perfusion. These degenerative changes affect the distensibility, contractility, and size of the heart, as well as the operation of the heart valves that control blood flow through the chambers. We now examine these changes to understand their impact on overall cardiac performance.

COMPLIANCE AND CONTRACTILITY OF THE HEART

Degenerative changes in the fibrous skeleton of the heart over time result in the elastic tissue being replaced by fibrotic tissue, which resembles scar tissue and is not capable of stretching to any great degree (Martini, 1998; Thibodeau and Patton, 1996). Decreased elasticity of the fibrous skeleton causes decreased *compliance* and distensibility of the heart, thus reducing diastolic filling, stroke volume, and cardiac output, at a given heart rate. Similarly, the replacement of damaged cardiac muscle cells by nonfunctional fibrotic tissue decreases myocardial *contractility*, thus reducing systolic ejection, stroke volume, and cardiac output at a particular heart rate. In addition, fibrosis of cardiac muscle may affect the nodes of the intrinsic conduction system, leading to conduction problems.

In general, age brings a gradual decrease in the size of myocardial muscle fibers and a decline in muscle strength (Tortora and Grabowski, 1996). Recall that the inability of the heart to generate sufficient force to overcome ventricular afterload may contribute to a low-output condition called congestive heart failure (CHF). Overall, the cumulative effects of senescence on the myocardium decrease cardiac output. However, because general levels of physical activity and metabolism also decline with advancing age, the reduction in maximum cardiac output in a healthy older person is not necessarily an impediment to an active lifestyle.

HEART VALVES

With age, heart valves undergo degenerative changes similar to those described for heart muscle. Valve cusp tissue becomes replaced by fibrotic tissue that causes the valves to lose flexibility, becoming hardened, distorted, and less effective. This increase in rigidity of the valves reduces pumping efficiency and also contributes to a decrease in the heart's ability to maintain adequate cardiac output (Thibodeau and Patton, 1996). Sclerosis and thickening of valve cusps is greatest at points in the heart where blood flow velocity and stresses are greatest. Consequently, fibrotic changes and heart murmurs are commonly associated with the mitral valve (Marieb, 1998).

Cardiac Output, Cardiac Index, and Cardiac Reserve

CARDIAC OUTPUT AND CARDIAC INDEX

For a variety of reasons previously discussed, such as reduced myocardial compliance and contractility, *cardiac output* (C.O.), expressed as the *cardiac index* (CI), steadily declines as we get older. Recall from Chapter 20 that cardiac index is a convenient hemodynamic measurement that allows the cardiac output of different-sized people to be compared by relating cardiac output to *body surface area* (BSA). With advancing age, the cardiac index falls from a value of approximately 4.2 L/min per m^2 at age 10, to about 2.4 L/min per m^2 by age 80 (Guyton and Hall, 1996). Cardiac output is regulated in proportion to overall *basal metabolic rate* (BMR); therefore, a declining cardiac index parallels declining activity with age.

Recall that cardiac output is controlled by venous return. That is, the various factors that affect peripheral circulation, such as local vasomotor effects caused by tissue oxygen levels, affect the volume of blood returning to the heart. This returning volume causes passive stretch of the myocardial wall, directly stimulating (1) the *rhythmicity* of the sinoatrial node, (2) the *Frank-Starling mechanism*, and (3) the *Bainbridge reflex* (see Chap. 19). These mechanisms, in turn, cause the heart to contract with sufficient force to eject the returning blood into the arteries.

Venous return is determined, in part, by the cumulative blood flow of all the local blood flows from the different regions of peripheral circulation. As discussed in Chapter 21, much of the control of local blood flow is accomplished via the vascular response to tissue hypoxia. Local tissue needs for oxygen are determined by the metabolic activity of the tissue. Therefore, cardiac output is determined by the sum of the factors throughout circulation that control local blood flow. The different local blood flows summate to form the venous return, which then causes the heart to match its output to this volume, thus pumping the returning blood into circulation again. Therefore, as BMR declines with advancing age, cardiac output is automatically adjusted downward by the declining local blood flow and venous return.

CARDIAC RESERVE

The maximum percentage that cardiac output can increase above normal is called the *cardiac reserve* (see Chap. 19). In a normal young adult the cardiac reserve is approximately three times to four times normal, a value often expressed as 300% to 400%. Endurance-trained athletes may have a cardiac reserve as high as 500% to 600% (Guyton and Hall, 1996).

In the elderly, cardiac reserve may be as low as 200%. Although this level of reserve may *appear* to be adequate (10 L/min compared with 5 L/min at rest), the output can easily be surpassed. For instance, physiologic stress such as moderate exercise encountered by an older person when climbing stairs can cause this cardiac reserve to quickly disappear, resulting in acute dyspnea and fatigue. The heart in an older person is less able to respond to stressors that demand increased output (Carola, Harley and Noback, 1990; Marieb, 1998). Part of the reason for this decline in response is that sympathetic control of heart rate becomes less efficient, resulting in a heart rate that gradually becomes lower, but more variable (Marieb, 1998). Maximum heart rate is also reduced in elderly persons (Marieb, 1998; Tortora and Grabowski, 1996). Reduction of cardiac reserve in an older person is a result of the cumulative effect of degenerative changes in the cardiovascular system. These changes include reduced myocardial strength, reduced compliance of the heart wall, atherosclerotic changes in blood vessels, and reduced elasticity of blood vessels—all of which reduce pumping efficiency, cardiac output, and cardiac reserve.

Coronary Circulation

Maximum blood flow through the *coronary arteries* is about 35% lower at the age of 60 than in a person at age 30 (Van de Graff and Fox, 1989). In fact, by age 60, almost all persons will have had at least one coronary vessel close, usually due to *thrombosis*, or clot formation (Guyton and Hall, 1996). Most people will be unaware of this event because of rapid development of *collateral circulation*. Recall that the *coronary circulation* is composed of an extensive collateral circulatory system formed by several *arterial anastomoses* of the coronary arteries (see Chap. 17 and 21). This collateral system provides alternative routes for blood flow through *large* blood vessels in the heart. At a tissue level, however, *small* blood vessels must quickly develop to supply a myocardial region that has become deprived of blood because of blockage of a small blood vessel.

Occlusion of an artery or vein causes a new vascular channel to develop around the obstruction, thus partially restoring blood flow. Briefly, the stages in such revascularization are as follows: (1) minute vascular loops, already present in the tissue proximal and distal to the blockage, undergo vascular relaxation and dilatation; (2) continued relaxation of smooth muscle fibers in the collateral blood vessels causes increased vasodilation and blood flow to the affected region; and (3) finally collateral blood vessels grow into the region, forming multiple collateral channels via the mechanism of *angiogenesis,* or the development of new blood vessels. In this process, tissue oxygen deficiency, nutrient deficiency, or both, trigger the formation of *angiogenesis factors* that promote new vessel growth into the tissue being revascularized.

In patients in whom thrombosis occurs too rapidly to permit the development of collateral circulation through the process of vascular relaxation and angiogenesis, cardiac ischemia becomes widespread, and serious heart attacks may occur (Guyton and Hall, 1996). With age, there is an increase in the incidence of such *coronary artery disease* (CAD), the major cause of heart disease and death in older persons (Tortora and Grabowski, 1996).

Cardiac Conduction System

As pointed out in the preceding section covering degenerative changes in myocardium and valves, fibrosis of heart muscle may adversely affect the conducting tissue of the heart (Marieb, 1998). These fibrotic changes may increase the incidence of cardiac arrhythmias in the older heart. Electrocardiographic (ECG) changes include slower and more erratic depolarization within the conduction system (Van de Graff and Fox, 1989).

Summary

This chapter focused on age-related changes in structure and function of the cardiovascular system. The chapter explored the effects that arteriosclerosis has on compliance and resistance of blood vessels, the effects that degenerative renal changes have on long-term control of blood pressure, the effects of anemia on blood viscosity, blood flow, and ventricular loadings, and the effects that fibrotic changes in heart muscle and heart valves have on distensibility, contractility, blood flow, and conduction of electrical impulses in the heart.

BIBLIOGRAPHY

Carola R, Harley JP, and Noback CR: Human Anatomy and Physiology, ed 2. McGraw-Hill, New York, 1992.

Guyton AC and Hall JE: Textbook of Medical Physiology, ed 9. WB Saunders, Philadelphia, 1996.

Guyton AC: Textbook of Medical Physiology, ed 8. WB Saunders, Philadelphia, 1991.

Marieb EN: Human Anatomy and Physiology, ed 4. Benjamin/Cummings, Menlo Park CA, 1998.

Martini FH: Fundamentals of Anatomy and Physiology, ed 4. Prentice Hall, Upper Saddle River, NJ, 1998.

Saladin KS: Anatomy and Physiology: The Unity of Form and Function. WCB/McGraw-Hill, Boston, 1998.

Shier D, Butler J, and Lewis R: Hole's Human Anatomy and Physiology, ed 7. Wm C Brown, Dubuque, IA, 1996.

Thibodeau GA and Patton KT: Anatomy and Physiology, ed 3. Mosby–Year Book, St Louis, 1996.

Thomas CL (ed): Taber's Cyclopedic Medical Dictionary, ed 18. FA Davis, Philadelphia, 1997.

Tortora GJ and Grabowski SR: Principles of Anatomy and Physiology, ed 8. HarperCollins, New York, 1996.

Van De Graaff KM and Fox SI: Concepts of Human Anatomy and Physiology, ed 2. Wm C Brown, Dubuque, IA, 1989.

UNIT THREE

The Urinary System and Acid-Base Balance

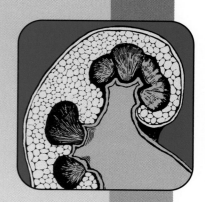

This unit emphasizes integration and connective issues among the respiratory, cardiovascular, and renal systems. In this unit we assimilate much of the information already covered in the textbook and add the functions of the urinary system to the mix of concepts and mechanisms. For example, the term *blood gases* perfectly describes the inseparable connection between respiratory and cardiovascular system function. But how do *renal functions,* far removed from the actual workings of the heart and lungs, influence blood gases?

Interestingly, many examples of interrelationships among the respiratory, cardiovascular, and renal systems have already been studied in preceding chapters. These include mechanisms such as long-term blood pressure control via the renin-angiotensin-aldosterone mechanism, the erythropoietin response to hypoxia, and the diuresis response to elevated plasma volume, to name a few. This unit briefly reviews these mechanisms and adds a few more topics to help the reader integrate the functions of the renal system with those of the combined cardiopulmonary system.

CHAPTER 23

Renal Structure and Function

chapter objectives

After studying this chapter the reader should be able to:

☐ List the functions carried out by the kidneys.
☐ Describe the location of the kidneys an describe the location and function of the following structures:
   Renal artery, renal vein, hilum, ureter, bladder, urethra.
☐ Describe the location of the renal cortex and renal medulla and differentiate between renal columns and renal pyramids.
☐ Describe the structural relationships among the renal papilla, minor calyx, and major calyx.
☐ Differentiate between cortical and juxtaglomerular nephrons.
☐ Trace the flow of blood through the vascular components of the nephron.
☐ Describe the differences between glomerular capillaries and peritubular capillaries.
☐ Explain how the efferent arteriole raises blood pressure within the glomerular.
☐ Describe the structure and function of the glomerular (Bowman's) capsule.
☐ Trace the flow of glomerular filtrate through the tubular components of the nephron.
☐ Describe the following stages in diuresis:
   Glomerular filtration, tubular reabsorption, tubular secretion.

☐ Explain how the stages of diuresis differ in regards to *selectivity* of substances added to, or subtracted from, the glomerular filtrate.

☐ Describe net filtration pressure (NFP) by explaining the interactions of glomerular filtration pressure, capsular hydrostatic pressure, and colloid osmotic pressure.

☐ Describe glomerular filtration rate (GFR) by explaining how the filtration coefficient and the net filtration pressure affect the volume of urine formed per unit time.

☐ Define the following terms:
Osmole (osm), osmolality, osmolarity.

☐ Describe, in general terms, how the concentration of wastes in the kidney helps conserve fluid and maintain the osmolarity of the extracellular fluid.

☐ Explain how a salinity gradient from the renal cortex to the renal medulla develops by describing the permeability of the collecting ducts.

☐ Define a countercurrent mechanism.

☐ Explain how the high salt concentration of the renal medulla is *produced* by describing the operation of the countercurrent multiplier.

☐ Explain how the high salt concentration of the renal medulla is *maintained* by describing the operation of the countercurrent exchanger.

☐ Explain how changes in blood pressure, plasma volume, and vasomotion affect diuresis.

☐ Describe the mechanism of action of the following hormones in regards to their effect on diuresis:
Antidiuretic hormone (ADH), aldosterone, atrial natriuretic peptide (ANP).

☐ Describe the role of the kidney as a secretory organ by explaining the mechanism of action of the following:
Erythropoietin, renin.

key terms

afferent arteriole
aldosterone
antidiuretic hormone (ADH)
atrial natriuretic peptide (ANP);
  atriopeptin
bladder
collecting duct (CD)
countercurrent exchanger
countercurrent multiplier
distal convoluted tubule (DCT)
diuresis (dī″ ū-rē′ sis)
  glomerular filtration
  tubular reabsorption
  tubular secretion
efferent arteriole
erythropoietin (EPO)
glomerular capsule (glō-mer′ ū-lar);
  Bowman's capsule
glomerular filtrate; ultrafiltrate
glomerular filtration rate (GFR)
glomerulus; glomerular capillary loops;
  glomerular capillary tuft
hilum

juxtaglomerular apparatus (JGA)
loop of the nephron; loop of Henle
major calyx (kā′ lix)
minor calyx
nephrons
  cortical nephrons
  juxtamedullary nephrons
net filtration pressure (NFP)
  capsular hydrostatic pressure
  colloid osmotic pressure (COP)
  glomerular filtration pressure
osmolality
osmolarity
osmole (Osm)
peritubular capillaries
proximal convoluted tubule (PCT)
renal artery
renal columns
renal cortex
renal medulla
renal papilla
renal pelvis
renal pyramids

renal vein
renin
ureter

urethra
vasa rectae

To understand how the kidneys regulate the normal acid-base status of the bloodstream, we must first have a solid understanding of the normal structure and function of the kidneys. That understanding begins with a brief review of the gross and microscopic anatomy of the kidney, and continues with a discussion of the stages of diuresis, including the concept of osmolarity, countercurrent mechanisms, and the factors that modify diuresis. The chapter concludes with a review of the hormonal and enzymatic actions of the kidney.

Maintenance of the Internal Environment

Although the kidneys are most often associated with the mechanism of filtration, several other renal functions of equal importance are performed by the paired organs. These functions are effectively carried out, in part, because the kidneys are exposed to a large total volume of blood on a continual basis 24 hours a day. The mechanism of filtration is outlined below. For the time being, it is sufficient to point out that filtration of blood allows substances of a certain size to be removed from the blood. These substances collectively form *glomerular filtrate,* the precursor of urine. (The term *filtrate* refers to substances that pass through a filter.) Nitrogenous waste products such as ammonia, urea, and uric acid are constituents of glomerular filtrate, and are eliminated with urine. Of course, not everything filtered from the plasma is a waste product. Substances such as water, glucose, vitamins, and amino acids are filtered from the plasma and then recovered from the glomerular filtrate and reintroduced into the bloodstream; therefore, recovery of valuable substances for reuse is an important renal function associated with filtration and excretion of wastes.

In addition to these familiar renal functions—filtration, excretion, and recovery—the kidney also functions as an endocrine gland, secreting the hormone *erythropoietin (EPO)* that regulates red blood cell production and, hence, the oxygen-carrying capacity of the bloodstream. The kidneys also secrete *renin.* This enzyme catalyzes the production of angiotensin, a powerful vasoactive substance that constricts blood vessels and stimulates the release of *aldosterone.* Aldosterone, in turn, helps in the regulation of electrolyte and fluid levels in the plasma, and in the long-term control of fluid volumes and blood pressure. Finally, the kidneys assist in the maintenance of the pH of the bloodstream by regulating the concentration of hydrogen ions eliminated in the urine and the amount of bicarbonate retained in the bloodstream. This mechanism helps compensate for respiratory and nonrespiratory (metabolic) disturbances that may affect the acid-base balance of the blood.

As can be seen by the foregoing description, renal functions play an integral role in the maintenance of the internal environment of the body. Homeostasis of fluids, electrolytes, and hydrogen ions, as well as oxygen transport status, plasma volume, and blood pressure, are affected by different renal functions.

Macroscopic Anatomy

The paired kidneys are situated on the posterior wall of the peritoneal cavity, approximately at the level T12-L3. Each kidney is protected by a fibrous tissue capsule and is surrounded by an insulating layer of adipose tissue. This location posterior to the peritoneal cavity is described as *retroperitoneal.* Each kidney is supplied with blood by a **renal artery** that branches off the abdominal aorta and enters the medial side of the organ; blood returns from each kidney to the inferior vena cava through a **renal vein** (Fig. 23–1; see also Color Plate 15). Branches of these blood vessels are described in the next section. The concave medial side of the kidney is pierced by a fissure called the **hilum,** which allows the **ureter** to exit. The upper expanded part of the ureter is known as the **renal pelvis,** a funnellike structure that collects urine in the interior of the kidney before passing through the hilum. The paired ureters carry urine from the kidneys to the **bladder,** where it is temporarily stored before passing out of the body through the **urethra.**

Although the kidneys have a small hollow space in their interior where urine is collected, they are considered solid, rather than hollow, organs. Consequently, they have a thin exterior veneer called the **renal cortex** that overlies a central core called the **renal medulla.** The medulla is composed of a variable number of triangular-shaped units called **renal pyramids.** Thin pillars of cortical material called **renal columns** extend from the outer cortex into the medulla, separating individual

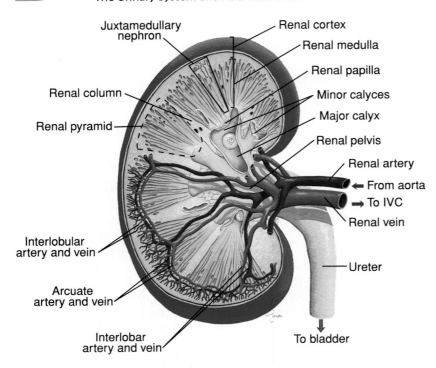

Juxtamedullary nephron
Renal cortex
Renal medulla
Renal papilla
Renal column
Minor calyces
Major calyx
Renal pyramid
Renal pelvis
Renal artery
From aorta
To IVC
Renal vein
Interlobular artery and vein
Ureter
Arcuate artery and vein
Interlobar artery and vein
To bladder

FIGURE 23–1. Structural features of the kidney. Frontal section of the right kidney showing internal structure and blood vessels. An individual *nephron* is outlined in the upper part of the kidney. Dotted lines outline the triangular-shaped renal pyramids comprising the renal medulla. Afferent arterioles branch from the interlobular arteries. Several minor calyces open into larger major calyces that connect with the renal pelvis. The renal pelvis opens to the ureter through the medial fissure, called the *hilum*. (Adapted from Scanlon VC and Sanders T: Essentials of Anatomy and Physiology, ed. 3. FA Davis, Philadelphia, 1999, p 405, with permission.) (See also Color Plate 15.)

renal pyramids. A **minor calyx** is a hollow, cup-shaped structure that fits over the apical (medullary) end of the renal pyramid and collects urine in a dropwise fashion from the **renal papilla** of the renal pyramid. Renal papillae receive urine from thousands of *collecting ducts* and convey it into the minor calyx through small openings (see Fig. 23–1). Urine collected from several minor calyces moves into a **major calyx** before being transported into the renal pelvis. To understand how urine is formed before it passes through these different gross anatomical structures, we need to examine the microscopic anatomy of the kidney, particularly the structure of the functional units known as *nephrons.*

Microscopic Anatomy

Each renal pyramid is composed of thousands of functional units known as **nephrons** (Fig. 23–2; see also Color Plate 16). It is within nephrons that plasma is filtered and glomerular filtrate converted to urine. Two morphologic types of nephrons are recognized: *cortical nephrons* and *juxtamedullary nephrons.* **Cortical nephrons** are located entirely within the renal cortex. These nephrons are oriented perpendicular to the long axis of the renal pyramids. They are relatively small and compact and are found directly beneath the surface of the kidney. **Juxtamedullary nephrons** are much longer than the cortical variety. Approximately one-third of a juxtamedullary nephron is found in the cortex, with the remainder extending as a long loop into the medulla. All the nephrons connect with collecting ducts

that convey urine to the renal papillae. The collecting ducts and the loops of the juxtamedullary nephrons are arranged in a parallel array formed by microtubules. Together, these structures give a faintly striated (striped) appearance to the renal pyramids. Individual nephrons consist of two types of structures: *vascular components* that convey blood and *tubular components* that convey glomerular filtrate, the precursor of urine.

VASCULAR COMPONENTS OF THE NEPHRON

The blood supply to the kidney provides about 1 to 1.5 L of blood per minute. This flowrate represents approximately 20% to 25% of the cardiac output. Because the kidneys are relatively small, a flowrate of 1 to 1.5 L/min translates into perfusion of about 420 mL/min per 100 g of tissue (Ganong, 1995). Such a rate of perfusion ensures that the kidney cells are exposed to a large volume of blood in a given time. In fact, renal perfusion moves as much as 1500 L of blood through the kidneys in a single day, a volume that would fill 10 40-gal oil drums! With such exposure, the kidneys have ample opportunity to process plasma and convert it into urine.

Upon entering the hilum of the kidney, the renal artery branches into successively smaller vessels: *interlobar arteries, arcuate arteries,* and *interlobular arteries.* For the purposes of this discussion, we do not need to examine the detailed distribution of these arteries within the kidney. Instead, we can begin our study with smaller

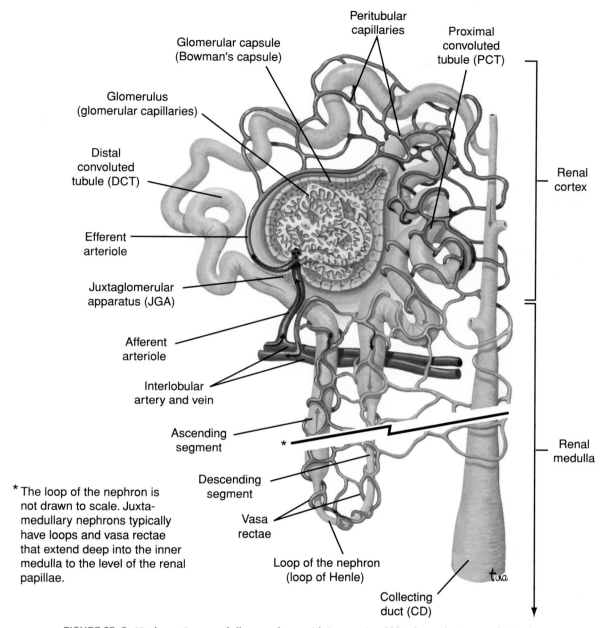

FIGURE 23–2. Nephron. Juxtamedullary nephron with its associated blood vessels. Arrows depict the direction of flow of blood and of glomerular filtrate. (Adapted from Scanlon VC and Sanders T: Essentials of Anatomy and Physiology, ed. 3. FA Davis, Philadelphia, 1999, p 406, with permission.) (See also Color Plate 16.)

branches of the interlobular arteries known as *afferent arterioles* (see Fig. 23–2). The **afferent arterioles** carry a large quantity of blood under relative high pressure to a capillary structure known as the **glomerular capillary loops,** or **glomerular capillary tuft.** This bundle of capillaries is also known simply as the **glomerulus.** Unlike other capillaries in the body designed for nutrient, gas, and waste exchange, the glomerular capillaries function in *glomerular filtration,* a mechanism explained in a later section.

Glomerular capillaries are fenestrated—that is, they have prominent openings between adjacent endothelial cells that allow small-diameter substances to exit freely from the vascular compartment. The pores are covered by a thin glycoprotein membrane. Substances filtered from the bloodstream include *electrolytes* such as sodium, potassium, chlorine, calcium, bicarbonate, and hydrogen ions, *nutrients* such as glucose and amino acid molecules, *vitamins* such as vitamin C, and *metabolic wastes* such as urea and ammonia. In addition, large volumes of *water* leave the glomerular capillaries under pressure. The resulting fluid is produced at a rate of about 170 to 180 L per day, and is known as glomerular filtrate. Substances such as large plasma proteins and red blood cells are not normally filtered at the glomerulus. Consequently, they remain in the bloodstream and exert an osmotic pressure on the glomerular filtrate that tends to draw some fluid back into the glomerular capillaries.

Blood leaving the glomerular capillaries continues into the **efferent arteriole.** This blood vessel has a lumen diameter smaller than that of the glomerular capillaries. Consequently, because the efferent arteriole is located "downstream" from the glomerulus, its restricted orifice reduces blood flow and effectively raises blood pressure within the glomerular capillary loops (see Fig. 23–2).

Note that blood entering the kidney travels first through a unique vascular system composed of special high-pressure capillaries supplied by an arteriole on the proximal side, and drained by an arteriole on the distal side (afferent arteriole → glomerular capillaries → efferent arteriole). Because these special capillaries do not function in gas, nutrient, and waste exchange, they are not drained by venous structures that return blood directly to general circulation. Instead, blood leaving the efferent arterioles enters the **peritubular capillaries,** a network of low-pressure capillaries in close proximity to the tubular components of the nephron (see Fig. 23–2). It is here that various exchanges take place that alter the physical and chemical composition of glomerular filtrate. The efferent arterioles of juxtaglomerular nephrons also give rise to long, straight blood vessels called the **vasa rectae.** These blood vessels supply the renal medulla and function to maintain the osmotic concentration of the extracellular fluid of the medulla, a mechanism described more fully in a later section.

Blood is collected from the peritubular capillaries and directed into *venules* that drain into progressively larger veins—*interlobular veins, arcuate veins,* and *interlobar veins.* The renal vein receives blood from these veins and returns it to the inferior vena cava, thus completing the circuit of the kidney.

TUBULAR COMPONENTS OF THE NEPHRON

Distinct from the blood-transporting vascular structures discussed previously, the tubular portions of the nephron carry glomerular filtrate that is being processed into urine. Figure 23–2 shows the transfer of fluid out of the glomerular capillaries (vascular component) into a spherical structure known as the **glomerular capsule** or **Bowman's capsule** (tubular component). The glomerular capsule is a porous, double-walled structure that completely surrounds the ball of capillaries forming the glomerulus. The function

of the glomerular capsule is to collect the fluid that has been forced out of the glomerular capillaries. A useful analogy here is the image of a hollow, collapsible ball such as a tennis ball, with one side pushed in by a deep depression. If the depression is filled with a bundle of porous capillaries leaking fluid, and the inner wall of the ball's depression is equipped with pores, fluid will be able to stream out of the porous capillaries and pass through the porous inner wall of the ball. The fluid will be "trapped," however, in the narrow space between the inner and outer layers of the ball where it will exit from the ball via a narrow tube. This analogy can be quite helpful in understanding the role of the different vascular and tubular structures involved in the mechanism of glomerular filtration.

Glomerular filtrate leaving the glomerular capsule enters the **proximal convoluted tubule (PCT),** a small-diameter tube that twists and turns on itself before continuing into the renal medulla as the descending segment of the **loop of the nephron,** also known as **loop of Henle** (see Fig. 23–2). Although tubular structures are common to both cortical and juxtamedullary nephrons, loops of the nephron reaching deep into the renal pyramids of the medulla are characteristic of the juxtamedullary type of nephron. Cortical nephrons are much more compact and do not possess long loops of Henle. The loop turns sharply and continues back toward the glomerulus as the ascending segment of the loop of the nephron, becoming the **distal convoluted tubule (DCT)** at approximately the level of the proximal convoluted tubule (see Fig. 23–2). Numerous **collecting ducts (CDs)** receive urine from distal convoluted tubules, and convey it to the renal papilla for release into the calyces and the renal pelvis (see Fig. 23–1).

Diuresis—Stages in the Formation of Urine

Under pressure, fluid exuded out of glomerular capillaries enters the glomerular capsule where it is referred to as **glomerular filtrate** or **ultrafiltrate.** Samples of this fluid drawn from tubular structures proximal to the glomerulus bear a close resemblance to plasma, the fluid from which glomerular filtrate is made. Further along the tubular system of the nephron, however, striking changes occur to the physical and chemical makeup of the fluid. In fact, samples of glomerular filtrate drawn from tubular structures distal to the glomerulus closely resemble urine. The basic difference between the physical and chemical composition of plasma and urine is found in the *concentrations* of the various substances found in the two fluids. The concentration of electrolytes, waste products, and nutrients found in the glomerular filtrate reflects the various stages of urine formation as the makeup of the fluid progressively changes from the glomerular capsule to the collecting duct. Three different, but interrelated, stages of diuresis are recognized: **glomerular filtration, tubular reabsorption**, and **tubular secretion.** We now examine each of these processes that contribute to **diuresis,** the process of urine formation.

GLOMERULAR FILTRATION

As explained previously, the blood pressure within glomerular capillaries is relatively high because of the restriction to outflow caused by the narrowed lumen of the efferent arteriole. This elevated pressure causes plasma, along with substances dissolved and suspended in plasma, to be forced out of the capillaries into the glomerular capsule. This stage of diuresis is called glomerular filtration (Fig. 23–3). Because selection is on the basis of physical size, glomerular filtration is considered a *nonselective mechanism*—waste products as well as valuable substances of a certain size are filtered from the blood. In later stages of diuresis, valuable substances such as glucose molecules, which are relatively small, are recovered and re-enter the

bloodstream. On the other hand, large-diameter, high-molecular-weight substances such as plasma proteins and red blood cells are not normally found in the glomerular filtrate. In fact, their presence in the filtrate may indicate a defect in the filtration membrane formed by the endothelial cells of the glomerular capillaries and the epithelial cells of the glomerular capsule. For instance, sustained high blood pressure may rupture the delicate membranes of the filtration units, resulting in *proteinuria* (proteins in the urine) or *hematuria* (blood in the urine).

TUBULAR REABSORPTION

As pointed out previously, the protein- and erythrocyte-free fluid that enters the glomerular capsule is a mixture of both valuable and waste products. A *selective mechanism* called tubular reabsorption is responsible for moving valuable substances such as glucose molecules from the tubular parts of the nephron into the peritubular capillaries, thus recovering them prior to elimination (see Fig. 23–3). In simple terms, if a substance is *not* reabsorbed after being filtered, it becomes a part of urine and is eliminated.

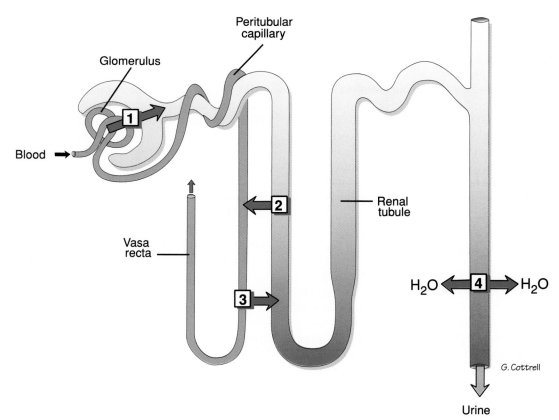

FIGURE 23–3. Steps in the formation of urine: (1) *Glomerular filtration*—a plasmalike substance called filtrate is produced from the blood. (2) *Tubular reabsorption*—valuable substances, including water, are removed from the filtrate and returned to the blood. (3) *Tubular secretion*—additional waste products are removed from the blood and added to the filtrate. (4) *Concentration*—additional water is removed from the filtrate, further concentrating the fluid.

An important constituent of the glomerular filtrate is the large volume of water filtered at the glomerulus during a 24-hour period. For instance, of the 170 to 180 L of glomerular filtrate produced each day, more than 99% of the fluid is reabsorbed from the tubules, leaving about 1.7 to 1.8 L of concentrated urine. The actual amount of urine produced each day varies and is dependent on factors such as blood pressure, exercise, perspiration, defecation, and water vapor loss from the alveoli. Through alteration in the amount of fluid reabsorbed from the tubules, the kidneys help maintain fluid homeostasis.

Other substances in the filtrate altered by the mechanism of tubular reabsorption include glucose, vitamins, amino acids, sodium ions, and bicarbonate ions. Both active and passive reabsorption mechanisms move substances through the tubule cells. These mechanisms are dependent upon the operation of various ion pumps in the tubule cells. Because bicarbonate ions (HCO_3^-) are among the most important acid buffers in the body, the number of bicarbonate ions returned to the bloodstream helps regulate the pH of the plasma. These mechanisms, as well as the acidification of urine via the elimination of hydrogen ions (H^+), are discussed in the next chapter.

Diuretics are therapeutic agents that increase the rate of urine formation. Several different classes of diuretics are recognized on the basis of their mechanism of action. A common mechanism involves the inhibition of the tubular reabsorption of water, either through direct or indirect means. By increasing the rate of formation of urine, diuretic drugs decrease the volume of plasma remaining in circulation. This plasma-depleting action of diuretics has the overall effect of lowering total body water and is especially useful in pathophysiologic states such as congestive heart failure and hypertension. These clinical conditions are aggravated by high plasma volumes and thus respond favorably to the use of diuretics.

TUBULAR SECRETION

The substances to be eliminated by the kidneys do not necessarily enter the ultrafiltrate during glomerular filtration. In a first pass through the glomerular capillaries, some waste products in the blood may simply not be filtered. Renal perfusion is so great, however, that there is a good chance that a waste product will be filtered on another circuit through the kidney. Certain waste products can also be *selectively removed* from the peritubular capillaries and transferred into the kidney tubules for elimination. Tubular secretion involves the movement of substances such as hydrogen ions, potassium ions (K^+), and ammonia from the plasma into the filtrate (see Fig. 23–3). This stage in diuresis occurs independently of glomerular filtration

and tubular reabsorption, and represents the last opportunity for nephrons to rid the body of wastes or make adjustments in the concentration of plasma constituents such as hydrogen ions. Acidification of urine and pH regulation is discussed in the following chapter.

Filtration Pressure and Filtration Rate

NET FILTRATION PRESSURE

Systemic blood pressure determines renal pressure, and it is this driving pressure, called the **glomerular filtration pressure,** that forces fluid into the glomerular capsule (Fig. 23–4). Normal glomerular filtration pressure is about 60 to 75 mm Hg, a value more than twice that of systemic capillaries. As blood pressure falls, glomerular filtration pressure, glomerular filtration, and diuresis decrease. Conversely, an increase in blood pressure causes an increase in glomerular filtration pressure, glomerular filtration, and diuresis.

As can be seen in Figure 23–4, two different pressures *oppose* this driving pressure. The glomerular capsule, as well as the entire tubular system of the nephron, is always full of fluid, which exerts a pressure called the **capsular hydrostatic pressure.** The opposing pressure of this fluid must be overcome by the glomerular filtration pressure for more fluid to enter the glomerular capsule and diuresis to proceed. If an obstruction restricts any part of the tubular system, the capsular hydrostatic pressure increases above a normal value of approximately 20 to 25 mm Hg and starts to decrease the rate of glomerular filtration.

Recall that large-molecular-weight substances such as red blood cells and plasma proteins are not normally filtered. Consequently, these large colloidal substances remain in the glomerular capillaries and exert an osmotic pressure on the fluid that has entered the glomerular capsule. (*Osmosis* refers to the tendency of water to move through a semipermeable membrane to a region of higher solute concentration.) The higher concentration of solutes in the bloodstream moves water back into the glomerular capillaries. The pressure created by this osmotic effect is approximately 30 mm Hg and is called the **colloid osmotic pressure (COP).** The COP represents another opposing pressure that must be overcome by the glomerular filtration pressure for filtration to proceed.

Overall, the relationships among the three pressures acting at the glomerular capsule can be summarized as the **net filtration pressure (NFP).** As this effective filtration pressure decreases, the rate of urine formation decreases. Therefore:

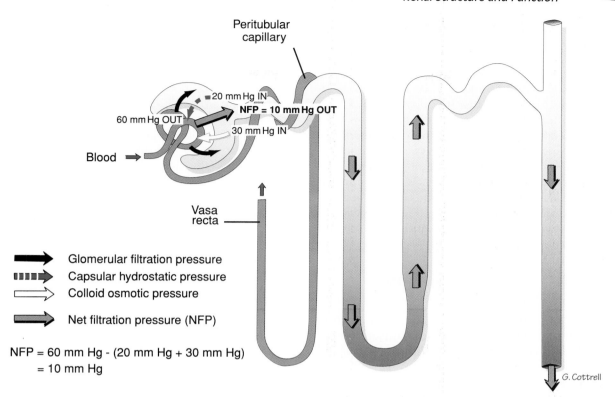

Peritubular
capillary

20 mm Hg IN
NFP = 10 mm Hg OUT
60 mm Hg OUT
30 mm Hg IN

Blood ⟶

Vasa
recta

⟶ Glomerular filtration pressure
⟶ Capsular hydrostatic pressure
⟶ Colloid osmotic pressure
⟶ Net filtration pressure (NFP)

NFP = 60 mm Hg - (20 mm Hg + 30 mm Hg)
   = 10 mm Hg

G. Cottrell

FIGURE 23–4. Net filtration pressure. Several forces are involved in glomerular filtration. Glomerular filtration pressure provides the driving force to force fluid out of the glomerular capillaries and into the glomerular capsule. Capsular hydrostatic pressure and colloid osmotic pressure oppose this driving force. Urine continues to be formed if the net filtration pressure (NFP) is positive. (See text for details.)

$$
\begin{aligned}
\text{Net filtration} &= \text{glomerular} - (\text{capsular} + \text{colloid} \\
\text{pressure} &\quad \text{filtration} \quad\ \text{hydrostatic} \quad \text{osmotic} \\
&\quad\ \text{pressure} \quad\ \text{pressure} \quad\ \text{pressure}) \\
&= 60 \text{ mm Hg} - (20 \text{ mm Hg} + 30 \text{ mm Hg}) \\
&= 10 \text{ mm Hg}
\end{aligned}
$$

As can be seen in this equation, diuresis continues as long as the net filtration pressure remains positive.

GLOMERULAR FILTRATION RATE

The volume of glomerular filtrate formed per minute by the two kidneys is known as the **glomerular filtration rate (GFR).** Approximately 12.5 mL of filtrate per minute is formed for every 1 mm Hg of net filtration pressure (Saladin, 1998). This value is known as the *filtration coefficient* (K_f). Both the filtration coefficient and the net filtration pressure affect the GFR, as shown by the following example for an adult man:

$$
\begin{aligned}
\text{GFR} &= K_f \times NFP \\
&= \frac{12.5 \text{ mL/min}}{1 \text{ mm Hg}} \times 10 \text{ mm Hg} \\
\therefore \text{ GFR} &= 125 \text{ mL/min}
\end{aligned}
$$

Osmolarity and Countercurrent Mechanisms

UNITS OF OSMOTIC CONCENTRATION

Maintenance of the osmotic concentration of body fluids is one of the many important functions of the kidney. Osmotic concentration is expressed in different ways, including *osmolality* and *osmolarity*. One **osmole (Osm)** is equal to 1 mole of dissolved solute particles. If the solute does not undergo ionization in water, then 1 mol of solute yields 1 Osm of dissolved particles. For example, a 1-molar (mol/L) solution of glucose is also 1 Osm/L. On the other hand, if a solute *does* ionize, it yields 2 or more moles of dissolved particles in solution. All the ions in a solution composed of different substances affect osmosis and contribute to the total osmotic concentration of the solution. Thus, a 1 mol/L solution of sodium chloride (NaCl) = 2 Osm/L, because NaCl ionizes into 1 mol of sodium ions (Na^+) and 1 mol of chloride ions (Cl^-) in solution.

Osmolality refers to the number of osmoles of solute per kilogram of water, whereas **osmolarity** is the number of osmoles of solute per liter of solution. Because it is easier to measure the volume of a solution than it is to determine the mass of water it contains, most clinical calculations of osmotic concentration are based on osmolarity (Saladin, 1998). At the concentrations found in human body fluids, there is very little concentration difference between the two terms; therefore, osmolality and osmolarity are used nearly interchangeably. Physiologic concentrations, being relatively dilute, are typically expressed in *milli*osmoles per liter (1 mOsm = 1 $\times$ 10^{-3} Osm). Most body fluids such as plasma, intracellular fluid, and interstitial fluid have similar osmotic concentrations of approximately 300 mOsm/L. Urine, on the other hand, may have an osmotic concentration as high as 1200 mOsm/L. In the next section we discuss the significance of differing osmotic concentrations found in different parts of the nephron.

CONCENTRATION OF WASTES AND CONSERVATION OF FLUID

Overall, renal function aids in the conservation of fluid and the maintenance of isotonic conditions in the extracellular fluid (ECF). First, the production of a hypertonic solution of urine (1200 mOsm/L) allows a large quantity of waste to be eliminated without the loss of large volumes of fluid. Second, the ability of the kidneys to maintain the osmolarity of extracellular fluid (300 mOsm/L) provides osmotic conditions that are physiologically compatible with the ECF, thus ensuring that a net loss or gain of fluid in the cells of the body does not occur.

SALINITY GRADIENT

The osmolarity of the ECF in the cortical region is approximately 300 mOsm/L, increasing to approximately 1200 mOsm/L at the renal papillae (Fig. 23–5). One of the reasons the osmotic concentration of the ECF deep in the medulla is four times greater than that in the cortex is that the collecting ducts are permeable to water but are impermeable to NaCl. As a result of this permeability difference, a salinity gradient develops from the cortex to the medulla, as water continually leaves the collecting ducts. The shift of water out of the collecting ducts by osmosis produces urine that is increasingly concentrated from the cortical to the medullary regions of the kidney. This account helps explain *how* the medulla becomes salty, but *why* does it remain so? What keeps salt from simply diffusing throughout the kidney from regions of high salt concentration to those of lower salt concentration? The mechanism that resists this diffusion tendency is described in the next section.

COUNTERCURRENT MULTIPLIER

A *countercurrent mechanism* is one in which fluids influence each other in some way as a result of moving in opposite directions through parallel tubes that are close together. Such a mechanism generally increases the efficiency of the overall process. Arteries and veins are often arranged in such a fashion; their close proximity to each other allows heat to exchange between the vessels, thus minimizing the effect of a low blood temperature as blood returns to the warm core of the body from the relatively cooler extremities. In the kidney, the descending segment and the ascending segment of the loop of the nephron lie very close to each other as they pass through regions of the kidney having differing salt concentrations.

The permeability of the two segments differs. The descending limb is permeable to water but not to NaCl. On the other hand, the ascending limb is impermeable to water but permeable to NaCl, actively transporting Na^+, K^+, and Cl^- from the tubule into the surrounding ECF (see Fig. 23–5). From the ECF, electrolytes can enter the peritubular capillaries. The **countercurrent multiplier** is the mechanism that occurs in the descending and ascending limbs of the loops of the nephron that functions to amplify, or *multiply*, the high concentration of salt in the medulla. This mechanism helps prevent the diffusion of salt as a result of the salinity gradient.

Because the descending segment is permeable to water, more and more water leaves the tubule as the segment penetrates into the increasingly concentrated salt regions of the renal medulla. Of course, as more water leaves the filtrate, the fluid left behind becomes more concentrated, reaching a peak of 1200 mOsm/L in the loops of the nephron in the inner medulla (see Fig. 23–5). Recall that the ascending limb of the loop of the nephron is relatively impermeable to water, but that electrolytes are readily transported out of the filtrate into the surrounding ECF. Because the osmolarity of the filtrate in the first part of the ascending segment is high, ions rapidly move into the ECF according to their concentration gradient. Water, however, cannot follow the ions because the tubule cells are impermeable to water. The shift of ions into the ECF simultaneously raises the osmolarity of the renal medulla and reduces the osmolarity of the glomerular filtrate. The multiplier process thus maintains the high salt concentration of the medulla. As filtrate moves through the ascending segment toward the renal cortex, however, the transport of ions into the surrounding tissue fluid decreases, resulting in a dilute filtrate and a dilute ECF in the cortical region (see Fig. 23–5). The osmolarity of the glomerular filtrate is reduced to approximately 100 mOsm/L as the ascending segment nears the renal cortex (Saladin, 1998).

COUNTERCURRENT EXCHANGER

The peritubular capillaries continue as microscopic blood vessels called the vasa rectae (see Fig. 23–2). These blood vessels are closely aligned with the loops of the nephrons and extend into the inner portion of the renal

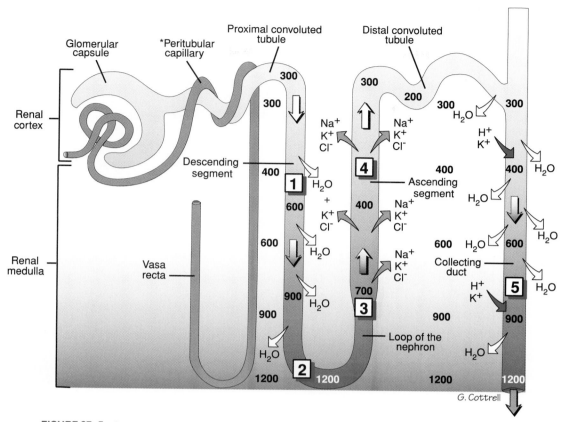

FIGURE 23–5. Countercurrent multiplier. All numerical values are in mOsm/L. In this renal mechanism involving the loop of the nephron, several steps occur that *increase* the osmolarity of the glomerular filtrate. The descending segment is permeable to water but impermeable to salt, whereas the ascending segment is impermeable to water but permeable to salt. The collecting duct is permeable to water. (1) The high osmolarity of the extracellular fluid causes water to leave the descending segment. (2) As more and more water leaves by osmosis, the salt concentration of the fluid in the loop increases. (3) The increased salt concentration in the ascending limb causes more salt to be transported to the extracellular fluid. (4) The transfer of more salt increases the osmolarity of the extracellular fluid in the renal medulla, thus attracting more water from the descending segment. (5) Water continues to leave the collecting duct as hydrogen ions and potassium ions are added, thus further concentrating the filtrate.

*Peritubular capillaries also wrap around the distal convoluted tubule and the loop of the nephron and continue as the vasa rectae extending into the deeper parts of the renal medulla.

medulla. Vasa rectae are arranged in a parallel array with blood flowing through them in opposite directions (Fig. 23–6). The resulting countercurrent mechanism operates to *maintain* the high osmolarity of the medulla. This mechanism, called the **countercurrent exchanger,** does not multiply, or increase, the salinity of the renal medulla. Instead, it prevents the osmotic concentration of the medulla from decreasing. Without such a mechanism, the salt concentration gradient between the ECF and the bloodstream would continually load electrolytes into the blood vessels, thus decreasing the salinity of the medulla. The countercurrent exchanger allows blood vessels descending into the high salt concentration of the medulla to unload water because of osmosis, and to take on salt because of the concentration gradient (see Fig. 23–6). However, as the blood vessels emerge from the medulla and travel up toward the renal cortex, the reverse process occurs. In other words, osmosis causes wa-

ter to move from the ECF into the blood vessels, and salt diffuses from the blood vessels into the ECF along a concentration gradient (see Fig. 23–6). Thus there is no net gain or loss of salt or water in the renal medulla or the bloodstream. Salt and water merely *exchange* by moving into and out of the adjacent parallel blood vessels of the renal medulla.

Factors Affecting Diuresis

BLOOD PRESSURE, PLASMA VOLUME, AND VASOMOTOR EFFECTS

Because glomerular filtration is directly affected by glomerular filtration pressure, the control of diuresis is linked to systemic blood pressure. As blood pressure rises, the kidneys produce more urine, which lowers

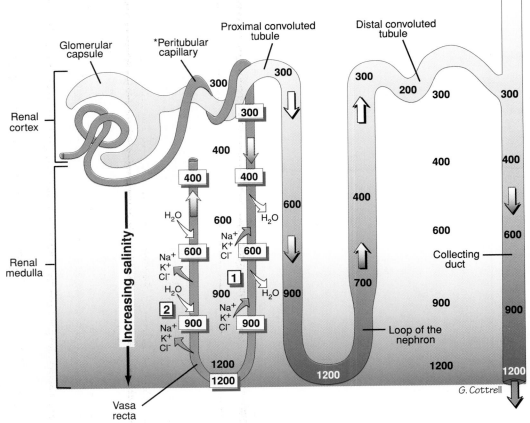

FIGURE 23–6. Countercurrent exchanger. All numerical values are in mOsm/L. In this countercurrent mechanism involving the vasa rectae, the metabolic needs of the cells of the renal medulla are met without disruption of the osmolarity of either the blood or the extracellular fluid. Several steps occur that *maintain* the osmolarity of the extracellular fluid surrounding the loops of the nephrons. Essentially, the vasa rectae absorb as much water on their way out of the medulla as they unload on the way in, thus preserving the salinity gradient of the medulla. (1) As the vasa rectae descend into the medulla, water diffuses out of the blood vessels and salt diffuses in, according to their respective concentration gradients. (The blood becomes nearly isotonic with the extracellular fluid in the medulla.) (2) As blood flows back toward the renal cortex through parallel blood vessels, salt diffuses out and water diffuses in, according to their concentration gradients. (The blood becomes nearly isotonic with the extracellular fluid in the cortex.)

*Peritubular capillaries also wrap around the distal convoluted tubule and the loop of the nephron and continue as the vasa rectae extending into the deeper parts of the renal medulla.

the plasma volume and decreases blood pressure. Conversely, as blood pressure decreases, in response to severe hemorrhage for example, diuresis decreases and the kidneys form less urine. This mechanism conserves fluid and helps restore plasma volume so that venous return and cardiac output can be maintained.

Diuresis is affected by a variety of factors including changes in total body water brought about by losses associated with perspiration, defecation, vomiting, and respiration. As water is lost through these other routes, plasma volume decreases and diuresis slows.

Changes in external temperature dramatically affect the rate of urine formation. For example, when the ambient temperature decreases, the thermoregulatory center in the hypothalamus signals the vasomotor cen-

ter of the medulla. This medullary center responds by initiating vascular shunting in the form of simultaneous vasoconstriction of superficial blood vessels supplying the skin and extremities *and* vasodilation of blood vessels supplying the internal organs, including the kidneys. The increase in renal perfusion results in the production of large quantities of dilute urine.

HORMONAL EFFECTS

Antidiuretic Hormone

The hypothalamus responds to increases in the osmotic pressure of blood. Such an increase may be brought about by an increase in salt concentration associated with a loss of fluid accompanying dehydration. Secretory cells in the hypothalamus synthesize **antidiuretic hormone (ADH),** which is released into the bloodstream from the posterior pituitary (neurohypophysis). ADH targets the collecting ducts, where it increases their permeability to water, causing more water to be reabsorbed. Consequently, less fluid remains in the glomerular filtrate and urine output declines.

Aldosterone

The adrenal cortex releases the steroid hormone **aldosterone** in response to the arrival of angiotensin II in the bloodstream (see Chap. 21). Like ADH, aldosterone exhibits an antidiuretic effect in the kidney tubules by restricting the volume of fluid recovered from the glomerular filtrate. Unlike ADH, aldosterone increases water reabsorption by first increasing the reabsorption of minerals such as sodium ions from the glomerular filtrate. As the rate of sodium ion reabsorption in the kidney increases, the sodium ion concentration in the peritubular capillaries exerts an osmotic effect on water in the glomerular filtrate. Because water moves toward a region of higher solute concentration, water is reabsorbed, thus reducing the volume of glomerular filtrate and the volume of urine produced.

There is an obligatory loss of potassium ions into the filtrate and urine when sodium ions are reabsorbed.

Atrial Natriuretic Peptide

In Chapter 21 we discussed the unique action of **atrial natriuretic peptide (ANP),** also known as **atriopeptin,** in regard to the regulation of blood pressure. Recall that this substance is a naturally occurring *diuretic* hormone.

> **NOTE:** The term *natriuretic* refers to substances that increase the rate of excretion of sodium in the urine.

ANP is released from the wall of the right atrium in response to stretching of the heart wall as blood returns to the heart. The degree of stretch is proportional to venous return. Various antidiuretic mechanisms are halted by the action of ANP, thus bringing about an increase in diuresis:

- The release of renin from the kidney is inhibited; therefore, angiotensin is not produced and aldosterone is not released from the adrenal cortex.
- Antidiuretic hormone from the hypothalamus is inhibited.

TABLE 23-1	**Factors Affecting Diuresis**		
Factor		**Increased Diuresis**	**Decreased Diuresis**
Blood Pressure, Plasma Volume, and Vasomotor Effects			
Blood pressure			
Increased		√	
Decreased			√
Plasma volume and total body water			
Increased (e.g., increased water intake)		√	
Decreased (e.g., hemorrhage, perspiration, defecation, vomiting, respiratory losses)			√
Hormonal Effects			
Antidiuretic hormone (ADH, antidiuretic vasopressin)			
Increases permeability of collecting ducts to water, increasing the reabsorption of water			√
Aldosterone			
Increases reabsorption of sodium into peritubular capillaries, which increases the reabsorption of water			√
Atrial natriuretic peptide (ANP, atriopeptin)			
Inhibits renin, thus inhibiting aldosterone; inhibits aldosterone action at tubule cells; inhibits antidiuretic hormone		√	
Diuretic Drugs (many different drugs; different mechanisms of action)			
Furosemide (Lasix)			
Inhibits the reabsorption of electrolytes		√	
Spironolactone (Aldactone)			
Antagonizes aldosterone at tubule cells		√	

- The action of aldosterone at the kidney tubule cells is blocked.

Table 23–1 summarizes the factors affecting diuresis.

Hormonal and Enzyme Actions of the Kidney

In addition to being a filtration and excretion organ, the kidney functions in a secretory role, producing hormones such as *erythropoietin* that are released into the bloodstream to produce their effects at other organs, and enzymes such as *renin* that function as biological catalysts to enhance biochemical reactions.

ERYTHROPOIETIN

Hypoxia causes specialized kidney cells to secrete the enzyme **erythropoietin (EPO)**. Erythropoietin is distributed throughout the circulatory system, where it stimulates stem cells in the bone marrow to increase the rate of maturation of red blood cells. As the number of red blood cells increases, the total amount of hemoglobin and the oxygen-carrying capacity of the blood increase, thus relieving hypoxia. Within homeostatic limits, this erythropoietic response to hypoxia is effective, but as the *packed cell volume* (PCV) increases, the viscosity of the blood increases, thus increasing resistance, pressure, and the workload on the heart.

RENIN

Modified distal convoluted tubule cells comprising the **juxtaglomerular apparatus (JGA)** are located adjacent to the afferent arteriole of the nephron (see Fig. 23–2). In this strategic location, the juxtaglomerular cells are stimulated by mechanical stretching of the afferent arteriole wall in response to changes in renal (and systemic) blood pressure. The operation of the JGA is the basis of the renal mechanism and the release of the enzyme **renin** discussed in Chapter 21 in conjunction with the long-term control of blood pressure.

Summary

In keeping with the preclinical and preparatory nature of the text and its emphasis on the normal anatomy and physiology of the cardiopulmonary system, this chapter did not provide *in-depth* coverage of related pathophysiologic and clinical topics affecting the kidney, such as acute and chronic renal failure, or the differential diagnosis of acid-base disturbances. Instead, the chapter reinforced many of the relationships among the respiratory, cardiovascular, and renal systems already encountered in the book. The chapter began with a review of the macroscopic and microscopic anatomy of the kidney, and followed with a discussion of diuresis, osmolarity, and countercurrent mechanisms. In addition, factors affecting the formation of urine were examined, and a brief review of the hormonal and enzymatic functions of the kidney was presented. This chapter serves as an introduction to renal processes such as active transport pumps and compensation mechanisms. These processes are discussed in the following chapter, which covers the role of the kidney in the maintenance of acid-base levels in the bloodstream.

BIBLIOGRAPHY

Cottrell GP and Surkin HB: Pharmacology for Respiratory Care Practitioners. FA Davis, Philadelphia, 1995.

Ganong WF: Review of Medical Physiology, ed 17. Appleton & Lange, Norwalk, CT, 1995.

Guyton AC and Hall JE: Textbook of Medical Physiology, ed 9. WB Saunders, Philadelphia, 1996.

Martini FH: Fundamentals of Anatomy and Physiology, ed 4. Prentice Hall, Upper Saddle River, NJ, 1998.

Saladin KS: Anatomy and Physiology: The Unity of Form and Function. WCB/McGraw-Hill, Boston, 1998.

Shier D, Butler J, and Lewis R: Hole's Human Anatomy and Physiology, ed 7. Wm C Brown, Dubuque, IA, 1996.

Thibodeau GA and Patton KT: Anatomy and Physiology, ed 3. Mosby–Year Book, St Louis, 1996.

Tortora GJ and Grabowski SR: Principles of Anatomy and Physiology, ed 8. HarperCollins, New York, 1996.

CHAPTER 24

Acid-Base Balance

chapter objectives

After studying this chapter the reader should be able to:

☐ Define the following terms:
   Active transport pump, cotransport (symporter) mechanism,
      countertransport (antiporter) mechanism.

☐ Describe how the reabsorption of electrolytes and water in the tubules is
   affected by the operation of the Na^+/K^+ pump, Na^+-K^+-$2Cl^-$ symporters, and
   Na^+-Cl^- symporters.

☐ Describe how the tubule cells adjust the pH of urine and blood by explaining
   the operation of the Na^+/H^+ antiporters and HCO_3^-/Cl^- antiporters.

☐ Explain how conditions of hypochloremia or hypokalemia may upset normal
   acid-base balance by describing the involvement of Cl^- and K^+ with
   symporter and antiporter mechanisms in the tubule cells.

☐ Describe the concept of pH and explain why the maintenance of a stable pH
   environment is essential to normal function.

☐ Differentiate between volatile and nonvolatile acids.

☐ Define an acid and a base according to the Brønsted-Lowry theory.

☐ Describe the general function of a buffer pair.

☐ Define the dissociation constant (K_a) of an acid.

☐ State the general form of the Henderson-Hasselbalch equation.

☐ Explain the isohydric principle as it relates to the pH of blood that contains
   multiple buffer systems.

☐ Explain why the bicarbonate buffer system is commonly used to assess the
   acid-base status of the bloodstream.

☐ Define the apparent pK (pK') used in the determination of acid-base levels in
   the bloodstream.

☐ Explain the origin of the 20:1 ratio between bicarbonate ion concentration
   and carbon dioxide concentration.

☐ Define the following terms:
   Acidemia, acidosis, alkalemia, alkalosis.

- ☐ Describe the operation of the phosphate and protein buffer system in the bloodstream.
- ☐ Describe the four classic, or "pure," types of acid-base disturbances: Respiratory acidosis, respiratory alkalosis, metabolic acidosis, metabolic alkalosis.
- ☐ Explain why the term "nonrespiratory" is more accurate than "metabolic" in regard to acid-base disturbances.
- ☐ Describe respiratory acidosis and respiratory alkalosis, in general terms, by explaining shifts in the equilibrium reaction involving carbon dioxide and water.
- ☐ Describe the changes in H_2CO_3, HCO_3^-, and H^+ produced by the following respiratory conditions: Acute ventilatory failure, chronic ventilatory failure, acute alveolar hyperventilation, chronic alveolar hyperventilation.
- ☐ Explain how the kidneys help restore a respiratory acid-base disturbance to normal.
- ☐ Describe how chronic metabolic acidosis occurs and explain how the lungs help restore the acid-base disturbance to normal.
- ☐ Describe how chronic metabolic alkalosis occurs and explain how the lungs help restore the acid-base disturbance to normal.
- ☐ Compare and contrast the activities of renal compensation mechanisms and respiratory compensation mechanisms in acid-base disturbances.

key terms

acidemia
acidosis
active transport pump
   Na^+/K^+ pump
   Na^+-K^+-$2Cl^-$ symporter
   Na^+-Cl^- symporter
   Na^+/H^+ antiporter
   HCO_3^-/Cl^- antiporter
acute alveolar hyperventilation
acute ventilatory failure
alkalemia
alkalosis
apparent pK (pK')
buffer; buffer system
   bicarbonate buffer system
   phosphate buffer system
   protein buffer system

chronic alveolar hyperventilation
chronic metabolic acidosis; chronic nonrespiratory acidosis
chronic metabolic alkalosis; chronic nonrespiratory alkalosis
chronic ventilatory failure
cotransport mechanism; symporter mechanism
countertransport mechanism; antiporter mechanism
dissociation constant (K_a) of acid
Henderson-Hasselbalch equation
isohydric principle
nonvolatile acid; fixed acid
respiratory acidosis
respiratory alkalosis
volatile acid

The focus of this chapter is the interaction of the kidneys and lungs in the maintenance of acid-base balance. To understand renal and respiratory compensatory mechanisms involved in acid-base balance, information regarding active transport pumps is presented, along with a review of acids, bases, and buffers. Although the chapter is not designed to provide comprehensive coverage of acid-base topics, it introduces the reader to the fundamentals underlying renal pathophysiology and related clinical applications.

Active Transport Pumps

To understand the role of the kidney in the regulation of acid-base levels in the bloodstream, we first need to discuss how the cells of the kidney move substances through cell membranes by means of *active transport pumps*. An **active transport pump** is a mechanism that transfers electrolytes through cell membranes against concentration gradients. Different active transport pumps operate in different parts of the nephrons of the kidney. The *primary active transport pump* in the tubule cells of the nephron is the **Na$^+$/K$^+$ pump.** This exchange mechanism uses the energy derived from splitting adenosine triphosphase (ATP) to transport sodium ions (Na$^+$) into extracellular fluid and potassium ions (K$^+$) into intracellular fluid, thus creating ionic concentration gradients on respective sides of the tubule cell membrane. By contrast, *secondary active transport pumps* rely indirectly on ATP to move substances through cell membranes. In a secondary active transport mechanism, stored energy is represented by the Na$^+$ concentration gradient established by the activity of the primary Na$^+$/K$^+$ pump. Although cell membranes are only slightly permeable to Na$^+$, secondary active transport pumps provide special pathways for Na$^+$ movement. Sodium ions then follow these pathways, creating conditions that result in the transport of other substances through the membrane in an *indirect* manner. Several examples of these transport pumps are discussed below.

Two types of active transport mechanisms are responsible for moving substances through cell membranes: *cotransport mechanisms* and *countertransport mechanisms.* In **cotransport** or **symporter mechanisms,** Na$^+$ and other substances move together in the same direction through the membrane. Recovery of filtered substances such as glucose from the glomerular filtrate is accomplished by symporter mechanisms operating in the tubule cells. **Countertransport** or **antiporter mechanisms** move Na$^+$ and another substance in opposite directions through the cell membrane. Such an exchange between Na$^+$ and hydrogen ions (H$^+$) in the tubule allows H$^+$ to be expelled in the urine at the same time that Na$^+$ is recovered.

On the basis of these mechanisms, it can be seen that Na$^+$ availability in the kidney affects the operation of both symporter and antiporter mechanisms. Therefore, any condition or drug that affects sodium ion concentration will influence the level of electrolytes that normally interact with Na$^+$ in transport mechanisms. For instance, some diuretics interfere with Na$^+$ symporters and antiporters, thus influencing active transport of electrolytes through the membrane of tubule cells. The electrolyte levels, in turn, influence the fluid levels in the kidney. We now examine the fate of electrolytes in the kidney and the resulting effect on *acid-base balance* when these electrolyte levels are altered.

Electrolytes and Blood pH

REABSORPTION OF ELECTROLYTES AND WATER

As we have seen, sodium ions are a major constituent of glomerular filtrate—that is, they are found in high concentration in the fluid that has been filtered from the blood. Within the *intracellular* fluid of proximal and distal convoluted tubule cells, however, the concentration of Na$^+$ is relatively low. In addition, the interior of the tubule cells is negative with respect to the outside. As a result of these gradient conditions, Na$^+$ in the ultrafiltrate passively diffuse into the tubule cells (Fig. 24–1). From the interior of the tubule cells, primary active transport via the sodium pump (also known as Na$^+$-K$^+$-ATPase) moves Na$^+$ from the tubule cells into the interstitial fluid bathing the peritubular capillaries (see Fig. 24–1). From here, Na$^+$ is reabsorbed into the blood vessels. Meanwhile, potassium ions are transported by the Na$^+$/K$^+$ pump into the tubule cells as Na$^+$ is expelled. Numerous leakage channels for K$^+$ exist, however, thus allowing K$^+$ to passively diffuse out of the tubule cells into the filtrate and be excreted. Therefore, reabsorption of Na$^+$ is the overall effect of primary active transport in the tubules.

Following the reabsorption of Na$^+$ via primary active transport, passive reabsorption of water by osmosis occurs, causing water to move from the glomerular filtrate into peritubular capillaries. The movement of water from the filtrate, however, merely increases the concentration of solutes left behind, creating a concentration gradient for ions such as K$^+$, chloride ions (Cl$^-$), and bicarbonate ions (HCO$_3^-$). The concentration gradient, in turn, promotes the reabsorption of such ions into blood vessels via passive diffusion (see Fig. 24–1).

A secondary active transport mechanism called the **Na$^+$-K$^+$-2Cl$^-$ symporter** is responsible for the reabsorption of ions in the loop of the nephron. This symporter is a cotransport system that simultaneously moves one Na$^+$, one K$^+$, and two Cl$^-$ from the glomerular filtrate into the interstitial fluid and the peritubular capillaries (Fig. 24–2). This symporter, like other secondary active transport pumps, depends on the sodium pump to maintain a low Na$^+$ concentration within tubule cells. As explained above, leakage channels allow K$^+$ to pass back into the filtrate; therefore, the net effect of Na$^+$-K$^+$-2Cl$^-$ symporter activity is reabsorption of Na$^+$ and Cl$^-$. Potent diuretics such as *furosemide* inhibit the Na$^+$-K$^+$-2Cl$^-$ symporter, resulting in the excretion of multiple ions and a powerful diuretic effect as water passively "follows" the ions and is eliminated from the body. Mechanisms such as these that promote Cl$^-$ and K$^+$ loss decrease the plasma concentration of chloride ions and potassium ions, leading to acid-base disturbances that

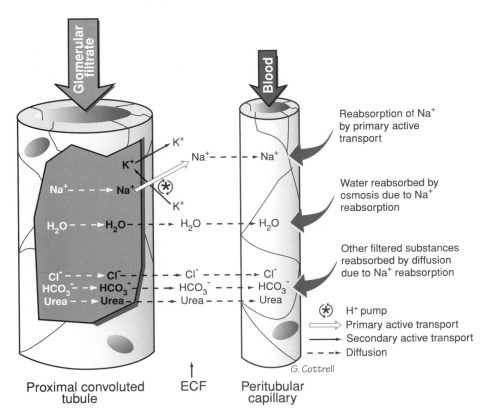

FIGURE 24–1. Primary active transport of Na$^+$ in the proximal convoluted tubule. Note: Reactions occurring in the filtrate are labeled in white; those occurring in the tubule cells are labeled in black. Substances in the filtrate enter tubule cells before being transported to the extracellular fluid and capillaries for reabsorption. (ECF = extracellular fluid; CA = carbonic anhydrase.) (Adapted from Cottrell GP and Surkin HB: Pharmacology for Respiratory Care Practitioners. FA Davis, Philadelphia, 1995, p 277, with permission.)

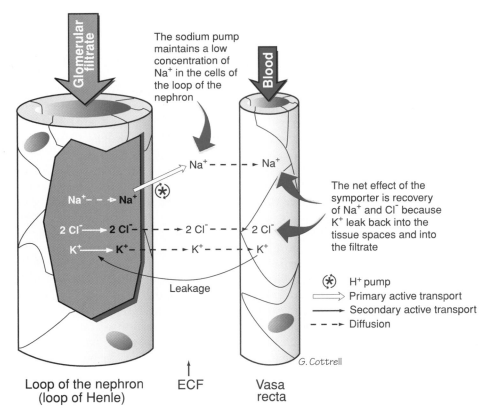

FIGURE 24–2. Na$^+$-K$^+$-2Cl$^-$ symporter in the loop of the nephron. Note: Reactions occurring in the filtrate are labeled in white; those occurring in the tubule cells are labeled in black. Substances in the filtrate enter tubule cells before being transported to the extracellular fluid and capillaries for reabsorption. (ECF = extracellular fluid; CA = carbonic anhydrase.) (Adapted from Cottrell GP and Surkin HB: Pharmacology for Respiratory Care Practitioners. FA Davis, Philadelphia, 1995, p 278, with permission.)

are discussed below. Similarly, mechanisms or conditions that result in elimination of large numbers of Na⁺ may indirectly cause *metabolic alkalosis*. Briefly, metabolic alkalosis, more correctly called *nonrespiratory alkalosis*, may occur when the Na⁺ remaining in the ultrafiltrate exchange for H⁺ via a countertransport mechanism. The hydrogen ions in the filtrate are then excreted, making the urine more acidic and the blood more alkaline.

In the distal portions of the nephron, **Na⁺-Cl⁻ symporters** continue the reabsorption of Na⁺, Cl⁻, and water. As explained previously, diuretic mechanisms that inhibit such symporters promote Cl⁻ depletion, leading to hypochloremia. Inhibition of the Na⁺-Cl⁻ symporters may also cause metabolic alkalosis caused by excessive H⁺ excretion following the reabsorption of large numbers of Na⁺.

Table 24–1 summarizes the percentages of filtered substances reabsorbed in different parts of the nephron.

SECRETION OF ELECTROLYTES AND CONTROL OF BLOOD pH

Although the concentration of K⁺ in the glomerular filtrate is continually changed throughout the tubular system, final adjustments to K⁺ levels in the filtrate are made by the cells of the collecting ducts. At these distal locations, an exchange with Na⁺ occurs. In other words, as the concentration of Na⁺ increases, more K⁺ are secreted into the filtrate to be eliminated with the urine. This mechanism explains why many common diuretics exhibit an unwanted side effect of K⁺ depletion. As mentioned earlier, most diuretics promote water loss from the kidney by inhibiting Na⁺ reabsorption from the filtrate. Once this filtrate reaches the collecting ducts, the high Na⁺ concentration triggers the secretion (and loss) of K⁺ (Cottrell and Surkin, 1995).

The kidney is capable of adjusting urine pH over a wide range (5.0 to 8.0). This broad range of values, in turn, helps maintain normal blood pH within its relatively narrow numeric range (7.35 to 7.45), thus minimizing the disruptive effects of excess acid or base in the bloodstream. Tubule cells regulate blood pH through the secretion of hydrogen ions, the reabsorption of bicarbonate ions, or a combination of the two processes. We now examine these renal mechanisms and their role in homeostasis of blood pH.

First, the tubule cells *acidify* the urine by secreting H⁺ directly into the filtrate by means of a countertransport mechanism. **Na⁺/H⁺ antiporters** are secondary active transport pumps that move one H⁺ into the filtrate in exchange for one Na⁺ that moves into the bloodstream (Fig. 24–3). The hydrogen ions are liberated within tubule cells through the dissociation of carbonic acid (H_2CO_3). Diuretics that inhibit Na⁺ reabsorption produce a filtrate rich in sodium ions that promotes secretion of H⁺ through this countertransport mechanism. As a result of the ion exchange, the urine becomes acidic and the blood pH increases. Such a mechanism may result in *nonrespiratory alkalosis*. Hydrogen ions that enter the filtrate are normally buffered by HCO_3^- to form H_2CO_3. Figure 24–3 shows the pathway whereby HCO_3^- is reabsorbed by the peritubular capillaries.

Within the distal convoluted tubules, H_2CO_3 dissociates into HCO_3^- and H⁺. The hydrogen ions are secreted directly into the filtrate by a primary active transport pump (Fig. 24–4). Normally, most of the H⁺ would simply recombine with HCO_3^- in the filtrate, but recall that nearly all the HCO_3^- has already been reabsorbed. Therefore, H⁺ combine with other buffers present in the filtrate. These H⁺ buffers include ammonia and monohydrogen phosphate. Ammonia (NH_3) is converted to ammonium ion (NH_4^+) by the addition of H⁺ ($NH_3 + H^+ \rightarrow NH_4^+$); monohydrogen phosphate (HPO_4^{2-}) is converted to dihydrogen phosphate ($H_2PO_4^-$) by the addition of H⁺ ($HPO_4^{2-} + H^+ \rightarrow H_2PO_4^-$) (see Fig. 24–4). In the tubule cells, HCO_3^- from the dissociation of H_2CO_3 is reabsorbed through the action of a **HCO_3^-/Cl⁻ antiporter;** therefore, Cl⁻ exchange with HCO_3^- and enter the filtrate to be eliminated from the body (see Fig. 24–4).

TABLE 24-1	**Reabsorption of Filtered Substances**			
Filtered Substance	**Proximal Convoluted Tubule**	**Loop of the Nephron**	**Distal Convoluted Tubule**	**Collecting Ducts**
Na⁺	65%	25%	5%	*
K⁺	50%	40%	5%	*
Cl⁻	50%	25%	20%	*
HCO_3^-	80%–90%	0%	5%	*
Water	65%	15%	15%	*
Nutrients	100%	0%	0%	0%

*Approximately 95% of all filtered solutes have been returned to the bloodstream. Final adjustments are made in the collecting ducts, including fine adjustments to sodium water levels by the action of aldosterone and antidiuretic hormone.

Source: Data from Tortora and Grabowski (1996).

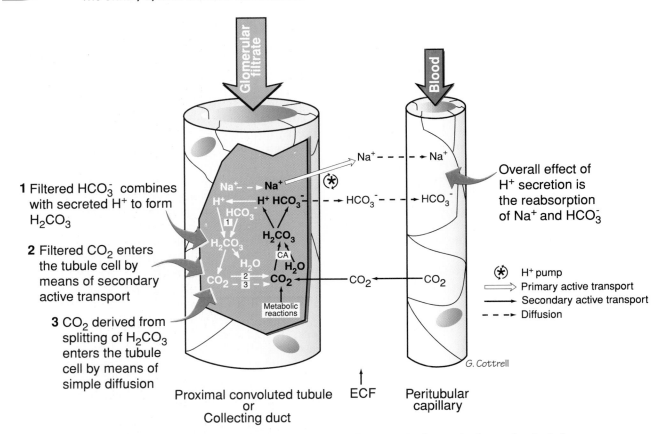

1 Filtered HCO_3^- combines with secreted H^+ to form H_2CO_3

2 Filtered CO_2 enters the tubule cell by means of secondary active transport

3 CO_2 derived from splitting of H_2CO_3 enters the tubule cell by means of simple diffusion

Overall effect of H^+ secretion is the reabsorption of Na^+ and HCO_3^-

(✱) H^+ pump
⟹ Primary active transport
→ Secondary active transport
- - -▸ Diffusion

Metabolic reactions

Proximal convoluted tubule or Collecting duct   ECF   Peritubular capillary

G. Cottrell

FIGURE 24–3. Na^+/H^+ antiporter and reabsorption of the HCO_3^- in the proximal convoluted tubules or collecting ducts. Note: Reactions occurring in the filtrate are labeled in white; those occurring in the tubule cells are labeled in black. Substances in the filtrate enter tubule cells before being transported to the extracellular fluid and capillaries for reabsorption. (ECF = extracellular fluid; CA = carbonic anhydrase.) (Adapted from Cottrell GP and Surkin HB: Pharmacology for Respiratory Care Practitioners. FA Davis, Philadelphia, 1995, p 279, with permission.)

In addition to secretion of hydrogen ions into the glomerular filtrate, tubule cells raise blood pH through the reabsorption of HCO_3^- that has been filtered. Bicarbonate is generated through the dissociation of H_2CO_3, an acid formed when CO_2 from metabolic reactions in the tubule cells or CO_2 in the filtrate combines with H_2O in the presence of carbonic anhydrase (see Fig. 24–3). Thus, for each H_2CO_3 molecule that dissociates, one HCO_3^- can be reabsorbed and one H^+ can be secreted. This dual action allows HCO_3^- to buffer the blood and H^+ to exchange with Na^+ to acidify the urine (see Fig. 24–3).

Through an indirect mechanism, acid-base balance can be disturbed by decreased levels of chloride ions in the blood (*hypochloremia*), and by decreased levels of potassium ions in the blood (*hypokalemia*):

- In conditions of hypochloremia, relatively few Cl^- enter the glomerular filtrate from the bloodstream. Therefore, fewer Cl^- are available for cotransport with Na^+ by the Na^+-K^+-2Cl^- symporter in the

loop of the nephron and the Na^+-Cl^- symporter in the distal parts of the nephron. As a result of the scarcity of Cl^-, large numbers of Na^+ remain in the glomerular filtrate. Recall that the countertransport action of the Na^+/H^+ antiporter in the collecting ducts normally reabsorbs Na^+ and moves H^+ from the bloodstream into the filtrate, acidifying the urine. Thus, hypochloremia indirectly causes *nonrespiratory alkalosis* in the body by promoting the excretion of H^+.

- Through a mechanism very similar to the one associated with hypochloremia, conditions of hypokalemia result in fewer K^+ available for cotransport out of the filtrate with Na^+ by the Na^+-K^+-2Cl^- symporter. Consequently, the Na^+ concentration of the filtrate remains high. In addition, the exchange of Na^+ with K^+ in the collecting ducts decreases because K^+ levels are depressed. The Na^+/H^+ antiporter, as described previously, exchanges large numbers of Na^+ for H^+, thus producing an acidic

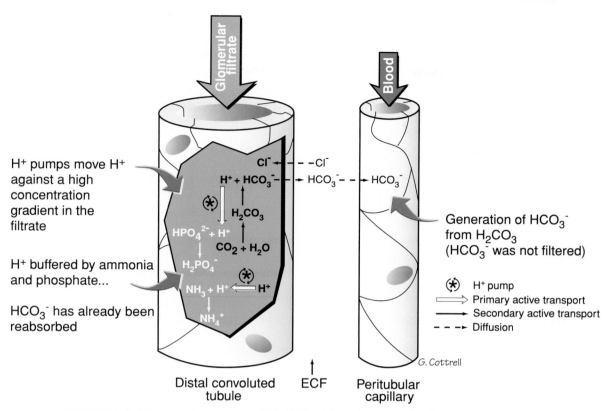

FIGURE 24–4. Primary active transport of H^+, HCO_3^-/Cl^- antiporter, and reabsorption of the HCO_3^- in the distal convoluted tubule. Note: Reactions occurring in the filtrate are labeled in white; those occurring in the tubule cells are labeled in black. Substances in the filtrate enter tubule cells before being transported to the extracellular fluid and capillaries for reabsorption. (ECF = extracellular fluid; CA = carbonic anhydrase.) (Adapted from Cottrell GP and Surkin HB: Pharmacology for Respiratory Care Practitioners. FA Davis, Philadelphia, 1995, p 280, with permission.)

urine and raising blood pH. Therefore, in an indirect way, hypokalemia can bring about *nonrespiratory alkalosis.*

Plasma Buffers

HYDROGEN ION CONCENTRATION

The normal pH of the bloodstream is about 7.40, with a physiologic range of 7.35 to 7.45. This range of pH values is usually perceived as being extremely "narrow." In this section we examine how the blood, lungs, and kidneys work together to maintain the homeostatic range of pH in the plasma. But is a pH range of 7.40 ± 0.05 really all that narrow? To answer this question we must remember two important concepts related to pH: (1) the pH scale is *inverted;* that is, small numerical values on the scale represent large concentrations of hydrogen ions and large numbers represent small concentrations of hydrogen ions; and (2) pH values are points on a *logarithmic scale* representing the hydrogen ion concentration of a solution. The explanation of these concepts follows.

Logarithms are used so that we may work more easily with large ranges of numbers. In the case of hydrogen ion concentration in solutions such as plasma, scientists found that the actual number of hydrogen ions in solution is quite small, typically measured in *billionths* of equivalents of H^+ per liter, or *nano*equivalents per liter (nEq/L). To work conveniently with such unwieldy numbers (1 nEq = 1×10^{-9} Eq), pH was defined as the negative, or inverse, logarithm of the hydrogen ion concentration. Thus:

$$pH = -\log[H^+]$$

Two important goals are accomplished with this definition of pH. First, a large range of values can be represented by using the logarithmic scale. Second, by utilizing the inverse logarithm of the hydrogen ion concentration, the pH value itself is always positive. (As an added "bonus," the awkward scientific notation used with very small numbers is eliminated.) The pH value simply represents the *power,* or *exponent,* to which the base 10 is raised to arrive at the hydrogen ion concentration of the solution, expressed in nEq/L. With this conceptual background in mind, it can be seen that a pH value of 7.6 represents a smaller concentration of H^+ than does a pH value of 7.1.

By convention, the pH scale extends from 0 to 14. Values less than 7.0 on the pH scale are considered acidic; those greater than 7.0 are basic. Keep in mind, however, that the pH scale itself is a *relative* scale, meaning that the acidity or alkalinity of different substances can be compared with each other by comparing their respective pH values. For example, pure distilled water has a pH of 7.0, making it far more acidic than blood, which has a pH of 7.4, even though the value 7.4 is decidedly alkaline on the *overall* pH scale.

The normal pH range (7.35 to 7.45) of arterial blood of a healthy person at sea level represents a much larger difference in the concentration of hydrogen ions than the numerical values suggest (Box 24–1). In fact, the absolute range of pH consistent with human life is about 6.8 to 7.8, representing a 10-fold variation in hydrogen ion concentration (Levitsky, 1995; Mines, 1993). Very few important substances in the plasma exhibit change of this magnitude without causing serious homeostatic upset. In the following section we examine how *plasma buffers, alveolar ventilation,* and changes in *hydrogen ion secretion* and *bicarbonate ion retention* in the kidney operate to minimize the damage to the internal environment that would be caused by large-scale changes in the hydrogen ion concentration of the plasma.

IMPORTANCE OF A STABLE pH ENVIRONMENT

Hydrogen ions are highly reactive and capable of combining with anions as well as with negatively charged regions of large complex molecules such as proteins. When functional groups of important proteins react with H^+, conformational changes in protein structure often occur, resulting in changes in protein activity. Proteins affected by interaction with hydrogen ions include hemoglobin, structural proteins, and enzymes. For example, acidic conditions in the tissues are associated with increased metabolic activity. As we saw in Chapter 13, a decrease in pH resulting from such conditions causes a right shift in the oxyhemoglobin dissociation curve, a phenomenon known as the *Bohr effect.* The cause of the decreased oxygen loading of the hemoglobin molecule is the conformational change in hemoglobin produced by the increase in the concentration of H^+ (Levitsky, 1995). Changes in enzyme activity caused by alterations of pH can be especially damaging because many essential bio-

P E R S P E C T I V E S

BOX 24–1

How Close Is a Blood pH of 7.3 to a Blood pH of 7.6?

With all common *logarithmic scales,* each whole number increment represents a 10-fold change in whatever is being measured. Recall that a logarithm represents the power to which the base 10 is raised. Consider the following example to decide if a small change in a logarithmic value represents a small change in what is actually being measured.

EXAMPLE

The *Richter Scale,* named after the American seismologist Charles Richter (1900–1985), is a logarithmic scale developed by Richter in 1935. It is used to measure the magnitude of the seismic sound waves generated by an earthquake. The scale provides an *indirect way* of comparing the destructive forces generated during earthquakes. An earthquake measuring 7.6 on this scale is almost *twice* as powerful as an earthquake that measures "only" 7.3, as shown by the following calculation.

Earthquake measuring 7.3: $1 \times 10^{7.3} = 19,952,624$

Earthquake measuring 7.6: $1 \times 10^{7.6} = 39,810,717$

Although the force of an earthquake measuring 7.3 on the Richter Scale is capable of causing enormous and widespread destruction in populated areas, the potential for damage is clearly greater with an earthquake measuring 7.6. From this example, it can be seen that small changes in logarithmic measurements—whether of seismic activity or hydrogen ion concentration—are often deceptive!

chemical reactions are totally dependent on an optimal pH environment. When this environment changes significantly, critical reactions may fail, producing an irreversible state that may be incompatible with life. Clearly, maintenance of the pH of body fluids, especially that of the blood, is crucial to our well-being. In the following section we examine several mechanisms designed to maintain the pH of the internal environment.

SOURCES OF ACIDS

Cellular metabolism is responsible for generating large amounts of carbon dioxide (CO_2). The gas is produced as an end-product of the aerobic metabolism of ingested substances such as glucose. In previous chapters we discussed the fate of CO_2 in the tissues and the bloodstream as it is hydrated to form carbonic acid (H_2CO_3). Carbonic acid, in turn, dissociates into a hydrogen ion and a bicarbonate ion:

$$CO_2 + H_2O \leftrightarrow H_2CO_3 \leftrightarrow H^+ + HCO_3^-$$

In the pulmonary capillaries the process reverses; thus CO_2 enters the alveoli and is eliminated via alveolar ventilation. Because H_2CO_3 can be converted to a gas and removed from the body by the lung, it is said to be a **volatile acid.**

Small amounts of **nonvolatile,** or **fixed, acids** are also produced in the tissues during normal cellular metabolism. These fixed acids include *sulfuric acid, phosphoric acid, hydrochloric acid,* and *lactic acid.* Fixed acids may also be ingested or formed during pathophysiologic processes such as *cardiac arrest* or *diabetic ketoacidosis.* The kidneys normally function to remove fixed acids from the body.

ACIDS AND BASES

To discuss the role of the plasma, the lungs, and the kidneys in the maintenance of blood pH, it is useful to review some of the essential terminology associated with acids and bases. This information is usually presented in chemistry courses, introductory physiology courses, or both. The reader is encouraged to consult appropriate texts listed in this chapter's bibliography to review important terms and concepts in further detail, if desired.

Although several different ways exist to describe acids and bases, the most useful definition for physiologic purposes involves the *Brønsted-Lowry theory* of acids (Beachey, 1998; Cottrell and Surkin, 1995; Levitsky, 1995). In this description, an acid is defined as any substance that donates a hydrogen ion (a proton) in aqueous solution. A base is a substance that accepts a proton from another substance. This concept of *proton donor* and *proton acceptor* is helpful in understanding the important reactions involving acids and bases in the body. The *strength* of an acid or a base is related to the extent that the substance dissociates, or ionizes, in solution. The strength of an acid or base has nothing to do with its concentration. A *strong acid* is one that dissociates almost completely into hydrogen ions and its *conjugate base;* whereas, a *weak acid* only slightly dissociates in aqueous solutions.

BUFFERS

A **buffer,** or **buffer system,** is a combination of substances in aqueous solution that resists changes in the hydrogen ion concentration when a strong acid or a strong base is added to the mixture. A buffer pair is generally composed of a weak acid and its conjugate base. The activity of the buffer system results in a small fluctuation in pH but prevents a large change in the pH of a fluid when the solution is exposed to large numbers of either hydrogen ions (H^+) or hydroxyl ions (OH^-). Several different physiologic buffers exist in the body. These typically are buffer pairs that function in the physiologic range of pH values found in the bloodstream. These buffers include *bicarbonate, phosphate,* and *protein,* and are discussed subsequently. The effectiveness of buffers in neutralizing H^+ in solution can be assessed through a determination of the **dissociation constant (K_a) of acid,** a measure of how readily an acid ionizes in aqueous solution.

Consider the following: in aqueous solution, an acid (HA) dissociates into a hydrogen ion (H^+) and its conjugate base, an anion (A^-). Thus:

$$HA \leftrightarrow H^+ + A^-$$

The relationship among the undissociated acid, the hydrogen ions, and the base at equilibrium can be shown by the following ratio:

$$\frac{[H^+][A^-]}{[HA]} = K_a$$

where:
K_a = dissociation constant for acid

This equation can be rearranged in the following way:

$$[H^+] = \frac{K_a[HA]}{[A^-]}$$

The pH can be obtained by taking the logarithm of both sides of the equation and multiplying each side by -1:

$$\log[H^+] = \log K_a + \log \frac{[HA]}{[A^-]}$$

$$-\log[H^+] = -\log K_a + \log \frac{[A^-]}{[HA]}$$

Therefore:

$$pH = pK_a + \log \frac{[A^-]}{[HA]}$$

This relationship is the general form of the classic **Henderson-Hasselbalch equation.** The equation relates the pH of a solution with the pK_a of its dissociated $[A^-]$ and undissociated $[HA]$ components when the system is at equilibrium. Two important considerations follow from the Henderson-Hasselbalch equation:

- For any buffer system, the ratio of dissociated to undissociated forms, $[A^-]/[HA]$, defines a *unique* pH.
- In a solution such as blood that contains several different buffers, the various $[A^-]/[HA]$ ratios must *all* be consistent with the pH of the solution. In other words, all of the buffer pairs are in equilibrium with the same hydrogen ion concentration *and will behave similarly.*

This relationship among buffer pairs is known as the **isohydric principle,** and can be shown by the following example:

$$pH = pK_1 + \log \frac{[A_1^-]}{[HA_1]} = pK_2 + \log \frac{[A_2^-]}{[HA_2]}$$

$$= pK_3 + \log \frac{[A_3^-]}{[HA_3]}$$

With the equivalence of the isohydric principle in mind, it can be seen that assessment of the acid-base status of a fluid sample can be effectively carried out by a detailed analysis of the $[A^-]$ and $[HA]$ of a *single* buffer pair such as the bicarbonate buffer system. With several buffers such as bicarbonate, phosphate, and proteins operating within the bloodstream, why choose to analyze the *bicarbonate/carbonic acid buffer system?* What is special about the pK_a and the ratio of the concentration of HCO_3^- to the concentration of H_2CO_3 that makes this buffer pair the most widely studied *and* the most effective physiologic buffer in the body?

Bicarbonate

Assessment of the acid-base status of the blood is most often carried out through a study of the **bicarbonate buffer system** (HCO_3^-/H_2CO_3). According to Mines (1995), there are at least three reasons for the study of this particular buffer system. First, the members of the buffer pair are present in relatively high concentration in the blood and are, therefore, relatively easy to analyze. Second, metabolism continually adds large quantities of CO_2 to the body; therefore, any dysfunction in the mechanisms that normally remove

CO_2 from the body immediately results in significant acid-base disturbances. Finally, the overall acid-base balance of the body is maintained primarily through regulation of the two members of the buffer pair—the renal system controls the concentration of HCO_3^-, and the respiratory system controls PCO_2 through control of alveolar ventilation. *Conceptually,* the Henderson-Hasselbalch equation can be rewritten to reflect this important fact:

$$pH = pK + \log \frac{[kidneys]}{[lungs]}$$

Clearly, the functional form of the Henderson-Hasselbalch equation has no practical value. However, it can be expressed in a useful *quantitative* form as:

$$pH = pK' + \log \frac{[HCO_3^-]}{[(0.03 \text{ mM/L})/\text{mm Hg}]PCO_2}$$

In this common form of the Henderson-Hasselbalch equation, the numerator has units of *mEq/L* (the concentration of HCO_3^- in plasma), and the denominator has units of *mM/L* (the concentration of CO_2 in plasma). Note also that the **apparent pK (pK')** is specific to this equation that uses the concentration of CO_2 in the denominator rather than the concentration of H_2CO_3. The pK' of this system is 6.1. Why is the concentration of H_2CO_3 not used in this common version of the Henderson-Hasselbalch equation? After all, H_2CO_3 *is* the undissociated form of the solution at equilibrium. The primary reason is that the quantities of undissociated acid (H_2CO_3) in the plasma are normally very small and difficult to analyze (Mines, 1995). However, the equilibrium relationship between CO_2 and H_2CO_3 in the plasma ($CO_2 + H_2O \leftrightarrow H_2CO_3 \leftrightarrow H^+ + HCO_3^-$) is a *quantitative* relationship, allowing us to replace $[H_2CO_3]$ in the denominator of the classic Henderson-Hasselbalch equation with a term composed of $PCO_2 \times$ solubility constant of (0.03 mM/L)/mm Hg. At 37°C, there is about 1000 times as much dissolved CO_2 in the plasma as there is H_2CO_3, but since both the dissolved carbon dioxide and carbonic acid are in equilibrium, they are both treated as undissociated HA in the modified Henderson-Hasselbalch equation (Levitsky, 1995). This consideration applies only to the bicarbonate buffer system. Interestingly, the bicarbonate system functions effectively as a buffer of fixed acids mainly because the lungs, as an *open system,* continually remove CO_2 from the body. In a *closed system,* that is, a system that does not communicate with the external environment, the bicarbonate buffer system is not nearly as effective.

Recall that the normal carbon dioxide tension in arterial blood is approximately 40 mm Hg and that the pK' (apparent pK) of the $[HCO_3^-]/[CO_2]$ system is equal to 6.1. Using a $[HCO_3^-]$ of 24 mEq/L, we can calculate the pH of the arterial blood:

$$pH = pK' + \log \frac{[HCO_3^-]}{[(0.03 \text{ mM/L})/\text{mm Hg}]PCO_2}$$

$$= 6.1 + \log \frac{24 \text{ mEq/L}}{[(0.03 \text{ mM/L})/\cancel{\text{mm Hg}}] \times 40 \cancel{\text{mm Hg}}}$$

$$= 6.1 + \log \frac{24 \text{ mEq/L}}{1.2 \text{ mM/L}}$$

$$= 6.1 + \log 20/1$$

$$\therefore pH = 6.1 + 1.3 = 7.4$$

The pH of this plasma will be 7.4 as long as the ratio of $[HCO_3^-]/[CO_2]$ is 20:1. This relationship is independent of the values of the numerator and denominator and provides a convenient way of assessing arterial blood samples. If the pH of the plasma is 7.4 and the bicarbonate/carbon dioxide concentration ratio is 20:1, the sample is indicative of normal, sea-level arterial blood. On the other hand, an acidic blood sample is characterized by an arterial pH less than 7.4 and a ratio less than 20:1; an alkaline sample is marked by an arterial pH greater than 7.4 and a bicarbonate/carbon dioxide ratio greater than 20:1. **Acidemia** refers to a condition where the pH of the blood sample is less than 7.4, whereas, **alkalemia** exists when the pH of the blood sample is greater than 7.4. **Acidosis** and **alkalosis** are *general* terms referring to acidic and alkaline conditions, respectively, and are often used to describe the acid-base status of the blood.

Phosphate

The **phosphate buffer system** $(H_2PO_4^-/HPO_4^{2-})$ consists of a buffer pair made up of dihydrogen phosphate $(H_2PO_4^-)$ and monohydrogen phosphate (HPO_4^{2-}):

$$H_2PO_4^- \leftrightarrow H^+ + HPO_4^{2-}$$

The pK of the acid form of the buffer is 6.8; therefore, at pH values close to 7.0, the acid form donates a proton, and the base form accepts a proton (Levitsky, 1995).

Proteins

Some proteins in the body possess buffering groups on their amino acids. Collectively, these substances form a **protein buffer system.** The various plasma proteins have pKs ranging from approximately 5.5 to 8.5, thus a large range of buffering capacity is provided by the plasma proteins. Hemoglobin is present in large quantities in the blood, and possesses amino acids having pKs ranging from about 7 to 8 (Levitsky, 1995).

Compensation in Respiratory and Nonrespiratory Disturbances

OVERVIEW OF "PURE" ACID-BASE DISORDERS

Although this text does not focus on pathophysiologic changes affecting body systems, the intimate connection between alveolar ventilation and blood pH, and between renal mechanisms and blood pH, means that abnormalities in either the lungs or the kidneys, or both, may result in significant acid-base disturbances. The acid-base status of normal arterial blood can be changed by altering the amount of volatile and nonvolatile acids in the body. The resulting pH disturbances are classically described as four major categories of acid-base disorders—the so-called pure acid-base disturbances (Table 24–2). In actual fact, "pure" acid-base disorders are rare. More often, acid-base upsets are caused by a mix of different initiating events. For the sake of simplicity, however, single causes are described with the four types of disturbance. In general, *respiratory acidosis* is caused by an increase in the P_{ACO_2}, *respiratory alkalosis* results from a decrease in the P_{ACO_2}, *metabolic acidosis* is caused by the addition of nonvolatile acids, and *metabolic alkalosis* develops when nonvolatile acids are removed from the body. It should be noted that the term "nonrespiratory" is more accurate than the term "metabolic" when describing the addition or removal of acids other than H_2CO_3. Stated another way, some acid-base disturbances involving nonvolatile, or fixed, acids have nothing to do with *metabolism.* For instance, the accumulation of organic acids in the tissues of a person with diabetes during an episode of acute ketoacidosis has the potential to lower the pH of the blood, but is not the result of normal *metabolic* processes. Nevertheless, we will use the term "metabolic" interchangeably with "nonrespiratory" to describe acid-base disturbances that do not initially involve changes in CO_2 and carbonic acid levels.

RESPIRATORY ACIDOSIS AND ALKALOSIS

The hydration of carbon dioxide to form carbonic acid, and the resulting dissociation of the acid into bicarbonate ions and hydrogen ions, immediately affects the pH of the plasma, as shown by the following equation:

$$CO_2 + H_2O \leftrightarrow H_2CO_3 \leftrightarrow H^+ + HCO_3^-$$

$$|\xleftarrow{\hspace{1cm}} A \xrightarrow{\hspace{1cm}}|$$

$$|\xleftarrow{\hspace{1cm}} B \xrightarrow{\hspace{1cm}}|$$

| TABLE 24-2 | Changes in CO_2, H^+, and HCO_3^- Levels during "Pure" Acid-Base Disturbances |

	Change (Stimulus)			Effect on Plasma Components			Compensatory Response		
							Respiratory Compensation	Renal Compensation	
Acid-Base Disturbance	P_{ACO_2}	Volatile Acid (H_2CO_3)	Nonvolatile Acid (e.g., lactic acid)	$[H^+]$	pH	HCO_3^+	Alveolar Ventilation	$NaHCO_3$ Reabsorption	H^+ Secretion
Respiratory Acidosis	↑	↑		↑	↓	↑			
Acute ventilatory failure							↑		
Chronic ventilatory failure								↑	↑
Respiratory Alkalosis	↓	↓		↓	↑	↓			
Acute alveolar hyperventilation							↓		
Chronic alveolar hyperventilation								↓	↓
Nonrespiratory Acidosis			↑	↑	↓	(↓)			
Chronic metabolic acidosis with respiratory compensation							↑	↑	↑
Nonrespiratory Alkalosis			↓	↓	↑	(↑)			
Chronic metabolic alkalosis with respiratory compensation							↓	↓	↓

↓ = Decreased.
↑ = Increased.
(↓) = The decrease in plasma bicarbonate is *less than* the usual response to respiratory acidosis caused by chronic ventilatory failure.
(↑) = The increase in plasma bicarbonate is *greater than* the usual response to respiratory alkalosis caused by chronic alveolar hyperventilation.

It is convenient to view this equilibrium reaction as being made up of a series of two interrelated reactions: Reaction A—the *hydration* of CO_2 to form H_2CO_3; and Reaction B—the *dissociation* of H_2CO_3 to bicarbonate and hydrogen ions. The *law of mass action* describes chemical reactions in equilibrium. Such reactions are affected by variables such as temperature, as well as the concentration of *reactants* and *products* taking part in the reaction. Using the hydration of CO_2 that occurs in the plasma, consider the following examples that illustrate shifts in the equilibrium reaction among the components:

EXAMPLE 1

When the concentration of reactants increases, chemical reactions are driven toward the creation of additional product—in other words, the reaction shifts toward the production of more product to restore the equilibrium among the various components. For example, excess CO_2 combines with water (which is assumed to be unlimited), thus forming a large amount of H_2CO_3. Carbonic acid, therefore, is both the *product* of the hydration reaction (Reaction A), and the *reactant* of the ionization reaction (Reaction B) going "to the right." In the ionization reaction, the increased

concentration of H_2CO_3 acts as excess reactant, thus further driving the equilibrium reaction to the right, and increasing the hydrogen ion concentration in the plasma:

$$CO_2 + H_2O \rightarrow \underset{\text{(excess)}}{H_2CO_3} \rightarrow H^+ + HCO_3^-$$

Respiratory acidosis results from the accumulation of CO_2 as shown in the previous equation. Such a condition is marked by a fall in the pH of the plasma as the hydrogen ion concentration increases (see Table 24–2).

EXAMPLE 2

According to the law of mass action, the removal of product causes a shift in an equilibrium reaction. Because equilibrium reactions shift "to the right" as well as "to the left," we now consider the changes that result when CO_2 is removed from a system that is in equilibrium. As CO_2 product is removed, the reaction shifts to the left to replace the product being exhaled. Of course, the reduction in carbonic acid causes a further leftward shift, resulting in the association of H^+ and HCO_3^- in the plasma. As the two ions combine to replace the carbonic acid being converted into CO_2 and H_2O, the hydrogen ion concentration of the bloodstream decreases:

$$CO_2 + H_2O \leftarrow H_2CO_3 \leftarrow H^+ + HCO_3^-$$
(removal)

Respiratory alkalosis results from the depletion of carbon dioxide as shown above. Such a condition is marked by a rise in the pH of the plasma as the hydrogen ion concentration decreases. Note also the *volatile* nature of H_2CO_3, meaning that it can be converted to CO_2, and subsequently removed from the body as exhaled carbon dioxide.

The following section describes different kinds of acid-base disturbances that result in respiratory acidosis and respiratory alkalosis. Note that in acute disturbances, changes in alveolar ventilation, or *respiratory compensation*, help restore pH homeostasis, whereas in chronic acid-base disturbances, *renal compensation* helps re-establish the normal pH of the bloodstream. Acute changes in ventilation and blood pH are controlled through the central chemoreceptor (hypercapnic drive) mechanism (see Chap. 10). Chronic adjustments to blood pH are brought about through changes in the amount of HCO_3^- reabsorbed by the kidney, and the amount of H^+ secreted by the kidney.

Acute Ventilatory Failure

Respiratory acidosis begins with an increase in the concentration of CO_2, an increase that normally results from a rise in the carbon dioxide tension. **Acute ventilatory failure,** an abrupt decrease in the respiratory minute volume, may be caused by acute hypoventilation. Such a condition accompanies central nervous system (CNS) depressant toxicity resulting from barbiturate or narcotic overdose. The sudden onset of ventilatory failure causes the alveolar ventilation ($\dot{V}A$) to abruptly decline, thus elevating the PA_{CO_2}, Pa_{CO_2}, and P_{CO_2} throughout the body. As a result of these changes, the concentration of CO_2 increases in the tissue fluid, plasma, and elsewhere in the body. Through hydration and ionization, CO_2 molecules form additional H_2CO_3, HCO_3^-, and H^+. Acute changes in H_2CO_3 are more significant than acute changes in HCO_3^-; therefore, the $[HCO_3^-]/[CO_2]$ ratio decreases to a value less than 20:1, thus lowering the pH of the plasma. In cases of respiratory acidosis, the plasma concentrations of CO_2, HCO_3^-, and H^+ are higher than normal, as shown in Table 24–2.

Chronic Ventilatory Failure with Renal Compensation

Prolonged hypoventilation (for more than 24 hours) is indicative of **chronic ventilatory failure,** a condition

that results in respiratory acidosis. In this condition, the kidneys attempt to restore homeostasis by increasing their reabsorption of HCO_3^- from the glomerular filtrate (see Table 24–2). As additional HCO_3^- enters the bloodstream, the buffering capacity of the plasma increases, thus raising the pH back toward normal. Renal compensation accompanying chronic ventilatory failure is responsible for HCO_3^- and pH values that are *greater than* those produced by the usual respiratory response to acidosis.

Renal compensation to a respiratory acid-base disturbance helps restore the normal arterial pH. Although the process of renal compensation helps move the *arterial pH* back toward a "normal" of 7.4, it should be pointed out that the acid-base *disturbance* itself is far from normal. In fact, during renal compensation to a respiratory acidosis, the partial restoration of blood pH toward normal actually moves the $[HCO_3^-]$ further from normal (Mines, 1993). What then, is considered "normal" in these instances?

When discussing compensatory mechanisms in cases of acidosis and alkalosis, many sources describe "partial" or "complete" compensation, meaning that the respiratory or renal compensatory mechanism has partially or completely restored arterial blood pH to a "normal" of 7.4. This accomplishment, while important to the overall stability of the system, is not the same as restoration of the acid-base disturbance to normal. The Pa_{CO_2} as well as the $[HCO_3^-]/[CO_2]$ ratio can be decidedly abnormal in spite of a normal blood pH. Ultimately, the $[HCO_3^-]/[CO_2]$ ratio must be restored to 20:1 to produce an arterial blood pH of 7.4. Assuming the lungs provide adequate ventilation to prevent hypoxia, the kidneys will generate new HCO_3^- over a period of days or weeks, thus raising the $[HCO_3^-]$ and restoring the 20:1 ratio (Mines, 1993).

The kidneys alone cannot completely restore a respiratory acid-base disturbance to normal; that is, complete renal compensation does not occur, even though the arterial blood pH may be restored. A respiratory disturbance can be completely restored to normal only when the ventilatory response restores the P_{CO_2} to normal.

Acute Alveolar Hyperventilation

In **acute alveolar hyperventilation,** or an abrupt increase in the respiratory minute volume, the concentration of CO_2 decreases. Such a change in breathing activity may accompany anxiety. As the CO_2 concentration decreases, so does the carbon dioxide tension. The decline in PA_{CO_2}, in turn, causes a decrease in the Pa_{CO_2}, thus causing depletion of more H_2CO_3 as the equilibrium reaction shifts to the left. This shift causes more HCO_3^- and H^+ to associate into H_2CO_3. The resulting decrease in plasma $[HCO_3^-]$ and $[H^+]$ raises the pH of the bloodstream, causing respiratory alkalosis. As pointed out previously, acute changes in the levels of H_2CO_3 are more significant than acute changes in the levels of HCO_3^-. In the case of acute alveolar hyperventilation, the $[HCO_3^-]/[CO_2]$ ratio increases to a value greater than 20:1, and the blood becomes alkalotic (pH greater than 7.4). The rise in pH causes a decrease in medullary chemoreceptor activity; that is, respiratory compensation in cases of acute respiratory alkalosis takes the form of reduced rate and depth of breathing to restore pH homeostasis in the short term (see Table 24–2).

Chronic Alveolar Hyperventilation with Renal Compensation

Hyperventilation persisting for more than 24 hours is termed **chronic alveolar hyperventilation,** a condition that results in respiratory alkalosis. The kidneys attempt to correct the increased pH of the plasma by excreting additional HCO_3^- from the body (see Table 24–2). As HCO_3^- leaves the bloodstream, the buffering capacity of the plasma decreases, lowering the pH back toward the homeostatic range.

NONRESPIRATORY ACIDOSIS AND ALKALOSIS

Chronic Metabolic Acidosis with Respiratory Compensation

When the accumulation of hydrogen ions from nonrespiratory sources exceeds the buffering capacity of the plasma, a state of *nonrespiratory acidosis* exists. Because the accumulation of hydrogen ions often occurs over time, the condition is considered *chronic,* compared to the *acute* changes associated with minute-to-minute fluctuations in carbon dioxide partial pressure and concentration. Thus, the condition is referred to as **chronic metabolic acidosis** or **chronic nonrespiratory acidosis.** The concentration of H^+ in the tissues and the bloodstream builds up as the production of fixed acids increases, overwhelming the plasma buffers. It should be pointed out that the rise in hydrogen ion concentration occurs rapidly once the buffering capability of the bloodstream is surpassed, resulting in an abrupt fall in pH.

The accumulation of H^+ from fixed acid sources can result from either normal metabolic processes or from abnormal disease processes. It is for this reason that the term "nonrespiratory" is preferred over "metabolic" when describing acid-base disturbances that are not CO_2-induced. For example, lactic acid temporarily accumulates in the muscles as a result of normal *metabolic* processes associated with strenuous exercise. On the other hand, conditions such as cardiac arrest result in the tissue accumulation of acidic by-products of anaerobic metabolism, including lactic acid and pyruvic acid.

Severe diarrhea results in the massive loss of both fluid and electrolytes from the intestine, including the loss of a large quantity of sodium bicarbonate ($NaHCO_3$), an important buffer required for the normal functioning of pancreatic and intestinal enzymes. With the loss of $NaHCO_3$ the overall acid-buffering capacity of the body is reduced, resulting in acidosis. Clearly, a rise in H^+ concentration can be the result of processes that are not truly "metabolic." In spite of this conceptual limitation, the term "metabolic" is commonly used to describe acidotic conditions that are not the result of CO_2 excess.

Conditions of "pure" metabolic acidosis and alkalosis do not exist in subjects having a normal respiratory response to changing H^+ concentration. Changes in ventilation rapidly occur, resulting in a degree of respiratory compensation. The change in ventilation and the resulting change in P_{CO_2} move the pH back *toward* normal; that is, the respiratory system partially compensates for the metabolic acid-base disturbance. As discussed with renal compensation to respiratory acidosis, the process of respiratory compensation to metabolic acidosis helps push the arterial pH back toward a "normal" of 7.4, but the arterial acid-base status itself is decidedly abnormal. During respiratory compensation to a metabolic acidosis, there is an immediate increase in alveolar ventilation as the blood pH decreases (see Table 24–2). The increase in ventilatory rate lowers the Pa_{CO_2}, thus moving the blood pH back toward normal, and offsetting the metabolic acidosis. The partial restoration of blood pH toward normal moves the $[HCO_3^-]$ even further from normal. Respiratory compensation to a metabolic acid-base disturbance cannot restore the system to normal—such restoration requires the action of the kidney (Mines, 1993).

During such compensation, the kidney secretes additional H^+ to reduce the concentration of fixed acids, thus raising the blood pH. Urine pH can decrease from a high of 8 to as low as 5 under such conditions, representing a 1000-fold increase in H^+ concentration. The kidney also increases the reabsorption of $NaHCO_3$, thus augmenting the buffering capacity of the plasma.

Chronic Metabolic Alkalosis with Respiratory Compensation

The depletion of H^+ or the build-up of base from nonrespiratory sources, that is, from sources unrelated to a decrease in the P_{CO_2} level, may exceed the buffering capacity of the plasma, causing the arterial pH to increase. When this condition occurs, a state of *nonrespiratory alkalosis* is said to exist. Because the accumulation of base or the elimination of H^+ may occur over time, the condition is considered *chronic,* compared with rapid changes in pH brought about by *acute* changes in carbon dioxide partial pressure and concentration. The term, **chronic metabolic alkalosis** or

chronic nonrespiratory alkalosis, is used to describe this type of acid-base disturbance.

Nonrespiratory alkalosis describes acid-base disturbances whereby the blood pH is elevated by conditions that do not involve CO_2. These conditions include *hypokalemia, hypochloremia, vomiting,* and the *administration of sodium bicarbonate.* A decreased plasma concentration of potassium or chloride ions may lead to an alkalotic condition in the bloodstream, as described previously.

Severe vomiting (emesis) or prolonged gastric suctioning depletes hydrogen ions through the removal of gastric juice. This fluid contains large amounts of hydrochloric acid (HCl); therefore, its loss from the body upsets the acid-base balance, elevating the pH of the bloodstream. Finally, administration of $NaHCO_3$ carries with it the risk for producing metabolic alkalosis because the bicarbonate ion (HCO_3^-) is an effective buffer of H^+ wherever they are found, thus effectively raising the pH. Clearly, the causes of metabolic alkalosis briefly outlined previously are independent of the partial pressure of carbon dioxide in the bloodstream. How is normal blood pH restored under such alkalotic conditions?

The normal compensatory response to nonrespiratory (metabolic) alkalosis involves an immediate decrease in alveolar ventilation, mediated through the central respiratory control mechanism (see Table 24–2). The decrease in ventilatory rate increases the Pa_{CO_2} and H^+ concentration. This change helps shift the blood pH back toward normal, thus offsetting metabolic alkalosis. During alkalotic conditions, the kidney compensates by secreting fewer H^+, thus raising the urine pH and lowering the blood pH. The kidney also decreases the reabsorption of $NaHCO_3$. As a result of this mechanism, $NaHCO_3$ is eliminated with the urine, thereby reducing the acid-buffering capability of the plasma. In general, during conditions of chronic metabolic alkalosis accompanied by respiratory compensation, both the HCO_3^- and pH values are higher than those produced by the usual response to alkalosis.

COMPENSATORY MECHANISMS— SIMILARITIES AND DIFFERENCES

Certain similarities and differences exist between the two types of compensation—renal and respiratory. For example, both renal compensation and respiratory compensation push $[HCO_3^-]$ further from normal during the process of restoring blood pH toward normal. The renal compensation to respiratory acid-base disturbances is much slower than the respiratory compensation to metabolic acid-base disturbances, taking days or weeks to reach completion (Mines, 1993). In contrast, respiratory compensation occurs almost immediately.

The two mechanisms also differ in their relative abilities to restore the arterial pH completely to normal. For instance, renal compensation can restore the pH completely to normal, whereas respiratory compensation only partially restores pH back to normal.

Summary

The focus of this chapter was the reinforcement of the functional relationships that exist among the respiratory, cardiovascular, and renal systems. Some of these relationships were introduced in previous chapters. Because the text has consistently emphasized preclinical and preparatory topics, this chapter did not provide *in-depth* coverage of related pathophysiologic and clinical topics such as acute and chronic renal failure, differential diagnosis of acid-base disturbances, or the treatment of mixed acid-base disturbances. Instead, it provided a detailed examination of active transport pumps operating in the kidney tubule cells and a brief review of acids, bases, and buffers. This essential information was followed by an introduction to compensation mechanisms involved in respiratory and nonrespiratory acid-base disturbances, and a discussion of the role played by various processes in the maintenance of blood pH. Armed with this basic knowledge of renal function, the reader can more easily master the technical application of the information in the clinical setting.

BIBLIOGRAPHY

Beachey W: Respiratory Care Anatomy and Physiology: Foundations for Clinical Practice. Mosby–Year Book, St. Louis, 1998.

Cottrell GP and Surkin HB: Pharmacology for Respiratory Care Practitioners. FA Davis, Philadelphia, 1995.

Des Jardins T: Cardiopulmonary Anatomy and Physiology: Essentials for Respiratory Care, ed 3. Delmar Publishers, Albany, NY, 1998.

Ganong WF: Review of Medical Physiology, ed 17. Appleton & Lange, Norwalk, CT, 1995.

Guyton AC and Hall JE: Textbook of Medical Physiology, ed 9. WB Saunders, Philadelphia, 1996.

Levitzky MG: Pulmonary Physiology, ed 4. McGraw-Hill, New York, 1995.

Malley WJ: Clinical Blood Gases: Application and Noninvasive Alternatives. WB Saunders, Philadelphia, 1990.

Mines AH: Respiratory Physiology, ed 3. Raven Press, New York, 1993.

Shapiro BA, Peruzzi WT, and Kozelowski-Templin R: Clinical Application of Blood Gases, ed 5. Mosby–Year Book, St. Louis, 1994.

Tortora GJ and Grabowski SR: Principles of Anatomy and Physiology, ed 8. HarperCollins, New York, 1996.

West JB: Respiratory Physiology: The Essentials, ed 6. Williams & Wilkins, Baltimore, 1998.

Cardiopulmonary Physiology—Symbols and Abbreviations

The following groupings and subgroupings into primary symbols and secondary modifiers, along with the symbols and abbreviations used in spirometry, are consistent with the approved nomenclature of the Committee on Respiratory Physiology of the International Union of Physiological Sciences (IUPS). Main symbols are usually capital letters set on the line with modifiers set as lowercase letters or as small capitals, as in $PaCO_2$, which stands for *partial pressure of carbon dioxide, arterial*. Note that a dot placed above a letter indicates flow, and that the same letter may refer to one entity in pulmonary mechanics, another in gas exchange, and in some cases, different entities. For example, capital C stands for *compliance, capacity,* or *closing* in pulmonary mechanics and for *concentration* or *content* in the context of gas exchange. The other symbols and abbreviations listed in the appendix are derived from a variety of cardiopulmonary physiology sources (see references).

General Symbols and Measurements

cm H_2O	centimeters of water pressure
mm Hg	millimeters of mercury pressure
P	partial pressure, pressure (gas or blood)
$\overline{X}$	dash above a symbol indicates mean value
$\dot{X}$	dot above a symbol indicates volume per unit time
f	frequency per unit time
[x]	square brackets around symbol indicate concentration

Primary Gas Symbols— Capital Letters

P	partial pressure; gas tension; pressure
V	volume
$\dot{V}$	gas flow rate (volume per unit time, as in L/min)
F	fractional concentration in a dry gas, FGAS (expressed as a decimal fraction)

Secondary Gas Symbols— Small-Capital Modifiers of the Primary Symbol*

A	alveolar
B, BAR	barometric
D	dead space
E	expired, expiratory
ET	end-tidal
I	inspired, inspiratory
L	lung
T	tidal

Primary Blood Symbols— Capital Letters

C	content
Q	volume of blood
$\dot{Q}$	perfusion, blood flow (volume of blood per unit time)
S	saturation (decimal fraction or percentage)

Secondary Blood Symbols— Lowercase Modifiers of the Primary Symbol†

a	arterial
b	blood, in general

*Not subscript, e.g., PB = barometric pressure
†Not subscript

c   capillary
c′   pulmonary end-capillary
i   ideal
max   maximum
v   venous
$\bar{v}$ mixed venous

Gas Abbreviations*

CO   carbon monoxide
CO_2 carbon dioxide
H_2O water vapor
N_2 nitrogen
O_2 oxygen

Pulmonary Function Testing/Spirometry

CC   closing capacity
CV   closing volume
ERV   expiratory reserve volume
$FEF_{25\%-75\%}$ forced expiratory flow, midexpiratory phase; the average flow during the middle 50% of the FVC (formerly known as the midexpiratory flow rate [MEFR])
$FEF_{200-1200}$ forced expiratory flow between 200 and 1200 mL of FVC
FEV   forced expiratory volume
FEV_1 forced expiratory volume in 1 second; forced expiratory volume in the first second
FEV_1/FVC   percentage of the FVC exhaled in the first second
FRC   functional residual capacity
FVC   forced vital capacity
IRV   inspiratory reserve volume
IVC   inspiratory vital capacity
MVV   maximum voluntary ventilation; ventilatory capacity
PEF, PEFR   peak expiratory flow rate
RV   residual volume
TLC   total lung capacity
VC   vital capacity

Volumes and Ventilation

R   respiratory exchange ratio (carbon dioxide elimination divided by oxygen uptake)
RQ   metabolic respiratory quotient (carbon dioxide production divided by oxygen consumption)

*Appear as the last element of the symbol, usually as small capitals, but may occasionally appear as subscript

VA   alveolar volume
$\dot{V}A$ alveolar ventilation
$\dot{V}_{CO_2}$ carbon dioxide production per minute
VD   dead space volume
$\dot{V}D$ anatomical dead space ventilation
$\dot{V}E$ minute ventilation; minute volume; total ventilation
$\dot{V}_{O_2}$ oxygen consumption per minute

Pulmonary Mechanics

P_{alv}, PA   alveolar pressure
P_{aw} airway pressure
P_{bs} pressure at the body surface (usually atmospheric pressure, PB)
P_m mouth pressure
P_{pl} pleural pressure; intrapleural pressure
P_{ta} transairway pressure
P_{tp} transpulmonary pressure
P_{tt} transthoracic pressure
Re   Reynold's number
T_C time constant
WOB   work of breathing

Flow, Pressure, Volume, and Diffusion Relationships

C   compliance (volume/pressure)
C_{cw} chest wall compliance
C_L lung compliance
C_{dyn} dynamic lung compliance
C_{st} static lung compliance
C/FRC   specific lung compliance
DLCO   diffusing capacity of the lung for carbon monoxide (mL/min per mm Hg)
E   elastance (pressure/volume)
R   resistance (pressure/flow)
R_{aw} airway resistance

Blood Contents

Ca_{O_2} arterial oxygen content (mL/dL)
$C(a-\bar{v})_{O_2}$ arterial-mixed venous oxygen content difference
Cc'_{O_2} pulmonary end-capillary oxygen content (mL/dL)
$C\bar{v}_{O_2}$ mixed venous oxygen content (mL/dL)
HCO_3^- blood bicarbonate ion concentration (mEq/L)
pH   potency of hydrogen, a measure of the hydrogen ion concentration ($pH = -\log[H^+]$)

Blood Gases

The main symbols and modifiers are combined to derive common terms used in cardiopulmonary physiology, as shown by the following examples:

$P(A\text{-}a)O_2$	alveolar-arterial oxygen tension gradient
PAO_2	partial pressure of oxygen, alveolar (alveolar oxygen tension)
PaO_2	partial pressure of oxygen, arterial (arterial oxygen tension)
$PACO_2$	partial pressure of carbon dioxide, alveolar (alveolar carbon dioxide tension)
$PaCO_2$	partial pressure of carbon dioxide, arterial (arterial carbon dioxide tension)
$P\bar{v}O_2$	partial pressure of oxygen, mixed venous (mixed venous oxygen tension)
$P\bar{v}CO_2$	partial pressure of carbon dioxide, mixed venous (mixed venous carbon dioxide tension)
$Pc'O_2$	partial pressure of oxygen, pulmonary end-capillary (pulmonary end-capillary oxygen tension)
SaO_2	arterial oxygen saturation
SpO_2	oxygen saturation as measured by pulse oximetry
$S\bar{v}O_2$	mixed venous oxygen saturation

Ventilation-Perfusion Relationships

$\dot{V}A/\dot{Q}$	alveolar ventilation divided by blood flow (expressed as a decimal fraction such as 0.8); ventilation-perfusion ratio
$\dot{Q}s$	shunted cardiac output
$\dot{Q}T$	total cardiac output
$\dot{Q}s/\dot{Q}T$	shunt fraction or shunted cardiac output ratio (fraction of the cardiac output perfusing non-ventilated regions of the lung)
VD/VT	dead space to tidal volume ratio; dead space fraction (fraction of the tidal volume ventilating nonperfused regions of lung)

Hemodynamic Measurements—Direct

BP	blood pressure (assume systemic pressure unless stated otherwise)
C.O., $\dot{Q}$	cardiac output (total cardiac output, $\dot{Q}T$, is also used)
CVP	central venous pressure
EDP	end-diastolic pressure
EDV	end-diastolic volume
ESP	end-systolic pressure
ESV	end-systolic volume
HR	heart rate
MAP	mean arterial pressure (assume systemic pressure unless stated otherwise)
MPAP	mean pulmonary artery pressure
PAP	pulmonary artery pressure
PCWP	pulmonary capillary wedge pressure
RAP	right atrial pressure

Hemodynamic Measurements—Derived

Measurements that include an *index* are based on a calculation of body surface area, or BSA, as in CI = C.O./BSA.

CI	cardiac index
LVSW	left ventricular stroke work
LVSWI	left ventricular stroke work index
PVR	pulmonary vascular resistance
PVRI	pulmonary vascular resistance index
RVSW	right ventricular stroke work
RVSWI	right ventricular stroke work index
SV	stroke volume
SVI	stroke volume index
SVR	systemic vascular resistance
SVRI	systemic vascular resistance index

Gas Measurements

ATPD	gas at ambient temperature and pressure, dried
ATPS	gas at ambient temperature and pressure, saturated with water vapor
BTPD	gas at body temperature and pressure, dried
BTPS	gas at body temperature and pressure, saturated with water vapor

Starling Forces

π_c	plasma colloidal osmotic pressure; plasma colloidal oncotic pressure
π_i	interstitial fluid colloidal osmotic pressure; interstitial fluid colloidal oncotic pressure
P_c	capillary pressure; capillary hydrostatic pressure
P_i	interstitial fluid hydrostatic pressure

Other Useful Symbols and Abbreviations

2,3-DPG	2,3-diphosphoglycerate
$\alpha_1\text{-AT}$	α_1-antitrypsin; α_1-protease inhibitor (α_1-PI)

ACE	angiotensin-converting enzyme	JGA	juxtaglomerular apparatus
ACh	acetylcholine	L:S	lecithin:sphingomyelin ratio
ADH	antidiuretic hormone	LT	leukotriene
ALS	amyotrophic lateral sclerosis	LA	left atrium
ANP	atrial natriuretic peptide; atriopeptin	LV	left ventricle
ANS	autonomic nervous system	MG	myasthenia gravis
AP	action potential	MI	myocardial infarction
A-P	anterior-posterior	NANC	nonadrenergic noncholinergic
ATP	adenosine triphosphate	NE	norepinephrine
AV	atrioventricular	NCF-A	neutrophil chemotactic factor of anaphylaxis
BSA	body surface area		
BMR	basal metabolic rate	NFP	net filtration pressure
bpm	beats per minute	P_{50}	partial pressure of oxygen at 50% hemoglobin saturation
CD	collecting duct		
CF	cystic fibrosis		
CHF	congestive heart failure	PAF	platelet-activation factor
CNS	central nervous system	PCT	proximal convoluted tubule
COP	colloid osmotic pressure	PFT	pulmonary function testing
COPD	chronic obstructive pulmonary disease	PRG	pontine respiratory group
CPG	central pattern generator	PG	prostaglandin
CSF	cerebrospinal fluid	RA	right atrium
CVA	cerebral vascular accident	RAR	rapidly adapting receptor; irritant receptor
DCT	distal convoluted tubule	RBC	red blood cell
DRG	dorsal respiratory group	RMP	resting membrane potential
ECF-A	eosinophil chemotactic factor of anaphylaxis	RV	right ventricle
		SA	sinoatrial
ECG, EKG	electrocardiogram	SL	semilunar
ECMO	extracorporeal membrane oxygenation	SRG	spinal respiratory group
		ST	surface tension
EPO	erythropoietin	SVC	superior vena cava
GFR	glomerular filtration rate	VRG	ventral respiratory group
Hb	hemoglobin	WBC	white blood cell
HbA	adult hemoglobin		
HbCO	carboxyhemoglobin		
$HbCO_2$	carbaminohemoglobin		
HbF	fetal hemoglobin		
HbS	sickle cell hemoglobin		
Hbmet	methemoglobin		
Hct	hematocrit		
HMD	hyaline membrane disease		
IVC	inferior vena cava		

- American Medical Association Manual of Style, ed 8. Williams & Wilkins, Baltimore, 1989.
- Beachey W: Respiratory Care Anatomy and Physiology: Foundations for Clinical Practice. Mosby–Year Book, St. Louis, 1998.
- Guyton AC and Hall JE: Textbook of Medical Physiology, ed 9. WB Saunders, Philadelphia, 1996.
- West JB: Respiratory Physiology: The Essentials, ed 6. Williams & Wilkins, Baltimore, 1998.

DuBois Body Surface Area Chart

Nomogram for the Assessment of Body Surface Area*

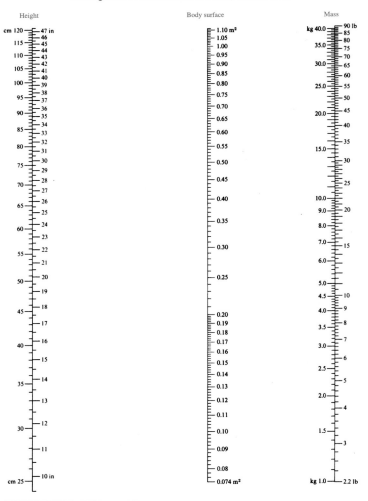

Source: Lentner, C (ed): Geigy Scientific Tables, ed 8. Ciba Geigy, Basle, Switzerland, 1981.

*The body surface area is given by the point of intersection with the middle scale of a straight line joining height and weight.

APPENDIX B–1. Nomogram for the assessment of body surface area. (From: Lentner, C (ed): Geigy Scientific Tables, ed. 8. Ciba Geigy, Basle, Switzerland, 1981. As published in Thomas, CL (ed): Taber's Cyclopedic Medical Dictionary, ed. 18. FA Davis, Philadelphia, 1997, pp 246–247, with permission.) (*continued*)

Nomogram for the Assessment of Body Surface Area* (Continued)

Height	Body surface	Mass
cm 200 — 79 in	2.80 m²	kg 150 — 330 lb
78	2.70	145 — 320
195 — 77		140 — 310
76	2.60	135 — 300
190 — 75		130 — 290
74	2.50	— 280
185 — 73		125 — 270
72	2.40	120 — 260
180 — 71		115 — 250
70	2.30	110 — 240
175 — 69	2.20	105 — 230
68		100 — 220
170 — 67	2.10	95 — 210
66		
165 — 65	2.00	90 — 200
64	1.95	85 — 190
160 — 63	1.90	80 — 180
62	1.85	
155 — 61	1.80	75 — 170
60	1.75	70 — 160
150 — 59	1.70	65 — 150
58	1.65	60 — 140
145 — 57	1.60	
56	1.55	55 — 130
140 — 55	1.50	50 — 120
54	1.45	
135 — 53	1.40	45 — 110
52	1.35	40 — 100
130 — 51	1.30	35 — 90
50	1.25	30 — 80

*The body surface area is given by the point of intersection with the middle scale of a straight line joining height and weight.

APPENDIX B–1. (*continued*)

abdominothoracic pump mechanism SEE: respiratory pump.

accessory expiratory group Respiratory muscles used when ventilatory effort is increased beyond normal, resting values. These respiratory muscles bring about expiration by (1) assisting the upward movement of the diaphragm as it relaxes (e.g., abdominal group) or (2) actively moving the ribs downward and inward to decrease the thoracic volume (e.g., internal intercostal group).

accessory inspiratory group Respiratory muscles used when ventilatory effort is increased beyond normal, resting values. These respiratory muscles assist the inspiratory effort of the diaphragm to bring about inspiration by (1) elevating the ribs to increase the lateral diameter of the thorax or (2) moving the sternum forward to increase the anteroposterior (A-P) diameter of the thorax. Accessory inspiratory muscles include the external intercostal group, internal intercostals–interchondral parts, levator costae, pectoralis major, pectoralis minor, scalenus, serratus anterior, sternocleidomastoids, subcostals, and trapezius.

acidemia A condition in which the blood pH is less than 7.4.

acidosis A general term referring to acidic conditions; often used to describe the acid-base status of the blood.

acinus (as' i-nus) singular; **acini** (as' i-n ī) plural 1. The smallest division of a gland; a group of secretory cells surrounding a cavity. 2. The terminal respiratory gas exchange unit of the lung, composed of airways and alveoli distal to a terminal bronchiole. SYN: primary lobule; terminal respiratory unit.

acquired resistance The development of specific antibodies to offending substances called antigens. Resistance develops as a result of initial exposure ("sensitizing dose"); subsequent exposure to the same antigen ("shocking dose") results in the rapid production of large numbers of antibodies and an antigen-antibody reaction that neutralizes the offending substance.

active expiration SEE: triphasic pattern of breathing.

active transport pump A mechanism that transfers electrolytes through cell membranes against concentration gradients. The following active transport pumps operate in different parts of the nephron:

Na⁺/K⁺ pump The primary active transport pump in kidney tubule cells; the mechanism moves sodium ions into the extracellular fluid and potassium ions into the intracellular fluid, thus establishing concentration gradients across the cell membrane.

Na⁺-Cl⁻ symporter A secondary active transport mechanism that operates in the distal portions of the nephron to cotransport one sodium ion and one chloride ion from the glomerular filtrate into the interstitial fluid and peritubular capillaries surrounding the loops.

Na⁺/K⁺-2Cl⁻ symporter A secondary active transport mechanism that operates in the loop of the nephron to cotransport one sodium ion, one potassium ion, and two chloride ions from the glomerular filtrate into the interstitial fluid and peritubular capillaries surrounding the loops.

Na⁺/H⁺antiporter A secondary active transport mechanism that countertransports one sodium ion and one hydrogen ion. The secondary active transport pumps move one H^+ into the filtrate in exchange for one Na^+ that moves into the bloodstream.

HCO₃⁻/Cl⁻ antiporter A secondary active transport mechanism that countertransports one bicarbonate ion and one chloride ion. The secondary active transport pumps move one Cl^- into the filtrate in exchange for one HCO_3^- that moves into the bloodstream.

acute alveolar hyperventilation A condition characterized by an abrupt increase in the respiratory minute ventilation, and a decrease in carbon dioxide concentration.

acute ventilatory failure An abrupt decrease in the respiratory minute ventilation caused by conditions such as acute hypoventilation.

adenoid (ad' e-noyd) Lymphoid tissue forming a prominence on the roof of the posterior superior wall of the nasopharynx. SYN: pharyngeal tonsil (far in' jē al).

adrenergic receptors Cell membrane receptors activated by noradrenaline (norepinephrine) and catecholaminelike chemical messengers; antagonized by specific adrenergic-blocking agents. SYN: adrenoreceptors.

α₁-adrenergic receptors When activated, these postjunctional adrenoceptors trigger an "excitatory" change in effectors (e.g., vasoconstriction). SYN: α_1-adrenoceptors.

β₁-adrenergic receptors These postjunctional adrenoceptors are found primarily on cardiac muscle cell membranes; when activated, they trigger an increase in the heart rate (positive chronotropism), an increase in the force of contraction (positive inotropism), and an increase in conduction velocity (positive dromotropism). SYN: β_1-adrenoceptors.

β₂-adrenergic receptors When activated, these postjunctional adrenoceptors trigger an "inhibitory" change in effectors (e.g., vasodilation). SYN: β_2-adrenoceptors.

adrenoreceptors SEE: adrenergic receptors.

afferent arteriole A small branch of the interlobular arteries within the kidney. Afferent arterioles convey a large volume of blood under relatively high pressure toward the glomerulus of the nephrons. SEE: glomerulus.

air vesicle SEE: alveolus.

airway resistance (R_aw) A measurement of resistance in a conducting passage calculated by dividing the transairway pressure (mouth pressure minus alveolar pressure) by the flowrate of the gas.

alar cartilages (a' lar) Wing-shaped cartilages (greater and lesser alar cartilages) forming the broad lateral wall of each nostril.

aldosterone Adrenocortical steroid hormone that promotes the reabsorption of sodium ions and the retention of water. Aldosterone release is caused by the presence of angiotensin II. SEE: angiotensin II.

alkalemia A blood condition in which the pH is greater than 7.4.

alkalosis A general term referring to alkaline conditions; often used to describe the acid-base status of the blood.

allergen SEE: antigen.

α₁-antitrypsin A low-molecular-weight glycoprotein that inhibits proteolytic enzymes such as neutrophil elastase. Deficiency of α_1-antitrypsin in the serum is associated with early-onset emphysema in some patients. SYN: α_1-protease inhibitor. SEE: neutrophil elastase (NE).

alveolar-arterial oxygen tension gradient [P(A-a)o₂] The difference between alveolar and arterial partial pressures of oxygen. The value is the difference between the theoretical and actual values for oxygen tension and is calculated by subtracting the arterial value from the ideal alveolar value obtained from the ideal alveolar oxygen equation. SEE: ideal alveolar oxygen equation.

alveolar-capillary membrane The structures and substances through which gases must pass as they diffuse from air to blood (oxygen) or blood to air (carbon dioxide). These include the alveolar fluid and surfactant, cell of the alveolar wall, interstitial space (tissue fluid), and cell of the capillary wall. SYN: respiratory membrane.

alveolar dead space The volume of gas entering alveoli that are underperfused or unperfused.

alveolar duct A branch of a respiratory bronchiole that leads to the alveolar sacs of the lungs. Alveolar ducts are composed entirely of alveoli.

alveolar macrophage A macrophage is a monocyte that has left the circulation and settled and matured in a tissue. Along with neutrophils, macrophages are the major phagocytic cells of the immune system. Alveolar macrophages reside in the alveoli of the lung, where they ingest foreign material that has evaded clearance mechanisms in the proximal parts of the respiratory system.

alveolar period The final period in the development of the tracheobronchial tree, characterized by final structural development of the respiratory zone of the immature lung. It extends from approximately 24 weeks to birth at 38 to 41 weeks; however, alveoli continue to form for approximately 8 years. SYN: terminal sac period.

alveolar pressure (P_alv, P_a) The pressure at the distal end of the conducting "tube" of the airways.

alveolar sac The terminal portion of an air passageway within the lung. Its wall is made of simple squamous epithelium and is surrounded by pulmonary capillaries. This is the site of gas exchange. Each alveolar sac is connected to a respiratory bronchiole by an alveolar duct.

alveolar septal capillaries Pulmonary capillaries located in the walls of alveoli, with a large surface area relative to their volume. Alveolar septal capillaries are affected by the degree of stretch of the alveoli and by the pressure within the capillaries. Any decrease in pressure inside the alveolar septal capillaries, or increase in pressure outside them, occludes the vessels, increases the pulmonary vascular resistance, and reduces pulmonary perfusion.

NOTE: The lung effects responsible for dilation and constriction of alveolar septal capillaries produce *opposing* effects in extra-alveolar blood vessels.

alveolar ventilation (V̇A) That portion of the minute ventilation reaching alveoli involved in gas exchange. SEE: minute ventilation.

alveolus (al-vē′ ō-lus) singular; **alveoli** (al-vē′ ō-ī) plural. One of the terminal saccules of an alveolar duct where gases are exchanged in respiration. SYN: air vesicle.

anastomosis (a-nas″ tō-mō′ sis) A natural communication between blood vessels, either directly or by means of connecting channels. Various anastomoses in coronary circulation provide collateral circulatory routes so that blood can reach a particular part of the heart through alternate pathways.

anatomical dead space ventilation (VD) The portion of minute ventilation that does not contribute to alveolar ventilation. The value can be calculated as (1) the product of dead space volume and respiratory rate or (2) the product of the total ventilation and the dead space to tidal volume ratio.

angiogenic clusters SEE: blood islands.

angiotensin II A powerful vasoactive substance produced from a precursor called angiotensin I. Angiotensin II promotes widespread vasoconstriction of blood vessels and stimulates the secretion of aldosterone from the adrenal cortex. In general, angiotensin II actions are responsible for elevating blood pressure.

angiotensin-converting enzyme (ACE) An enzyme produced by pulmonary endothelial cells. ACE catalyzes the conversion of angiotensin I to the powerful vasoactive substance angiotensin II as pulmonary blood passes through the lung.

angle of Lewis SEE: sternum.

anion shift SEE: chloride shift.

anoxia Complete lack of oxygen.

anterior interventricular sulcus (sul′-kus) External landmark of the heart; a shallow groove separating the right and left ventricles on the anterior surface.

antibody Naturally produced protein (immunoglobulin) that neutralizes a specific antigen; antibodies consist of complex glycoproteins produced by B lymphocytes in response to the presence of an antigen. A single antibody molecule consists of four polypeptide chains that provide binding sites for (1) complement (used to inactivate invading microorganisms) and (2) the specific antigen.

antidiuretic hormone (ADH) Hypothalamic hormone released from the posterior pituitary in response to increased osmotic concentration of the blood; targets the kidney tubules to promote increased water reabsorption. SYN: vasopressin.

antigen A protein or oligosaccharide marker on the surface of cells that identifies the cell as self or non-self. The production of antibodies by B lymphocytes neutralizes or destroys the cell if necessary and stimulates cytotoxic responses by granulocytes, monocytes, and lymphocytes. Inflammation occurs when neutrophils, monocytes, and macrophages encounter an antigen from any source during bodily injury. Reactions to antigens by T and B cells are part of the specific immune response. SYN: allergen.

autoantigens Antigens on the body's own cells.

foreign antigens Antigens on all other cells. If an autoantigen has been damaged, it may appear to be a foreign antigen.

antiporter mechanism SEE: countertransport mechanism.

aortic body One of two small bodies located in the arch of the aorta and containing the endings of the aortic nerve.

apex The pointed extremity of a conical structure; the apex of the heart is the inferior end facing the diaphragm.

apex of the lung The superior, subclavicular portion of the lung.

apnea Temporary cessation of breathing activity, as occurs in non-respiratory activities such as speaking, sneezing, and coughing.

apparent pK (pK′) A specific factor (6.1) used in the quantitative form of the Henderson-Hasselbalch equation used with the bicarbonate buffer system. (See text for the form of the equation.) SEE: buffer; Henderson-Hasselbalch equation.

arrhythmias Irregular heart action caused by physiological or pathological disturbances in the discharge of cardiac impulses from the sinoatrial node or their transmission through conductile tissue of the heart. SYN: dysrhythmias.

arteries Blood vessels that carry blood away from the heart; structural characteristics are designed to withstand relative high blood pressure and include thick muscular layers and elastic connective tissue of the tunica media.

conducting arteries Larger arteries proximal to the heart (e.g., aorta, pulmonary arteries); prominent amounts of elastic tissue are present in the walls to damp, or absorb, pulsatile blood flow. SYN: elastic arteries.

distributing arteries Smaller branches of the conducting arteries that function to distribute blood to specific regions (e.g., radial artery, femoral artery); prominent amounts of smooth muscle found in the walls. SYN: muscular arteries.

resistance arteries Small-diameter arteries with a thick tunica media in proportion to the lumen diameter; resistance arteries are capable of changing their diameters in response to various stimuli (e.g., neural). SEE: tunica media.

arterioles Thin-walled, small-diameter resistance vessels that are branches of small-diameter arteries; a high proportion of their walls are composed of smooth muscle and are capable of rapidly changing their diameters to affect vascular resistance.

arteriosclerosis (ar- tē″ rē-ō-skle-rō′ sis) A disease of blood vessels characterized by thickening, hardening, and loss of elasticity of the arterial wall.

arteriovenous pressure gradient The pressure differential between the proximal and distal parts of a blood vessel.

arytenoid cartilages (ar″ i-tē′ noyd) Paired cartilages that articulate with the cricoid cartilage of the larynx. The posterior ends of the vocal cords attach to the arytenoids. Tension on the cords is altered by inward and outward rotation of the arytenoids. SEE: larynx.

atherosclerosis (ath″ er-o-‴-skle-ro‴′ sis) A disease of blood vessels characterized by the deposition of fatty, plaquelike material on the luminal wall of blood vessels. (Atherosclerosis is a type of arteriosclerosis, but the terms are not interchangeable.)

atrial natriuretic peptide (ANP) A diuretic hormone secreted by the right atrium in response to stretching of the atrial wall caused by elevated venous return volumes; inhibits antidiuretic substances such as renin, aldosterone, and antidiuretic hormone. SYN: atriopeptin.

atriopeptin SEE: atrial natriuretic peptide (ANP).

atrioventricular bundle A bundle of fibers of the impulse-conducting system of the heart. From its origin in the atrioventricular node, the bundle enters the interventricular septum, where it divides into two branches whose fibers pass to the right and left ventricles, respectively. The fibers of each branch become continuous with the conduction myofibers (Purkinje fibers) of the ventricles. SYN: bundle of His.

atrioventricular node Specialized cardiac muscle fibers, located near the lower interatrial septum, that receive impulses from the sinoatrial node and transmit them to the atrioventricular bundle.

atrioventricular sulcus External landmark of the heart; a shallow groove that encircles the heart, separating the atria from the ventricles. SYN: coronary sulcus.

atrioventricular valves Valves that control the movement of blood from the atria to the ventricles; atrioventricular valves prevent reflux of blood into the atria when the powerful ventricles contract.

left atrioventricular valve The valve that closes the orifice between the left atrium and left ventricle of the heart. SYN: bicuspid valve; mitral valve.

right atrioventricular valve The valve that closes the orifice between the right atrium and right ventricle of the heart. SYN: tricuspid valve.

auditory tube The tube extending from the middle ear to the nasopharynx, 3 to 4 cm long and lined with mucous membrane. Occlusion of the tube leads to the development of otitis media. SYN: eustachian tube.

auscultation (aws″ kul-tā′ shun) Process of listening for sounds within the body, usually sounds of thoracic or abdominal viscera, to detect abnormalities or fetal heart sounds.

autacoid Tissue hormone released from, or produced as a result of, an antigen-antibody reaction. Autacoids produce highly localized effects close to the point where they are produced. In general, autacoids are formed rapidly, act, and then decay or are destroyed enzymatically.

eicosanoids A family of autacoids synthesized from inactive arachadonic acid precursors released from target cell membranes. Prostanoids such as prostaglandins (PGs) and thromboxane (TXA) are produced through the cyclo-oxygenase enzyme pathways; leukotrienes (LTs) are produced through the lipoxygenase enzyme pathway, as follows:

LTB_4	leukocyte attractant
LTC_4	histaminelike actions
LTD_4	histaminelike actions
LTE_4	histaminelike actions
$PGF_{2\alpha}$ and PGD_2	smooth muscle contraction
TXA_2	smooth muscle contraction; platelet aggregation
PGE_2 and PGI_2	smooth muscle relaxation

eosinophil chemotactic factor of anaphylaxis (ECF-A) Autacoid that induces eosinophils to migrate to an area of tissue damage.

histamine Autacoid responsible for contraction of nonvascular smooth muscle, relaxation of vascular smooth muscle, increased capillary permeability, and increased glandular secretion.

kinins Autacoids such as bradykinin that produce powerful histaminelike effects in damaged tissue.

neutrophil chemotactic factor of anaphylaxis (NCF-A) Autacoid that induces neutrophils to migrate to an area of tissue damage.

platelet activation factor (PAF) Autacoid that causes platelets to aggregate, or accumulate, in damaged tissue.

autonomic nervous system (ANS) The portion of the peripheral nervous system that provides motor control of the viscera; composed of two antagonistic divisions.

parasympathetic division Functionally opposes the sympathetic division of the ANS; returns organ function to baseline levels during "rest and relaxation" conditions (e.g., decreased gastrointestinal activity).

sympathetic division Functionally opposes the parasympathetic division of the ANS; alters organ function to meet a stress situation encountered during "fight or flight" conditions (e.g., elevated heart rate)

autoregulation Self-governing blood-flow control mechanism operating in systemic capillary beds that responds to accumulated carbon dioxide, hydrogen ions, and lactic acid by promoting vasodilation and increased local blood flow.

autorhythmic Pertaining to an intrinsic rhythm; rhythm that is self-generating. In cardiology, the term autorhythmic implies that a tissue is capable of spontaneous depolarization.

Bainbridge reflex An increase in heart rate caused by an increase in blood pressure or distention of the heart.

baroreceptor reflex Changes in heart rate, force of contraction, and rate of ventilation caused by the degree of stimulation of the aortic arch and carotid sinus baroreceptors, which are special mechanoreceptors that detect the degree of stretch of major arterial walls. Systemic hypertension and an *increase* in baroreceptor stimulation results in a reduction in heart rate, force of contraction, and ventilatory rate; systemic hypotension and a *decrease* in baroreceptor stimulation causes an increase in heart rate, force of contraction, and ventilatory rate.

baroreceptors Sensory nerve endings that are stimulated by changes in pressure. Baroreceptors are found in the walls of the atria of the heart, vena cava, aortic arch, and carotid sinus.

base In general, the lower part of anything; the supporting part; the base of the lung is the inferior or diaphragmatic part; the base of the heart is the superior part where the great vessels enter and exit the heart.

base of the lung The inferior or diaphragmatic surface of the lung.

Biot's breathing A pattern of breathing characterized by short periods of rapid breathing at uniform depth, followed by periods of apnea. Biot's breathing is sometimes associated with cases of increased intracranial pressure.

bicuspid valve SEE: atrioventricular valves.

bladder A muscular, membranous, distensible reservoir that holds urine. The urinary bladder is situated in the pelvic cavity, where it receives urine from the kidneys through the ureters and discharges urine from the body through the urethra.

blood flow The volume of blood flowing through a vessel in a given time; in the resting state total blood flow is equal to cardiac output (approximately 5 L/min in an adult). SEE: cardiac output ($\dot{Q}$).

blood islands Masses and cords of undifferentiated mesenchymal cells in the developing embryo that are the precursors of future blood vessels. SYN: angiogenic clusters.

blood vessel length The total length of a vascular channel; changes in blood vessel length occur very slowly and can affect vascular resistance.

blood vessel radius The radius of a blood vessel; changes in vessel radius occur rapidly and can affect vascular resistance.

blood viscosity A measure of the resistance of blood to flow. Blood viscosity can be affected by the number of cells, plasma proteins, and plasma in circulation.

body cavity SEE: coelom.

body surface area (BSA) The external surface area of the body (approximately 1.5 to 2 m² for an adult); use of BSA data in various hemodynamic indices allows calculated measurements to be compared among persons of differing sizes.

Bohr dead space The physiologic dead space volume (i.e., the total volume of air in the respiratory system that is nonfunctional in terms of gas exchange). Bohr dead space consists of the volume of the anatomical dead space plus the volume of the alveolar dead space, and represents the total wasted ventilation in the respiratory system.

Bohr effect The effect of an acid environment on hemoglobin; hydrogen ions alter the structure of hemoglobin and increase the release of oxygen. It is especially important in active tissues producing carbon dioxide and lactic acid. (It is the opposite of the Haldane effect.)

bony palate SEE: hard palate.

Bowman's capsule SEE: glomerular capsule.

bradycardia (brad″ ē-kar′ dē-a) A slow heartbeat characterized by a pulse rate below 60 beats per minute.

bronchial buds (brong′ kē-al) Right and left bronchial buds form as outpouchings of the single lung bud. Bronchial buds are the precursors of the right and left mainstem (primary) bronchi.

bronchiole (brong′ kē-ol) One of the smaller subdivisions of the bronchial tubes.

bronchoconstriction reflex Protective reflex of the tracheobronchial tree that restricts entry of potentially damaging substances into the deeper and more vulnerable parts of the respiratory system. Subepithelial irritant receptors are stimulated by inhaled noxious gases, particulate matter, allergens, or pathogens. The motor response resulting from the stimulation results in rapid bronchospasm, glandular secretion, and histamine release. SYN: irritant reflex. SEE: rapidly adapting receptor (RAR).

bronchopulmonary segments A small subdivision of the lobes of the lung.

buccal cavity SEE: oral cavity.

bucket-handle movement Rib cage movement in which the downward-slung ribs are pivoted upward by rotating about an axis of rotation that passes through the head of the rib at the costovertebral joint and the costal cartilage of the rib that articulates with the sternum at the costosternal joint. The upward movement brings the ribs into a more horizontal position that increases the lateral diameter of the thorax during forced inspiration.

buffer A combination of substances in aqueous solution that resists changes in hydrogen ion concentration when a strong acid or a strong base is added to the mixture. A buffer pair is generally composed of a weak acid and its conjugate base. Buffer systems prevent large fluctuations in the pH of a solution. Important physiologic buffers include the bicarbonate buffer system, phosphate buffer system, and protein buffer system.

bulbus cordis (bul′ -bus kŏr′-dus) Cranial extension of the embryonic heart that gives rise to the pulmonary trunk, ascending aorta, and a portion of the right atrium.

bundle branches (right and left) Branches of the atrioventricular bundle that travel down the interventricular septum toward the apex of the heart and transmit electrical impulses into the conduction myofibers of the ventricles.

bundle of His SEE: atrioventricular bundle.

C-fiber afferents Terminal endings of unmyelinated nerve fibers. SYN: juxtacapillary receptors; juxtapulmonary capillary receptors; juxta-alveolar receptors; J receptors.

    bronchial C fibers C-fiber afferents located near bronchi; stimulated by lung hyperinflation and chemicals.

    pulmonary C fibers C-fiber afferents located near blood vessels in the lung; stimulated by lung hyperinflation and chemicals.

canalicular period (kan" a-lik' ū-lar) A transitional period in the development of the tracheobronchial tree, characterized by development of both the terminal bronchioles and the respiratory bronchioles of the lung. Canalicular period extends from approximately 17 weeks to 24 weeks.

canals of Lambert One of several bronchoalveolar communications in the lung. These canals may help to prevent atelectasis. SEE: pores of Kohn.

capacitance vessels Blood vessels such as medium- and large-diameter veins that have a large lumen diameter and the capability of storing or accommodating a large volume of blood, thus affecting the returning volume of blood to the heart and the blood pressure.

capillaries Very small-diameter blood vessels that connect the arterial to the venous system; composed of a single layer of squamous epithelial cells to aid in the transfer of substances into and out of the vascular compartment.

capillary bed A group of 10 to 100 capillaries supplied by a single metarteriole; capillary beds provide the exchange "membrane" for the transfer of substances into and out of the bloodstream.

capillary pressure (Pc) Outward Starling force acting upon capillaries, which causes fluid and dissolved substances to be forced out of the vascular compartment. The force is produced by the pumping action of the ventricles of the heart. SYN: capillary hydrostatic pressure. SEE: Starling forces.

capsular hydrostatic pressure The pressure in the nephrons exerted by the presence of fluid in the tubular system. This pressure opposes the glomerular filtration pressure and helps determine the net filtration pressure. SEE: glomerular filtration pressure; net filtration pressure (NFP).

capsule cells SEE: type II cells.

carbon dioxide transport The transfer of carbon dioxide within the bloodstream by different transport mechanisms. The following three main mechanisms are responsible for transporting most of the carbon dioxide produced in the tissues:

    bicarbonate transport Mechanism of carbon dioxide transport in which CO_2 diffuses into red blood cells, combines with water, and is converted to carbonic acid. Carbonic acid ionizes into hydrogen ions and bicarbonate. Bicarbonate ions diffuse out of the red blood cells into the plasma, where they combine with sodium ions to form sodium bicarbonate, which is carried to the lungs.

    carbaminohemoglobin transport Mechanism of carbon dioxide transport in which CO_2 diffuses into red blood cells, where it combines with hemoglobin to form carbaminohemoglobin, which is transported to the lungs.

    plasma dissolution Mechanism of carbon dioxide transport in which CO_2 combines with water in the plasma to form carbonic acid, which ionizes to bicarbonate, which is then transported to the lungs.

carboxyhemoglobin A compound formed by carbon monoxide and hemoglobin in carbon monoxide poisoning.

cardiac accelerator nerve A collection of sympathetic adrenergic nerve fibers that originates in the cardioacceleratory center of the medulla and transmits electrical impulses to the heart.

cardiac action potential The series of electrical changes that occur at the cell membrane of a myocardial cell. Several different phases of the action potential are recognized, and not all phases are seen in all parts of the heart.

    Phase 0 (depolarization) Loss of the polarized state across the membrane when a stimulus is applied or threshold is reached. Some myocardial tissues, such as the sinoatrial node, depolarize slowly when voltage-gated slow Na^+ channels and voltage-gated slow Ca^{2+} channels open; others, such as ventricular fibers depolarize quickly as voltage-gated fast Na^+ channels open.

    Phase 1 (transient repolarization) A brief repolarization phase that is halted by the plateau phase.

    Phase 2 (plateau phase) A period of extended depolarization (200 to 400 milliseconds), caused by the opening of voltage-gated slow Ca^{2+} channels that delays the repolarization process. The plateau phase interrupts repolarization, and is thus responsible for the short period characteristic of transient repolarization.

    Phase 3 (repolarization) Re-establishment of the polarized state as voltage-gated Na^+ channels close and voltage-gated slow K^+ channels open.

    Phase 4 (polarization) Baseline electrical activity in a cell membrane produced by the action of active transport pumps that maintain electrical concentrations across the membrane (e.g., -70 mV). SYN: resting membrane potential.

NOTE: In certain cardiac cells such as cells of the sinoatrial node, Phase 4 is characterized by a slow rise to threshold called the pacemaker potential.

cardiac center A neuronal pool in the medulla made up of a *functional* collection of nerve cells that control cardiac activity. The following two antagonistic centers are recognized:

    cardioacceleratory center A functional grouping of nerve cells in the medulla that sends excitatory impulses to the heart by means of adrenergic fibers in the cardioaccelerator nerve.

    cardioinhibitory center A functional grouping of nerve cells in the medulla that sends inhibitory impulses to the heart by means of cholinergic fibers in the vagus nerve.

cardiac conduction system A system of specialized myocardial tissues that initiates electrical impulses, distributes them throughout the myocardium, and synchronizes the various parts of the heart so their activity is unified and coordinated. This system consists of two specialized nodes of tissue and a system of high-speed muscle pathways (i.e., the Purkinje system). SYN: intrinsic conducting system. SEE: Purkinje system.

cardiac electrophysiology The study of the electrical events associated with contraction and relaxation of the heart.

cardiac index (CI) Cardiac output divided by body surface area. SEE: cardiac output (Q); body surface area.

cardiac myocytes Heart muscle cells; these fibers contain one nucleus per cell and are branched and generally shorter and thicker than skeletal muscle fibers. SYN: cardiac muscle cells.

cardiac notch The concavity on the anterior border of the left lung into which the heart projects.

cardiac output (C.O., Q) A measure of the amount of blood pumped by the heart per unit time; calculated as the product of the stroke volume and the heart rate, and usually expressed as "milliliters per minute" or "liters per minute."

cardiac reserve A measure of the functional reserve of the heart, usually expressed as multiples of the resting cardiac output (e.g., 2X, 3X), or as a percentage of the resting cardiac output (e.g., 300%, 400%). SEE: cardiac output (Q̇).

carina (ka-rī'-na) The ridge at the lower end of the trachea separating the openings of the two mainstem bronchi.

carotid body A sensory structure at the bifurcation of the common carotid artery that contains chemoreceptors and pressoreceptors.

cartilaginous airways Airways of the conducting zone that have cartilage supporting elements in their walls. Cartilaginous airways include the trachea, mainstem bronchi, lobar bronchi, segmental bronchi, and subsegmental bronchi.

central pattern generator (CPG) A centrally located network of nerve cells that generates a patterned motor output that results in rhythmic, repetitive behaviors such as respiration or locomotion. The respiratory CPG not only controls respiratory activity but also coordinates respiratory activity with nonrespiratory activities, such as swallowing, yawning, and coughing.

central venous pressure (CVP) The initial blood pressure recorded when a pulmonary artery catheter is initially inserted into a systemic vein; peripheral venous pressure (PVP) correlates well with CVP. CVP is used in hemodynamic calculations to represent right ventricular end-diastolic pressure. SEE: right ventricular stroke work index (RVSWI); pulmonary artery catheter.

chemoreceptor A sense organ or sensory nerve ending that is stimulated by and reacts to certain chemical stimuli such as heart rate, force of contraction, and ventilatory rate (e.g., carotid and aortic bodies, medullary chemoreceptors, taste buds, olfactory cells of the nose).

chemosensitive area The area of the medulla containing chemoreceptors sensitive to hydrogen-ion concentration in the cerebrospinal fluid (CSF); the concentration of hydrogen ions is proportional to the amount of carbon dioxide diffusing into the CSF from cerebral blood vessels.

Cheyne-Stokes breathing A pattern of breathing characterized by a period of apnea lasting 10 to 60 seconds, followed by a period of increasing depth and rate of breathing, followed by a period of decreasing depth and frequency until another period of apnea develops. Cheyne-Stokes breathing is sometimes associated with central nervous system depressant drug overdoses, or reduced cerebral blood flow.

chief cells SEE: type I cells.

chloride shift The shift of chloride ions from the plasma into the red blood cells upon the addition of carbon dioxide from the tissues, and the reverse movement when carbon dioxide is released in the lungs. It is a mechanism for maintaining constant pH of the blood. SYN: anion shift.

choana (kō′ a-na) A funnel-shaped opening, especially of the posterior nares; one of the communicating passageways between the nasal fossae and the nasopharynx. SYN: internal naris.

choke points A location within an airway that is prone to collapse during forced exhalation.

cholinergic receptors Cell membrane receptors activated by acetylcholine (ACh) and other choline ester chemical messengers; antagonized by specific cholinergic-blocking agents. SYN: cholinoceptors.

M$_3$-muscarinic cholinergic receptors Postjunctional receptors located at the parasympathetic postganglionic-neuroeffector synapses (e.g., myocardial cell membranes). SYN: M$_3$-muscarinic receptors.

N$_1$-nicotinic cholinergic receptors Postjunctional receptors located at the autonomic ganglia (i.e., at the synapse between preganglionic and postganglionic fibers of both ANS divisions). SYN: N$_1$-nicotinic receptors.

N$_2$-nicotinic cholinergic receptors Postjunctional receptors located at the neuromuscular junctions of the somatic nervous system (i.e., at the synapse between somatic motoneurons and skeletal muscle fibers). SYN: N$_2$-nicotinic receptors.

chordae tendineae (kor′ dēten-din′ ēē) One of several small, tendinous cords that connect the free edges of the atrioventricular valves to the papillary muscles and prevent inversion of these valves during ventricular systole.

chorionic villi (kō-rē-on′-ik vil′ē-) Vascular projections from the chorion that help increase the surface area of the blood-blood interface.

chronic alveolar hyperventilation A condition of hyperventilation lasting for more than 24 hours. The condition results in respiratory alkalosis. Renal compensation includes the excretion of additional bicarbonate from the body.

chronic metabolic acidosis A condition resulting from the chronic accumulation of fixed acids in the tissues that overwhelms the buffering capacity of the plasma and causes a decrease in the pH of the plasma. SYN: chronic nonrespiratory acidosis.

chronic metabolic alkalosis A condition resulting from the chronic depletion of hydrogen ions or the accumulation of base from nonrespiratory sources that overwhelms the buffering capacity of the plasma and causes an increase in the pH of the plasma. SYN: chronic nonrespiratory alkalosis.

chronic ventilatory failure A condition resulting from prolonged hypoventilation (for more than 24 hours); the condition results in respiratory acidosis and generally involves renal compensation as the kidneys attempt to reabsorb additional bicarbonate from the glomerular filtrate.

chronotropic (kron″ ō-trop′ ik) Influencing the rate of occurrence of an event, such as the heartbeat.

ciliary transport mechanism SEE: mucociliary escalator.

Clara cells One of the secreting cells in the surface epithelium of the bronchioles. These cells, along with goblet cells, provide secretions for the respiratory tract. The secretion is a mucus-poor protein that coats the epithelium.

classic shunt equation Equation used to calculate the ratio of blood flow through a shunt compartment to the total cardiac output when the end-capillary ideal oxygen content, the oxygen content of arterial blood, and the oxygen content of mixed venous blood are known (see text for the form of the equation). SEE: cardiac output ($\dot{Q}$).

closing volume The lung volume at which a critical collapse of air-

ways begins to occur during exhalation. The collapse is due to the combined effect of (1) increased intrapleural pressure and (2) decreased radial traction of small airways at lower lung volumes.

coelom (sē′ lom) The cavity in an embryo between the split layers of lateral mesoderm. In mammals it develops into the pleural, peritoneal, and pericardial cavities. SYN: body cavity.

extraembryonic coelom In humans, the cavity in the developing blastocyst that lies between the mesoderm of the chorion and the mesoderm covering the amniotic cavity and yolk sac.

intraembryonic coelom One of the paired cavities that extends longitudinally through the embryo. Fusion of the paired intraembryonic coeloms ultimately forms the pericardial, pleural, and peritoneal cavities.

pleuroperitoneal coelom The common body cavity extending from the paired pleural canals into the peritoneal cavity. (Development of the diaphragm ultimately partitions this coelom into paired pleural cavities and a single peritoneal cavity.) SEE: pleural canals.

collecting duct Small-diameter tubular structures that receive urine from several distal convoluted tubules and convey it to the renal papillae for release into the calyces and renal pelvis.

colloid osmotic pressure The pressure in the nephrons created by the presence of proteins in the blood within the glomerular capillaries. This pressure opposes the glomerular filtration pressure and contributes to the net filtration pressure. SEE: glomerular filtration pressure; net filtration pressure (NFP).

compliance The property of altering size and shape in response to application of force, weight, or release from force. The lung and thoracic cage of a child may have a high degree of compliance as compared with that of an elderly person. SEE: elastance.

dynamic compliance A measure of the ease of lung inflation with positive pressure.

static compliance A volume-to-pressure measurement of lung distensibility with exhalation against a closed system, taken under conditions of no airflow.

compliance work SEE: elastic work.

conductance The measure of flow through a tube for a given pressure difference; conductance is the reciprocal of resistance.

conducting zone The part of the respiratory system consisting of all the generations of air passages, extending from the trachea to the terminal bronchioles; no gas exchange occurs in the conducting zone.

conduction myofibers Fine terminal branches of the right and left bundle branches that form an elaborate electrical distribution network within the ventricles. SYN: Purkinje fibers.

convective acceleration (Bernoulli effect) In pulmonology, convective acceleration refers to the inverse variation in pressure with gas velocity. The velocity of a gas must increase to maintain the same flowrate when a gas flows from a large-diameter tube into a small-diameter tube. As gas enters the narrower tube, pressure energy is converted to kinetic energy, and a greater proportion of the total energy is made up of kinetic energy, hence the higher velocity of the gas. (These fundamentals generally refer to *fluids*, which consist of gases as well as liquids.)

corniculate cartilages (kōr-nik′ ū-lāt) Small, paired, horn-shaped cartilages. SEE: larynx.

coronary circulation The system of blood vessels that supplies blood to the myocardium of the heart. Blood leaves the aorta through the right and left coronary arteries, which supply the myocardium. Blood passes through capillaries and is collected in veins, most of which empty into the coronary sinus, which opens into the right atrium. A few of the small veins open directly into the atria and ventricles. SEE: thebesian veins.

coronary sinus A thin-walled, venous structure on the posterior wall of the right atrium that collects venous blood from the coronary circulation and returns it to the right atrium.

coronary sulcus SEE: atrioventricular sulcus.

costal cartilage Hyaline cartilage that connects the osseous part of a true rib to the sternum, or the osseous part of a false rib to the costal cartilage of the rib above.

costal impressions Shallow indentations on the lateral surface of the lungs caused by contact with the ribs.

costal margin The inferior edge, or margin, of the costal cartilages of the rib cage. The right and left costal margins meet at the infrasternal angle (T10–11), which ranges from 70 to 110 degrees.

costal pleura SEE: pleura.

costal (lateral) surface The lateral surface of the lungs that contacts the inside of the thoracic cage.

costochondral junction The articulation formed between the osseous and cartilaginous parts of a rib. SYN: costrochondral joint.

cotransport mechanism A type of active transport mechanism in which sodium ions and other substances move together in the same direction through a cell membrane. SYN: symporter mechanism.

cotyledon (cot-i-lē′ -don) 1. A mass of villi on the chorionic surface of the placenta. 2. Any of the rounded portions into which the placenta's uterine surface is divided.

countercurrent exchanger The mechanism that maintains the high osmolarity of the renal medulla; blood vessels descending into the high salt concentration of the medulla are allowed to unload water because of osmosis and to take on salt because of the concentration gradient, thus preventing the osmotic concentration of the medulla from decreasing.

countercurrent multiplier The mechanism that occurs in the descending and ascending segments of the loop of the nephron that amplifies the high concentration of salt in the medulla to prevent the diffusion of salt as a result of the salinity gradient in the deeper parts of the medulla.

countertransport mechanism A type of active transport mechanism in which sodium ions and other substances move in opposite directions through a cell membrane. SYN: antiporter mechanism.

cribriform plate (krib′ ri-fōrm) Small, horizontally oriented thin plate of the ethmoid bone. It forms the roof of the nasal cavity and a small portion of the cranial floor. The sievelike appearance is due to the olfactory foramina that perforate the plate and transmit branches of the olfactory nerves. SYN: horizontal plate.

cricoid cartilages (krī′ koyd) The lowermost cartilage of the larynx; shaped like a signet ring, with the broad portion or lamina being posterior, the anterior portion forming the arch. SEE: larynx.

critical flowrate The critical flow velocity at which a laminar flow pattern begins to break up and become less uniform and more chaotic.

cuneiform cartilages (kū-nē′ i-fōrm) One of two small pieces of yellow elastic cartilage that lie in the aryepiglottic fold of the larynx immediately anterior to the arytenoid cartilage. SEE: larynx.

cusps One of the leaflike divisions or parts of the valves of the heart.

Dalton's law of partial pressures The total pressure of a mixture of gases is equal to the sum of the individual partial pressures of the gases comprising the mixture.

dead space to tidal volume ratio (V_D/V_T) A measure of the amount of minute ventilation wasted ventilating the conducting zone of the lung.

desmosomes Structures within intercalated discs of myocardial tissue that bind adjacent cardiac myocytes together and stabilize them by means of interlocking filaments.

diaphragm The dome-shaped skeletal muscle separating the abdomen from the thoracic cavity. It contracts with each inspiration, flattening out downward, permitting the bases of the lungs to descend. It relaxes with each expiration, elevating itself and restoring the inverted basin shape.

  central tendon Tough, membranous, flattened tendon surrounded by radially oriented striated muscle fibers that contract or relax, thus changing its tension.

  crura Columnlike masses of muscle fibers that arise from the lumbar vertebrae, to connect the vertebral column with the central tendon. The right and left crura fuse together at the aorta.

  hemidiaphragm Half of the diaphragm; the muscular portion of the right and left hemidiaphragms is divided into three parts: costal part (lateral), lumbar/vertebral part (posterior), and sternal part (anterior).

diastolic pressure The blood pressure recorded during ventricular diastole.

diffusing capacity of the lung for carbon monoxide (D_{LCO}) A measure of the ability of the lung to diffuse gases, using carbon monoxide (CO) as a test gas, and using Fick's law for the calculations. (Carbon monoxide is used because of its remarkable ease of diffusion through the alveolar-capillary membrane and its extremely slow rate of equilibration along the pulmonary capillary.)

diffusion-limited gas exchange Gas transfer at the alveolar-capillary membrane that is determined by the diffusing capacity, or conductance properties of the membrane itself, rather than the delivery of pulmonary blood to the membrane.

diffusivity The rate of diffusion of a gas through a membrane along a partial pressure gradient.

2,3-diphosphoglycerate (2,3-DPG) An organic phosphate in red blood cells that alters the affinity of hemoglobin for oxygen. This intermediate compound accumulates within red blood cells under anaerobic conditions (e.g., strenuous exercise) and causes hemoglobin molecules to become less flexible and less able to bind oxygen.

dissociation constant (K_a) of acid A measure of how readily an acid ionizes in aqueous solution. The effectiveness of buffers in neutralizing hydrogen ions in solution can be assessed through a determination of the dissociation constant.

distal convoluted tubule A small-diameter tube of the nephron that is located distal to the glomerular capsule; receives glomerular filtrate from the ascending segment of the loop of the nephron and conveys it to the collecting ducts of the nephron. SEE: glomerular filtrate.

disturbed flow SEE: transitional flow.

diuresis (dī″ ū-rē′ sis) The process of urine formation. The following stages of diuresis are recognized:

  glomerular filtration The nonselective process of removing particles from the bloodstream by allowing the liquid portion to pass through a membrane formed by the endothelial cells of the glomerular capillaries and the epithelial cells of the glomerular capsule. The pore spaces allow the liquid (glomerular filtrate) to pass but are too small to permit passage of larger particles such as red blood cells and larger plasma proteins. SEE: glomerulus; glomerular capsule.

  tubular reabsorption The movement of selective substances from the glomerular filtrate into the bloodstream (i.e., from the tubular component to the vascular component of the nephron). SEE: glomerular filtrate.

  tubular secretion The movement of selective substances from the bloodstream into the glomerular filtrate (i.e., from the vascular component to the tubular component of the nephron). SEE: glomerular filtrate.

diving reflex Apnea and bradycardia caused by stimulation of nasal or facial receptors with cold water.

dorsal respiratory group (DRG) Medullary respiratory center located in the nucleus of the solitary tract. Inspiratory neurons of the DRG stimulate phrenic motoneurons to bring about contraction of the diaphragm, which initiates inspiration.

dromotropic (drōm″ ō-trop′ ik) Affecting the conductivity of nerve or muscle fibers.

dry gas fraction (F_{GAS}) The percentage composition of the gases of respiratory importance found in a mixed sample of dry ambient air. The dry gas fractions in the mixture total 100%.

ductus arteriosus (duk′ tus ar-tēr′-i-ō-sus) A channel of communication between the pulmonary trunk and the aorta of the fetus.

ductus venosus (duk′ tus ven-ō′-sus) The smaller, shorter, and posterior of two branches into which the umbilical vein divides after entering the abdomen. It empties into the inferior vena cava.

dynamic compression The external compression effect that causes collapse of an airway due to the production of a choke point. At a critical transmural pressure, the external collapse pressure overcomes the internal distending pressure, causing a critical narrowing of the tube.

dynamic lung compliance (C_{dyn}) A measurement of how readily a lung region fills during a period of gas flow. The ratio of dynamic compliance to static compliance is about the same (1:1) throughout all breathing frequencies in a normal lung. In a *partially obstructed lung*, however, the ratio of dynamic compliance to static compliance decreases as the rate of breathing increases because of the effect of obstructed regions with longer time constants.

dynamics The science of bodies in motion and their forces.

dyspnea A symptom caused by shortness of breath that results from the increase in the work of breathing in response to an increase in airway resistance.

dysrhythmias: SEE: arrhythmias.

ectopic focus Electric stimulation of cardiac contractions beginning at a location other than the sinoatrial node.

effective solubility The volume of gas that combines with a given volume of blood at a particular partial pressure, usually expressed as mL of gas per 100 mL of blood, or as mL/dL.

efferent arteriole The small-diameter blood vessel that carries blood away from the glomerulus after it has been filtered. Efferent arterioles connect with peritubular capillaries, where various exchanges take place. SEE: pertibular capillaries; glomerulus.

effort-dependent flowrate That part of the flow-volume loop determined by the degree of respiratory effort expended; peak expiratory flow and peak inspiratory flow are proportional to ventilatory effort.

effort-independent flowrate That part of the flow-volume loop not determined by the degree of respiratory effort expended. After lung volume has fallen by about 20%, expiration becomes flow-limited (i.e., effort-independent) by the structural and dynamic characteristics of the lung itself, not by the expiratory effort expended (e.g., increased intrapleural pressure and decreased radial traction of small airways at lower lung volumes contribute to the effort-independent portion of forced expiration).

ejection fraction The volume of blood pumped by the heart with one contraction (stroke volume), expressed as a percentage of the total volume of blood in the chamber (end-diastolic volume).

elastance The tendency of a material to return to its original form after having been deformed; the character or quality of such a material. Elastance is the reciprocal of compliance. SEE: compliance.

elastic arteries SEE: arteries.

elastic forces Forces that promote collapse of the alveoli and lung, thus contributing to instability. Elastic forces are due to the elastic connective tissue of the lung interstitium and to surface tension caused by the fluid lining the alveoli.

elastic resistance Impedance produced by the static elastic recoil of the lung and thorax (e.g., elasticity of the lung interstitium, surface tension effects of alveolar fluid, and elasticity of the chest wall).

elastic work The work of breathing that must be expended to overcome the static resistance factors that make up elastic resistance. SYN: compliance work.

elasticity A measurement of the ability of a solid to deform when a force is applied; the energy of deformation is temporarily stored, and the solid returns to its original shape when the force is removed.

electrocardiogram (ECG, EKG) A record of the electrical activity of the heart. The electrocardiogram provides important information concerning the spread of excitation to the different parts of the heart, and is of value in diagnosing cases of abnormal cardiac rhythm and myocardial damage. Several different components of the normal ECG are recognized, including:

P wave Electrical activity caused by depolarization of the atria; atrial systole begins.

P-Q interval The period extending from the start of the P wave to the start of the QRS complex. SYN: P-R interval.

QRS complex Electrical activity caused by depolarization of the ventricles.

S-T segment The period of time extending from the end of the S wave to the beginning of the T wave; ventricular systole begins.

T wave Electrical activity caused by repolarization of the ventricles.

embryology The science that deals with the origin and development of an individual organism.

end-diastolic pressure (EDP) The blood pressure in the left ventricle at the end of the diastolic period.

end-diastolic volume (EDV) The volume of blood in the left ventricle at the end of diastole, just prior to ventricular contraction. The EDV represents the maximum amount of blood held by the chamber following diastolic filling.

end-systolic volume (ESV) The volume of blood remaining in the left ventricle at the end of systole, following ventricular contraction.

endocardium The endothelial membrane that lines the chambers of the heart and is continuous with the tunica intima (the lining of arteries and veins).

endothelial (endocardial) tubes Paired, primitive, tubelike muscular structures in the embryo that are the precursors of the primitive heart tube, an early undifferentiated pump.

epicardium The serous membrane on the surface of the myocardium. SYN: visceral pericardium.

epiglottis cartilage (ep" i-glot' is) The uppermost cartilage of the larynx, located immediately posterior to the root of the tongue. It covers the entrance of the larynx when the individual swallows, thus preventing food or liquids from entering the airway. SEE: larynx.

equal pressure point The pressure in an airway immediately before critical closure occurs (i.e., the transmural pressure equals zero at the equal pressure point immediately before a choke point develops).

equilibration of gases The process by which gas partial pressure equalization occurs on both sides of the alveolar-capillary membrane during the transit time through a pulmonary capillary.

erythrocyte A mature red blood cell (RBC), or corpuscle. Each is an anucleated, biconcave disk averaging 7 μm in diameter. An RBC has a typical cell membrane and an internal stroma, or framework, made of lipids and proteins to which more than 200 million molecules of hemoglobin are attached. SYN: red blood cell (RBC).

erythropoietin A hormone produced by the kidney in response to hypoxemia. Erythropoietin targets bone marrow to accelerate the production and maturation of red blood cells, which increase the hematocrit, viscosity of blood, and the oxygen-transporting capability of the blood.

estimated shunt equations Modified versions of the classic shunt equation used when sampling of mixed venous blood is unavailable or impractical. These derived equations assume a given arteriovenous oxygen content difference in their calculations (e.g., 3.5 vol% or 5 vol%). (See text for the form of the equation).

ethmoid bone (eth' moyd) A sievelike, spongy bone that forms a roof for the nasal fossae and part of the floor of the anterior fossa of the skull. It permits passage of the olfactory nerves to the brain and also contains three groups of air cavities—the ethmoid sinuses—that open into the nasal cavity.

eupnea Normal, spontaneous breathing resulting in the movement of the tidal volume of air (approximately 500 mL) by the gentle movement of the diaphragm.

eustachian tube SEE: auditory tube.

expiratory compliance curve A measure of the elastic properties of the lung generated during expiration; the curve is produced when the transpulmonary pressure (or distending pressure) is plotted against the lung volume during deflation.

external naris SEE: nostril.

extra-alveolar blood vessels Blood vessels found in the lung parenchyma, but outside the alveoli. Extra-alveolar blood vessels are tethered to connective tissue elements and are alternatively expanded and squeezed during lung inflation and deflation, respectively.

NOTE: The lung effects responsible for dilation and constriction of extra-alveolar blood vessels produce *opposing* effects in the alveolar septal capillaries.

extra-alveolar capillaries Small pulmonary blood vessels located outside the alveoli in the interstitium of the lung.

extrapulmonary shunting A type of shunt in which a portion of desaturated blood enters the systemic arteries without first passing through the pulmonary arteries (i.e., the shunt mechanism itself is found outside the lung). Examples are bronchial and thebesian vein drainage into the pulmonary veins and left ventricle, respectively.

extrinsic laryngeal muscles One of two muscle groups of the larynx. These muscles include the infrahyoid, suprahyoid, omohyoid, sternohyoid, sternothyroid, and other muscle groups. SEE: larynx intrinsic laryngeal muscles.

faucial tonsil SEE: palatine tonsils.

fetal hemoglobin The type of hemoglobin found in the erythrocytes of the normal fetus. It is capable of taking up and giving off oxygen at lower oxygen tensions than can the hemoglobin in adult erythrocytes.

fibrous skeleton The spiral arrangement of myocardial fibers interwoven with collagenous and elastic connective tissue fibers. The fibrous skeleton provides structural support for the heart, provides something against which the myocardial fibers can pull, and electrically isolates the atria from the ventricles.

Fick's law of diffusion The gas law relationship that states that the volume of gas diffusing across a membrane or liquid film per unit time is directly proportional to the area of the membrane, the diffusivity of the gas, and the gas partial pressure gradient, but inversely proportional to the thickness of the membrane.

fixed acid SEE nonvolatile acid.

flow-resistive pressure loss The decrease in pressure caused by the nature of fluids in motion (e.g., flow pattern of a gas, effect of friction on moving gas molecules).

flow-volume curve The curve produced when the instantaneous flowrate of air (y-axis) is plotted against the volume of air moved (x-axis); *expiratory* flow-volume curves are generated above the x-axis; *inspiratory* flow-volume curves are generated below the x-axis.

flow-volume loop Continuous loop formed by the combined expiratory flow-volume curve and the inspiratory flow-volume curve. SEE: flow-volume curve.

fluid dynamics The study of the behavior of fluids (gases and liquids) in motion.

foramen ovale The opening between the two atria of the fetal heart. It usually closes shortly after birth as a result of hemodynamic changes related to respiration.

forced expiratory flow between 25% and 75% of FVC (FEF$_{25\%-75\%}$) Spirometric measurement of exhalation occurring in the middle half of a forced expiratory maneuver. This region of a forced vital capacity curve is flow-limited.

forced expiratory volume in 1 second (FEV$_1$) The volume of air (in liters) exhaled in the first 1 second of a forced expiration.

forced vital capacity (FVC) The change in lung volume from total lung capacity (TLC) to residual volume (RV) during a forced expiration. SEE: lung capacities; lung volumes.

fossa ovalis (fah'-sa ō-val'-iss) The remnant of the embryonic foramen ovale in the interatrial septum of the heart.

Frank-Starling law The length-tension relationship of myocardial tissue that determines how forcefully the heart wall contracts when it is passively stretched by a returning volume of blood. Within physiologic limits the heart tends to pump all of the blood returning to it without allowing excessive damming of blood to occur in the veins. SYN: Starling's law of the heart.

frontal bone The forehead bone; also forms the lateral part of the bridge of the nose.

functional syncytium A collection of cells connected by gap junctions in an intricate way, thus allowing them to function as a single unit. In the heart, two such functional syncytia are found, separated by a fibrous band of nonconducting fibrous tissue:

atrial syncytium The collection of atrial muscle cells that are bound together mechanically, chemically, and electrically so that they function as a single atrial "cell," or atrial pump.

ventricular syncytium The collection of ventricular muscle cells that are bound together mechanically, chemically, and electrically so that they function as a single ventricular "cell" or ventricular pump.

gamma globlin (γ-globulin) SEE: immunoglobulin.

gap junctions Electrical synapses within intercalated discs of myocardial tissue that permit rapid distribution of electrical impulses between cells without the use of neurochemicals.

glandular period The initial period in the development of the tracheobronchial tree, extending from gestation to approximately 16 weeks. It can be divided into two stages: The embryonic period and the pseudoglandular period.

glomerular capsule (glō-mer' ū-lar) A spherical structure that surrounds the glomerulus. The glomerular capsule has a porous, double-walled structure that allows it to filter and collect the fluid (glomerular filtrate) that has been forced out of the glomerular capillaries under pressure. SYN: Bowman's capsule. SEE: glomerulus; glomerular filtrate.

glomerular filtrate The fluid that has been forced out of the glomerular capillaries under pressure. In the proximal regions of the nephron, glomerular filtrate resembles plasma from which it is derived; in the distal portions of the nephron, the glomerular filtrate resembles urine in its physical and chemical makeup. Samples of filtrate from intermediate parts of the urine show a transitional state from plasma to urine. SYN: ultrafiltrate.

glomerular filtration pressure The driving pressure in the nephrons that pushes fluid into the glomerular capsule from the glomerular capillaries; contributes to the net filtration pressure in the nephrons and is due to the blood pressure generated by the left ventricle. SEE: glomerulus; glomerular capsule; net filtration pressure (NFP).

glomerular filtration rate (GFR) The volume of glomerular filtrate formed per minute by the pair of kidneys, typically 125 mL/min for an adult man.

glomerulus A compact bundle of capillaries in the nephron that are specialized for glomerular filtration. The glomerular capillaries receive blood from afferent arterioles and convey it to efferent arterioles. SYN: glomerular capillary loops; glomerular capillary tuft.

glomus cells SEE: type I cells.

glottis (glot' is) The sound-producing apparatus of the larynx consisting of the two vocal cords and the intervening space, the rima glottidis. A leaf-shaped lid of fibrocartilage (the epiglottis) protects this opening. SEE: larynx.

Graham's law The gas law relationship that states that the diffusion rate of a gas is inversely proportional to the square root of the gram molecular weight of the gas.

great cardiac vein Located within the anterior interventricular sulcus; drains blood from the anterior side of the heart.

great vessels Collective term given to the large-diameter blood vessels that enter and exit the heart at its base.

aorta Large artery that originates in the left ventricle and carries oxygenated blood to all parts of the body except the blood going to the lungs for gas exchange.

inferior vena cava (IVC) Large vein carrying deoxygenated blood to the right atrium from regions that are inferior to the heart.

pulmonary trunk Large-diameter arterial trunk that exits from the right ventricle and bifurcates into the right and left pulmonary arteries that carry deoxygenated blood to the lungs. SYN: pulmonary arteries.

pulmonary veins One of four veins that carry oxygenated blood from the lungs to the left atrium.

superior vena cava (SVC) Large vein carrying deoxygenated blood to the right atrium from regions that are superior to the heart.

Hagen-Poiseuille law SEE: Poiseuille's law.

Haldane effect The oxygenation of hemoglobin, which lowers its affinity for carbon dioxide. (It is the opposite of the Bohr effect.)

hard palate The anterior part of the palate supported by the maxillary and palatine bones. SYN: bony palate.

heart sounds Sounds produced by turbulence in the heart:

first heart sound (S1) The sound associated with ventricular systole and the turbulence created when the atrioventricular valves close.

second heart sound (S2) The sound associated with ventricular diastole and the turbulence created when the semilunar valves close.

third heart sound (S3) The faint sound associated with rapid ventricular filling during diastole; sometimes heard in children and adolescents.

fourth heart sound (S4) The sound associated with atrial systole; sometimes faintly audible just before the first heart sound of the next cycle. The sound is rare in normal hearts but may occur when atrial pressure is high or the ventricle is stiff in conditions such as ventricular hypertrophy.

hematocrit (Hct) 1. A centrifuge for separating solids from plasma in the blood. 2. The volume of erythrocytes packed by centrifugation in a given volume of blood. The hematocrit is expressed as the percentage of total blood volume that consists of erythrocytes or as the volume in cubic centimeters of erythrocytes packed by centrifugation of blood.

hemodynamics The study of the fluid dynamics principles that influence the circulation of blood through the heart and blood vessels.

hemoglobin (Hb) The iron-containing pigment of the red blood cells, which carries oxygen from the lungs to the tissues. The amount of hemoglobin in the blood averages 12 to 16 g/100 mL of blood in women, 14 to 18 g/100 mL in men, and somewhat less in children. Hemoglobin is a conjugated protein consisting of a colored iron-containing pigment called *heme* and a simple protein, *globin*.

hemoglobin P$_{50}$ The partial pressure of oxygen at which hemoglobin is 50% saturated (approximately 27 mm Hg). The value is used to produce a standard oxyhemoglobin dissociation curve that is used for assessment of oxygen transport status in patients.

Henderson-Hasselbalch equation Mathematical relationship that relates the pH of a solution with the dissociation constant of its dissociated and undissociated ionic components when the system is at equilibrium. (See text for the form of the equation.)

Henry's law The relationship that states that, at a given temperature, the volume of gas that dissolves in a liquid is directly proportional to the partial pressure of the gas.

Hering-Breuer deflation reflex A reflex mediated by a slowly adapting receptor known as a pulmonary stretch receptor. The reflex provides expiratory facilitation by reducing the period of expiration following marked deflation of the lung. SEE: slowly adapting receptor.

Hering-Breuer inflation reflex A reflex mediated by a slowly adapting receptor known as a pulmonary stretch receptor. The reflex provides inspiratory inhibition and is triggered by steady lung inflation to limit excessive lung expansion. SEE: slowly adapting receptor.

hilum Medial fissure found on the surface of solid organs that allows structures to enter and exit the organ. The hilum of the lung allows passage of the root, which consists of the mainstem bronchus, pulmonary blood vessels, nerves, and lymphatics; the hilum of the kidney allows passage of the ureter, renal blood vessels, nerves, and lymphatics.

His-Purkinje system SEE: Purkinje system

homogeneous lung SEE: ideal lung.

horizontal plate SEE: cribriform plate.

hydrostatic effect The effect produced by gravity that assists the return of blood draining from regions superior to the heart (e.g., head and neck).

hydrostatic pressure gradient Regional difference in intrapleural pressure resulting from the effect of gravity and the weight of lung tissue. Intrapleural pressures become progressively greater going down through the mass of tissue from the apex to the base of the lung.

hypercapnic drive Respiratory control based on the *indirect* detection of arterial hypercapnia by central chemoreceptors. An increase in arterial carbon dioxide tension causes the chemoreceptors to send sensory impulses to the medullary respiratory center SEE: medullary chemoreceptors.

hyperpnea An increase in the depth of breathing, with or without an increase in the rate of breathing.

hyperventilation An increase in ventilation reaching the alveoli that results from an increase in the depth of breathing, the rate of breathing, or both.

hypoventilation A decrease in ventilation reaching the alveoli that results from a decrease in the depth of breathing, the rate of breathing, or both.

hypoxemia A condition of low oxygen tension in arterial blood.

hypoxia Low or inadequate oxygen or a relative deficiency of oxygen for cellular metabolism. Several types of hypoxia are recognized:

anemic hypoxia Hypoxia caused by a reduction in the amount of hemoglobin available for gas transport, because of reduced production of red blood cells, increased loss of red blood cells, or the presence of defective hemoglobin (e.g., methemoglobin, carboxyhemoglobin).

histotoxic hypoxia Hypoxia caused by disruption of cellular enzyme systems by poisons (e.g., cyanide) that impair cellular respiration. Cells are unable to utilize the oxygen delivered to them despite adequate arterial oxygen tension, hemoglobin concentration, and flowrates.

hypoxic hypoxia Hypoxic hypoxia is commonly referred to as hypoxemic hypoxia (or relative deficiency in the bloodstream), but is described accurately as a condition of relative oxygen deficiency in the tissues caused by low arterial oxygen tension. (Causes include low alveolar oxygen tension, diffusion impairment, intrapulmonary shunting, and extrapulmonary shunting.) SYN: hypoxemic hypoxia.

stagnant hypoxia Hypoxia caused by conditions of extremely low blood flowrates to the tissues despite adequate arterial oxygen tension and hemoglobin concentration. SYN: ischemic hypoxia.

hypoxic drive Respiratory control based on the *direct* detection of arterial hypoxemia by peripheral chemoreceptors located in the aortic and carotid bodies. A decrease in arterial oxygen tension below the range of 80 to 100 mm Hg activates the chemoreceptors, which cause sensory impulses to be sent to the medullary respiratory area.

hypoxic pulmonary vasoconstriction The response of pulmonary arterioles to depressed alveolar oxygen tension. The vascular response shunts pulmonary blood flow *away from* alveoli that are underventilated, toward lung regions that are better ventilated, thus minimizing ventilation-perfusion inequalities in the lung.

hysteresis (Gr. *a coming too late*) A disparity in which the appearance of an effect fails to keep up to keep pace with its cause. In pulmonary mechanics, hysteresis is the difference between inflation and deflation of the lung, as shown on a static volume-pressure curve, where the shape of the inflation curve differs from that of the deflation curve. Hysteresis is caused by the gradual opening of alveoli at different volumes and by changes in surface tension that occur as the volume of the lung changes.

ideal alveolar oxygen equation Equation used to calculate the alveolar oxygen tension when the alveolar carbon dioxide tension, the inspired oxygen fraction, the barometric pressure, the water vapor partial pressure, and the respiratory exchange ratio are known (see text for the form of the equation).

ideal lung A fictitious model in which the lung is considered homogenous with respect to ventilation-perfusion ratios, which are assumed to be identical for each alveolus. The alveolar oxygen tension (P_{AO_2}) is the same in each alveolus, the capillary blood oxygen tension and content are the same for blood exiting from each alveolus, and the systemic arterial oxygen tension (Pa_{O_2}) is equal to the P_{AO_2} because the blood flowing out of the lung is a mixture of end-capillary blood from each identically perfused and ventilated alveolus. SYN: homogeneous lung.

immunoglobulin (Ig) A plasma protein that is converted into a specific antibody by immune system cells. IgE is the specific protein converted into antibody in allergic reactions. SYN: gamma globulin (γ-globulin).

inferior nasal conchae (kong' kē) One of the three scroll-like bones (turbinates) that project medially from the lateral wall of the nasal cavity. Each overlies a meatus. The inferior nasal conchae are paired facial bones. (The superior and middle nasal conchae are processes of the lateral mass of the ethmoid bone.) SEE: ethmoid bone.

inferior thoracic aperture SEE: thoracic outlet.

inotropic (in" ō-trop' ik) Influencing the force of muscular contractility.

inspiratory compliance curve A measure of the elastic properties of the lung generated during inspiration; the curve is produced when the transpulmonary pressure or distending pressure) is plotted against the lung volume during inflation.

interatrial band High-speed bundle of atrial muscle fibers that rapidly spread electrical impulses through the walls of the atria to distribute signals to the left atrium.

interatrial septum The wall in the heart separating the two atria.

interbronchial connections Small anastamoses between adjacent bronchi providing collateral ventilation to distal parts of the lung.

intercalated disc A modification of the cell membrane of adjacent cardiac muscle cells made up of interdigitating margins; it contains intercellular junctions for electrical and mechanical linkage of contiguous cells.

interdependence of alveoli The communal structural and functional arrangement of alveoli, resulting from the elastic tissue that supports and maintains the patency of alveoli, and the shared septa between alveoli. The collapse of an alveolus is opposed by the adjacent alveoli, thus adding to the stability of the lung.

interlobar fissures (horizontal, oblique) Deep grooves or folds separating the lobes of the lung; the visceral pleura extends into the recesses of the interlobar fissures.

internal naris SEE: choana.

internodal pathways High-speed bundles of atrial muscle fibers that rapidly spread electrical impulses from the sinoatrial node to the atrioventricular node.

interstice SEE: interstitium.

interstitial fluid colloid osmotic pressure (π_I) Outward Starling force that draws fluid out of the capillaries because of the presence of high-molecular-weight substances (colloids) found in the tissue spaces. SYN: interstitial fluid colloid oncotic pressure. SEE: Starling forces.

interstitial fluid pressure (P_I) Outward Starling force acting on the capillary wall that draws fluids into the tissue spaces because of the negative pressure maintained by the "pumping" action of lymph capillaries that scavenge fluid from the interstitial spaces. SYN: interstitial fluid hydrostatic pressure. SEE: Starling forces.

interstitium (in" ter-stish' ē-um) The space or gap in a tissue or structure of an organ, in contradistinction to its functional parts, or parenchyma. SYN: interstice. The interstitium of the lung consists of supporting elements, such as collagen and elastin fibers. SEE: parenchyma.

interventricular septum The wall in the heart separating the two ventricles.

intervillous spaces The spaces located between chorionic villi of the placenta.

intra-alveolar pressure The pressure within the alveoli of the lungs. SYN: alveolar pressure; intrapulmonary pressure.

intrapleural pressure The pressure within the pleural cavity, a potential space between the visceral and parietal pleurae; a negative pleural pressure (approximately −7 mm Hg relative to atmospheric pressure) is maintained by the continual drainage of lymph out of the pleural space, and counteracts the tendency of the lung to collapse. SYN: pleural pressure.

intrapleural space SEE: pleural cavity.

intrapulmonary shunting The effect produced when blood is delivered to alveoli that are underventilated or unventilated, resulting in the production of a venous admixture that has an oxygen tension and oxygen content close to that of mixed venous blood entering the alveolar-capillary system. SYN: pulmonary shunting.

intrinsic conducting system SEE: cardiac conducting system.

intrinsic laryngeal muscles One of two muscle groups of the larynx. These muscles include the cricothyroid, external and internal thyroarytenoid, transverse and oblique arytenoid, and external and internal thyroarytenoid muscle groups. SEE: larynx; extrinsic laryngeal muscles.

intrinsic oscillator A functional area of the brainstem involved in the control of ventilation. This control area receives afferent impulses from peripheral receptors, integrates them with the functional state of the controlling neurons, and sends integrated command signals to the muscles of breathing. Ventilatory control *oscillates*, or alternates, between mutually antagonistic groups of nerve cells controlling the various muscles of breathing.

irritant relfex SEE: bronchoconstriction reflex.

ischemic hypoxia SEE: hypoxia.

isohydric principle The relationship in which all the buffer pairs in a system are in equilibrium with the same hydrogen ion concentration and thus behave similarly. SEE: buffer.

J receptors, juxtacapillary receptors, juxtapulmonary capillary receptors, juxta-alveolar receptors SEE: C-fiber afferents.

juxtaglomerular apparatus (JGA) Modified distal convoluted tubule cells of the nephrons that monitor the degree of stretch of the walls of the afferent arteriole supplying a glomerulus. Low blood pressure causes the juxtaglomerular apparatus to release renin, which initiates the renin-angiotensin-aldosterone mechanism for the long-term control of blood pressure.

Kussmaul's breathing A pattern of breathing characterized by an increase in the rate and depth of breathing, resulting in a deep, gasping type of respiratory pattern. Kussmaul's breathing sometimes accompanies severe nonrespiratory acidosis, as occurs in severe salicylate toxicity.

lacrimal bones Small, paired facial bones forming part of the medial orbit and the lateral walls of the nasal cavity.

laminar flow An orderly type of flow pattern in which the fluid molecules move in a parallel fashion along the walls of the conducting tube. The flow pattern is perfectly uniform, with the velocity profile assuming a parabolic shape because the higher-velocity molecules move along the central core and the slower-velocity molecules move at the periphery. (The molecules in contact with the tube wall have zero velocity.)

laryngopharynx (lar-in″ gō-far′ inks) The lowest part of the pharynx, the laryngopharynx is lined with stratified squamous epithelium and opens inferiorly to the larynx anteriorly and the esophagus posteriorly. The laryngopharynx is located below the hyoid bone. SEE: pharynx.

laryngotracheal tube (la-ring″ gō-trā′ kē-al) Primitive tube that develops from the floor of the pharynx. The cranial portion gives rise to the larynx; the caudal portion develops into the trachea and forms an outpouching called the lung bud.

larynx (lar′ inks) A musculocartilaginous organ at the upper end of the trachea below the root of the tongue, lined with ciliated mucous membrane; part of the airway and the organ of voice. The larynx consists of nine cartilages bound together by an elastic membrane and moved by muscles.

lateral cartilages Paired supporting cartilages of the external nose that extend from the nasal bones to the alar cartilages. SEE: alar cartilages.

left atrium (LA) Left superior chamber of the heart, which receives blood from the pulmonary veins and pumps blood to the left ventricle.

left coronary artery Branch of the aorta supplying the myocardium; divided into two major branches:

  anterior interventricular branch Located in the anterior interventricular sulcus; supplies blood to the interventricular septum and the anterior wall of both ventricles.

  circumflex branch Located in the coronary sulcus; supplies blood to the left atrium and the posterior wall of the left ventricle.

left ventricle (LV) Left inferior chamber of the heart, which receives blood from the left atrium and pumps blood into the systemic circuit through the aorta.

left ventricular stroke work index (LVSWI) Hemodynamic measurement of contractility, or work performed by the left ventricle. LVSWI is calculated as the product of the stroke volume index and the difference between the mean arterial pressure and the left ventricular end-diastolic pressure (represented by the pulmonary capillary wedge pressure). See text for equation with appropriate conversion factor. SEE: stroke volume index (SVI); mean arterial pressure (MAP); pulmonary capillary wedge pressure (PCWP).

ligamentum arteriosum (lig″ a-men′-tum ar-tēr′-i-ō-sum) The fibrous band that is the remnant of the embryonic ductus arteriosus. SEE: ductus arteriosus.

ligamentum teres (lig″ a-men′-tum tare′-ēz) A fibrous cord extending upward from the umbilicus and enclosed in the lower margin of the falciform ligament of the liver; represents the remnant of the umbilical vein external to the liver in the fetus. SYN: round ligament of the liver.

ligamentum venosum (lig″ a-men′-tum ven-ō′-sum) The fibrous band that is the remnant of the embryonic ductus venosus. SEE: ductus venosus.

lines of defense A system of barriers and mechanisms that prevents or minimizes the entry or effect of potentially damaging substances or pathogens.

  first line of defense Mechanical and chemical barriers (e.g., skin, epithelial layers, mucous membranes, gastric juice).

  second line of defense Phagocytic cells of the body (e.g., neutrophils, alveolar macrophages).

  third line of defense Specific antibodies produced by the immune system.

lingua A "tongue-shaped" strip of tissue located at the lower margin of the cardiac notch of the left lung.

lingual tonsils (ling′ gwal) A mass of lymphoid tissue located in the root of the tongue.

lobar bronchi Subdivisions of the mainstem bronchi that supply the individual lobes of the lung. The right mainstem bronchus branches into the right superior and right intermediate lobar bronchus; the intermediate bronchus splits into the right middle lobar bronchus and the right inferior lobar bronchus. The left mainstem bronchus branches into the left superior lobar bronchus and the left inferior lobar bronchus. SYN: secondary bronchi.

lobar buds Outpouchings from the right and left mainstem bronchi. Lobar buds are the precursors of the lobar (secondary) bronchi supplying lobes of the lungs.

lobes of the lung One of the large divisions of the lungs: superior and inferior lobes of the left lung; superior, middle, and inferior lobes of the right lung.

loop of the nephron A long, tubular component of the nephron that *loops*, or turns 180 degrees, upon itself; it consists of a *descending segment* that extends from the proximal convoluted tubule and an *ascending segment* that extends toward the distal convoluted tubule. SYN: loop of Henle.

lower respiratory tract The part of the respiratory system that begins with the larynx and continues as several generations of airways supplying the alveoli.

lung bud A single outpouching from the caudal end of the laryngotracheal tube. The lung bud is the precursor of the right and left bronchial buds. SEE: laryngotracheal tube.

lung capacities Lung spirometric measurements composed of two or more lung volumes:

  functional residual capacity (FRC) The amount of air (approximately 2.4 L) remaining in the lungs at the end of a normal expiration; FRC consists of the expiratory reserve volume and the residual volume. (The residual volume cannot be voluntarily exhaled; therefore, only part of the FRC is functional in terms of gas exchange.) SEE: lung volumes.

inspiratory capacity (IC) The amount of air (approximately 3.6 L) brought into the lungs by a maximal inspiratory effort following a normal expiration; IC equals the tidal volume plus the inspiratory reserve volume. SEE: lung volumes.

total lung capacity (TLC) The total amount of air that can be held by the lungs with a maximal inspiratory effort (approximately 6 L); TLC consists of the vital capacity plus the residual volume. SEE: lung volumes.

vital capacity (VC) A measure of the total amount of *usable* air available in the lungs following a maximal inspiratory effort and a maximal expiratory effort (approximately 4.8 L); VC equals the sum of the inspiratory reserve volume, tidal volume, and the expiratory reserve volume. SEE: lung volumes.

lung resistance The impedance (resistance) encountered when the lung volume changes over time (as opposed to lung inflation and deflation under static conditions). A rapid change in lung volume requires a greater pleural pressure gradient than that required to change the lung volume *slowly*. Lung resistance is due to nonelastic resistance caused by the combined effect of airway resistance and tissue viscous resistance.

lung surfactant SEE: pulmonary surfactant.

lung volumes Lung spirometric measurements, as follows:

expiratory reserve volume (ERV) The amount of air (approximately 1.2 L) that can be expelled at the end of normal tidal breath through forceful contraction of the accessory expiratory group of muscles.

inspiratory reserve volume (IRV) The amount of air (approximately 3.1 L) that can be inhaled beyond the normal tidal volume; the IRV is attained by the combined activity of the diaphragm and the accessory inspiratory group of muscles.

residual volume (RV) The amount of air (approximately 1.2 L) remaining in the lungs after the most forceful expiration.

tidal volume (V_t) The amount of air moved by diaphragmatic activity during normal, relaxed, quiet breathing (approximately 0.5 L in an average young adult man).

mainstem bronchi Large cartilaginous airways that bifurcate from the trachea at the carina to supply each lung. The right mainstem bronchus is usually shorter, more vertical, and larger in diameter than the left mainstem bronchus. SYN: primary bronchi.

major calyx (kā′ lix) Hollow, branched "extensions" of the renal pelvis that branch into several minor calyces that contact the renal papillae of the renal pyramids.

marginally laminar flow SEE: transitional flow.

maxilla A single bone formed by the fusion of right and left maxillary bones. It contains several processes that form the skeletal base of most of the upper face, roof of the mouth, sides of the nasal cavity, and floor of the orbit. The alveolar process of the maxilla supports the teeth.

maximal voluntary ventilation (MVV) Maximal volume of air moved by strenuous breathing for a period of 15 seconds. SYN: ventilatory capacity.

mean arterial blood pressure (MABP) The sum of the diastolic pressure and one-third the pulse pressure.

mean pulmonary artery pressure (MPAP) Blood pressure recorded within the pulmonary artery.

meatus A passage or opening. The nasal meatuses are found on the side walls of the nasal cavity between the nasal conchae. SEE: ethmoid bone; inferior nasal conchae.

medial umbilical ligaments Fibrous cords that are the remnants of the embryonic umbilical arteries.

mediastinal (medial) surface The surface of the lungs that faces inward, toward the mediastinum. SEE: mediastinum.

mediastinum (mē″ dē-as-tī′ num) 1. A septum or cavity between two principal portions of an organ. 2. The mass of organs and tissues separating the lungs. It contains the heart and its large vessels, trachea, esophagus, thymus, lymph nodes, and connective tissue.

medullary chemoreceptors Chemoreceptors located on the ventrolateral surface of the medulla near the medullary respiratory center. Carbon dioxide diffuses from the bloodstream into the cerebrospinal fluid (CSF), where it combines with water to form carbonic acid. Carbonic acid ionizes to generate hydrogen ions,

which are detected by the central chemoreceptors to result in stimulation of the medullary respiratory center.

medullary ischemic reflex Reflex vasoconstriction of blood vessels in the lowermost part of the body that causes blood to be redistributed to the upper part of the body. This reflex is initiated by the medullary vasomotor center in response to hypoxia and hypercapnia resulting from inadequate perfusion of the brainstem.

metabolic respiratory quotient (RQ) The number of carbon dioxide molecules produced by the tissues relative to the oxygen molecules consumed by the tissues. (In the homeostatic state, the respiratory exchange ratio is normally equal to the metabolic respiratory quotient.)

metarterioles Small-diameter branches of arterioles that possess circularly arranged individual smooth muscle cells, rather than a continuous muscular layer within the tunica media; they function to connect arterioles directly with capillary beds and control the flow of blood into the capillary beds.

middle cardiac vein A vein located in the posterior interventricular sulcus; drains blood from the posterior aspect of the myocardium.

minor calyx A hollow, cup-shaped structure that is immediately adjacent to the renal papilla of a renal pyramid. Minor calyces collect urine and convey it into major calyces.

minute ventilation The volume of air moved per unit time, calculated as the product of the tidal volume and the respiratory rate (in breaths per minute). SYN: minute volume; total ventilation ($\dot{V}E$). SEE: lung volumes.

mitral valve SEE: atrioventricular valves.

mouth pressure (P_m) The pressure at the proximal end of the conducting "tube" of the airways.

mucociliary escalator Clearance mechanism in the airways that moves bronchial mucus upward toward the oropharynx; propulsion of mucus is provided by the rhythmic beating action of cilia, which contact and stretch bronchial mucus, thus overcoming its natural viscosity. SYN: ciliary transport mechanism. SEE: oropharynx.

mucus Complex fluid composed of water, glycoprotein, carbohydrates, lipids, DNA, and cellular debris.

gel phase The relatively viscous and elastic layer at the luminal surface of the airways.

sol phase The thinner, watery layer that contacts the beating cilia of the epithelial lining cells.

muscular arteries SEE: arteries.

myelinated fibers Nerve fibers that possess a myelin sheath; myelinated fibers involved in respiratory functions include slowly adapting receptors (SARs) and rapidly adapting receptors (RARs).

myocardium The middle layer of the wall of the heart, composed of cardiac muscle.

myogenic origin The initiation of electrical impulses in the myocardium itself, rather than in pacemaker tissue located extrinsic to the heart.

N_1, N_2 nicotinic receptors SEE: cholinergic receptors.

nasal bones Small, paired facial bones that form the medial part of the bridge of the nose.

nasal cavity One of two cavities between the floor of the cranium and the roof of the mouth, opening to the nose anteriorly and the nasopharynx posteriorly. Its lining of highly vascularized, ciliated epithelium warms and moistens inhaled air, and traps dust and pathogens on mucus that is then swept toward the pharynx. The nasal septum (ethmoid and vomer) separates the nasal cavities.

nasal fossa The cavity between the anterior opening to the nose and the nasopharynx.

nasolacrimal duct A duct that conveys tears from the lacrimal sac to the nasal cavity. It opens beneath the inferior nasal concha.

nasopharynx (nā zō-far-inks) The upper portion of the pharynx, the nasopharynx is located above the soft palate, lined with pseudostratified ciliated epithelium, and has openings to the posterior nares and eustachian tubes. SEE: pharynx.

natural resistance The naturally occurring nonspecific resistance factors that provide defense for the body (e.g., mechanical, chemical, and cellular lines of defense).

nephrons Functional units of the kidney where urine is formed. Two types of nephrons are recognized on the basis of their location:

cortical nephrons Relatively small and compact nephrons located entirely within the renal cortex.

juxtamedullary nephrons Relatively long nephrons with their proximal elements located in the renal cortex and their distal structures extending downward into the renal medulla.

net filtration pressure (NFP) The effective filtration pressure is determined by the difference between the glomerular filtration pressure and the sum of the capsular hydrostatic pressure and colloid osmotic pressure. If the NFP is positive, diuresis occurs and urine is formed; if the value is negative, urine is not formed.

neural net An elaborate network of interconnected neurons that provides complex pathways for the distribution of nerve impulses among nerve cells and between nerve cells and effectors.

neutrophil elastase (NE) A specific protease produced by neutrophils; NE is capable of destroying elastin in the lung, thus reducing the lung's resiliency. NE also damages bronchial epithelium, reduces ciliary beating, and promotes mucous gland hyperplasia. Anti-NE defenses include inhibitors with antielastase properties such as α_1-antitrypsin, secretory leukoprotease inhibitor, and α_2-macroglobulin.

nodal rhythm The regular electrical rhythm generated by the firing of the atrioventricular node.

nonadrenergic noncholinergic (NANC) neurotransmission Neural control of airway diameter not dependent on either the sympathetic or the parasympathetic division of the autonomic nervous system (ANS). Inhibitory NANC (i-NANC) transmitters such as nitric oxide functionally oppose the bronchoconstriction produced by parasympathetic (vagal) stimulation of airway smooth muscle. (Vasoactive intestinal peptide and adenosine triphosphate presumably play a moderator role in the i-NANC mechanism.)

noncartilaginous airways Airways of the conducting zone of the lung that do not contain supporting cartilage in their walls. Noncartilaginous airways continue from the subsegmental bronchi and include several generations of bronchioles and terminal bronchioles.

nonelastic resistance Collective term referring to the combined effect on lung resistance of airway resistance and tissue viscous resistance, factors affected by the dynamics of breathing.

nonelastic work The work of breathing that must be expended to overcome nonelastic resistance factors such as airway resistance and tissue viscous resistance. At higher breathing frequencies, nonelastic work must increase dramatically to overcome greatly increased airway resistance caused by chaotic air flow patterns.

nonideal lung Description of the normal lung in which significant differences in both ventilation and perfusion are seen in different regions. SYN: nonhomogeneous lung.

nonvolatile acid An acid that is produced in the tissues during normal cellular metabolism, ingested as part of the diet, or formed during pathophysiologic processes; fixed acids are normally removed from the body by the kidneys. SYN: fixed acid.

nostril One of the external apertures of the nose. SYN: external naris.

obstructive disease Pulmonary disease marked by pathophysiologic changes that limit expiratory flow at relatively low flowrates (e.g., asthma, chronic bronchitis, emphysema, cystic fibrosis).

oral cavity The cavity of the mouth. It includes the vestibule and oral cavity proper. SYN: buccal cavity.

oropharynx (ōr″ ō-far-inks) The middle part of the pharynx, the oropharynx is lined with stratified squamous epithelium and has an opening to the oral cavity. The oropharynx lies between the soft palate and the hyoid bone. SEE: pharynx.

orthopnea Respiratory condition in which there is breathing difficulty in any but an erect sitting or standing position. The muscles of respiration are forcibly used in the struggle to inhale and exhale. A sitting or standing posture is necessary to ease breathing.

osmolality The number of osmoles of solute per kilogram of water.

osmolarity The number of osmoles of solute per liter of solution. (Most clinical calculations of osmotic concentration are based on osmolarity.)

osmole (osm) A unit of osmotic concentration equal to 1 mole of dissolved solute particles.

oxygen consumption ($\dot{V}_{O_2}$) The amount of oxygen utilized by the tissues, calculated as the difference between systemic oxygen delivery and systemic oxygen return.

oxyhemoglobin An unstable compound formed by the combination of hemoglobin and oxygen. Hemoglobin with oxygen is found in arterial blood and is the oxygen carrier to the body tissue.

oxyhemoglobin dissociation curve A curve that shows the relationship between the partial pressure of oxygen and the percentage of saturation of hemoglobin with oxygen (i.e., the proportion of oxyhemoglobin to reduced hemoglobin). SEE: hemoglobin saturation curve.

left shift Factors that shift the curve to the left include a decrease in temperature, a decrease in carbon dioxide tension, and an increase in pH. Such factors cause an increase in affinity of hemoglobin for oxygen, and increased oxygen-binding capacity.

right shift Factors that favor a shift of the curve to the right, accelerating the release of oxygen from oxyhemoglobin, are a rise in temperature, an increase in carbon dioxide tension, and a decrease in pH. These factors cause a decrease in the affinity of hemoglobin for oxygen, and decreased oxygen-binding capacity.

P-R interval SEE: electrocardiogram.

pacemaker potential The gradual depolarization toward threshold seen in some self-excitatory tissues such as the sinoatrial node. The mechanism is spontaneous and autorhythmic, but is not fully understood.

pain reflex Apnea caused by sudden pain.

palate The bony and soft tissue partition separating the oral and nasal cavities. SEE: hard palate; soft palate.

palatine bones Paired facial bones that form the posterior part of the hard, or bony, palate. SEE: hard palate.

palatine tonsils A mass of lymphoid tissue that lies in the tonsillar fossa on each side of the oropharynx between the glossopalatine and pharyngopalatine arches. SYN: faucial tonsil.

papillary muscles (pap′ i-lar-ē) Short, blunt, pillarlike extensions on the lining of the heart that serve to anchor the chordae tendineae.

paranasal ducts Small ducts that drain the paranasal sinuses; the orifices open into the meatuses on the side walls of the nasal cavity.

paranasal sinuses Any of the anterior accessory nasal sinuses (frontal, ethmoidal, sphenoidal, and maxillary) that open into the nasal cavities. All are lined with a ciliated mucous membrane continuous with that of the nasal cavities.

parenchyma (par-en′ ki-ma) The essential parts of an organ that constitute its function, in contrast to its framework, or interstitium. The parenchyma of the lung is composed of the alveoli. SEE: interstitium.

parietal pericardium The outermost layer of the pericardial sac, composed of an inner serous layer and an outer fibrous layer; the parietal pericardium is continuous with the visceral pericardium.

partial pressure The pressure exerted by an individual gas in a mixture of gases; partial pressure of a gas is the product of the dry gas fraction and the barometric pressure of the mixture. SYN: tension (PGAS).

perfusion The rate of blood flow per given mass of tissue.

perfusion-limited gas exchange Gas exchange at the alveolar-capillary membrane that is determined by the rate of movement of blood through the pulmonary capillaries, rather than the rate of diffusion of gas across the membrane. The transfer of high-solubility gases such as nitrous oxide is limited by cardiac output, and is said to be perfusion limited. SEE: cardiac output ($\dot{Q}$).

pericardial cavity The narrow space found between the visceral and parietal layers of the pericardial sac; the cells that line the cavity secrete a serous (watery) fluid that lubricates the layers during the pumping action of the heart.

peripheral vascular resistance The resistance that blood encounters within blood vessels, subdivided into two categories: pulmonary vascular resistance (PVR) within the pulmonary circuit and systemic vascular resistance (SVR) within the systemic circuit. SEE: systemic vascular resistance (SVR); pulmonary vascular resistance (PVR).

peritubular capillaries A network of capillaries in close proximity to the tubular components of the nephron. Peritubular capillaries receive blood from the efferent arterioles and allow various exchanges (e.g., wastes, nutrients, electrolytes, water) to occur between the bloodstream and the glomerular filtrate. SEE: efferent arterioles; glomerular filtrate.

perpendicular plate (of ethmoid bone) Thin, midline plate of the ethmoid that projects inferiorly from the cribriform plate. The perpendicular plate forms the upper part of the nasal septum.

pharyngeal tonsil SEE: adenoid.

pharynx (far′ inks) A musculomembranous tube extending from the base of the skull to the level of the sixth cervical vertebra, where it becomes continuous with the esophagus. It consists of an upper (nasopharynx), middle (oropharynx), and lower (laryngopharynx) portion. The pharynx communicates with the posterior nares, eustachian tube, mouth, esophagus, and larynx. It provides a passageway for air from the nasal cavity to the larynx and for food from the mouth to the esophagus. It also acts as a resonating cavity.

phases of the cardiac cycle The sequence of events that occurs during one cycle of contraction of the heart. The following periods occur chronologically:

phase 1 (quiescent period) The interval between beats characterized by the lack of contraction of the chambers of the heart; atrial and ventricular pressures are zero; no sounds are produced; blood flows into the ventricles through open atrioventricular valves.

phase 2 (atrial systole) Contraction of the atria, which primes the ventricles so that they contain an end-diastolic volume prior to ventricular systole.

phase 3 (isovolumetric contraction) Extremely brief contractile activity in the ventricles, which generates tension in the ventricular muscle fibers without causing ejection of blood.

phase 4 (ventricular ejection) Contraction of the ventricular fibers, which causes an increase in intraventricular pressure such that it exceeds vascular pressure in the pulmonary trunk and aorta, thus allowing blood to be ejected into the pulmonary and systemic circuits, respectively.

phase 5 (isovolumetric relaxation) The first part of ventricular diastole; ventricular pressures decrease, but the volume of the ventricles does not immediately rise; all heart valves are closed; blood does not enter the ventricles.

ventricular filling Continuation of ventricular diastole; decrease in ventricular pressure allows atrioventricular valves to open and blood to enter the ventricles. NOTE: Three subphases overlap with both phase 1 and phase 2: rapid ventricular filling, diastasis (period of slower filling of the ventricles), and ventricular priming.

physiologic dead space ventilation The total amount of wasted ventilation in the lungs, composed of ventilation of (1) the anatomical dead space and (2) the alveolar dead space (i.e., excessive ventilation of alveoli that are not adequately perfused).

physiologic oxygen-binding capacity The *actual volume* of oxygen transport by 1 g of hemoglobin when the arterial oxygen saturation is 100%. The value is approximately 1.34 mL oxygen per gram of hemoglobin. (This value is less than the theoretical binding capacity because not all of the oxygen-binding sites on hemoglobin are available at a given time.)

physiologic shunt A venous admixture of blood coming from shunt compartments in the lung that have low ventilation-perfusion ratios. The blood exiting from the compartments is known as wasted blood flow. Two types of physiologic shunt are seen:

absolute shunt A physiologic shunt in which desaturated blood mixes with oxygenated blood without contacting the pulmonary blood stream. These shunts are refractory to supplemental oxygen therapy. SYN: true shunt. Two types of absolute shunt are recognized:

anatomic shunt An absolute shunt caused by a structure that allows blood to bypass the lungs. A small amount of anatomical shunting is caused by venous return through bronchial and thebesian veins; a large amount of anatomical shunting may be caused by congenital heart defects such as a patent ductus arteriosus, or by a vascular lung tumor.

capillary shunt A absolute shunt caused by severe pathophysiologic conditions, such as alveolar consolidation or atelectasis that totally block gas exchange in the alveolar-capillary system.

relative shunt A type of intrapulmonary shunt in which a portion of the pulmonary blood enters the lung but is not saturated with oxygen from the alveoli because of a high degree of ventilation-perfusion inequality in certain lung regions. This type of physiologic shunt is called a *shuntlike* effect because the results are similar to those produced by an actual anatomical shunt that diverts blood away from the lungs.

placenta The spongy structure in the uterus from which the fetus derives its nourishment and oxygen. The placenta consists of a fetal portion bearing many chorionic villi that interlock with corresponding structures on the lining of the uterus, which constitutes the maternal portion. The chorionic villi lie in spaces in the uterine endometrium, where they are bathed in maternal blood and lymph. Groups of villi are separated by placental septa, forming about 20 distinct lobules called cotyledons. When expelled following parturition, the placenta is known as the afterbirth. SEE: cotyledon.

plasma colloid osmotic pressure (π_c) Inward Starling force acting on the capillary that attracts fluid from the extravascular compartment into the capillary because of the presence of high-molecular-weight substances (colloids) in the blood vessel. SYN: plasma colloid oncotic pressure. SEE: Starling forces.

pleura (ploo′ ra) singular; **pleurae** (ploo′ r̄i) plural A serous membrane that enfolds both lungs and is reflected upon the walls of the thorax and diaphragm. The pleurae are moistened with a serous secretion that reduces friction during respiratory movements of the lungs. SEE: mediastinum; thorax.

parietal pleura The portion of the pleura that extends from the mediastinal roots of the lungs and covers the sides of the pericardium to the chest wall and backward to the spine. The visceral and parietal pleural layers are separated only by a lubricating secretion. These layers may become adherent or separated by fluid or air in diseased conditions. SYN: costal pleura.

visceral pleura The pleura that covers the lungs and lines the interlobar fissures. It is loose at the base and at sternal and vertebral borders to allow for lung expansion.

pleural canals Body cavities that are subdivisions of the intraembryonic coeloms. Pleural canals, as the precursors of the pleural cavities, receive the growing lungs as the lungs undergo continued embryonic development. SEE: pleuroperitoneal coelom.

pleural cavity The potential space between the parietal pleura that lines the thoracic cavity and the visceral pleura that covers the lungs. It contains pleural fluid, the serous fluid that prevents friction. SYN: pleural space; intrapleural space.

pleural fluid A monolayer of viscous, lubricating fluid that occupies the pleural space to reduce friction between the visceral and parietal pleurae; the fluid is derived from interstitial fluid and contains tissue proteins, which give it a slippery, mucoid consistency.

pleural pressure SEE: intrapleural pressure.

pleuropericardial folds Projections of tissue from the lateral body wall that fuse in the midline to form the pericardial cavity, and thus separate the heart from the paired pleural canals that contain the developing lungs.

pleuroperitoneal folds Projections of tissue from the dorsolateral body wall that fuse with the transverse septum to form the lateral elements of the future diaphragm. SEE: transverse septum.

Poiseuille's law A law that states that the rapidity of the capillary current is directly proportional to the fourth power of the radius of the capillary tube and the pressure on the fluid, and inversely proportional to the viscosity of the liquid and the length of the tube. SYN: Hagen-Poiseuille law.

pontine respiratory group (PRG) A respiratory center located in the dorsolateral pons in the parabrachial nuclei and the Kölliker-Fuse nucleus. The neurons of the PRG are not essential for respiratory rhythm generation, but they may modify the basic medullary rhythm. The precise nature of the interactions is unclear.

pores of Kohn (kōn) A passageway for gas from one alveolus of the lung to an adjacent one. These may be of assistance in preventing atelectasis.

posterior interventricular sulcus External landmark of the heart; a shallow groove separating the right and left ventricles on the posterior surface.

precapillary sphincter Small, circular ring of smooth muscle at the origin of a capillary branching from a metarteriole; contraction of precapillary sphincters directs blood from the metarteriole into the thoroughfare channel and venule; relaxation of precapillary sphincters allows blood to enter the capillaries making up the capillary bed. SEE: capillary; capillary bed; metarteriole; thoroughfare channel.

primary bronchi SEE: mainstem bronchi.

primary lobule SEE: acinus.

primary pacemaker SEE: sinoatrial node.

primitive heart tube Undifferentiated pump formed by the fusion of paired endocardial tubes in the embryo; the primitive heart tube ultimately differentiates into future pumping chambers.

primitive respiratory tube Embryonic precursor of the tracheobronchial tree, characterized by sequential development of the conducting and respiratory zones of the respiratory system, and divided into several developmental periods: glandular period, canalicular period, and alveolar period.

principal cells SEE: type I cells.

proprioceptors Receptors that respond to stimuli originating within the body itself, especially stimuli that respond to pressure, position, or stretch.

proximal convoluted tubule A small-diameter tube of the nephron located close to the glomerular capsule that conveys glomerular filtrate into the descending segment of the loop of the nephron. SEE: glomerular filtrate; loop of the nephron.

pulmonary artery catheter A balloon-tipped, flexible catheter with multiple recording capabilities and separate injection ports; used in right heart catheterization studies of cardiac activity.

pulmonary capillary wedge pressure (PCWP) The pressure in the pulmonary artery recorded with a special balloon-tipped catheter. The PCWP provides *an indirect measurement* of the pressure in the left ventricle because a static column of blood extends distally from the tip of the catheter occluding the pulmonary artery, through the pulmonary capillaries and pulmonary veins, and into the left atrium and left ventricle. PCWP is used in hemodynamic measurements to represent the left ventricular end-diastolic pressure. SEE: left ventricular stroke work index (LVSWI).

pulmonary chemoreflex Respiratory response produced by activation of C-fiber afferents by stimuli (e.g., apnea [induced by inhaling cold air], rapid breathing, bronchoconstriction, bradycardia, hypotension). The role of this reflex in breathing is not fully understood.

pulmonary circulation The flow of blood from the right ventricle of the heart to the lungs for exchange of oxygen and carbon dioxide in the pulmonary capillaries, then through the pulmonary veins to the left atrium.

pulmonary ligament A fold of pleura that extends from the hilus (hilum) of the lung to the base of the medial surface of the lung.

pulmonary mechanics The study of the volume and pressure changes produced in the thorax and lungs by the muscles of breathing; the muscles of ventilation generate the pressures that overcome the natural elasticity, or static properties, of the respiratory system during conditions of zero gas flow.

pulmonary shunting SEE: intrapulmonary shunting.

pulmonary surfactant A complex phospholipid substance in the lung that regulates the amount of surface tension of the fluid lining the alveoli. Exogenous lung surfactant from natural and artificial sources is available for treating patients with respiratory distress syndrome. SYN: lung surfactant.

pulmonary vascular resistance (PVR) The peripheral resistance against which the right ventricle must work in order to eject its volume of blood into the pulmonary circuit; PVR indicates the magnitude of the right ventricular afterload; calculated as the pressure difference between the proximal blood pressure (pulmonary artery pressure) and the distal blood pressure (left atrial pressure), divided by the cardiac output ($\dot{Q}$). SEE: cardiac output ($\dot{Q}$).

pulmonary vascular resistance index (PVRI) The pulmonary vascular resistance divided by the body surface area. SEE: pulmonary vascular resistance (PVR); body surface area (BSA).

pulse pressure The difference between systolic pressure and diastolic pressure.

pump-handle movement Rib-cage movement in which the pivoting action of the rib occurs about an axis of rotation that passes through the head and the tubercle of the rib. The rotation involves the joint between the head of the rib and the superior and inferior facets of two adjacent vertebrae, and the costovertebral joint formed by the costal facet on the tubercle of the rib and the costal facet on the transverse process of a corresponding vertebra. Rib rotation causes a slight anterior displacement of the sternum, which increases the anteroposterior diameter of the thorax during forced inspiration.

Purkinje fibers SEE: conduction myofibers.

Purkinje system (per kin'-jē) That part of the cardiac conduction system consisting of the conduction pathways (atrioventricular bundle, bundle branches, conduction myofibers). SYN: His-Purkinje system (hiss' per kin'-jē).

rapidly adapting receptor (RAR) A sensory receptor of the myelinated fiber type that accommodates rapidly to a sustained stimulus to result in the slow firing of impulses to the central nervous system as part of the bronchoconstriction reflex; commonly found among epithelial cells of large airways and are stimulated by inhaled irritants or noxious substances (e.g., particulate matter). SYN: subepithelial irritant receptor. SEE: bronchoconstriction reflex.

red blood cell (RBC) SEE: erythrocyte.

renal artery The main blood vessel that branches from the abdominal aorta to supply the kidney.

renal columns Thin pillarlike extensions of the renal cortex that protrude into the renal medulla and separate adjacent renal pyramids.

renal cortex The outermost layer of the kidney.

renal mechanism SEE: renin-angiotensin-aldosterone mechanism.

renal medulla The innermost core of the kidney, composed of numerous renal pyramids.

renal papilla Finger-shaped structure located at the apical (medullary) end of the renal pyramids. Renal papillae convey urine into the minor calyces.

renal pelvis The upper expanded part of the ureter. The funnel-shaped renal pelvis collects urine and directs it into the urine for transport to the bladder.

renal pyramids Triangular-shaped structures composed of numerous collecting ducts and loops of nephrons arranged in a parallel fashion. The renal pyramids comprise the renal medulla.

renal vein The main blood vessel that returns blood to the inferior vena cava from the kidney.

renin The enzyme secreted by the juxtaglomerular apparatus (JGA) in the kidney in response to low blood pressure; renin brings about the conversion of the inactive plasma precursor angiotensinogen into angiotensin I, a mild vasoconstrictor.

renin-angiotensin-aldosterone mechanism Mechanism providing long-term control of blood pressure; conditions of hypoxia stimulate the juxtaglomerular cells of the kidney to secrete renin, which converts angiotensinogen in the plasma into angiotensin I. Pulmonary endothelial cells secrete angiotensin-converting enzyme (ACE), which transforms angiotensin I into angiotensin II, a powerful vasoactive substance that promotes widespread vasoconstriction and also stimulates the secretion of aldosterone. SYN: renal mechanism. SEE: aldosterone; angiotensin II; angiotensin-converting enzyme (ACE).

resistance vessel A blood vessel (e.g., arteriole) that is capable of dramatically changing its diameter to alter vascular resistance and blood pressure.

respiratory acidosis A condition resulting from the accumulation of carbon dioxide; blood pH falls markedly as the hydrogen ion concentration increases.

respiratory alkalosis A condition resulting from the depletion of carbon dioxide; blood pH rises markedly as the hydrogen ion concentration decreases.

respiratory bronchiole The proximal structure of the acinus of the respiratory zone; a tubelike structure characterized by the presence of alveoli arranged as small outpouchings from the tube.

respiratory center A functional collection of nerve cells in the brainstem that control ventilatory activity. The cells are linked together to form a neural net that includes the motoneurons innervating respiratory muscles. Three distinct neuronal complexes comprise the respiratory center in the brainstem: dorsal respiratory group (DRG), ventral respiratory group (VRG), and the pontine respiratory group (PRG). The spinal respiratory group (SRG) is located in the spinal cord.

respiratory exchange ratio (R) The ratio of carbon dioxide eliminated from the tissues relative to the oxygen taken up by the lungs. (In the homeostatic state, the respiratory exchange ratio is normally equal to the metabolic respiratory quotient.)

respiratory membrane SEE: alveolar-capillary membrane.

respiratory pump The venous return mechanism that operates because a high and low pressure is alternatively produced on each side of the diaphragm by its vertical movement. Blood flowing in the inferior vena cava is affected by the pressure difference caused by the up and down excursion of the diaphragm. (Venous valves prevent backflow.) SYN: abdominothoracic pump mechanism.

respiratory tree SEE: tracheobronchial tree.

respiratory zone The portion of the respiratory system consisting of gas-exchange units called alveoli, organized into respiratory bronchioles, alveolar ducts, and alveolar sacs. Such structures make up an acinus, or functional unit of the lung, collectively forming the parenchyma of the organ. SEE: acinus; parenchyma.

resting membrane potential SEE: cardiac action potential Phase 4 (polarization).

restrictive disease Pulmonary disease marked by pathophysiologic changes that limit the amount of lung inflation (e.g., pulmonary interstitial fibrosis).

Reynolds' number (Re) A measurement of gas flow used to predict whether the gas flow in a system will exhibit laminar or turbulent characteristics. It is *directly proportional* to the diameter of the tube, the average velocity of the gas, and density of the gas, and *inversely proportional* to the viscosity of the gas. Reynolds' numbers greater than 2000 indicate that the gas flow will be turbulent.

rheology The study of the deformation and flow of matter when forces are applied and removed; the characteristics of *elasticity* and *viscosity* are studied when considering the rheologic properties of matter. SEE: elasticity; viscosity.

rhythmogenesis The generation of rhythmic neuronal impulses that are intrinsic in a particular tissue. The kernel of the respiratory central pattern generator is composed of ventral medullary neurons in the pre-Bötzinger complex (pre-BÖTC) that exhibit rhythmogenesis.

ribs Curved, flattened bones of the thorax that provide protection for thoracic vertebrae and serve as sites of hemopoiesis. All 12 pairs of ribs have thoracic (T1 to T12) attachments posteriorly but exhibit different anterior attachments. The two basic classifications recognized on the basis of anterior attachments are (1) true ribs (ribs 1 through 7), which attach directly to the sternum by means of costal cartilages; and (2) false ribs (ribs 8–12), which do not have direct sternal attachments. Instead, the cartilages of ribs 8, 9, and 10 attach to the cartilage of the rib immediately above (suprajacent rib), and attach indirectly to the sternum through the cartilage of rib 7; ribs 10 and 11 (floating ribs) do not have any sternal attachments, but attach to the musculature of the ventrolateral abdominal wall.

  angle Intersection of the body and the neck of the rib; the point where the shaft turns forward, just distal to the tubercle.

  body The curved portion of the rib distal to the angle. SYN: shaft.

  costal groove Shallow groove on the inferior margin of the shaft of the rib; protects the intercostal neurovascular bundle composed of the intercostal nerve, artery, and vein.

  neck Narrowed portion of the rib between the head and the tubercle.

  tubercle Knoblike protrusion distal to the neck of the rib; forms the costovertebral joint with corresponding thoracic vertebrae.

right atrial pressure (RAP) Blood pressure recorded within the right atrium.

right atrium (RA) Right superior chamber of the heart that receives blood from the superior vena cava, inferior vena cava, and coronary sinus and pumps blood to the right ventricle.

right coronary artery Branch of the aorta supplying the myocardium; divided into two major branches:

  marginal branch Supplies blood to the lateral walls of the right atrium and right ventricle.

  posterior interventricular branch Located in the posterior interventricular sulcus; supplies blood to the posterior walls of both ventricles.

right heart catheterization Procedure by which a balloon-tipped pulmonary artery catheter with recording electrodes is passed through different heart chambers by being carried downstream by the flow of blood through the chambers. SEE: pulmonary artery catheter.

right ventricle (RV) Right inferior chamber of the heart that receives blood from the right atrium and pumps blood into the pulmonary circuit through the pulmonary trunk and pulmonary arteries.

right ventricular stroke work index (RVSWI) Hemodynamic measurement of contractility, or work performed by the right ventricle. It is calculated as the product of the stroke volume index and the difference between the mean pulmonary artery pressure and the right ventricular end-diastolic pressure (represented by the central venous pressure). See text for equation with appropriate conversion factor. SEE: stroke volume index (SVI); mean pulmonary artery pressure (MPAP); central venous pressure (CVP).

rima glottidis (rī'ma glot' id-is) The opening between the true vocal cords. SEE: larynx.

round ligament of the liver SEE: ligamentum teres.

SA node SEE: sinoatrial node.

secondary bronchi SEE: lobar bronchi.

segmental bronchi The third generation of airway in the conducting zone of the respiratory system. These branches of the lobar bronchi give rise to the subsegmental bronchi. SYN: tertiary bronchi.

semilunar valves Heart valves that control the flow of blood out of the ventricles, as follows:

  aortic semilunar valve Controls the flow of blood into the systemic circuit through the aorta. The valve is located at the junction of the left ventricle and the ascending aorta and is composed of three segments (semilunar cusps). The aortic valve prevents regurgitation at the entrance of the aorta to the heart.

  pulmonary semilunar valve Controls the flow of blood into the pulmonary circuit through the pulmonary trunk. The valve is located at the junction of the right ventricle and pulmonary artery. It is composed of three cusps and prevents regurgitation of blood from the pulmonary artery to the right ventricle.

senescence (se-nes'-ens) The process of growing old or the period of old age.

septal cartilage The anterior cartilaginous division between the right and left nasal fossae, or air channels.

shaft SEE: ribs.

sheath cells SEE: type II cells.

shunt compartment A group of alveoli in the lung that are underventilated or unventilated. Blood shunted to such a compartment exits and mixes with blood coming from properly ventilated compartments. The venous admixture that results has an oxygen tension that is greater than that of mixed venous blood but less than that of arterial blood coming from normally ventilated compartments.

sinoatrial node A specialized group of cells in the right atrium near the entrance of the superior vena cava into the right atrium that automatically generates impulses that spread to other regions of the heart. The normal cardiac pacemaker is the sinoatrial node. SYN: SA node; primary pacemaker.

sinus rhythm The normal cardiac rhythm, the stimulus for which begins at the sinoatrial node.

sinus venosus (sī-nus ven-ō'-sus) Embryonic heart structure that is the precursor of the great veins, the sinoatrial node, and portions of the right atrium.

skeletal muscle pump The mechanism that squeezes thin-walled veins and passively "pumps" blood toward the heart during skeletal muscle contraction. (The operation of venous valves prevents backflow.)

slowly adapting receptor A sensory receptor of the myelinated fiber type that accommodates *slowly* to a sustained stimulus. These receptors are found among airway smooth muscle cells and are involved in the Hering-Breuer reflexes. SEE: Hering-Breuer deflation reflex; Hering-Breuer inflation reflex.

soft palate The posterior musculomembranous fold partly separating the mouth and pharynx; located posterior to the hard palate. SYN: velum palatinum.

specific lung compliance A measure of lung compliance that "normalizes" the measurement to the same part of the volume-pressure curve, thereby permitting comparison of different respiratory systems. Specific lung compliance is calculated when the static lung compliance is divided by the functional residual capacity. The effect of different lung capacities on lung compliance is eliminated because the static transpulmonary pressures at total lung capacity and at residual volume are the same regardless of lung size.

spinal respiratory group A respiratory center composed of interneuronal pools found in the cervical and thoracic spinal cord; probably shapes the respiratory pattern in some way through inhibitory synaptic connections to respiratory motoneurons. The details of the interaction are not fully understood.

spirometry Measurement of the air capacity of the lungs; spirometry deals with the recording of air moved into and out of the lungs during different conditions of breathing.

stage I expiratory inhibition SEE: triphasic pattern of breathing.

stage II expiration SEE: triphasic pattern of breathing.

Starling forces The four primary fluid dynamic forces that act on the inside and the outside of capillaries to cause fluid to be transferred into and out of the vascular compartment. The forces acting inside the capillary are the capillary pressure and the plasma colloid osmotic pressure; the forces acting on the outside of the capillary are the interstitial fluid pressure and the interstitial fluid colloid osmotic pressure.

Starling's law of the heart SEE: Frank-Starling law.

static lung compliance (C$_{st}$, C$_L$) The change in lung volume per unit change in pressure under conditions of no flow. Lungs with increased static compliance are very distensible; lungs with low compliance are stiff and expand with difficulty.

sternocostal joints SEE: thoracic joints.

sternum The narrow, flat bone in the median line of the thorax in front. It consists of the following parts:

body The largest part of the sternum; the body possesses lateral costal notches that articulate with the costal cartilages of ribs 2 through 7.

clavicular notches Shallow notches located on the upper margin of the manubrium that articulate with the medial ends of the clavicles at the sternoclavicular joints.

costal notches Shallow notches on the lateral margins of the manubrium and body of the sternum that articulate with the costal cartilages of ribs 1 through 7 (sternoclavicular joints).

infrasternal angle Angle formed by the right and left costal margins.

jugular notch Midline notch on the superior margin of the manubrium, located at approximately the level of T3. SYN: suprasternal notch.

manubrium Superior part of the sternum that articulates with the clavicles and ribs 1 and 2.

sternal angle Articulation formed by the junction of the manubrium and the body of the sternum (T4–5), approximately 5 cm below the jugular notch. SYN: angle of Lewis.

xiphoid Inferior process of the sternum, located at the lower end of the body at approximately the level of T10 or T11.

stroke volume (SV) The amount of blood ejected by the heart with one contraction (usually left ventricle), calculated as the difference between the end-diastolic volume and the end-systolic volume. SEE: end-diastolic volume (EDV); end-systolic volume (ESV).

stroke volume index (SVI) Stroke volume divided by the body surface area. SYN: stroke index (SI). SEE: body surface area (BSA); stroke volume (SV).

subepithelial irritant receptor SEE: rapidly adapting receptor.

subsegmental bronchi The fourth generation of airway in the conducting zone of the respiratory system. These branches of the segmental bronchi give rise to the bronchioles.

superior thoracic aperture SEE: thoracic inlet.

suprasternal notch SEE: sternum.

surface tension The force resulting from the mutual attraction of a liquid's molecules to each other, which produces a cohesive state that causes that liquid to assume a shape that presents the smallest surface area to the surrounding liquid or gas. This phenomenon accounts for the spherical shape assumed by fluids, such as drops of oil or water.

sustentacular cells SEE: type II cells.

symporter mechanism SEE: cotransport mechanism.

systemic circulation The general circulation through the whole body except the lungs.

systemic oxygen delivery The amount of oxygen delivered to the tissues, calculated as the product of the total cardiac output and the arterial oxygen content.

systemic oxygen return The amount of oxygen not used by the tissues and thus returned to circulation, calculated as the product of total cardiac output and the mixed venous blood oxygen content.

systemic vascular resistance (SVR) The peripheral resistance against which the left ventricle must work to eject its volume of blood into systemic circulation; SVR indicates the magnitude of the left ventricular afterload.

systemic vascular resistance index (SVRI) Systemic vascular resistance divided by the body surface area. SEE: systemic vascular resistance (SVR); body surface area (BSA).

systolic pressure The peak arterial blood pressure recorded during ventricular systole.

tachycardia (tak″ē-kar′ dē-a) An abnormal rapidity of heart action, usually defined as a heart rate greater than 100 beats per minute in adults.

tachypnea Abnormally rapid respiratory rate.

target cells Cells that synthesize and store allergic mediators or their immediate precursors, and serve as the target site for anti-

gen-antibody reactions that take place at the surface of the target cell membranes.

basophils Basophilic leukocytes of the granulocytic series serving as target cells.

eosinophils Eosinophilic leukocytes of the granulocytic series serving as target cells; normally present in relatively small numbers. An increase in numbers (eosinophilia) is indicative of allergic or parasitic tissue reactions. Eosinophils are attracted to areas of tissue damage by chemoattractants such as ECF-A. SEE: eosinophil chemotactic factor of anaphylaxis (ECF-A), under autacoid.

mast cells Large population of target cells residing in the tissues; especially numerous near the airways and small blood vessels of the lung. SYN: tissue basophils.

neutrophils Neutrophilic leukocytes of the granulocytic series serving as target cells; an increase in numbers (neutrophilia) often accompanies inflammatory conditions. Neutrophils are attracted to areas of tissue damage by chemoattractants such as NCF-A. SEE: neutrophil chemotactic factor of anaphylaxis (NCF-A), under autacoid.

platelets Cells that consist of small fragments of cytoplasm derived from large precursor stem cells; they act as target cells of antigen-antibody reactions and also produce thromboxane. Platelets are attracted to areas of tissue damage by chemoattractants such as PAF. SYN: thrombocytes. SEE: platelet activation factor (PAF), under autacoid.

tension (P$_{GAS}$) SEE: partial pressure.

terminal bronchiole Small-diameter branches of the bronchioles. These noncartilaginous airways are the last elements of the conducting zone, and give rise to the respiratory bronchioles of the respiratory zone.

terminal respiratory unit SEE: acinus.

terminal sac period SEE: alveolar period.

tertiary bronchi SEE: segmental bronchi.

thebesian veins (thē-bē′ zē-an) Small venules that convey blood from the myocardium to the left heart (left atrium and ventricle).

theoretical oxygen-binding capacity The *theoretical volume* of oxygen transport by 1 g of hemoglobin when the arterial oxygen saturation is 100%. The value is approximately 1.39 mL oxygen per gram of hemoglobin. (The physiologic oxygen-binding capacity of 1.34 mL/g is slightly less than the theoretical oxygen-binding capacity.)

thermodilution studies Studies done with a multilumen pulmonary artery catheter to estimate cardiac output (see text for full explanation of the procedure). SEE: cardiac output (Q̇).

thoracic inlet Narrow, superior opening into the thorax; bounded by the sternum anteriorly, the first pair of ribs laterally, and T1 dorsally. SYN: superior thoracic aperture.

thoracic joints Numerous articulations that provide the means for the dimensions of the thorax to be changed in several different ways. Thoracic joints include the following:

costochondral joints Articulation between the osseous part of the rib and the hyaline cartilage forming the costal cartilage of the rib.

costovertebral joints Articulations between the rib and the thoracic vertebrae; the two types are (1) articulation between head of the rib and the superior and inferior articular facets and (2) costotransverse joints between the tubercle of the rib and the transverse facet of the corresponding thoracic vertebra.

interchondral joints Hyaline cartilage articulations between the costal cartilages of ribs 5 through 8 or 9.

intervertebral joints Fibrocartilaginous joints of the vertebral column that provide a slight range of motion between adjacent vertebrae at the intervertebral discs.

manubriosternal joint A sternal joint formed by the articulation between the manubrium and the body of the sternum.

sternochondral joints Articulation between the sternum and the costal cartilages of ribs 1 through 7. SYN: sternocostal joints.

xiphisternal joint A sternal joint formed by the articulation between the body and the xiphoid process of the sternum.

thoracic outlet Inferior opening of the thorax; bounded by the costal cartilages, anterolateral abdominal wall, and the lower thoracic vertebrae. SYN: inferior thoracic aperture.

thoracic vertebrae One of the 12 vertebrae that connect the ribs and form part of the posterior wall of the thorax.

thorax That part of the body between the base of the neck superiorly and the diaphragm inferiorly. The thorax includes the thoracic vertebrae (T1 to T12), 12 pairs of ribs, sternum, costal cartilages, muscles, mediastinal structures, heart and pericardium, and the lungs and pleurae.

thoroughfare channel A blood vessel serving as the continuation of the metarteriole and connecting the metarteriole with a venule; blood entering a thoroughfare channel is routed directly into the venule without flowing through a capillary bed.

thrombocytes SEE: target cells.

thyroid cartilage The largest cartilage of the larynx, a shield-shaped cartilage that forms the prominence known as the Adam's apple.

thyroid notch The characteristic indentation on the anterior surface of the thyroid cartilage of the larynx.

time constant (T_c) The time (in seconds) required to inflate a particular lung region. The time constant is the product of airway resistance (R_{aw}) and static lung compliance (C_{st}). Lung regions with long time constants take longer to fill (because of increased airway resistance or compliance), whereas lung regions with short time constants fill in a shorter time (because of decreased airway resistance or decreased static lung compliance).

tissue basophils SEE: target cells.

tissue viscous resistance Impedance to air flow caused by the movement of lung structures such as pleural membranes, lung parenchyma, and lung interstitium as they slide past one another during lung inflation and deflation; this component of nonelastic resistance increases as the frequency of breathing increases.

total carbon dioxide content The sum volume of the carbon dioxide transported in its various modes: carbon dioxide in a *dissolved form* in the plasma and red blood cells, combined with hemoglobin or plasma proteins as carbamino compounds; and in a *bicarbonate form* carried by red blood cells and the plasma.

total ventilation (V_E) SEE: minute ventilation.

trabeculae carneae (tra-bek'-ū-lēcar' nē-ē) Any of the thick muscular tissue bands attached to the inner walls of the ventricles of the heart.

trachea (trā' kē-a) A cylindrical cartilaginous tube, approximately 4 in (11.3 cm) long, that originates at the larynx. It extends to the fifth dorsal vertebra, where it divides at a point called the carina into two bronchi, one leading to each lung. SYN: windpipe. SEE: bronchi.

tracheobronchial tree The trachea, bronchi, and their terminal arborizations (branches). SYN: respiratory tree.

transairway pressure (P_{ta}) The pressure difference ($P_1 - P_2$) along the conducting "tube" of the airways; it is the pressure difference between the mouth pressure (P_m) at the proximal end and the alveolar pressure (P_{alv}) at the distal end of the conducting tube.

transit time The length of time it takes for a red blood cell to pass an alveolus at the alveolar-capillary membrane (approximately 0.75 s). Transit time in pulmonary capillaries is affected by the driving pressure in the pulmonary circuit and the pulmonary vascular resistance.

transitional flow An uneven and mixed pattern of parallel flow lines and eddies that occurs at lower flowrates in larger-diameter passageways that branch, converge, or narrow because of an obstruction. SYN: marginally laminar flow; disturbed flow.

transmural pressure (P_{tm}) The pressure across the wall of a conducting tube or container.

P_{tm} across the chest wall The pressure difference, or transthoracic pressure (P_{tt}), between the pleural pressure (P_{pl}) and the atmospheric pressure (P_{atm}), or pressure at the surface of the body.

P_{tm} across the wall of an airway The pressure difference between the outward elastic recoil pressure of the airway and the pleural pressure pressing inward on the airway.

P_{tm} across the wall of an alveolus The pressure difference, or transpulmonary pressure (P_{tp}), between the alveolar pressure (P_{alv}) and the pleural pressure (P_{pl}).

transplacental barrier The series of membranes serving as the interface between fetal and maternal circulatory systems; it restricts the entry of red blood cells and large molecules, and provides the exchange structure for the transfer of gases, nutrients, and wastes between the bloodstream of the mother and that of the fetus.

transpulmonary pressure (P_{tp}) The pressure difference between the intra-alveolar pressure and the intrapleural pressure. The transpulmonary pressure is a measure of the collapse tendency, or recoil pressure, of the lung at each point of its expansion. SEE: transmural pressure.

transthoracic pressure (P_{tt}) The pressure difference between the pleural pressure and the atmospheric pressure, or pressure at the surface of the body. The transthoracic pressure is a measure of the elasticity of the chest wall, and reflects the applied pressure at the chest wall. (Transthoracic pressure is also a type of transmural pressure because it is a measure of the pressure *across* the chest wall itself.) SEE: transmural pressure.

transverse septum The lateral projection of tissue from the anterior body wall that fuses with the right and left pleuroperitoneal folds to form the diaphragm. SEE: pleuroperitoneal folds.

tricuspid valve SEE: atrioventricular valves.

triphasic pattern of breathing A three-phase sequence of neuronal control of the muscles of breathing, dependent on reciprocal inhibitory interactions between phase-specific groups of neurons. The following sequence occurs in the three phases:

early inspiration Ramplike depolarization of brainstem inspiratory interneurons following release from expiratory inhibition drives phrenic motoneurons to result in contraction of the diaphragm.

expiration Respiratory network released from postinspiratory inhibition; elastic recoil of lungs and thorax initiates passive expiration; expiratory neurons activate expiratory muscles during periods of increased respiratory activity. SYN: stage II expiration; active expiration.

postinspiratory inhibition Reactivation of the inspiratory neurons is prevented; vagal motoneurons in the rostral ventral respiratory group (rVRG) discharge to cause contraction of laryngeal adductors and an increase in expiratory airflow resistance; nonvagal motoneurons (postinspiratory interneurons) in the Bötzinger complex (BÖTC) depolarize to prevent additional inspiratory activity. SYN: stage I expiratory inhibition.

true shunt SEE: physiologic shunt.

truncus arteriosus The arterial trunk from the embryonic heart.

tunica externa The outermost layer of arteries and veins; composed of loose connective tissue that anchors the blood vessel to surrounding tissues. SYN: tunica adventitia.

tunica interna The innermost layer of arteries and veins. Composed of squamous epithelium called endothelium; the endothelium is supported by the basement membrane and the lamina propria (a thin layer of smooth muscle and connective tissue). SYN: tunica intima.

tunica media Middle layer of arteries and veins composed of smooth muscle, elastic tissue, and collagen; important in the control of vessel diameter and vascular resistance.

turbinates Collective name given to the superior and middle nasal conchae of the ethmoid bone, and the paired inferior nasal conchae. The turbinates disrupt the airflow in the nasal cavity, creating turbulent flow, and causing heavier particulate matter to be removed. SEE: ethmoid bone; inferior nasal conchae.

turbulent flow A characteristic flow pattern of fluids in which all the molecules (gas or liquid) do not travel in a straight-line axial direction. Instead, some move in the radial direction, causing a chaotic flow pattern with eddies and vortices that mix the molecules and cause the velocity of those moving along the tube wall to be the same as the velocity of those moving in the central, axial location. (Velocity profile is blunt.)

type 1 pneumocyte One of the two types of cells that form the alveoli of the lung. Type 1 cells consist of simple squamous epithelium that permits gas exchange. Type 1 cells are not numerous but form most of the surface area of the alveoli because of their flattened shape. SYN: type 1 alveolar cell. SEE: type 2 pneumocyte.

type 2 pneumocyte One of the two types of cells that form the alveoli of the lung. Type 2 cells are rounded or cuboidal and produce pulmonary surfactant. Type 2 cells are more numerous than type 1 cells. SYN: type 2 alveolar cell. SEE: pulmonary surfactant; type 1 pneumocyte.

type I cells Parenchymal (functional) cells of the aortic and carotid bodies. The cell clusters are closely associated with nerve fiber bundles of the carotid sinus nerve and with sinusoidal fenestrated capillaries. Hypoxemia causes stored catecholamines in the type I cells to be released, stimulating carotid sinus nerve endings and causing stimulation of the medullary respiratory area. SYN: glomus cells; chief cells; principal cells.

type II cells Supporting cells found around clusters of type I cells within aortic and carotid bodies. SYN: capsule cells; sheath cells; sustentacular cells.

ultrafiltrate SEE: glomerular filtrate.

umbilical arteries Branches of the internal iliac arteries in the fetus; these paired arteries carry blood from the fetus to the placenta, where nutrients are obtained and carbon dioxide and oxygen are exchanged. SEE: placenta.

umbilical cord The attachment connecting the fetus with the placenta. It contains two arteries and one vein surrounded by a gelatinous substance. After birth, the stump of the umbilical cord shrivels and becomes the umbilicus or navel. The umbilical cord is delivered with the placenta as afterbirth. SEE: placenta.

umbilical vein The single vein through which oxygenated blood from the placenta returns to the fetus. SEE: placenta.

unmyelinated fibers (C-fiber afferents) Nerve fibers that do not posses a myelin sheath; unmyelinated fibers involved in respiratory functions include pulmonary C fibers and bronchial C fibers.

upper respiratory tract The part of the respiratory system consisting of the nasal cavity, oral cavity, and pharynx.

ureter The tubular structure that conveys formed urine from the kidney to the urinary bladder.

urethra The tubular structure that transports urine from the bladder to the outside of the body.

uvula (ū′ vū-la) A small, soft structure hanging from the free edge of the soft palate in the midline above the root of the tongue. It is composed of muscle, connective tissue, and mucous membrane.

vagus nerve The 10th cranial nerve. It is a mixed nerve, having motor and sensory functions and a wider distribution than any of the other cranial nerves. In the cardiopulmonary system, the vagus nerve carries cardioinhibitory impulses to the heart, as well as sensory impulses from subepithelial irritant receptors of the airways, and motor impulses to smooth muscle of the airways.

vasa rectae Long, relatively straight blood vessels in the medulla that receive blood from the efferent arterioles and maintain the concentration of the extracellular fluid of the medulla. SEE: efferent arterioles.

vasomotor center Functional grouping of nerve cells in the medulla that sends motor impulses through sympathetic fibers to blood vessels (especially the arterioles) that control vessel diameter and resistance.

vasopressin SEE: antidiuretic hormone.

veins Blood vessels that carry blood toward the heart. Veins have a relatively thin wall section and a large lumen diameter in proportion to their overall diameter.

velum palatinum SEE: soft palate.

venous return The returning volume of blood, affected by factors such as the arteriovenous pressure gradient, respiratory pump, skeletal muscle pump, and the hydrostatic effect.

venous sinus A thin-walled venous structure with a large lumen and no smooth muscle. Venous sinuses such as the coronary sinus function to collect blood from specific circulatory routes. SEE: coronary sinus.

venous valves Small, thin leaflets (or cusps) located in medium and small veins. Venous valves provide unidirectional blood flow through veins and work in conjunction with venous return mechanisms such as the respiratory pump and the skeletal muscle pump.

ventilation-perfusion ratio (VA/Q̇) The ratio of ventilation to blood flow in a single alveolus, a group of alveoli, or the entire lung. In a single alveolus, the ratio is determined by the ventilation of the alveolus divided by the capillary blood flow; for the entire lung, the ratio is determined by the total alveolar ventilation divided by the entire pulmonary blood flow.

ventilatory capacity SEE: maximal voluntary ventilation.

ventral respiratory group (VRG) Respiratory center of the medulla divided into three anatomical regions:

caudal VRG (cVRG) Located at the inferior end of the VRG between the spinal cord and the medulla, the cVRG is composed of the nucleus retroambigualis (NRA). The group consists mainly of expiratory neurons interspersed with a few inspiratory neurons.

intermediate VRG (iVRG) Located in the middle region of the VRG, the iVRG includes the nucleus ambiguus (NA) and paraambigual regions. The group contains both inspiratory and expiratory neurons and functions to control and coordinate valvular muscles (airway resistance) and respiratory pump muscles. The iVRG is an integral part of the respiratory central pattern generator (CPG).

rostral VRG (rVRG) Located at the superior end of the VRG, the region contains two distinct types of nerve cells: (1) pharyngeal motoneurons of the NA that exhibit inspiratory and expiratory discharge patterns and (2) interneurons that project to the caudal medulla and spinal cord and exhibit expiratory discharge patterns. These interneurons make up the Bötzinger complex (BÖTC) of the medulla.

ventricular afterload The vascular resistance against which the ventricles must work; this resistance opposes the opening of the semilunar valves.

ventricular folds SEE: vocal cords.

ventricular preload The filling pressure on the ventricles, caused by the pressure of returning blood in the atria.

venules Small-diameter venous structures that drain blood from capillary beds and thoroughfare channels and direct it into larger diameter veins.

vestibule The anterior part of the nostrils, containing the vibrissae.

vibrissae (vī-bris′ ē) Stiff hairs within the nostrils at the anterior nares.

visceral pericardium SEE: epicardium

viscosity Measurement of the resistance of a fluid to flow when a force is applied.

vocal cords Either of two thin, reedlike folds of tissue within the larynx that vibrate as air passes between them, producing sounds that are the basis of speech.

false vocal cords One of the folds of mucous membrane parallel to and above the true vocal cords. SYN: ventricular folds. SEE: larynx.

true vocal cords The thin edges of the vocal lips of the larynx, each of which encloses the vocal ligament which is involved in the production of sound. SYN: vocal folds. SEE: larynx; vocal ligament.

vocal ligament A strong band of elastic tissue lying within the vocal fold. Vocal ligaments form the medial edge of the rima glottidis.

volatile acid An acid that can be converted to a gas and removed from the body by the lungs (e.g., carbonic acid, H_2CO_3).

voltage-gated ion channels Channels formed through cell membranes by proteins; slight alterations in their shape allow them to act as "gates" to open or close an ion channel. Ions diffuse according to the concentration gradient established across the membrane. Voltage-gated channels in myocardial cells are altered by electrical impulses, and form the basis of cardiac electrophysiology, as follows:

voltage-gated fast Na^+ channels Respond to stimuli by rapidly opening to allow sodium ion influx.

voltage-gated slow Ca^{2+} channels Respond to stimuli by slowly opening to allow extracellular calcium ions to enter the cell.

voltage-gated slow K^+ channels Respond to stimuli by slowly opening to allow potassium ion efflux.

voltage-gated slow Na^+ channels Respond to stimuli by slowly opening to allow sodium ion influx.

vomer The plow-shaped bone that forms the lower and posterior portion of the nasal septum, articulating with the ethmoid, the sphenoid, the two palatine bones, and the palatine process of the maxilla.

water vapor partial pressure (P_{H_2O}) The partial pressure, or tension, exerted by water vapor in the inspired air stream. At 37°C, water vapor partial pressure is approximately 47 mm Hg; therefore, the partial pressures of other inspired gases are reduced before they reach the alveoli because of the addition of another gas (water vapor) to the mixture.

windpipe SEE: trachea.

work of breathing (WOB) The total amount of work that must be expended by the respiratory muscles to overcome the combined effect in the respiratory system of elastic resistance factors (static elastic recoil of the lungs and thorax), and nonelastic resistance factors (airway resistance plus tissue viscous resistance).

zone model of perfusion A model for predicting blood flow through different regions of the lung based on relative pressures in the pulmonary arterial system, pulmonary venous system, and the alveoli. Four different zones are recognized:

zone 1 Apical regions of the upright lung. Pulmonary arterial pressure is less than alveolar pressure; therefore, pulmonary capillaries are collapsed, restricting blood flow.

zone 2 Lung zone roughly on a level with the heart in the upright lung. Pulmonary artery pressure is greater than alveolar pressure, resulting in optimal perfusion.

zone 3 Lung zone slightly below the heart. Pulmonary artery pressure is higher than pulmonary venous pressure, and pulmonary venous pressure is higher than alveolar pressure, ensuring distention of capillaries and peak flow values.

zone 4 Basilar regions of the lung. Poorly inflated alveoli cause extra-alveolar blood vessels to collapse, increasing pulmonary vascular resistance and decreasing blood flow to the zone.

An "f" following a page number indicates a figure, a "t" indicates a table, and a "b" indicates a box.